CANCER IN THE SPINE

CURRENT CLINICAL ONCOLOGY

Maurie Markman, MD, Series Editor

CANCER IN THE SPINE

Comprehensive Care

Edited by

ROBERT F. MCLAIN, MD

*Lerner College of Medicine and The Cleveland Clinic Spine Institute
Department of Orthopaedic Surgery, The Cleveland Clinic Foundation
Cleveland, OH*

Section Editors

KAI-UWE LEWANDROWSKI, MD

The Cleveland Clinic Spine Institute, The Cleveland Clinic Foundation, Cleveland, OH

MAURIE MARKMAN, MD

University of Texas M. D. Anderson Cancer Center, Houston, TX

RONALD M. BUKOWSKI, MD

Taussig Cancer Center, The Cleveland Clinic Foundation, Cleveland, OH

ROGER MACKLIS, MD

Department of Radiation Oncology, The Cleveland Clinic Foundation, Cleveland, OH

EDWARD C. BENZEL, MD, FACS

The Cleveland Clinic Spine Institute, The Cleveland Clinic Foundation, Cleveland, OH

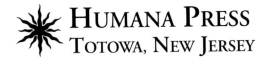

HUMANA PRESS
TOTOWA, NEW JERSEY

humanapress.com

For additional copies, pricing for bulk purchases, and/or information about other Humana titles, contact Humana at the above address or at any of the following numbers: Tel.: 973-256-1699; Fax: 973-256-8341; E-mail: orders@humanapr.com; or visit our website at www.humanapress.com

This publication is printed on acid-free paper. ∞
ANSI Z39.48-1984 (American National Standards Institute)
Permanence of Paper for Printed Library Materials.

Production Editor: Melissa Caravella

Cover design by Patricia F. Cleary

Cover illustration: From Fig. 4 in Chapter 21, "Primary Tumors of the Spine," by Rex C. Haydon and Frank M. Phillips and Fig. 3 in Chapter 26, "Spinal Metastasis: *Indications for Surgery*," by Iain H. Kalfas.

Printed in the United States of America. 10 9 8 7 6 5 4 3 2 1
eISBN 1-59259-971-0

Library of Congress Cataloging-in-Publication Data

Cancer in the spine : comprehensive care / edited by Robert F. McLain
  ; section editors, Maurie Markman ... [et al.].
    p. ; cm. -- (Current clinical oncology)
  Includes bibliographical references and index.
  ISBN 1-58829-074-3 (alk. paper)
  1. Spine--Cancer--Diagnosis. 2. Spine--Cancer--Therapy.   I. McLain,
Robert F. II. Series: Current clinical oncology (Totowa, N.J.)
  [DNLM: 1. Spinal Neoplasms--therapy. 2. Combined Modality Therapy.
3. Spinal Neoplasms--diagnosis.   WE 725 C215 2006]
RC280.S72C36 2006
616.99'4711--dc22   2005022738

Preface

Recent advances in medical treatment have dramatically changed our approach to many forms of cancer. Nowhere is this more apparent than in our approach to patients with cancer of the spinal column. A scant 30 years ago, spinal tumors were considered largely untreatable. Tumor resection was considered futile, if not mutilating, and radiotherapy was limited in dose and approach to what the spinal cord could bear. Diagnosis often came late, when treatment could only be brought to bear on the sequelae of tumor growth—spinal cord compression and mechanical instability and pain. The seemingly inevitable progression from spinal metastasis to fracture, intractable pain, cord compression, and paresis left the patient bedridden, malnourished, and narcotized, and easy prey for the bedsores, pneumonia, or urinary tract infections that would eventually take their lives. Even today many physicians quietly consider the appearance of a spinal metastasis to be the death knell for their patients with carcinoma.

Early diagnosis, improved screening, and better follow-up screening of those with known primary disease have improved our ability to recognize spinal tumors at an early and more manageable stage. Advances in imaging technology and histological techniques have improved diagnostic accuracy and reduced the need for more invasive techniques that carry greater cost, morbidity, and discomfort for the patient.

Although advances in chemotherapeutic and medical management regimens have improved long-term survival and cure rates for patients with many forms of cancer, advances in supportive medical care have reduced the impact of many attendant systemic problems that rendered patients "too sick" for aggressive therapy or surgery. Improved perioperative and intra-operative management now allows us to accomplish radical resection of spinal tumors considered inoperable just a decade ago.

Advances in radiotherapeutic modalities have simultaneously improved the efficacy of tumor treatment while reducing the collateral damage inherent in approaches of the past. The ability to focus therapy on the tumor itself reduces the risk of injury to the spinal cord and to the overlying skin, permitting more aggressive therapy with a lower complication rate. Newer therapeutic modalities such as brachytherapy and intra-operative radiotherapy allow us to precisely boost radiation doses to tumor foci without causing damage to the sensitive structures nearby.

Improvements in surgical technique have resulted in better survival and cure rates for patients with both primary and metastatic lesions. Prolonged bed rest, necessitated by surgical resection and spinal cord decompression, is largely a thing of the past. Advances in surgical technique, and a quantum leap in spinal instrumentation, now allow surgeons to radically resect lesions at any level of the spinal column with the full expectation that the patient will be up and out of bed within days of surgery. Rapid return to function and independence, combined with more reliable pain relief, makes surgical care a reasonable consideration for many patients previously thought beyond help. New, minimally invasive surgical techniques can provide dramatic pain relief, with greatly reduced morbidity, in even the sickest patients.

Advances in end-of-life care cannot be overlooked either. Patients with cancer fear pain and loss of independence. Improvements in medical pain management allow patients to function independently despite advanced disease, with less impairment of mental function.

More than ever before, care of the patient with cancer of the spinal column requires interdisciplinary cooperation and coordination. Injudicious use of one modality, even in terms of timing, can make it difficult or impossible to safely apply other treatment options in a given patient. A multidisciplinary team, with a broad perspective as to the relative value and risk associated with the many treatment options now available, has the best chance for coordinating care of these challenging patients so that treatment effect is maximized and complications and injury are avoided. Fortunately, the growing recognition that there is much to be gained—that these patients *will* benefit from an aggressive, coordinated approach to cancer management—has spurred greater interest in their care and the collaboration needed to provide that care.

The goal of *Cancer in the Spine: Comprehensive Care* is to provide an overview of the many disciplines involved in caring for patients with cancer of the spine, and to provide some guidance as to how these different modalities may be combined to provide the most effective treatment for today's patients. Although the chapters that follow are rich in technical descriptions and survival data, care and compassion remain the fundamental properties that any physician must bring to these cases. No patient is "too sick" to be helped. There is no such thing as "benign neglect." Sometimes, in the end, all we can offer is to be there, and sometimes, that is what our patients need the most.

Robert F. McLain, MD

Contents

Contributors

RONY ABOU-JAWDE, MD • *Hematology and Medical Oncology, Taussig Cancer Center, The Cleveland Clinic Foundation, Cleveland, OH*

HOWARD S. AN, MD • *Department of Orthopaedic Surgery, Rush-Presbyterian-St.Luke's Medical Center, Chicago, IL*

L. BRETT BABAT, MD • *The Cleveland Clinic Foundation, Cleveland, OH*

GORDON R. BELL, MD • *The Cleveland Clinic Spine Institute and the Department of Orthopaedic Surgery, The Cleveland Clinic Foundation, Cleveland, OH*

EDWARD C. BENZEL, MD • *The Cleveland Clinic Spine Institute, The Cleveland Clinic Foundation, Cleveland, OH*

MARK H. BILSKY, MD • *Department of Surgery, Neurosurgery Service, Memorial Sloan-Kettering Cancer Center, New York, NY*

PATRICK BOLAND, MD • *Department of Surgery, Orthopaedic Service, Memorial Sloan-Kettering Cancer Center, New York, NY*

G. THOMAS BUDD, MD • *Hematology and Medical Oncology, Taussig Cancer Center, The Cleveland Clinic Foundation, Cleveland, OH*

RONALD M. BUKOWSKI, MD • *Experimental Therapeutics Program, Taussig Cancer Center, The Cleveland Clinic Foundation, Cleveland, OH*

FRANK P. CAMMISA, JR., MD, FRCS • *Spine Care Institute, Spinal Surgical Service, The Hospital for Special Surgery, Department of Clinical Surgery, Weill Medical College of Cornell University, New York, NY*

JEAN-VALÉRY C. E. COUMANS, MD • *Department of Neurosurgery, Massachusetts General Hospital, Boston, MA*

RICHARD L. CROWNOVER, MD, PhD • *The Reading Hospital Regional Cancer Center, West Reading, PA*

MELLAR P. DAVIS, MD, FCCP • *Taussig Cancer Center, The Cleveland Clinic Foundation, Cleveland, OH*

THOMAS F. DELANEY, MD • *Department of Radiation Oncology, Harvard Medical School, Boston, MA; Department of Radiation Oncology, Northeast Proton Therapy Center, Massachusetts General Hospital, Boston, MA*

ROBERT DREICER, MD, FACP • *Genitourinary Medical Oncology and Experimental Therapeutics, Department of Hematology/Oncology and the Urologic Institute, The Cleveland Clinic Foundation, Cleveland, OH*

MOHAMED A. ELSHAIKH, MD • *Department of Radiation Oncology, University of Michigan School of Medicine, Ann Arbor, MI*

DARYL R. FOURNEY, MD, FRCSC • *Department of Neurosurgery, The University of Texas M.D. Anderson Cancer Center, Houston, TX*

FEDERICO P. GIRARDI, MD • *Orthopaedic Surgery, Spinal Surgical Service, The Hospital for Special Surgery, New York, NY*

ZIYA L. GOKASLAN, MD, FACS • *Department of Neurosurgery, The Spine Program, The University of Texas M.D. Anderson Cancer Center, Houston, TX*

GREGORY P. GRAZIANO, MD • *Department of Orthopaedic Surgery, University of Michigan School of Medicine, Ann Arbor, MI*

MICHAEL J. HARRIS, MD • *Arthritis Institute, Centinela-Freeman Medical Center, Inglewood, CA*

REX C. HAYDON, MD, PhD • *Section of Orthopaedic Surgery and Rehabilitation Medicine, Department of Surgery, University of Chicago Hospitals, Chicago, IL*

ANN M. HENWOOD, RN, MSN • *Department of Neurosurgery, The Cleveland Clinic Spine Institute, The Cleveland Clinic Foundation, Cleveland, OH*

DAVID G. HICKS, MD • *Department of Anatomic Pathology, The Cleveland Clinic Foundation, Cleveland, OH*

JOHN HILL, MD • *Mohamad Hussein Myeloma Research Program, Taussig Cancer Center, The Cleveland Clinic Foundation, Cleveland, OH*

FRANCIS J. HORNICEK, MD, PhD • *Center for Sarcoma and Connective Tissue Oncology, Massachusetts General Hospital and Department of Orthopedic Surgery, Harvard Medical School, Boston, MA*

MOHAMAD HUSSEIN, MD • *Taussig Cancer Center, The Cleveland Clinic Foundation, Cleveland, OH*

THOMAS E. HUTSON, DO, PharmD • *Genitourinary Oncology Program, Texas Oncology, Baylor Sammons Cancer Center, Dallas, TX*

IAIN H. KALFAS, MD • *Department of Neurosurgery, The Cleveland Clinic Foundation, Cleveland, OH*

SUJITH KALMADI, MD • *Department of Hematology and Medical Oncology, Taussig Cancer Center, The Cleveland Clinic Foundation, Cleveland, OH*

A. JAY KHANNA, MD • *Johns Hopkins Orthopaedic Surgery at Good Samaritan Hospital, Baltimore, MD*

FRANK LAMARCA, MD • *Department of Neurosurgery, University of Michigan School of Medicine, Ann Arbor, MI*

SUSAN B. LEGRAND, MD • *The Harry R. Horvitz Center for Palliative Medicine, The Cleveland Clinic Taussig Cancer Center, The Cleveland Clinic Foundation, Cleveland, OH*

MESFIN A. LEMMA, MD • *Johns Hopkins Orthopaedic Surgery at Good Samaritan Hospital, Baltimore, MD*

KAI-UWE LEWANDROWSKI, MD • *The Cleveland Clinic Spine Institute, The Cleveland Clinic Foundation, Cleveland, OH*

ISADOR H. LIEBERMAN, MD • *The Cleveland Clinic Spine Institute, The Cleveland Clinic Foundation, Cleveland, OH*

KEITH R. LODHIA, MD, MS • *Department of Neurosurgery, University of Michigan School of Medicine, Ann Arbor, MI*

ADIR LUDIN, MD • *Department of Radiation Oncology, The Cleveland Clinic Foundation, Cleveland, OH*

ROGER M. MACKLIS, MD • *Department of Radiation Oncology, The Cleveland Clinic Foundation, Cleveland, OH*

HENRY J. MANKIN, MD • *The Orthopaedic Research Laboratories, Massachusetts General Hospital, Boston, MA*

REX A. W. MARCO, MD • *Department of Orthopaedic Surgery and Department of Neurosurgery, University of Texas Medical School, Houston, TX*

MAURIE MARKMAN, MD • *University of Texas M. D. Anderson Cancer Center, Houston, TX*

ROBERT F. MCLAIN, MD • *Lerner College of Medicine and The Cleveland Clinic Spine Institute, Department of Orthopaedic Surgery, The Cleveland Clinic Foundation, Cleveland, OH*

ANIS O. MEKHAIL, MD • *Department of Orthopaedics, University of Illinois at Chicago, Chicago, IL*

TAREK MEKHAIL, MD, MSc, FRCSI, FRCSEd • *Lung Cancer Program, The Cleveland Clinic Taussig Cancer Center, The Cleveland Clinic Foundation, Cleveland, OH*

LEAH MOINZADEH, PT • *Department of Physical and Occupational Therapy, The Cleveland Clinic Foundation, Cleveland, OH*

PAUL PARK, MD • *Department of Neurosurgery, University of Michigan School of Medicine, Ann Arbor, MI*

SANDEE PATTI, OT • *Department of Physical and Occupational Therapy, The Cleveland Clinic Foundation, Cleveland, OH*

FRANK M. PHILLIPS, MD • *Department of Orthopaedic Surgery, Rush University Medical Center, Chicago, IL*

RICHARD PLACIDE, MD • *West End Orthopaedic Clinic Inc., Chippenham Medical Center, Richmond, VA*

ASHLEY R. POYNTON, MD, FRCSI, FRCS • *Spine Fellow, The Hospital for Special Surgery and Memorial Sloan-Kettering Cancer Center, New York, NY*

BRANCO PRPA, MD • *Department of Orthopaedic Surgery, The Cleveland Clinic Foundation, Cleveland, OH*

DEREK RAGHAVAN, MD • *Department of Hematology and Medical Oncology, Taussig Cancer Center, The Cleveland Clinic Foundation, Cleveland, OH*

S. SETHU REDDY, MD • *Department of Endocrinology, Diabetes and Metabolism, The Cleveland Clinic Foundation, Cleveland, OH*

JIGAR SHAH, MD • *Department of Hematology and Oncology, Taussig Cancer Center, The Cleveland Clinic Foundation, Cleveland, OH*

DANIEL SHEDID, MD • *The Cleveland Clinic Spine Institute, The Cleveland Clinic Foundation, Cleveland, OH*

MICHAEL K. SHINDLE, MD • *Department of Orthopaedic Surgery, Hospital for Special Surgery, New York, NY*

RONALD M. SOBECKS, MD • *Department of Hematology and Oncology, The Cleveland Clinic Foundation, Cleveland, OH*

AJAY SOOD, MD • *Department of Internal Medicine, The Cleveland Clinic Foundation, Cleveland, OH*

MICHAEL P. STEINMETZ, MD • *Department of Neurosurgery, The Cleveland Clinic Foundation, Cleveland, OH*

DAISUKE TOGAWA, MD, PhD • *The Cleveland Clinic Spine Institute and the Department of Orthopaedic Surgery, The Cleveland Clinic Foundation, Cleveland, OH*

EERIC TRUUMEES, MD • *William Beaumont Hospital, Royal Oak, Michigan; Wayne State University, Detroit, MI*

TODD VITAZ, MD • *Department of Neurological Surgery, University of Lousiville School of Medicine, Louisville, KY*

DECLAN WALSH, MD • *Palliative Medicine Program, The Harry R. Horvitz Center for Palliative Medicine, The Cleveland Clinic Taussig Cancer Center, The Cleveland Clinic Foundation, Cleveland, OH*

BRUCE A. WASSERMAN, MD • *Russell H. Morgan Department of Radiology and Radiological Science, Johns Hopkins Medical Institutions, Baltimore, MD*

1 Cancer of the Spine

How Big Is the Problem?

KAI-UWE LEWANDROWSKI, MD, GORDON R. BELL, MD,
AND ROBERT F. MCLAIN, MD

CONTENTS

1. US CANCER STATISTICS

For the second consecutive year, the Centers for Disease Control and Prevention (CDC) and the National Cancer Institute have released an annual US Cancer Statistics report (1). Published in collaboration with the North American Association of Central Cancer Registries, this report provides detailed information on cancer incidence, surveillance, epidemiology, and end results for 66 selected primary cancer sites and subsites for males (Table 1), 70 selected primary cancer sites and subsites for females (Table 2), and for all cancer sites combined (Figs. 1 and 2). In addition, these data have been analyzed with regard to geographic area, race, sex, and age (Table 3). According to the CDC and National Cancer Institute, 84% of the US population is covered in the 2000 surveillance report (1).

2. FREQUENCY OF SPINAL TUMORS

As indicated by the 2000 CDC US Cancer Statistics (1), the most common primary malignancies for men include prostate, lung, and colon with the incidence ranging from 160.4 to 65.0 cases per 100,000. For women, the leading primary malignancy is breast cancer followed by lung and colon cancer with the incidence ranging from 128.9 to 47.0 cases per 100,000. By comparison, spinal tumors are very rare. A review of data obtained from the Leeds Tumor Registry revealed that only 2.8% of the 1950 cases had tumors in the spine, which can arise from bone, cartilage, and rarely from other tissues (as is the case with lipomas, meningiomas, and neurofibromas) (2). Primary bone tumors in the spine are extremely rare as well. Of the 2000 sarcomas arising in bone each year in the United States,

only 10% are found in the spine (3). In fact, the incidence of primary tumors of the spine per 100,000 persons per year is estimated as between 2.5 and 8.5 (3).

In comparison, the vast majority (95%) of the clinically relevant spinal tumors are metastases (4). More than 60% of these metastases arise from myelomas, lymphomas, or adenocarcinomas of the breast, lung, and prostate (Table 4) (5). Metastases in the axial and appendicular skeleton are extremely common and may be present in up to 70% of the patients with advanced adenocarcinoma before death (4). With respect to breast cancer, this rate may be as high as 85% (5). These clinical observations are corroborated by autopsy studies, which showed that metastases are present in nearly 80% of advanced-stage cancer patients (6).

3. METASTATIC SPINE TUMORS: AGE AND GENDER

Visceral or bony metastases should be expected in the majority of patients with advanced-stage disease at some point during the course of their illness (7). This becomes particularly apparent in patients older than 40 yr. As shown in Table 3, the incidence of carcinomas, myelomas, and lymphoma is sharply increased (8). In general, spinal metastases are considered a preterminal event, which indicates that a cancer may no longer be curable. In other words, regional disease has become a systemic illness. Of the 18,000 patients in the United States diagnosed annually with vertebral metastases, men are disproportionately more affected, with a male to female ratio of 3:2 (9).

4. LOCATION OF SPINAL METASTASES

The spinal column is the most common site of skeletal or osseous metastases (10). Rates of metastatic spread to the spine

From: Current Clinical Oncology: Cancer in the Spine: Comprehensive Care.
Edited by: R. F. McLain, K-U. Lewandrowski, M. Markman, R. M. Bukowski,
R. Macklis, and E. C. Benzel © Humana Press, Inc., Totowa, NJ

Table 1
Invasive Cancer Incidence Rates for the 15 Primary Sites With the Highest Age-Adjusted Incidence Rates
Within Race-Specific Categories

	All races		White		Black		Asian/Pacific Islander	
1.	Prostate	160.4	Prostate	150.5	Prostate	233.8	Prostate	86.2
2.	Lung and bronchus	87.9	Lung and bronchus	86.8	Lung and bronchus	107.1	Lung and bronchus	54.6
3.	Colon and rectum	65.0	Colon and rectum	64.5	Colon and rectum	67.3	Colon and rectum	49.4
4.	Urinary bladder	37.8	Urinary bladder	39.9	Oral cavity and pharynx	18.2	Stomach	20.0
5.	Non-Hodgkin's lymphoma	21.6	Non-Hodgkin's lymphoma	22.0	Urinary bladder	17.4	Liver and IBD	19.0
6.	Melanomas of the skin	19.4	Melanomas of the skin	21.0	Kidney and renal pelvis	17.1	Urinary bladder	14.9
7.	Kidney and renal pelvis	16.4	Kidney and renal pelvis	16.4	Stomach	16.8	Non-Hodgkin's lymphoma	14.5
8.	Oral cavity and pharynx	15.7	Oral cavity and pharynx	15.3	Pancreas	15.4	Oral cavity and pharynx	11.2
9.	Leukemias	14.5	Leukemias	14.9	Non-Hodgkin's lymphoma	15.1	Pancreas	9.8
10.	Pancreas	12.1	Pancreas	11.8	Esophagus	12.1	Kidney and renal pelvis	8.4
11.	Stomach	10.5	Stomach	9.5	Larynx	12.0	Leukemias	8.3
12.	Esophagus	8.5	Brain and ONS	8.2	Multiple myeloma	10.9	Esophagus	3.9
13.	Larynx	7.8	Esophagus	8.2	Leukemias	10.5	Brain and ONS	3.5
14.	Brain and ONS	7.7	Larynx	7.4	Liver and IBD	9.5	Multiple myeloma	3.3
15.	Liver and IBD	7.4	Liver and IBD	6.5	Brain and ONS	4.5	Thyroid	3.3

Source: Center for Disease Control US Cancer Statistics, 2000 Incidence Report: Top 15 Cancer Sites.
US males by race, rates per 100,000.
ONS, other nervous system; IBD, interlobular bile ducts.

Table 2
Invasive Cancer Incidence Rates for the 15 Primary Sites With the Highest Age-Adjusted Incidence Rates
Within Race-Specific Categories

	All races		White		Black		Asian/Pacific Islander	
1.	Breast	128.9	Breast	131.4	Breast	108.3	Breast	77.9
2.	Lung and bronchus	52.5	Lung and bronchus	53.8	Colon and rectum	51.9	Colon and rectum	33.8
3.	Colon and rectum	47.0	Colon and rectum	46.2	Lung and bronchus	46.5	Lung and bronchus	26.0
4.	Corpus and uterus, NOS	23.5	Corpus and uterus, NOS	24.2	Corpus and uterus, NOS	18.4	Corpus and uterus, NOS	13.7
5.	Ovary	15.8	Ovary	16.4	Cervix uteri	12.9	Thyroid	11.9
6.	Non-Hodgkin's lymphoma	15.4	Non-Hodgkin's lymphoma	15.8	Pancreas	12.6	Stomach	11.7
7.	Melanomas of the skin	12.4	Melanomas of the skin	13.8	Ovary	10.5	Non-Hodgkin's lymphoma	10.5
8.	Thyroid	10.7	Thyroid	11.0	Non-Hodgkin's lymphoma	10.3	Ovary	10.4
9.	Urinary bladder	9.8	Urinary bladder	10.3	Stomach	8.8	Cervix uteri	8.7
10.	Pancreas	9.5	Pancreas	9.1	Kidney and renal pelvis	8.6	Pancreas	8.6
11.	Cervix uteri	9.2	Leukemias	8.9	Multiple myeloma	8.6	Liver and IBD	7.6
12.	Leukemias	8.7	Cervix uteri	8.6	Leukemias	7.0	Oral cavity and pharynx	5.9
13.	Kidney and renal pelvis	8.4	Kidney and renal pelvis	8.5	Thyroid	6.7	Leukemias	5.7
14.	Oral cavity and pharynx	6.0	Oral cavity and pharynx	6.0	Urinary bladder	6.5	Urinary bladder	3.9
15.	Brain and ONS	5.5	Brain and ONS	5.8	Oral cavity and pharynx	5.1	Kidney and renal pelvis	3.7

Source: Center for Disease Control United States Cancer Statistics, 2000 Incidence Report: Top 15 Cancer Sites.
US Females by race, rates per 100,000.
ONS, other nervous system.

vary widely according to the primary tumor of origin (Table 5). However, autopsy studies indicated that vertebral metastases increase in frequency in a caudal direction along the vertebral column *(11–14)*. This distribution appears to correlate with the increasing volume of bone marrow within the vertebral bodies from the cervical to the lumbar regions of the spine. For example, breast cancer metastases account for nearly 54% of all spine metastases among women *(15)*. The most frequent locations of tumors, in descending order, are the vertebrae (85%), the paravertebral spaces (10–15%), the epidural space (<5%), and intradural/intramedullary *(16)*. As demonstrated in a large series of 1585 patients with symptomatic epidural

deposits, the vast majority (70.3%) of lesions are located in the thoracic and thoracolumbar spine, 21.6% in the lumbosacral spine, and 8.1% in the cervical spine *(17)*. More recently, it has been suggested that as many as 20% of spinal metastases arise in the cervical segments *(16–18)*. Because 10 to 38% of patients have metastases in multiple noncontiguous spine sites *(7,18)*, skip lesions in other areas of the spine should be suspected particularly in patients with advanced-stage disease.

5. MAGNITUDE OF THE PROBLEM

Of the one million new cases of cancer diagnosed annually, metastases will develop in two-thirds of the patients *(11,20)*.

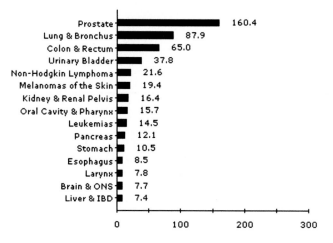

Fig. 1. Cancer incidence, males, all races, rate per 100,000. (Source: CDC US Cancer Statistics, 2000 Incidence Report, Top 15 Cancer Sites.)

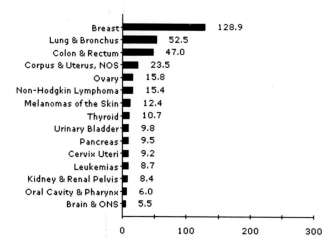

Fig. 2. Cancer incidence, females, all races, rate per 100,000. (Source: CDC US Cancer Statistics, 2000 Incidence Report, Top 15 Cancer Sites.)

Table 3
Age-Specific Invasive Cancer Incidence Rates[a] by Primary Site and Gender (All Races), United States: NPCR and SEER Registries That Meet Quality Criteria[b,c]

Age at diagnosis	Males	Females
<1	22.8 (20.5–25.2)	23.0 (20.7–25.6)
1–4	20.9 (19.8–22.0)	17.9 (16.9–19.0)
5–9	12.3 (11.6–13.1)	9.6 (9.0–10.3)
10–14	12.1 (11.4–12.9)	11.2 (10.5–11.9)
15–19	20.9 (19.9–21.8)	19.3 (18.3–20.2)
20–24	30.2 (29.0–31.4)	33.8 (32.5–35.1)
25–29	44.5 (43.0–45.9)	60.4 (58.7–62.2)
30–34	62.2 (60.6–63.9)	99.2 (97.1–101.3)
35–39	88.0 (86.1–89.9)	161.7 (159.1–164.2)
40–44	146.3 (143.9–148.8)	269.6 (266.3–272.9)
45–49	273.3 (269.8–276.9)	408.7 (404.4–413.0)
50–54	532.0 (526.7–537.4)	589.7 (584.2–595.2)
55–59	965.1 (956.9–973.4)	819.0 (811.7–826.4)
60–64	1542.3 (1530.6–1554.1)	1080.2 (1070.9–1089.5)
65–69	2258.1 (2242.9–2273.5)	1358.4 (1347.5–1369.4)
70–74	2806.0 (2788.1–2824.1)	1612.3 (1600.3–1624.5)
75–79	3071.5 (3050.3–3092.9)	1799.3 (1785.7–1812.9)
80–84	3160.2 (3132.6–3188.0)	1926.5 (1909.9–1943.2)
85+	3112.2 (3078.7–3146.0)	1809.3 (1793.0–1825.8)

Source: CDC United States Cancer Statistics, 2000 Incidence Report: Top 15 Cancer Sites.

[a]Rates are per 100,000 persons.

[b]Data are from selected statewide and metropolitan area cancer registries that meet the following data quality criteria: case ascertainment is at least 90% complete; ≥97% of cases pass a standard set of computerized edits; ≤5% of cases were ascertained by death certificate only; ≤3% of cases are missing information on sex; ≤5% of cases are missing information on race; ≤3% of cases are missing information on age. Rates cover approx 84% of the US population.

[c]Excludes basal and squamous cell carcinomas of the skin except when these occur on the skin of the genital organs, and in situ cancers except urinary bladder.

Data for specified races other than White and Black should be interpreted with caution.

NPCR, National Program of Cancer Registries; SEER, Surveillance Epidemiology and End Results.

Considering that 80% of these patients will be diagnosed with spinal metastases during the course of their disease, it is estimated that approx 500,000 patients will present with spinal metastases each year. Thirty-six percent of spinal metastases are asymptomatic and discovered incidentally (16). Symptomatic spinal cord involvement has been estimated to occur in 18,000 patients per year (21). With continued advances in the treatment of primary disease and local recurrences, patients are living longer and more frequently require treatment for symptomatic distant metastases. Bearing in mind that detection methods continue to improve, that patients survive longer, and that our population is aging, it is anticipated that the prevalence

Table 4
Prevalence and Prognosis of Metastatic Cancer

Primary tumor	Percent of total spine metastases (2748 cases)	Prevalence to bone in advanced disease (%)	Prevalence to spine in advanced disease (%)	Median survival (mo)	5-yr survival (%)
Breasts	21	65–75	16.5–37	24	20
Prostate	7.5	65–90	9.2–15	40	25
Lung	14	30–45	12–15	<6	<5
Kidney	5.5	20–30	3–6.5	6	10
Gastrointestinal (carcinoid)	5	–	4.7	–	–
Thyroid	2.5	60	4	48	40
Melanoma	–	14–55	1–2	<6	<5

Reproduced with permission from ref. *26*.

Table 5
Distribution of Metastases in the Spine

Primary tumor	Barron 1959	White 1971	Constans 1973	Paillas 1973	Chade 1976	Kretschmer 1979	Baldini 1979	Dunn 1980	Klein 1984	Knollmann 1984	Brihaye 1985	Total	%
Cervical and cervical thoracic	14	20	12	5	17	3	14	8	12	9	13	127	8.1
Thoracic and thoracic lumbar	83	186	87	50	108	90	83	75	116	74	163	1115	70.3
Lumbar and sacral	30	20	30	5	46	12	42	42	21	69	42	343	21.6
Total:	127	226	129	60	171	105	139	104	197	109	218	1585	

Reproduced with permission from ref. *27*.

of symptomatic spinal metastases is likely to increase substantially in the future, posing an ever growing challenge to the spine surgeon *(22)*.

6. THE CHALLENGE

The growing number of patients with metastatic processes in the spine requires application of sound oncological principles to reduce the morbidity and mortality associated with biopsies and surgical interventions. Continued advances in spinal instrumentation and perioperative supportive care are expected to permit more aggressive and effective surgical treatments, including the *en-bloc* removal of tumors. This will require a close working relationship between the patient, the oncologist, and the surgeon. A multidisciplinary oncology service is key to providing more effective palliation for advanced-stage cancer patients. Moreover, patient education is essential to allow the patient to make better informed, appropriate choices regarding his or her management.

REFERENCES

1. CDC United States Cancer Statistics, 2000 Incidence Report. Web site: http://www.seer.cancer.gov.
2. Dreghorn CR, Newman RJ, Hardy GJ, Dickson RA. Primary tumors of the axial skeleton—experience of the Leeds Regional Bone Tumor Registry. Spine 1990; 15:137–140.
3. Jaffe HL. Tumors and tumorous conditions of the bones and joints. Philadelphia, PA: Lea and Febiger; 1958.
4. McLain RF, Bell GR. Newer management options in patients with spinal metastasis. Cleve Clin J Med 1998; 65:359–367.
5. Harrington KD. Metastatic disease of the spine. J Bone Joint Surg Am 1986; 68:1110–1115.
6. Boriani S, Weinstein JN. Differential diagnosis and surgical treatment of primary benign and malignant neoplasms. In: Frymoyer JW, ed. The Adult Spine. Philadelphia, PA: Lippincott-Raven; 1997:951–987.
7. Asdourian PL. Metastatic disease of the spine. In: Bridwell KH, DeWald RL, eds. The textbook of spinal surgery. 2nd ed. Vol. 2. Philadelphia, PA: Lippincott-Raven; 1997:2007–2050.
8. Black P, Nair S, Giannakopoulos G. Spinal epidural tumors. In: Wilkins RH, Rengachary SS, eds. Neurosurgery. New York, NY: McGraw-Hill; 1996:1791–1804.
9. Constans JP. Divitiis ED, Donzelli R, et al. Spinal metastases with neurological manifestations. J Neurosurg 1983; 59:111–118.
10. Aaron AD. The management of cancer metastatic to bone. JAMA 1994; 15:1206–1209.
11. Nottebaert M, von Hochstetter AR, Exner GU, Schreiber A. Metastatic carcinoma of the spine. A study of 92 cases. Int Orthop 1987; 11:345–348.
12. Arseni CN, Simionescu MD, Horwath L. Tumors of the spine follow-up study of 350 patients with neurosurgical considerations. Acta Psychiatr Scand 1959; 34:398–410.
13. Bhalla SK. Metastatic disease of the spine. Clin Orthop 1970; 73:52–60.
14. Suen KC, Lau LL, Yermakov V. Cancer and old age. An autopsy study of 3,535 patients over 65 years old. Cancer 1974; 33:1164–1168.

15. Gilbert H, Apuzzo M, Marshall L, et al. Neoplastic epidural spinal cord compression. A current perspective. JAMA 1978; 240:2771–2773.
16. Byrne TN. Spinal cord compression from epidural metastases. N Engl J Med 1992; 327:614–619.
17. Brihaye J, Ectors P, Lemort M, Van Houtte P. The management of spinal epidural metastases. Adv Tech Stand Neurosurg 1988; 16:121–176.
18. Jenis LG. Dunn EJ, An HS. Metastatic disease of the cervical spine. A review. Clin Orthop 1999; (359):89–103.
19. Constans JP, de Divitiis E, Donzelli R,, Spaziante R, Meder JF, Haye C. Spinal metastases with neurological manifestations: review of 600 cases. J Neurosurg 1983; 59:111–118.
20. Schaberg J, Gainor BJ. A profile of metastatic carcinoma of the spine. Spine 1985; 10:19–20.
21. Rao S, Badani K, Schildhauer T, Borges M. Metastatic malignancy of the cervical spine. A nonoperative history. Spine 1992; 17:S407–S412.
22. Ruff RL, Lanska DJ. Epidural metastases in prospectively evaluated veterans with cancer and back pain. Cancer 1989; 63:2234–2241.
23. Shaw B, Mansfield FL, Borges L. One-stage posterolateral decompression and stabilization for primary and metastatic vertebral tumors in the thoracic and lumbar spine. (Comment: J Neurosurg 1990; 3:807), J Neurosurg 1989; 70:405–410.
24. Black P. Spinal metastasis: current status and recommended guidelines for management. Neurosurgery 1979; 5:726–746.
25. Gertzen PC, Welch WC. Current surgical management of metastatic spinal disease. Oncology 2000; 14:1013–1024.
26. Drury AB, Palmer AH, Highman WJ. Carcinomatous metastasis to the vertebral body. J Clin Pathol 1964; 17:448–457.
27. Brihaye J, Ectors P, LeMort M, Van Houtte P. The management of spinal epidural metastates. Adv Tech Stand Neurosurg 1988; 16:121–176.

2 Metastatic Disease to the Musculoskeletal System

David G. Hicks, MD

Contents

1. INTRODUCTION

Bone is a dynamic tissue that undergoes continuous remodeling. It goes through a balanced process that entails repeated cycles of bone resorption coupled with synthesis of new bone matrix (Fig. 1). These remodeling cycles are influenced by an individual's age, endocrine and nutritional status, and level of physical activity. This ongoing tissue turnover is important for meeting the often conflicting need of the skeleton to maintain structural support for the body while also providing a source of ions for mineral homeostasis. The maintenance of skeletal mass in the face of continuous bone remodeling requires the coordinated activities of osteoblasts and osteoclasts, the two cell types responsible for skeletal matrix formation and resorption *(1)* (Fig. 1). Advances in our understanding of the precise mechanisms that control the cellular interactions and coupled activities of these two cell types have provided new insight into a number of diseases affecting the skeleton. These disorders are characterized by an imbalance of remodeling with subsequent increase in bone resorption, decreased bone mass, and loss of skeletal stability and integrity. This is particularly true for neoplastic diseases, in which a number of common human malignancies have a propensity to spread to the skeleton, resulting in significant morbidity and mortality from bone destruction *(2)*.

1.1. METASTATIC DISEASE TO THE SKELETON

The strength and integrity of bone is dependent on the maintenance of this delicate balance between resorption and formation *(3)*. Complex regulatory interactions exist between a metastases and the host bone that disrupt this balance, facilitating dissemination and progression of certain types of tumors within the skeleton. Increasingly, evidence suggests that in order for tumors to successfully establish and grow in skeletal tissues, tumor cells must be able to interfere with normal bone cell function and indirectly tip the balance in favor of bone resorption *(4)*. Thus, it has become clear that in order for tumor cells to form a metastatic deposit and grow in the skeleton, bone resorption by osteoclasts must occur *(5)*. Recent research has provided new insights into osteoclast biology and the regulatory control of bone remodeling. This new knowledge has led to an increase in our understanding of the interactions between tumor cells and the bone microenvironment.

Tumor metastasis is the leading cause of death for patients with cancer, and the skeletal system is one of the most common sites to be affected by metastatic disease. However, not all tumors share the same likelihood of dissemination to the skeleton. Of the cancers that spread to bone, carcinomas of the breast and the prostate possess a special affinity, accounting for more than 80% of all cases of metastatic skeletal disease *(2)*. Other tumors that frequently spread to the skeleton include carcinomas of the lung, kidney, and thyroid *(2)*. This special osteotrophism or affinity to metastasize to bone involves characteristics of these tumors that allow them to establish and grow in bone, as well as unique features of the bone microenvironment, which makes the skeleton a particularly congenial place for these cells *(6)*. More than 100 yr ago, Stephen Paget referred to this as the "seed and soil" hypothesis, to explain the special affinity of breast cancer for the "fertile soil" of the bone microenvironment *(7)*.

1.2. CARCINOMA OF THE BREAST

Breast cancer is one of the most common malignancies in women. Up to one-third of women with early stage breast cancer will eventually succumb to their disease and many of them will have developed bone metastases during the course of their

From: *Current Clinical Oncology: Cancer in the Spine: Comprehensive Care.*
Edited by: R. F. McLain, K-U. Lewandrowski, M. Markman, R. M. Bukowski,
R. Macklis, and E. C. Benzel © Humana Press, Inc., Totowa, NJ

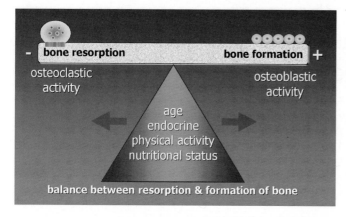

Fig. 1. Bone is a dynamic, metabolically active tissue. In order to maintain structural support for the body while providing a source of ions for mineral homeostasis, the skeleton must undergo continuous remodeling. This is a balanced process that entails repeated cycles of bone resorption by osteoclasts coupled with synthesis of new bone matrix by osteoblasts. An individual's age, endocrine and nutritional status, and level of physical activity influence these remodeling cycles. The maintenance of bone mass in the face of continuous bone remodeling requires the coordinated balanced activities of osteoblasts and osteoclasts in order to sustain the skeleton.

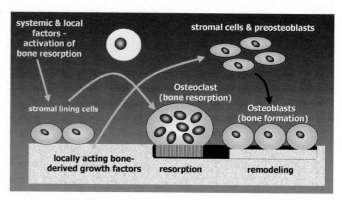

Fig. 2. The activities of the principal bone cells are highly regulated and link to maintain skeletal homeostasis. The temporal sequence in bone remodeling is initiated by osteoclastic bone resorption. The systemic (hormonal) or local (growth factor and cytokine) signals that activate bone resorption target the osteoblast/stromal cells, which regulate the activity of osteoclasts in a paracrine fashion. Osteoclasts are recruited from their hematopoietic/macrophage progenitors, to differentiate, attach to sites of bone resorption and develop a specialized ruffled border that facilitates transport of protons and proteases to degrade bone matrix. The microenvironment of the bone contains a rich supply of mitogenic growth factors synthesized by osteoblasts as part of the bone matrix, which are released by osteoclastic resorption. These osteoblast-derived growth factors funtion to regulate the proliferation and differentiation of osteoprogenitor into active osteoblasts, which then synthesize new matrix to replace the bone lost through resorption.

illness *(8)*. A significant percentage (50–70%) of patients with metastatic breast cancer will have skeletal involvement, contributing significantly to their morbidity *(9)*. In approx 50% of these patients, bone will be the predominant site of metastatic spread and in 20–25% of these patients the skeleton will be the only site of metastasis *(9)*. Approximately 80% of patients with bone-limited disease at the time of diagnosis developed skeletal complications (bone pain, fracture, and hypercalcemia), as will 60% of those with bone and visceral disease and 21% of those with no bone disease *(10)*.

1.3. CARCINOMA OF THE PROSTATE

Likewise, metastatic disease with bone loss and skeletal complications is common in patients with carcinoma of the prostate. Although relatively few patients will manifest bone metastases at initial diagnosis, a significant portion of these men will develop skeletal complications over the course of their disease *(11)*. One-third of patients will experience some adverse skeletal manifestation, including vertebral collapse requiring spinal orthosis, spinal cord compression, and pathological bone fracture *(12)*. Patients with high-grade tumors and those with progressive disease have the highest risk for bone metastases *(11)*. The tumor will have spread to the skeleton in 85–100% of patients who die of their disease *(13)*.

To help explain the interactions between tumor cells that metastasize to bone and the skeletal microenvironment, this chapter first reviews the biology of normal bone remodeling and some of the biological principles of metastasis. Some intriguing animal model studies that have added immensely to the understanding of this complex process are described. Finally, some of the current strategies used to treat this devastating complication of malignancy are briefly discussed.

2. THE BIOLOGY OF BONE REMODELING

Bone is a dynamic, metabolically active tissue throughout life. After skeletal growth is complete, remodeling of both cortical and trabecular bone is ongoing, and results in an annual turnover of approx 10% of the adult skeleton *(14)*. These bone-remodeling cycles are both temporally and spatially "coupled" and involve regulatory mechanisms that closely link the activities of these two cell types (Fig. 2). Bone resorption is, for the most part, a unique function of the osteoclast *(15)*, a specialized multinucleated polykaryon, which is derived from the hematopoietic monocyte/macrophage lineage *(16)*. The initial steps in this temporal sequence involve the proliferation of immature osteoclast precursors, differentiation into osteoclasts, matrix adherence, formation of a specialized ruffled border between the cell and the bone surface, and subsequent resorption *(1)*. The recognition and attachment of the osteoclast to bone matrix is controlled by specific integrin binding ($\alpha v\beta 3$) *(17)*. Integrin binding to the bone matrix signals the osteoclast to organize the cytoskeleton leading to polarization of the cytoplasm and the development of a specialized ruffled border that permits the establishment of an isolated space adjacent to the underlying bone surface *(18)*. The osteoclast then resorbs bone by the production of proteolytic enzymes and hydrogen ions, which are exported into the localized environment under the ruffled border of the cell *(19)*. A proton pump, similar to the vacuolar ATPase in the intercalated cells of the kidney, pumps hydrogen ions across the membrane of the cell, and lysosomal enzymes are also released creating the optimal conditions for the degradation of the matrix *(19)*. The conclusion of bone resorption is

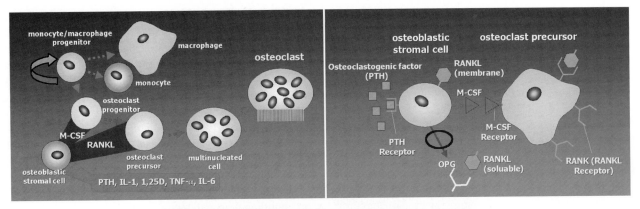

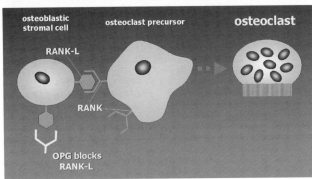

Fig. 3. Osteoclast commitment and differentiation are regulated by the expression of three critical molecules, macrophage colony-stimulating factor (M-CSF), receptor activator of nuclear factor (NF)-κB ligand (RANKL), and osteoprotegerin (OPG). Cells of the osteoblastic lineage play a paracrine role in the regulation of osteoclast formation and function. (A) The factors, which stimulate osteolytic bone resorption (e.g., parathyroid hormone [PTH], parathyroid hormone-related protein promoter [PTHrP], vitamin D3, interleukin [IL]-1, IL-6, tumor necrosis factor [TNF], and prostaglandins), interact with receptors on osteoblast/stromal cells stimulating the expression of M-CSF and RANKL. (B) M-CSF is a secreted protein, which interacts with its receptor on monocyte/macrophage progenitors causing these cells to become committed to the osteoclast lineage, creating a pool of osteoclastic precursors. RANKL is expressed on the cell membranes of osteoblasts/stromal cells. (C) When osteoclast precursors, which express the receptor RANK, are exposed to RANKL through cell-to-cell interaction with osteoblasts/ stromal cells, they will differentiate into mature activated osteoclasts. RANKL can also bind with OPG, which is a soluble receptor for RANKL, and acts as a decoy in the RANK–RANKL signaling system to inhibit osteoclastogenesis. M-CSF, RANKL, and OPG appear to be the molecular mediators of osteoclastogenesis, and provide a common pathway mediating the activation of bone resorption and controlling physiological bone turnover. The ratio of RANKL:OPG is an important determinant of osteoclast formation and activity and directly determines the rate of both physiological and pathological osteoclastic bone resorption.

most likely mediated by osteoclast apoptosis, however, the signals are still poorly understood. Drugs that inhibit bone resorption, such as bisphosphonates, induce osteoclast apoptosis, therefore, the cessation of osteoclast activity may be as important as their formation in the regulation of bone remodeling (20).

A large number of hormones, growth factors, inflammatory mediators, and cytokines are all known to stimulate osteolytic bone resorption through stimulation of osteoclast formation and function (21). How such a diverse group of factors (e.g., parathyroid hormone [PTH], parathyroid hormone-related protein promoter [PTHrP], vitamin D3, interleukin [IL]-1, IL-6, tumor necrosis factor [TNF], and prostaglandins) could all mediate the same important biological process has remained a mystery until recently, but this fact suggests some common pathway (22–24). It has long been known that cells of the osteoblastic lineage played an important paracrine role in the regulation of osteoclast formation and function (25). In cell culture studies, osteoclast formation from bone marrow requires the addition of 1,25(OH)2 vitamin D3, and the presence of stromal cells in the osteoblastic lineage that produce macrophage

colony-stimulating factor (M-CSF) as well as some other biological activity that has been recently identified (25). This activity has now been characterized with the discovery of three new family members of the TNF ligand and receptor signaling system, which have been shown to play a critical role in the control and regulation of bone turnover (26–30). These include the receptor activator of nuclear factor (NF)-κB ligand (RANKL) (29,30), its receptor, (RANK) (27,31), and its decoy receptor osteoprotegerin (OPG) (28,32). These three molecules appear to be the molecular mediators of osteoclastogenesis and provide a common pathway mediating the activation of bone resorption and controlling physiological bone turnover (Fig. 3).

Most of the previously mentioned factors, which stimulate osteoclasts, do so by upregulating the expression of RANKL mRNA in osteoblasts/stromal cells, which will then express RANKL on their cell membranes (25,27). Osteoclast precursors from the monocyte/macrophage lineage express the receptor RANK, and will differentiate into mature activated osteoclasts, when they are exposed to RANKL through cell-to-cell interaction with osteoblasts/stromal cells in the presence of

M-CSF *(27,28)*. RANKL can also bind with OPG, which is a soluble receptor for RANKL and acts as a decoy in the RANK–RANKL signaling system to inhibit osteoclastogenesis *(32)*. The ratio of RANKL:OPG is an important determinant of osteoclast formation and activity in vivo and directly determines the rate of bone turnover *(28)*. The process of the recruitment and differentiation of osteoclasts is shown schematically in Fig. 3.

During the process of resorption of bone, mitogenic growth factors stored within the matrix are released into the local microenvironments *(22–24)*. These osteoblast-derived growth factors, synthesized as a part of the extracellular matrix, function to regulate the proliferation of osteoprogenitor cells, causing them to differentiate into mature functional osteoblasts. These osteoblasts synthesize new bone matrix, replacing the bone that was lost through resorption, assuring a balance in skeletal remodeling (Fig. 2 *[33]*).

3. THE BIOLOGY OF METASTATIC DISEASE

In order for a tumor to metastasize, the cells must have the capacity to escape the primary site, travel via the circulatory system, and establish disease at a new distant site. To accomplish this formidable feat, a number of important molecular steps must take place, and this process is remarkably similar for the vast majority of different tumor types with the capacity for metastasis *(34)*.

The pattern of spread of metastasis is dependent both on the regional venous drainage of the primary organ, as well as selective characteristics of the target tissue resulting in homing of tumor cells to these preferential sites *(35)*. The propensity of tumors arising in the breast, prostate, and lung for bony metastasis suggests that there is selective homing of these tumor cells to the skeletal microenvironment. However, a comparison of prostate, breast, and lung tumors shows differences in the distribution of bony metastases, which are most likely explained by different patterns of regional venous drainage *(36,37)*. The high incidence of the spread of prostate cancer to the axial skeleton is partially explained by the drainage of Batson's plexus, where connections between the vertebral venous plexus and the marrow spaces allow metastases from prostate cancer to spread preferentially to the lower vertebrae *(36–38)*. This suggests that specific biological characteristics of the metastatic site and patterns of blood flow from the primary organ play a role in distant spread of disease. Additional evidence supporting this concept comes from animal model studies where the route of administration of tumor cells influences the occurance of bone metastases *(39)*. Intracardiac injection of tumor cells has been shown to consistently produce skeletal metastases in a number of animal models, whereas intravenous or subcutaneous injection does not produce bony lesions *(39–41)*. Other important biological factors for the dissemination of a malignancy involve angiogenesis, cell adhesion, invasion, and growth factors produced by tumor and host cells, as well as the local environment of the metastatic site *(34)*.

3.1. ANGIOGENESIS

A strong correlation has been observed between tumor aggressiveness and the degree of vascularization of a number of different types of cancers, including breast and prostate *(42–45)*. This data suggests that the capacity of a malignancy to generate new blood vessels (tumor angiogenesis) is important both in progressive growth of the primary tumor and its ability to form metastases *(46)*. A rich vascular bed not only increases the supply of nutrients to the primary tumor, but also increases the likelihood for dissemination. These newly formed vessels are, in all probability, more permeable to tumor cells facilitating entrance into the circulation *(47)*.

The balance between stimulatory and inhibitory growth factors regulates tumor angiogenesis, and a number of studies have demonstrated that metastatic potential directly correlates with tumor cell expression of several gene products, which function as pro-angiogenic molecules *(48)*. These factors include vascular endothelial growth factor (VEGF), basic fibroblast growth factor, IL-8, type IV collagenase (matrix metalloproteinases [MMP]2 and MMP9), and others *(34,47)*. The production of these growth factors leads to tumor growth and causes a concomitant increase in vascularization through stimulation of endothelial cell proliferation and migration, as well as a break down of extracellular matrix *(34)*. The proteolytic activity of type IV collagenase facilitates the migration of endothelial cells through the altered extracellular matrix toward the source of the angiogenic stimulus *(34,47,48)*. The expression of VEGF in Dunning prostatic adenocarcinoma has been shown to correlate with microvessel density and metastatic potential, where the highest mRNA and protein levels for VEGF were expressed by the most highly metastatic cell lines *(49)*. Recent studies have demonstrated that the pleiotropic transcription factor NF-kB regulates the expression of multiple genes including *IL-8* and *MMP-9*, and is constitutively actived in prostate cancer cells *(48)*. The blockade of NF-kB in the highly metastatic PC-3M human prostate cancer cell line resulted in significant inhibition of *VEGF*, *IL-8*, and *MMP-9* with subsequent inhibition of angiogenesis, invasion, and metastasis, in both cell culture and in animal models *(48)*. Additionally, angiogenesis in a metastatic focus probably plays a role in the establishment of tumor cells at sites of secondary disease. In an animal model of breast cancer, bone metastases contained large numbers of newly formed blood vessels at the periphery and within tumor tissue *(50)*. In cell culture studies, breast tumor cells stimulated proliferation, migration, and differentiation of bone marrow-derived endothelial cells *(50)*. Cytokine-stimulated endothelial cells may also participate in the establishment of a metastasis and help mediate bone destruction by targeting osteoclast precursors to sites of active bone resorption *(51)*.

3.2. CELL ADHESION

The establishment and subsequent growth of metastatic tumor cells in bone is also dependent on attachment to specific extracellular matrix components and to other cells (endothelial and stromal) in the skeletal microenvironment. Cell adhesion molecules (CAM) mediate several important cell-to-cell and cell-to-extracellular matrix interactions *(52,53)*. These attachments, through specific matrix binding, may signal tumor cell localization, migration, and proliferation and may also induce local expression of cytokines that stimulate bone resorption *(24,53)*.

A category of CAMs, the integrins, has been seen to play an important role in the metastasis of tumor cells to bone *(34)*. Integrins are a family of transmembrane receptors that bind to a variety of extracellular matrix proteins, are involved with cellular signal transduction and may be critical for the attachment of tumor cells to extracellular matrix (53,54). The $\alpha v \beta 3$ integrin, which mediates osteoclastic recognition and attachment to bone matrix, is also highly expressed in bone-residing breast carcinoma cells (55). Integrins interact with matrix through the Arg-Gly-Asp (RGD) peptide sequences present in extracellular matrix proteins (34). The addition of RGD peptides that compete with matrix constituents for integrin binding has been shown to inhibit metastasis of melanoma cells (56). Tumor cell attachment to vascular endothelium and to matrix constituents, such as laminin and fibronectin, are integrin-mediated (52). These proteins underlie endothelial cells and this binding may be an important initial step in tumor cell colonization of a metastatic site (53). Synthetic antagonists to laminin inhibit osteolytic bone metastasis formation by A375 cells in nude mice (57), supporting a role for matrix interactions in the establishment of tumor cells in the skeleton. The integrin $\alpha 4 \beta 1$ mediates cell–cell and cell–matrix interactions through adhesion to vascular cell adhesion molecule (VCAM)-1 and fibronectin (58). Transfection of Chinese hamster ovary cells with $\alpha 4 \beta 1$ resulted in bone and pulmonary metastases, whereas $\alpha 4 \beta 1$ negative cells yielded only pulmonary metastases (58). Antibodies against $\alpha 4$ or VCAM-1 inhibited bone metastasis, suggesting that $\alpha 4 \beta 1$ expression, can influence tumor cell trafficking and retention in skeletal tissues (58).

In addition to mediating the retention of tumor cells in bone, matrix interactions may also alter the cells' biological behavior, favoring proliferation and growth at the metastatic site (59). Bone extracts promote increases in chemotaxis and invasive ability of bone metastasizing prostate and breast cancer cells, but not that of non-bone metastasizing tumor cells (60). Exposure of certain types of tumor to growth factors that are found in the bone microenvironment might enhance their ability to adhere to bone matrix. Treatment of osteotropic PC-3 human prostatic carcinoma cells with transforming growth factor (TGF)-β (which is abundant in bone matrix and released in active form by osteoclastic resorption), causes an increase in synthesis of $\alpha 2 \beta 1$ integrin and promotes the adhesion and spreading of PC-3 cells on bone-derived collagen (24,61).

3.3. INVASION

The ability of tumor cells to invade tissues, with transversal of the extracellular matrix as well as angio-lymphatic channels, are critical early steps in the development of metastatic disease, and requires local proteolysis of matrix proteins and cell migration (62). The proteolytic breakdown of constituents of the extracellular matrix facilitates invasion and requires expression of specific proteases. The production of proteolytic enzymes aid tumor cells with detachment from the primary site, invasion of adjacent stroma, entrance and exodus from the circulation, and the establishment at a distant focus. The MMPs are a large family of proteolytic enzymes that are involved with the cleavage and turnover of many different components of the extracellular matrix and play an important role in physiological matrix remodeling (63). A large number of soluble MMPs have been characterized, which can be divided into three groups, including collagenases, stromelysins, and gelatinases, based on their in vitro substrate specificity (63). The production of

MMPs by many different tumor types has been demonstrated, and their expression levels have been shown to correlate with invasion, metastasis, and poor prognosis in several human cancers (34,64). Transfection of nonmetastatic cells with specific MMPs will produce a metastatic phenotype, and pharmacological agents, which act as specific MMP inhibitors, have been shown to inhibit metastasis in a number of animal models (64–67). In addition to playing a role in tumor invasion by facilitating extracellular matrix degradation, MMPs, through their proteolytic activity, may also help to maintain a microenvironment, which promotes tumor growth (63).

TNF-α is a key regulatory molecule in matrix catabolism, including the stimulation of osteoclastic bone resorption through the RANK–RANK-ligand signaling pathway (68). A number of different types of tumors have been shown to produce TNF-α, and its secretion by tumor cells is dependent on MMP activity (69). The inhibition of MMPs prevents activation and release of TNF-α from the plasma membrane of cells and results in a concomitant decrease in TNF-transcription and translation (70). Because TNF-α has been shown to increase the expression levels of MMPs (71), a vicious cycle could be set up where TNF-α stimulates MMP expression resulting in further TNF activity. This would simultaneously enhance tumor invasion and bone resorption, thus aiding in the establishment metastatic disease in the skeleton.

Tissue inhibitors of metalloproteinases (TIMPs) are produced by nearly all known cells that produce MMPs, bind with MMPs forming inactive complexes, and thus participate in the regulation of proteolysis and matrix turnover (72,73). These inhibitors, in addition to their physiological roles in the balance of matrix degradative activity, appear to be important as regulators of metastases (34). Transfection of metastatic cells with TIMPs or treatment with exogenously added TIMP has been shown to inhibit metastatic disease, including the development of osteolytic bone lesions (64,74,75).

Tumor invasion may involve the direct production of MMPs by tumor cells or, alternatively, induction of proteolytic enzyme expression by the host (52). Host fibroblasts and stromal cells associated with some invasive breast cancers express a gene that encodes stromelysin-3 (76). Stromelysis-3 RNA was found in 95% of invasive breast cancers, however, stromelysin protein and RNA were detected in the fibroblastic cells immediately surrounding the tumor, but not in the carcinoma cells or in stroma at a distance from the lesion (77).

3.4. THE ROLE OF GROWTH FACTORS IN TUMOR ESTABLISHMENT AND PROLIFERATION IN METASTATIC SITES

The establishment of metastatic disease requires tumor cell proliferation at the new site. Tumor cell products can impact the local environment of a metastasis in a reciprocal fashion, leading to a growth advantage in selective tissues. Such mechanisms appear to play a role in the case of metastatic disease to the skeleton. The microenvironment of the bone contains a rich supply of mitogenic growth factors (fibroblast growth factors 1 and 2, insulin-like growth factors (IGF)-1 and IGF-2, numerous bone morphogenetic proteins, TGF-βs, and others). These factors are stored within bone matrix and released by osteoclastic resorption (22–24) (Fig. 2). These osteoblast-derived growth factors function normally to regulate the differentiation and proliferation of indigenous bone cells (playing a physiological role in bone remodeling as previously described). However, these factors have also been shown to stimulate the growth of established cancer cell lines (24). Demineralized extracts of bone matrix and the conditioned media from resorbing bone cultures both contain growth stimulatory activity for several tumor cell lines with metastatic potential for the skeleton, and the extent of bone resorption correlates with this mitogenic effect (78). IGF-1 and IGF-2 have been shown to affect the growth of breast (79) and prostate (80) cancer cell lines. As a result, tumor cells with the capacity to stimulate osteoclastic bone resorption will enrich their local environment with the release of mitogenic factors, which can in turn, stimulate tumor proliferation and progression of disease.

3.5. THE INTERACTION OF METASTATIC TUMOR CELLS WITH OSTEOCLAST

Tumor cells utilize a number of different strategies to stimulate osteoclastic resorption, tipping the balance in normal bone remodeling in favor of bone destruction. By far, the most important of these mechanisms involves tumor cell production of factors that stimulate osteoclastic differentiation and activation. A number of different cytokines and growth factors capable of stimulating bone resorption by osteoclasts are expressed by metastatic as well as primary tumors of the skeleton. The list of factors includes most importantly, PTHrP (81,82), prostaglandin E (83), IL-1, IL-6, IL-11 (84–87), and TNF-α and -β (85,86,88). The activated osteoclast may participate in its own regulation in an autocrine/paracrine fashion by constitutively expressing pro-resorptive cytokines and, therefore, pathological bone lesions with large numbers of active osteoclasts may be, to a degree, self-perpetuating (85,86).

3.6. THE ROLE OF PTHRP

PTHrP is an autocrine/paracrine growth factor and a tumor product, which is homologous with the first 13 amino acid of PTH (89). This molecule shares a common receptor with PTH, was first identified for its role in hypercalcemia of malignancy, and, like PTH, is a potent activator of osteoclastic activity (89–91). PTHrP stimulates osteoclastic bone resorption by increasing osteoblast production of RANK-ligand and decreasing osteoblast production of OPG, (6), thereby tipping the balance of bone remodeling to favor bone breakdown.

3.6.1. PTHrP and Breast Cancer

Clinically, PTHrP has long been suspected to play a causal role in breast cancer-mediated osteolysis. In vivo studies have shown that breast cancer cell lines expressing PTHrP frequently metastasize to bone in nude mice (82). PTHrP is expressed in 50 to 60% of cases of human primary adenocarcinoma of the breast, and these patients are more likely to develop bone metastases (90,92). Of particular interest is the fact that PTHrP expression in bone metastases from breast cancer patients is higher than in the primary tumor, suggesting that the bone microenvironment has somehow enhanced tumor cell production of this factor (92–95). In an elegant series of experiments using an animal model of breast cancer metastasis to bone, it was shown that TGF-β released from bone by osteoclast resorption may feedback, and in a paracrine fashion upregulate PTHrP expression by the metastatic lesions in the

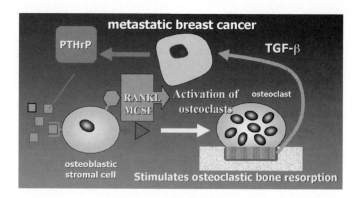

Fig. 4. The initial steps in the establishment of metastatic breast cancer in bone is the stimulation of osteoclastic resorption, tipping the balance in normal bone remodeling in favor of bone destruction. The secretion of tumor cell products, such as parathyroid hormone-related protein promoter (PTHrP), which stimulate osteoclastic differentiation and activation, mediates this process. Active transforming growth factor (TGF)-β released from bone matrix by osteoclast resorption will then feedback, and in a paracrine fashion upregulate PTHrP expression by the metastatic breast cancer cells. This positive feedback loop sets up a vicious cycle with the resultant osteolysis associated with metastatic breast carcinoma. PTHrP stimulates osteoclastic bone resorption by increasing osteoblast production of RANK-ligand and decreasing osteoblast production of OPG, thereby tipping the balance of bone remodeling to favor bone destruction.

skeleton (Fig. 4) (96). In vitro studies demonstrated that TGF-β significantly increased PTHrP production by human MDA-MB231 breast carcinoma cells (96). TGF-β signaling blockade using a dominant-negative mutant of the TGF-β type II receptor, rendered the cells unresponsive to this TGF-β effect in vitro, and likewise, the signaling blockade also cause significantly less bone destruction and formed fewer tumors in bone in an in vivo animal model (6,96). This intriguing data suggests that tumor cell stimulation of osteoclastic bone resorption by PTHrP, with subsequent release of TGF-β, can provide positive feedback, stimulating further production of PTHrP by tumor cells, setting up a paracrine loop with the resultant osteolysis associated with metastatic breast carcinoma (Fig. 4).

3.6.2. PTHrP and Prostate Cancer

The role of PTHrP in skeletal metastases from carcinoma of the prostate is less apparent. Although prostate cancer is characterized by metastases that are osteoblastic, histological and biochemical studies indicate an increase of both bone resorption and bone formation in these lesions, suggesting that the interactions between tumor cells and the bone microenvironment are quite multifaceted (97–100). Despite this, it seems clear that the stimulation of osteolysis is an important, and most likely, necessary component for the establishment of metastatic prostate cancer in bone (39). PTHrP is expressed and secreted by both normal and neoplastic prostatic epithelial cells, and a number of studies have provided evidence suggesting a role for PTHrP in the development of bone metastases (101–104). However, this association is complex and appears to be different from the observed role of PTHrP in breast cancer dissemination to the skeleton. PTHrP expression has been demonstrated in a number of prostatic carcinoma cell lines (105). However, transfection of a PTHrP expression vector into the rat prostate carcinoma cell line MATLyLu was not associated with any difference in the incidence of bone metastasis, size of metastatic foci, or tumor cell proliferation in an animal model *(106)*. Likewise, PTHrP protein was found to have a lower expression in the bone metastases than in the primary prostate tumor in human studies *(107)*, which is in contrast to the observations in breast carcinomas *(92–95)*. In vivo studies have shown that PTHrP expression does have a positive influence on prostate tumor growth and size when these cells were placed in the soft tissues of a rat hind limb, and also protected cells from apoptotic stimuli *(105)*.

3.7. RANK–RANKL SIGNALING PATHWAY: RELATIONSHIP TO PROSTATE AND BREAST

Recent reports have provided new insights into alternative molecular mechanisms whereby prostate carcinoma cells may directly mediate osteolysis. In vitro studies have shown that prostate tumor cells are capable of directly inducing osteoclastogenesis from osteoclast precursors in the absence of underlying bone stroma *(108)*. The malignant prostate cells were shown to produce a soluble form of RANKL, which accounted for the tumor-mediated stimulation of osteoclast formation *(108)*. Additionally, in vivo studies demonstrated that administration of OPG completely prevented the establishment of metastatic lesions in bone, emphasizing the important role that osteoclast activity plays in the establishment of skeletal metastases in cancer of the prostate *(108)*. Studies in human tissues have demonstrated the production of RANKL and OPG mRNA and protein in normal prostate and prostate cancer *(109)*, providing additional data supporting the concept of direct modulation of bone turnover. Of interest is the fact that RANKL and OPG expression was significantly increased in all of the bone metastases from prostate cancer compared with nonosseous metastases or the primary tumors in these studies *(109)*.

The significance of RANKL expression in the prostate gland is unclear at this time, but it seems likely that the RANK–RANKL signaling pathway will undoubtedly be found to play some role in normal prostatic physiology. Of interest in this regard is the fact that transgenic mice, which lack RANKL or RANK, demonstrate a mammary gland defect with the failure to form lobulo-alveolar mammary structures during pregnancy, resulting in the death of newborns *(110)*. RANKL-rescue experiments showed that RANKL acted directly on RANK-expressing mammary epithelial cells *(110)*. These findings suggest that this signaling pathway, which serves such a critical role in the regulation of bone remodeling, is also essential for normal mammary gland development. Further study will be needed to unravel the complex inter-relationships between the breast, prostate, and the skeletal system. However, it seems likely that such investigations will lead to new and novel paradigms in mammary and prostate glandular development and neoplasia, as well as an evolutionary rationale for the complex interactions and inter-relationships between hormonal regulation, gender, and the musculoskeletal system *(110)*.

3.8. ESTROGEN RECEPTOR AND BREAST CANCER METASTATSIS TO BONE

The hormone estrogen is a mitogen for breast tumor cells that express estrogen receptor. A role for estrogen in the dissemination of these carcinomas to the skeleton has been sug-gested, but the mechanism remains unclear *(6)*. For patients with cancer of the breast, bone metastasis is involved in nearly 50% of all distant recurrence events *(111)*. A higher rate of bone metastases is seen in lymph node positive compared with node negative patients, and, suprisingly, estrogen receptor positive tumors demonstrated a higher rate of bone recurrence than estrogen receptor negative carcinomas *(112–115)*. This is despite the fact that estrogen receptor positive patients have a lower overall rate of distant recurrence, and a better prognosis compared with estrogen receptor negative tumors *(115,116)*. Additionally, it seems likely that estrogen receptor signaling plays some role in bone metastasis, given that tamoxifen, an estrogen receptor antagonist, has been shown to help reduce bone recurrences in clinical studies *(112)*. The mechanism of this effect may be mediated at least in part by estrogen regulation of PTHrP expression. Estrogen has been shown to regulate the levels of PTHrP in early gestational tissues, as well as increase PTHrP expression in the estrogen receptor-positive breast carcinoma cell line MCF-7. Whether estrogen plays a role in enhanced PTHrP expression in the bone microenvironment remains unclear, but the clinical importance of these observations merits additional investigation, and it may enhance our understanding of tumor-induced osteolysis.

4. THERAPY FOR PATIENTS WITH METASTATIC BONE DISEASE

The development of enhanced methods for early detection along with better local treatment, has led to an improvement in outcome for many patients diagnosed with cancer. However, the treatment of patients who develop metastatic disease remains limited and, in many cases, palliative, despite the extensive use of radiation and chemotherapeutic agents. New or novel strategies that delay or prevent the development of metastatic disease would afford an opportunity to significantly improve both the quality and length of life for many patients diagnosed with a malignancy.

It seems clear that the resulting bone damage in metastatic disease to the skeletal system is because of osteoclastic bone resorption. Given that the rate-limiting step in bone destruction is the osteoclast, inhibiting the activity of these cells seems to be a reasonable primary therapeutic objective. Thus, the insights that have been gained in our understanding of osteoclast and bone biology have led to the development of new therapeutic approaches in the treatment of metastatic bone disease *(3)*. Effective anti-bone-resorptive agents are currently available, and continue to be developed, for the treatment of these patients.

Osteoclasts are inhibited by a class of drugs known as bisphosphonates, which are analogs of pyrophosphate, with a carbon atom replacing the oxygen and a variety of different side chains *(3)*. By inhibiting the osteoclast, bisphosphonates have been shown to reduce bone resorption regardless of cause. Thus, they have proved to be beneficial in the treatment of a number of conditions characterized by pathological bone loss including metastatic disease, osteoporosis, and inflammatory disorders like rheumatoid arthritis.

A number of clinical studies, as well as investigations in animal models, have documented the efficacy of bisphosphonates for the treatment of skeletal metastases in both breast and prostate cancer *(3)*. Through their inhibition of osteoclastic activity, possibly by inducing osteoclast apoptosis *(20)*, there appears to be a reduction in the skeletal events with bisphosphonate therapy, i.e., pain, fracture, and hypercalcemia, in patients with metastatic cancer. Despite what appears to be a clear benefit with bisphosphonate therapy, better treatments are still needed for patients with metastatic bone disease. Such improvements will most likely come with the development of new pharmacological agents that inhibit osteoclast function.

5. CONCLUSIONS

It is clear that the molecular mechanisms involved in osteolytic metastatic disease are multifaceted and complex involving bidirectional interactions between the metastasizing tumor cells and the bone microenvironment. What has emerged from the study of this process is a central role for the production of factors by specific bone-seeking tumor cells, which facilitate recruitment and activation of osteoclasts, leading to bone resorption, loss of matrix, and bone destruction. The subsequent release of mitogenic growth factors from the matrix would prove to be advantageous by altering tumor cells' behavior, aiding in their retension and colonization of the bone. These reciprical interactions could, in turn, set up a series of vicious paracrine cycles promoting the proliferation, adhesion, and invasion of cancer cells, as well as further bone resorption, supporting the establishment and progression of skeletal metastatic disease. The hope is that with a better understanding of the molecular mechanisms that mediate the loss of bone, more effective treatments will emerge, and ultimately, we will be able to prevent this devastating complication in patients with common malignancies who develop metastatic carcinoma.

REFERENCES

1. Masi L, Brandi ML. Physiopathological basis of bone turnover. Q J Nucl Med 2001; 45:2–6.
2. Coleman RE. Skeletal complications of malignancy. Cancer 1997; 80:1588–1594.
3. Rodan GA, Martin TJ. Therapeutic approaches to bone diseases. Science 2000; 289:1508–1514.
4. Goltzman D. Osteolysis and cancer. J Clin Invest 2001; 107:1219–1220.
5. Taube T, Elomaa I, Blomqvist C, Beneton MN, Kanis JA. Histomorphometric evidence for osteoclast-mediated bone resorption in metastatic breast cancer. Bone 1994; 15:161–166.
6. Guise TA. Molecular mechanisms of osteolytic bone metastases. Cancer 2000; 88:2892–2898.
7. Paget S. The distribution of secondary growths in cancer of the breast. Lancet 1889; 1:571–572.
8. Martin TJ, Moseley JM. Mechanisms in the skeletal complications of breast cancer. Endocr Relat Cancer 2000; 7:271–284.
9. Harvery HA. Issues concerning the role of chemotherapy and hormonal thereapy of bone metastases from breast carcinoma. Cancer 1997; 80:1646–1651.
10. Domchek SM, Younger J, Finkelstein DM, Seiden MV. Predictors of skeletal complications in patients with metastatic breast carcinoma. Cancer 2000; 89:363–368.
11. Carlin BI, Andriole GL. The natural history, skeletal complications, and management of bone metastases in patients with prostate carcinoma. Cancer 2000; 88:2989–2994.
12. Berruti A, Dogliotti L, Bitossi R, et al. Incidence of skeletal complications in patients with bone metastatic prostate cancer and hormone refractory disease: predictive role of bone resorption and formation markers evaluated at baseline. J Urol 2000; 164:1248–1253.
13. Whitmore WJ. Natural history and staging of prostate cancer. Urol Clin North Am 1984; 11:209–220.
14. Russell G, Mueller G, Shipman C, Croucher P. Clinical disorders of bone resorption. Novartis Found Symp 2001 232:251–267; discussion 267–271.
15. Teitelbaum SL. Bone resorption by osteoclasts. Science 2000; 289:1504–1508.
16. Athanasou NA, Sabokbar A. Human osteoclast ontogeny and pathological bone resorption. Histol Histopathol 1999; 14:635–647.
17. McHugh KP, Hodivala-Dilke K, Zheng MH, et al. Mice lacking beta3 integrins are osteosclerotic because of dysfunctional osteoclasts. J Clin Invest 2000; 105:433–440.
18. Teitelbaum SL, Tondravi MM, Ross FP. Osteoclasts, macrophages, and the molecular mechanisms of bone resorption. J Leukoc Biol 1997; 61:381–388.
19. Mundy GR. Bone-resorbing cells. In: Favus MJ ed. Primer on the Metabolic Bone Diseases and Disorders of Mineral Metabolism. 3rd ed. Philadelphia, PA: Lippincott-Raven; 1996:16–24.
20. Hughes DE, Wright KR, Uy HL, et al. Bisphosphonates promote apoptosis in murine osteoclasts in vitro and in vivo. J Bone Miner Res 1995; 10:1478–1487.
21. Canalis E. Regulation of bone remodeling. In: Favus MJ ed. Primer on the Metabolic Bone Diseases and Disorders of Mineral Metabolism. 3rd ed. Philadelphia, PA: Lippincott-Raven; 1996:29–34.
22. Hauschka PV, Mavrakos AE, Iafrati MD, Doleman SE, Klagsburn M. Growth factors in bone matrix: isolation of multiple types by affinity chromatography on heparin-sepharose. J Biol Chem 1986; 261:12,665–12,674.
23. Bautista CM, Mohan S, Baylink DJ. Insulin-like growth factors I and II are present in the skeletal tissue of ten vertebrates. Metabolism 1990; 39:96–100.
24. Orr FW, Lee J, Duivenvoorden WC, Singh G. Pathophysiologic interactions in skeletal metastasis. Cancer 2000; 88:2912–2918.
25. Boyce BF, Huges DE, Wright KR, Xing L, Dai A. Recent advances in bone biology provide insights into the pathogensis of bone disease. Lab Invest 1999; 79:83–94.
26. Chambers TJ. Regulation of the differentiation and function of osteoclasts. J Pathol 2000; 192:4–13.
27. Suda T, Takahashi N, Udagawa N, Jimi E, Gillespie MT, Martin TJ. Modulation of osteoclast differentiation and function by the new members of the tumor necrosis factor receptor and ligand families. Endocr Rev 1999; 20:345–357.
28. Hofbauer LC, Khosla S, Dunstan CR, Lacey DL, Boyle WJ, Riggs BL. The roles of osteoprotegerin and osteoprotegerin ligand in the paracrine regulation of bone resorption. J Bone Miner Res 2000; 15:2–12.
29. Takahashi N, Udagawa N, Suda T. A new member of tumor necrosis factor ligand family, ODF/OPGL/TRANCE/RANKL, regulates osteoclast differentiation and function. Biochem Biophys Res Commun 1999; 256:449–455.
30. Kong YY, Boyle WJ, Penninger JM. Osteoprotegerin ligand: a common link between osteoclastogenesis, lymph node formation and lymphocyte development. Immunol Cell Biol 1999; 77:188–193.
31. Anderson DM, Maraskovsky E, Billingsley WL, et al. A homologue of the TNF receptor and its lignad enhance T-cell growth and dentritic-cell function. Nature 1997; 390:175–179.
32. Simonet WS, Lacey DL, Dunstan CR, et al. Osteoprotegerin: a novel secreted protein involved in the regulation of bone density. Cell 1997; 89:309–319.
33. Puzas JE. Osteoblast cell biology-lineage and function. In: Favus MJ ed. Primer on the Metabolic Bone Diseases and Disorders of Mineral Metabolism. 3rd ed. Philadelphia, PA: Lippincott-Raven; 1996:29–34.
34. Woodhouse EC, Chuaqui F, Liotta LA. General mechanisms of metastasis. Cancer 1997; 80:1529–1537.
35. Nicolson GL. Organ specificity of tumor metastasis: role of preferential adhesion, invasion and growth of malignant cells at specific secondary sites. Cancer Metastasis Rev 1988; 7:143–188.

36. Cumming J, Hacking N, Fairhurst J, Ackery D, Jenkins JD. Distribution of bony metastases in prostatic carcinoma. Br J Urol 1990; 66:411–414.

37. Nishijima Y, Koiso K, Nemoto R. The role of the vertebral veins in the dissemination of prostate carcinoma. Nippon Hinyokika Gakkai Zasshi 1995; 86:927–932.

38. Batson OV. The function of the vertebral veins and their role in the spread of metastases. 1940; Ann Surg 112:138.

39. Goltzman D. Mechanisms of the development of osteoblastic metastases. Cancer 1997; 80:1581–1587.

40. Arguello F, Baggs RB, Frantz CN. A murine model of experimental metastasis to bone and bone marrow. Cancer Res 1988; 48:6876–6881.

41. Haq M, Goltzman D, Tremblay G, Brodt P. Rat prostate adenocarcimoma cells disseminate to bone and adhere preferentially to bone marrow-derived endothelial cells. Cancer Res 1992; 52:4613–4619.

42. Gasparini G. Clinical significance of the determination of angiogenesis in human breast cancer: update of the biological background and overview of the vicenza studies. Eur J Cancer 1996; 32A:2485–2493.

43. Karaiossifidi H, Kouri E, Arvaniti H, Sfikas S, Vasilaros S. Tumor angiogenesis in node-negative breast cancer: relationship with lapse free survival. Anticancer Res 1996; 16:4001–4002.

44. Heimann R, Ferguson D, Powers C, Recant WM, Weichselbaum RR, Hellman S. Angiogenesis as a predictor of long-term survival for patients with node-negative breast cancer. J Natl Cancer Inst 1996; 88:1764–1769.

45. Silberman MA, Partin AW, Veltri RW, Epstein JI. Tumor angiogenesis correlates with progression after radical prostatectomy but not with pathologic stage in Gleason sum 5 to 7 adenocarcinoma of the prostate. Cancer 1996; 79:772–779.

46. Saaristo A, Karpanen T, Alitalo K. Mechanisms of angiogenesis and their use in the inhibition of tumor growth and metastasis. Oncogene 2000; 19:6122–6129.

47. Denijn M, Ruiter DJ. The possible role of angiogenesis in the metastatic potential of human melanoma: clinicopathological aspects. Melanoma Res 1993; 3:5–14.

48. Huang S, Pettaway CA, Uehara H, Bucana CD, Fidler IJ. Blockade of NF-kB activity in human prostate cancer cells is associated with suppression of angiogenesis, invasion and metastasis. Oncogene 2001; 20:4188–4197.

49. Haggstrom S, Bergh A, Damber JE. Vascular endothelial growth factor content in metastasizing and nonmetastasizing Dunning prostatic adenocarcinoma. Prostate 2000; 45:42–50.

50. Winding B, Misander H, Sveigaard B, et al. Human breast cancer cells induced angiogenesis, recruitment, and activation of osteoclasts in osteolytic metastasis. J Cancer Res Clin Oncol 2000; 126:631–640.

51. McGowan NW, Walker EJ, Macpherson H, Ralston SH, Helfrich MH. Cytokine-activated endothelium recruits osteoclast precursors. Endocrinology 2001; 142:1678–1681.

52. Mundy GR. Mechanisms of bone metastasis. Cancer 1997; 80:1546–1556.

53. Albelda SM, Buck CA. Integrins and other cell adhesion molecules. FASEB 1990; 4:2868–2880.

54. Danen EH, vanMuijen GN, Ruiter DJ. Role of integrins as signal transducing cell adhesion molecules in human cutaneous melanoma. Cancer Surv 1995; 24:43–65.

55. Liapis H, Flath A Kitazawa S. Integrin avb3 expression by bone-residing breast cancer metastases. Diagn Mol Pathol 1996; 5:127–135.

56. Humphries MJ, Olden K, Yamada KM. A synthetic peptide from fibronectin inhibits experimental metastasis of murine melanoma cells. Science 1986; 233:467–470.

57. Nakai M, Mundy GR, Williams PJ, Boyce B, Yoneda TA. A synthetic antagonist to laminin inhibits the formation of osteolytic metastases by human melanoma cells in nude mice. Cancer Res 1992; 52:5395–5399.

58. Matsuura N, Puzon-McLaughlin W, Irie A, Morikawa Y, Kakudo K, Takada Y. Induction of experimental bone metastasis in mice by transfection of integrin α4B1 into tumor cells. Am J Pathol 1996; 148:55–61.

59. Sung JV, Stubbs JT, Fisher L, Aaron AD, Thompson EW. Bone sialoprotein supports breast cancer cell adhesion proliferationand migration through differential usage of the alpha(v)-beta3 and alpha(v)-beta5 integrins. J Cell Physiol 1998; 176:482–494.

60. Jacob K, Webber M, Benayahu D, Kleinman HK. Osteonectin promotes prostate cancer cell migration and invasion: a possible mechanism for metastasis to bone. Cancer Res 1999; 59:4453–4457.

61. Kostenuik PJ, Singh G, Orr FW. Transforming growth factor beta upregulates the integrin-mediated adhesion of human prostatic carcinoma cells to type I collagen. Clin Exp Metastasis 1997; 15:41–52.

62. Liotta LA. Tumor invasion and metastasis-role of the extracellular matrix. Cancer Res 1986; 46:1–7.

63. Curran S, Murray G. Matrix metalloproteinases in tumour invasion and metastasis. J Pathol 1999; 189:300–308.

64. DeClerck YA, Shimada H, Taylor SM, Langley KE. Matrix metalloproteinases and their inhibitors in tumor progression. Ann NY Acad Sci 1994; 732:222–229.

65. Masumori N, Tsukamoto T. Inhibitory effect of minocyclineon in vitro invasion and experimental metastasis of mouse renal adenocarcinoma. J Urology 1994; 151:1400–1404.

66. Davies B, Brown PD, East N, Crimmin MJ, Balkwill FR. A synthetic matrix metalloproteinase inhibitor decreases tumor burden and prolongs survival of mice bearing human ovarian carcinoma xenografts. Cancer Res 1993; 53:2087–2091.

67. Wang X, Fu X, Brown PD, Crimmin MJ, Hoffman RM. Matrix metalloproteinase inhibitor BB-94 (batimastat) inhibits human colon tumor growth and spread in a patient-like orthotopic model in nude mice. Cancer Res 1994; 54:4726–4728.

68. Zang YH, Heulsmann A, Tondravis MM, Mukherjee A, Abu-Amer Y. Tumor necrosis factor-α (TNF) stimulates RANKL-induced osteoclastogenesis via coupling of TNF type 1 receptor and RANK signaling pathways. J Biol Chem 2001; 276:563–568.

69. Gearing AJ, Beckett P, Christodouiou M, et al. Processing of tumour necrosis factor-a by metalloproteinases. Nature 1994; 370:555–557.

70. McGeehan GM, Becherer JD, Bast RC, et al. Regulation of tumour necrosis factor-a by a metalloproteinases inhibitor. Nature 1994; 370:558–561.

71. Mann EA, Hibbs MS, Spiro JD, et al. Cytokine regulation of gelatinase production by head and neck squamous cell carcinoma: the role of tumor necrosis factor-alpha. Ann Otol Rhinol Laryngol 1995; 104:203–209.

72. Stetler-Stevenson MG, Krutzsch HC, Liotta. Tissue inhibitor of metalloproteinase (TIMP-2): a new member of the metalloproteinase inhibitor family. J Biol Chem 1989; 264:17,374–17,378.

73. Murphy G, Willenbrock F, Crabbe T, et al. Regulation of matrix metalloproteinase activity. Ann NY Acad Sci 1994; 732:31–41.

74. DeClerck YA, Perez N, Shimada H, Boone TC, Langley KE, Taylor SM. Inhibition of invasion and metastasis in cells transfected with an inhibitor of metalloproteinases. Cancer Res 1992; 52:701–708.

75. Yoneda T, Sasaki A, Bunstan C, et al. Inhibition of osteolytic bone metastasis of breast cancer by combined treatment with the bisphosphonate ibandronate and tissue inhibitor of the matrix metalloproteinase-2. J Clin Invest 1997; 99:2509–2517.

76. Basset P, Bellocq JP, Wolf C, et al. A novel metalloproteinase gene specifically expressed in stromal cells of breast carcinomas. Nature 1990; 348:699–704.

77. Basset P, Wolf C, Rouyer N, Bellocq JP, Rio MC, Chambon P. Stromelysin-3 in stromal tissue as a control factor in breast cancer behavior. Cancer 1994; 74:1045–1049.

78. Manishen WJ, Sivananthan K, Orr FW. Resorbing bone stimulates tumor cell growth: a role for the host microenvironment in bone metastasis. Am J Pathol 1986; 123:39–45.

79. Reddy KB, Mangold GL, Tandon AK, et al. Inhibition of breast cancer cell growth in vitro by a tyrosine kinase inhibitor. Cancer Res 1992; 52:3636–3641.

80. Koutsilieris M, Frenette G, Lazure C, Lehoux JG, Govindan MV, Poychronakos C. Urokinase-type plasminogen activator: a paracrine factor regulating the bioavailability of IGFs in PA-III cell-induced osteoblastic metastases. Anticancer Res 1993; 13:481–486.

81. Rosol TJ, Capen CC, Horst RL. Effects of infusion of human parathyroid hormone-related protein-(1-40) in nude mice: histomorphometric and biochemical investigations. J Bone Miner Res 1988; 3:699–706.

82. Guise TA, Yin JJ, Taylorn SD, et al. Evidence for a causal role of parathyroid hormone-related protein in the pathogenesis of human breast cancer-mediated osteolysis. J Clin Invest 1996; 98:1544–1549.

83. Udagawa N, Takahashi N, Akatsu T, et al. The bone marrow-derived stromal cell lines MC3T3-G2/PA6 and ST2 support osteoclast-like cell differentiation in co-cultures with mouse spleen cells. Endocinology 125:1805–1813.

84. Jilka RL, Hamilton JW. Evidence for two pathways for stimulation of collagenolysis in bone. Calcif Tissue Int 1985; 37:300–306.

85. Hicks DG, Gokan T, O'Keefe RJ, et al. Primary lymphoma of bone. Correlation of magnetic resonance imaging features with cytokine production by tumor cells. Cancer1995; 75:973–980.

86. O'Keefe RJ, Teot LA, Singh D, Puzas JE, Rosier RN, Hicks DG. Osteoclasts constitutively express regulators of bone resorption: an immunohistochemical and in situ hybridization study Lab. Invest. 1997; 76:457–465.

87. Zhang Y, Fujita N, Oh-hara T, Morinaga Y, Nakagawa T, Yamada M Tsuruo T. Production of interleukin-11 in bone-derived endothelial cells and its role in the formation of osteolyti bone metastasis. Oncogene 1998; 16:693–703.

88. Thomson BM, Mundy GR, Chambers TJ. Tumor necrosis factor alpha and beta induce osteoblastic cells to stimulate osteoclastic bone resorption. J Immunol 1987; 138:775–779.

89. Suva LJ, Winslow GA, Wettenhall RE, et al. A parathyroid hormone-related protein implicated in malignant hypercalcemia: cloning and expression. Science 1987; 237:893–896.

90. Bundred NJ, Walker RA, Ratcliffe WA, Warwich J, Morrison JM, Ratcliffe JG. Parathyroid hormone related protein and skeletal morbidity in breast cancer. Eur J Cancer 1992; 28:690–692.

91. Abou-Samra A, Juppner H, Force T, et al. Expression cloning of a common receptor for parathyroid hormone and parathyroid hormone-related peptide from rat osteoblast-like cells: a single receptor stimulates intrcellular accumulation of both cAMP and inositol triphosphates and increases intracellular free calcium. Proc Natl Acad Sci USA 1992; 89:2732–2736.

92. Southby J, Kissin MW, Danks JA, et al. Immunohistochemical localization of parathyroid hormone-related protein in breast cancer. Cancer Res 1990; 50:7710–7716.

93. Powell GJ, Southby J, Danks JA, et al. Localization of parathyroid hormone-related protein in breast cancer metastasis: increased incidence in bone compared with other sites. Cancer Res 1991; 51:3059–3061.

94. Bundred NJ, Ratcliffe WA, Walker RA, Coley S, Morrison JM, Ratcliffe JG. Parathyroid hormone related protein and hypercalcaemia in breast cancer. Br Med J 1991; 303:1506–1509.

95. Guise TA. Parathyroid hormone-related protein and bone metastases. Cancer 1997; 80:1572–1580.

96. Yin JJ, Selander K, Chirgwin JM, et al. TGF-beta signaling blackade inhibits PTHrP secretion by breast cancer cells and bone metastases development. J Clin Invest 1999; 103:197–206.

97. Clarke NW, McClure J, George NJ. Morphometric evidence for bone resorption and replacement in prostate cancer. Br J Urol 1991; 68:74–80.

98. Urwin GH, Percival RC, Harris S, Beneton MN, Williams JL, Kanis JA. Generalised increase in bone resorption in carcinoma of the prostate. Br J Urol 1985; 57:721–723.

99. Garnero P. Markers of bone turnover in prostate cancer. Cancer Treat Rev 2001; 27:187–196.

100. Revilla M, Arribas I, Sanchez-Chapado M, Villa LF, Bethencourt F, Rico H. Total and regional bone mass and biochemical markers of bone remodeling in metastatic prostate cancer. Prostate. 1998; 35:243–247.

101. Iwamura M, Deftos LJ, Schoen S, Cocket ATK, Abrahamsson PA. Immunoreactive PTHrP is present in human seminal plasma and is of prostate origin. J Androl 1994; 15:410–414.

102. Iwamura M, Abrahamsson PA, Benning CM, Moynes RA, Gerhagen S, Cocket AT. Immunohistochemical localization of parathyroid hormone-related protein in prostatic intraepithelial neoplasia. Hum Pathol 1995; 26:797–801.

103. Rabanni SA, Gladu J, Harakidas P, Jamison B, GoltzmanD. Overproduction of parathyroid hormone-related peptide results in increased osteolytic skeletal metastasis by prostate cancer cells in vivo. Int J Cancer 1999; 18:257–264.

104. Deftos LJ. Prostate carcinoma: production of bioactive factors. Cancer 2000; 88:3002–3008.

105. Dougherty KM, Blomme EA, Koh AJ, et al. Parathyroid hormone-related protein as a growth regulator of prostate carcinoma. Cancer Res 1999; 59:6015–6022.

106. Blommme EAG, Dougherty KM, Pienta KJ, Capen CC, Rosol TJ, McCauley LK. Skeletal metastasis of prostate adenocarcinoma in rats: morphometeric analysis and role of parathyroid hormone-related protein. Prostate 1999; 39:187–197.

107. Iddon J, Bundred NJ, Hoyland J, et al. Expression of parathyroid hormone-related protein and its receptor in bone metastases from prostate cancer. J Pathol 2000; 191:170–174.

108. Zhang J, Dai J, Qi Y, et al. Osteoprotegerin inhibits prostate cancer-induced osteoclastogenesis and prevents prostate tumor growth in the bone. J Clin Invest 2001; 107:1235–1244.

109. Brown JM, Corey E, Lee ZD, et al. Osteoprotegerin and RANK ligand expression in prostate cancer. Urology 2001; 57:611–616.

110. Fata JE, Kong YY, Li J, et al. The osteoclast differentiation factor osteoprotegerin-ligand is essential for mammary gland development. Cell 2000; 103:41–59.

111. Paterson AH. The potential role of bisphosphonates as adjuvant therapy in the prevention of bone metastases. Cancer 2000; 88:3038–3046.

112. Smith R, Jiping W, Bryant J, et al. Primary breast cancer as a risk factor for bone recurrence: NSABP experience. Proc Am Soc Clin Oncol 1999; 18:457A.

113. Campbell FC, Blamey RW, Elston CW, Nicholson RI, Griffiths K, Haybittle JL. Oestrogen-receptor status and sites of metastasis in breast cancer. Br J Cancer 1981; 44:456–459.

114. Budd GT. Estrogen receptor profile of patients with breast cancer metastatic to bone marrow. J Surg Oncol 1983; 24:167–169.

115. Kamby C, Rasmussen BB, Kristensen B. Oestrogen receptor status of primary breast carcinomas and their metastases: relation to pattern of spread and survival after recurrence. Br J Cancer 1989; 60:252–257.

116. Coleman RE, Rubens RD. Clinical course and prognostic factors following bone recurrence from breast cancer. Br J Cancer 1998; 77:336–340.

3 The Pathophysiology of Spinal Metastases

Daisuke Togawa, MD, PhD and Kai-Uwe Lewandrowski, MD

Contents

1. INTRODUCTION

The American Cancer Society estimated that more Americans than ever, 1.33 million, were diagnosed with cancer in 2003 *(1)*. Reportedly, metastases develops in two-thirds of cancer patients *(2)*. After the lung and liver, the skeletal system is the third most common site of cancer metastasis *(3)*. These cancer metastases are also the most common skeletal tumors seen by orthopaedists, and the ratio of metastatic lesions to primary bone tumors is 25:1 *(4,5)*. Delamarter et al. *(6)* reported that only 29 (1.5%) cases had primary neoplasms of the lumbar spine in their study of 1971 patients with neoplastic disease. The prevalence of metastases increases with age. Patients who are 50 yr or older are at greatest risk for the development of metastatic disease. The gender ratio varies for each type of malignancy. However, when all neoplasms with the potential to metastasize are considered, men and women are equally at risk for metastatic lesions.

Sixty percent of all skeletal metastases *(7)* and 36% of vertebral lesions are asymptomatic *(8)* and discovered incidentally. Symptomatic spinal cord involvement has been estimated to occur in 18,000 patients per year *(9)*. Brihaye et al. *(10)* reviewed a total of 1477 cases and concluded that 16.5% of spinal metastases with epidural involvement arose from the breast, 15.6% from the lung, 9.2% from the prostate, and 6.5% from the kidney. The primary lesion remained unknown in 12.5% of patients. Metastatic lesions were seen in most patients between 50 and 60 yr of age, and there was no difference with regard to gender of the patient. They also analyzed 1585 cases of symptomatic epidural metastases and reported that 70.3% of the patients had involvement of both the thoracic and thora-

From: *Current Clinical Oncology: Cancer in the Spine: Comprehensive Care.*
Edited by: R. F. McLain, K-U. Lewandrowski, M. Markman, R. M. Bukowski, R. Macklis, and E. C. Benzel © Humana Press, Inc., Totowa, NJ

columbar regions of the spine, 21.6% had involvement of the lumbar and sacral regions, and 8.1% had involvement of both the cervical and cervicothoracic regions. Their findings confirmed that, although the lumbar spine is more frequently involved with metastatic disease, most patients with neurological dysfunction present with thoracic lesions.

Metastatic lesions in the spine represent the most common site of skeletal involvement *(11–15)*. This chapter focuses on the pathophysiology of tumor growth in the spine with particular consideration of tumor biology in the treatment of spinal metastases.

2. SPINAL METASTASES FROM VARIOUS TYPES OF CANCER

Skeletal metastases are produced by almost all forms of malignant disease, but are most often secondary to carcinomas of the breast, lung, prostate, or kidneys and less frequently from thyroid or gasterointestinal carcinomas *(8,9,16–21)*. The time interval between occurrence of the primary and spinal metastases varies according to the type and site of the primary tumor. In a review of 322 patients with documented metastatic bone disease, Schaberg and Gainor *(8)* determined that 80% of skeletal metastases arise from four major types of carcinoma (breast, lung, prostate, and renal cell). Breast cancer is the most common source of bony metastasis in women. Between 65 and 85% of women with breast cancer develop skeletal disease before death *(22)*. Among men, metastases from bronchogenic and prostatic carcinomas occur with the greatest frequency. Lymphoma and multiple myeloma are also a common source of disseminated skeletal lesions. However, there is some debate about whether multiple myeloma and lymphoma are considered metastatic or primary lesions of bone. Black et al. *(9)* estimated that for 9% of spinal metastases the primary source of the tumor could not be determined.

3. WAYS OF SPREADING: ANATOMICAL FACTORS

3.1. PAGET VS EWING

Two apparently opposing theories of patterns of tumor spread have long been discussed. In 1889, the English surgeon Stephen Paget published his observations from 735 autopsies of breast cancer patients. He noted that metastases were found more frequently in the liver and brain than in other organs, such as the kidneys and spleen. This led him to formulate the "seed and soil" hypothesis, which states that the process of metastatic spread depends on "cross-talk" between selected cancer cells (the "seeds") and specific organ microenvironments (the "soil") *(23)*. In 1928, James Ewing, an American pathologist, countered that there was no need to invoke mysterious "soil conditions," but that patterns of blood flow carrying cells from the primary tumor could account entirely for the unequal distribution of metastases. Hence, the first organ encountered in the circulation would harbor the greatest number. The observation that the lung, which was the first organ traversed by most breakaway tumor cells, has a high incidence of metastases supported this "mechanical" hypothesis *(24)*. In recent years, researchers have come to appreciate that both Paget and Ewing were partly correct, but neither hypothesis is thought to be entirely correct because predisposition to metastatic seeding is most probably multifactorial *(25)*.

Others have hypothesized that tumor cells lodge at sites of trauma, possibly attracted by a tumor growth-promoting factor released by dead or dying cells *(26)*. It has been observed that the vertebral body trabeculae routinely develop microfractures *(27)*, which may provide the microenvironment necessary for metastatic seeding. The host responds by producing bone in an attempt to repair the injury produced by the cancer invasion. Fast-growing aggressive lesions are associated with minimum reactive bone and radiographically appear purely lytic. Slow-growing or less aggressive metastases allow the formation of reactive bone to various degrees and appear radiographically blastic. Mixed areas can occur either within a single metastasis or at different sites *(28–31)*.

3.2. ROUTE OF SPREAD FROM THE PRIMARY SITE TO THE SPINE

Principle characteristics of malignant neoplastic lesions are the growth of tumor cells distant from the primary lesion. These distant lesions are referred to as metastases and are commonly found in the skeletal system. There are four potential pathways of metastasis: venous, arterial, direct extension, and lymphatic. It is thought that the most common pathway for metastatic embolization to the spine is through the venous system. To become established in the medullary canals of the spine, tumor emboli must first go through the capillary beds of the liver and lungs, often by establishing a metastasis at these locations. Alternatively, the tumor emboli may circumvent these filters and reach the medulla sinusoids by an entirely different route.

3.2.1. Venous Spread

After blood enters the vertebral body, it is drained by a large central basivertebral vein and smaller paraarticular veins *(32)*. Under normal conditions, 5 to 10% of the blood within the portal and caval systems is shunted into the vertebral venous system *(33)*. These venous channels connect with the epidural

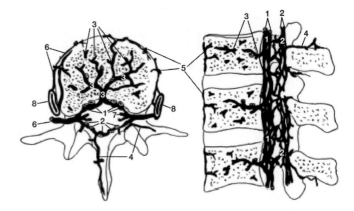

Fig. 1. Schematic representation of the vertebral venous system at the lumbar area (reproduced with permission from ref. *33a* showing the anterior internal vertebral venous plexus (1), posterior internal vertebral venous plexus (2), basivertebral veins (3), posterior external vertebral venous plexus (4), anterior external vertebral venous plexus (5), intervertebral vein (6), radicular vein (7), and the ascending lumbar vein (8).

venous plexus, a valveless system of veins within the spinal canal, first suggested to be a potential source of metastatic embolization by Batson *(34,35)*. Batson's plexus is a network of veins located in the epidural space between the bony spinal column and the dura mater covering the spinal cord. It is connected to the major veins that return blood to the heart and the inferior and superior vena cava. This plexus of vein is unique because there are no valves to control blood flow, and therefore any increased pressure in the vena cava system results in increased flow backward into Batson's plexus (Fig. 1).

In 1940, Batson *(34)* performed cadaveric studies in which he injected dye into either the penile dorsal vein of male specimens or the breast veins of female specimens. He discovered that the dye could be recovered in the vertebral veins. He postulated that any increase in intra-abdominal pressure would divert blood into the epidural venous plexus, thus providing a potential pathway of vertebral metastatic embolization for breast and prostate cancers *(34)*. The tendency of bone, and the axial skeleton in particular, to be a frequent site of skeletal metastases may be explained, at least in part, by the presence of Batson's plexus. Coman and Delong *(36)* provided additional evidence by first injecting tumor suspensions into the femoral veins of rats and then sacrificing the animals to determine the areas of embolization. They discovered that lung embolization occurred in 15 of 16 animals. When the same experiment was performed while the animal's intra-abdominal pressure was artificially increased, lumbar vertebral embolization developed in 12 of 14 animals. This provided in vivo evidence that Batson's epidural venous plexus is a potential pathway of metastatic embolization to the vertebral column.

3.2.2. Arterial Spread

Arterial embolization is another way of metastatic spread to the spine. Tumor cells may embolize through the arterial system and enter the vertebral bodies through the nutrient arteries.

For example, tumors of the lung may seed the vertebral column directly through the segmental arteries. This is believed to be another common mechanism of metastasis in lung cancer *(37)*.

3.2.3. Direct Extension

Direct extension has also been suggested as a potential pathway for prostate cancer *(38)*. Tumors located in either the retroperitoneum or the mediastinum may directly erode into the vertebral bodies as they expand, or they may enter the spinal canal through neural foramina. This explains why a prostate cancer metastasizes more often to the lumbar spine, whereas lung and breast cancers metastasize more often to thoracic spinal lesions.

3.2.4. Lymphatic Spread

Another route of metastatic spread to the spine is lymphogenous metastasis. Although lymphangiography has demonstrated lymph channels within bone, their clinical significance in providing a pathway for spinal metastatic embolization has not been defined.

3.3. SPINAL LEVELS OF DIFFERENT TYPES OF CANCER

Approximately 70% of symptomatic lesions are found in the thoracic spinal region and 20% in the lumbar region. Jaffe et al. *(39)* demonstrated that more than 70% of patients succumbing to cancer had evidence of vertebral metastases after careful postmortem examination. In his series, the thoracic spine was the most commonly involved segment of the vertebral column. Other investigators *(35,40,41)* have found that the lumbar spine was more frequently involved. Metastatic lesions affect the cervical spine less frequently than other portions of the axial skeleton (10%). Many large studies of metastatic disease of the spine do not include the cervical spine. One could argue that this is because of the relatively low incidence of cervical metastatic lesions *(42–44)*. More than 50% of patients with spinal metastases have multiple level involvement. Approximately 10 to 38% of patients have multiple, noncontiguous segment involvement. Gilbert et al. *(45)* found that tumors of the breast and lung usually metastasized to the thoracic area. However, the entire spine is often involved. Prostate carcinomas usually metastasize to the lumbar spine, sacrum, and pelvis *(45)*.

Venous drainage from the breast by the azygos veins communicates with the paravertebral venous plexus (Batson's plexus) in the thoracic region, and the prostate drains through the pelvic plexus in the lumbar region *(35)*. Retrograde flow through Batson's plexus has been shown to occur during Valsalva's maneuver and may allow direct implantation of tumor cells in the vascular sinusoids of the vertebral body without passing through the usual capillary networks. By contrast, blood from the lung drains principally via the pulmonary vein into the left heart and showers its tumor cells in a generalized fashion throughout the skeleton. Tumors of the colon and rectum, which drain through the portal system, tend to seed the liver and lung with metastases much earlier and more frequently than they do the axial skeleton.

4. PHYSIOLOGY OF SUCCESSFUL IMPLANTATION

For cancer cells to form viable metastatic foci, an exceedingly complex series of events must occur between those cells and the host environment *(46–48)*. The metastatic process is conventionally described as a five-step event: (1) release of cells from the primary tumor; (2) invasion of efferent lymphatic or vascular channels; (3) dissemination of these cells to tissues distant from their source; (4) endothelial attachment and invasion of the new host; and (5) growth of the original colony into a metastatic tumor focus *(49–51)*.

4.1. SEPARATION OF CELLS FROM THE PRIMARY TUMOR

The first stage, separation of tumor cells from the primary tumor, appears to be because of a combination of the loss of intercellular cohesiveness and subsequent transport within the original tumor interstitial tissue enhanced by a local collagen hydrolysis. The production of preteolytic enzymes aid tumor cells with detachment from the primary site and invasion of adjacent stroma. The matrix metalloproteinases are a large family of proteolytic enzymes that play an important role in physiologic matrix remodeling *(43)*. The production of matrix metalloproteinases by many different tumor types has been demonstrated, and their expression levels have been shown to correlate with invasion and metastasis *(44,45)*.

4.2. VASCULAR INVASION

Once tumor cells have escaped their parent they must invade local vessels to spread to distant sites as tumor emboli. Venous penetration appears to play a much more important role than lymphatic infiltration in the development of distant metastases. Spread by the lymphatic system is probably important only as far as the regional lymph nodes are concerned, from there the venous system is the carrier.

4.3. TRANSPORT

Once free in the circulation, cancer cells are able to migrate further depending on the local organ blood flow, general patterns systemic circulation, and perhaps a particular vulnerability of peripheral tissue (such as bone marrow) owing to peculiarities of sinusoidal permeability. The primary factor affecting migration, however, appears to be the ability of those cells to survive within the circulation during transport. Circulating tumor cells appear to be protected in part by a fibrin-platelet coagulum that surrounds the cells *(26,52,53)*. This coagulum isolates the circulating malignant cells from the hostile environment factors of the host, allowing them to multiply in some safety and to produce a small and protected colony *(15,54,55)*.

4.4. HOST ENDOTHELIAL ATTACHMENT

Once tumor cells have reached a peripheral site suitable for the development of a metastatic focus, direct attachment of these cells to vessel endothelium must occur before the tissues of the host organ can be invaded. The tendency of cancer cells to adhere to vascular endothelium is distinct from the mere formation of tumor emboli and provides the basis for establishing "beachheads" before interstitial invasion.

4.5. PROLIFERATION OF A METASTATIC FOCUS

Once a colony of tumor cells has become established within a peripheral site, it may be called a micrometastasis. In spinal metastases, the most common site of colony arrest is in the vascular end-loops adjacent to the vertebral end-plate. However, it will not become a clinically significant tumor focus unless it obtains its own vascular supply *(56)*. Secretion of "a tumor angiogenesis factor" was first demonstrated by Folkman *(57)*. The factor attracts vessels to a small tumor colony that would remain viable only through local tissue diffusion of nutrients and be incapable of subsequent invasion itself. The production of this angiogenesis factor appears to be blocked in part by postimmune responses, presumably mediated through lymphocytes. This phenomenon explains the late appearance of metastases long after resection of the original tumor focus. In such an instance, it can be postulated that a micrometastasis was established years earlier and attracted the vasculature required for growth much later. Adjuvant chemotherapy is probably most effective against such viable, yet poorly vascularized, peripheral tumor colonies.

In addition to a vascularizing factor, all tumors also appear to be able to secrete specific factors that enhance the establishment of their colonies in particular organs. Breast, prostatatic, lung, renal, and thyroid tumors all secrete osteoclast-activating factors that enhance their successful establishment in bone (58).

5. PROGRESSIVE GROWTH

The red bone marrow, located inside vertebral bodies, long bones, and flat bones, has a rich sinusoidal system. Sinusoidal vessels are usually under low pressure, thus allowing for the pooling of blood. This pooling of blood, along with other factors such as fibrin deposits and thrombosis, may encourage tumor growth. The red marrow of bone provides a biochemically and hemodyamically suitable environment for the implantation and proliferation of tumor cells. Because the capillary network of the vertebral red marrow is particularly susceptible to tumor implantation and invasion, tumor cells find it easier to escape from the circulation and multiply within the fine network of cancellous bone (18). The axial skeleton, which contains red marrow throughout a human's lifetime, is the most common site of skeletal metastasis. Finally, there are intrinsic factors inherent to the tumor cells themselves that may give one cell line a particular advantage in surviving and growing in the medullary space. Specifically, the elaboration of prostaglandins and the stimulation of osteoclast activating factors by breast cancer cells have been associated with the establishment of lytic metastases in bone (59). These cells may also produce a protective fibrin sheath, which further isolates them within the marrow.

After a metastasis is established within cancellous bone in vertebral bodies, it expands by producing a number of substances that either directly or indirectly cause bone resorption (60). Such chemical factors, including parathyroid hormone, osteoclast-activating factor, prostaglandins, and transforming growth factor related to metastases, have an effect on bone mineralization (61–70).

High levels of collagenase appear to correlate with tumor invasiveness, presumably the product of destroyed ground substance of bone (71). Tumor cells have been shown to secrete osteoclast-activating factor, which results in bone resorption through osteoclast stimulation (40,72). Tumors also are often associated with osteoblastic activity (prostate or breast cancers) release factors that stimulate osteoblasts to produce bone (73). Experimental studies involving breast and renal cancer have suggested that osteolysis may also be mediated by tumor prostaglandin secretion (74–76). Indomethacin, a prostaglan-

din inhibitor, has been shown to diminish, but not prevent, bone destruction in rats injected with tumor suspensions (77). In addition, as the neoplastic tissue envelops and applies direct pressure on the bony trabeculae, they become ischemic and are resorbed.

After cancellous bone in vertebral bodies is destroyed by metastases, cortical bone invasion occurs secondarily. This is consistent with the observation that metastatic involvement of a pedicle, which is composed of trabecular bone surrounded by cortical bone, is rarely observed alone, and is usually the result of direct extension from either the vertebral body or the posterior elements (78). Although the initial radiographic finding often will be destruction of a pedicle, the vertebral body typically is the first anatomic part to be affected (79) and is involved 20 times more often than the posterior elements (78) that is seen ranging from 14 to 30% of the cases. This is explained by the fact that in the absence of a blastic or sclerotic reaction from the vertebral cancellous bone, between 30 and 50% of the vertebral body must be destroyed before these changes can be recognized on a plain X-ray. However, with only minimum involvement, the pedicle exhibits early radiographic cortical changes that can be seen when the pedicle in cross-section is inspected on an antero-posterior radiographs (12). Thompson et al. (80) demonstrated by postmortem examination of patients who had died of metastatic disease that the posterior vertebral elements were significantly involved only one-seventh as often as was the vertebral body. Less often, the epidural space becomes the initial site of metastasis. In rare cases (3.4%), patients with neurological compromise may develop subdural or intramedullary metastases (10).

Each vertebra has barriers to the spread of tumor. The posterior longitudinal ligament is the weakest. Epidural metastasis is the most ominous complication of bone metastasis to the vertebral spine and is a surgical emergency. The most common path for tumor spread is through the posterior longitudinal ligament into the epidural space (81). The tumor enters the epidural space by contiguous spread from adjacent vertebral metastasis in the vast majority of cases. The remaining cases arise from the direct invasion of retroperitoneal tumor or tumor located in the posterior thorax through adjacent intervertebral foramina, or rarely from blood-borne seeding of the epidural space.

Besides mass effect, an epidural mass can cause cord distortion, resulting in demyelination or axonal destruction. Vascular compromise produces venous congestion and vasogenic edema of the spinal cord, resulting in venous infarction and hemorrhage. The relative importance of vascular factors as opposed to purely mechanical ones has been a subject of controversy for many years. The tempo of development of spinal compression is, perhaps, impossible to generalize. Once neurological symptoms become manifest, the condition is a surgical emergency.

6. SIGNIFICANT FACTORS FOR SUCCESSFUL TREATMENT

Treatment of patients with metastatic disease of the spine continues to be a challenging problem. With continued advances in the treatment of primary disease and local recurrences, patients are living longer and more frequently require treatment for symptomatic distant metastases. Additionally, the management of metastatic spinal disease has evolved considerably over the last decade, and several classification systems that may assist surgeons in determining appropriate surgical candidates have been proposed (16,62,68,69).

Surgical treatments should be tailored according to the patient's predicted survival period (1). Tokuhashi et al. (2) proposed an original scoring system for the preoperative evaluation of metastatic spine tumor prognosis. However, their scoring system is only applicable to the decision making between excisional or palliative procedures. Because aggressive surgery, such as total en-bloc spondylectomy, is now being more frequently advocated for spinal metastases, Tomita et al. (3,4) addressed the problem of appropriate surgical candidate selection with a more comprehensive classification system that is based on grouping tumors into intracompartmental, extracompartmental, and multiple lesions. Tomita's review clearly underlines the need for consideration of general oncological concepts to achieve successful local control of the spine lesion (82–85).

Recent advantages in spinal instrumentation and surgical approaches have enabled spine surgeons to treat these lesions more radically and to reconstruct the spinal column more effectively. The use of spinal stabilization in conjunction with the surgical treatment of these neoplasms has resulted in significant outcome-related improvements. Because significant advances have also occurred in the improved imaging techniques, diagnosis has become more accurate. It is desirable to establish newer ways of early detection of distant metastases to the spine, to predict biological behavior, and finally, to improve clinical management of spinal metastasis.

The inherent nature of specific primary and metastatic neoplasms determines their biological behavior and dictates which will have slow or rapid growth, which will be invasive, and which will produce metastases. Although metastatic lesions usually demonstrate behavior similar to their primary lesions, this is not always true; some metastases may be far more invasive or rapidly growing than the primary lesion of origin. It is this biological behavior of the primary or metastatic lesion that determines the likelihood and rate of spinal cord compression. Rapid tumor expansion may produce vertebral erosion, fracture, and result in acute cord compression with a poorer prognosis for improvement. Improved understanding of the tumor types and their biology will empower the surgeon to better define surgical indications and to predict successful clinical outcomes with surgical resection.

Currently, the treatment options available for metastatic spinal disease include radiation therapy, hormonal manipulation, chemotherapy, surgical resection, and most commonly, a combination of two or more of these treatment modalities. Reports of the success of various treatment protocols are contradictory because there is a lack of a standardized method for evaluating treatment success and there is a lack of understanding of the natural history of the metastatic disease process itself. Thus, current treatment options of patients with metastatic disease to the spine remain limited and in many cases are pallia-

tive. Several tumor-derived factors that stimulate bone resorption by osteoclastic activation have been recognized. Examples of such factors are parathyroid hormone related protein (70), prostaglandin E (71), Interleukin-1 (72), and tumor necrosis factor (73). Effective anti-bone-resorptive agents are currently available, and continue to be evaluated for the treatment of bone resorption owing to osteoclast activation (74).

From a surgical standpoint, it is important to consider that metastatic epidural compression in most instances develops ventral to the thecal sac. Therefore, studies describing the results of posterior decompression alone to treat neurological deterioration failed to show significant improvement of neurological deficit with surgical decompression alone. There is no advantage in the use of surgical laminectomy over radiation therapy alone for which reason laminectomy alone for decompression of neural elements has fallen out of favor (2,86–92).

Because of these poor results, many physicians have been taught that surgical intervention is not a viable addition to the treatment armamentarium and should be considered only as a last resort. However, anterior decompression, through removal of the vertebral body and any epidural tumor, has shown great benefit for the patients with spinal cord compression. Anterior surgical intervention is increasingly being accepted as a valuable component of the interdisciplinary treatment approach to the care of patients with symptomatic spinal metastases. Certain tumors (renal cell) with single metastatic foci without vertebral collapse are best treated by extirpation, when possible, and no irradiation, to allow the best long-term survival (46,48).

7. CONCLUSIONS

Despite recent advances in the treatment of spinal metastases, many problems remain making successful management of spinal metastases difficult. Early detection of small metastatic foci plays an important role. We anticipate that future advances in the understanding of molecular and cellular mechanisms in the various stages of carcinogenesis may provide the more effective clues to prevention and treatment of spinal tumors.

REFERENCES

1. American Cancer Society Cancer in America 2003. Web site: http://www.cancer.org/docroot/MED/content. Accessed September 30, 2004.
2. Shaw B, Mansfield FL, Borges L. One-stage posterolateral decompression and stabilization for primary and metastatic vertebral tumors in the thoracic and lumbar spine. J Neurosurg 1989; 70:405–410.
3. Boland PJ, Lane JM, Sundaresan N. Metastatic disease of the spine. Clin Orthop 1982; 169:95–102.
4. Francis KC, Hutter RV. Neoplasms of the spine in the aged. Clin Orthop 1963; 26:54–66.
5. Mirra JM. Bone Tumors: Clinical, Radiologic, and Pathologic Correlation. Philadelphia, PA: Lea and Febiger; 1989:1495–1517.
6. Delamarter RB, Sachs BL, Thompson GH, et al. Primary neoplasms of the thoracic and lumbar spine. An analysis of 29 consecutive cases. Clin Orthop 1990; 256:87–100.
7. Krishnamurthy GT, Tubis M, Hiss J, Blahd WH. Distribution pattern of metastatic bone disease. A need for total body skeletal image. JAMA 1977; 237:2504–2506.
8. Schaberg J, Gainor BJ. A profile of metastatic carcinoma of the spine. Spine 1985; 10:19–20.

9. Black P. Spinal metastasis: current status and recommended guidelines for management. Neurosurgery 1979; 5:726–746.

10. Brihaye J, Ectors P, Lemort M, Van Houtte P. The management of spinal epidural metastases. Adv Tech Stand Neurosurg 1988; 16:121–176.

11. Unni KK. Dahlin's Bone Tumors: General Aspects and Data on 11,087 Cases. 5th ed. Philadelphia, PA: Lippincott-Raven; 1996.

12. Harrington KD. Metastatic disease of the spine. In: Harrington KD, ed. Orthopaedic Management of Metastatic Bone Disease. St. Louis, MO: C. V. Mosby; 1988:309–383.

13. Berrettoni BA, Carter JR. Mechanisms of cancer metastasis to bone. J Bone Joint Surg Am 1986; 68:308–312.

14. Bhalla SK. Metastatic disease of the spine. Clin Orthop 1970; 73:52–60.

15. Johnston AD. Pathology of metastatic tumors in bone. Clin Orthop 1970; 73:8–32.

16. Clain A. Secondary malignant disease of bone. Br J Cancer 1965; 19:15–29.

17. Habermann ET, Sachs R, Stern RE, Hirsh DM, Anderson WJ. The pathology and treatment of metastatic disease of the femur. Clin Orthop 1982; 169:70–82.

18. Harrington KD. Metastatic disease of the spine. J Bone Joint Surg Am 1986; 68:1110–1115.

19. Milch RA, Changus GW. Response of bone to tumor invasion. Cancer 1956; 9:340–351.

20. Millburn L, Hibbs GG, Hendrickson FR. Treatment of spinal cord compression from metastatic carcinoma. Review of literature and presentation of a new method of treatment. Cancer 1968; 21:447–452.

21. Nottebaert M, Exner GU, von Hochstetter AR, Schreiber A. Metastatic bone disease from occult carcinoma: a profile. Int Orthop 1989; 13:119–123.

22. Viadana E, Cotter R, Pickren JW, Bross ID. An autopsy study of metastatic sites of breast cancer. Cancer Res 1973; 33:179–181.

23. Paget S. The distribution of secondary growths in cancer of the breast. Lancet 1889; 1:571–573.

24. Ewing J. Neoplastic Diseases. 6th ed. Philadelphia, PA: WB Saunders; 1928.

25. Onuigbo WI. Organ selectivity in human cancer metastasis. A review. Oncology 1974; 30:294–303.

26. Fisher B, Fisher ER, Feduska N. Trauma and the localization of tumor cells. Cancer 1967; 20:23–30.

27. Vernon-Roberts B, Pirie CJ. Healing trabecular microfractures in the bodies of lumbar vertebrae. Ann Rheum Dis 1973; 32:406–412.

28. Tanaka M, Fushimi H, Fuji T, Ford JM. Sclerosis of lytic metastatic bone lesions during treatment with pamidronate in a patient with adenocarcinoma of unknown primary site. Eur Spine J 1996; 5:198–200.

29. Aoki J, Yamamoto I, Hino M, et al. Sclerotic bone metastasis: radiologic-pathologic correlation. Radiology 1986; 159:127–132.

30. Jonsson B, Petren-Mallmin M, Jonsson H, Jr., Andreasson I, Rauschning W. Pathoanatomical and radiographic findings in spinal breast cancer metastases. J Spinal Disord 1995; 8:26–38.

31. Forbes GS, McLeod RA, Hattery RR. Radiographic manifestations of bone metastases from renal carcinoma. AJR Am J Roentgenol 1977; 129:61–66.

32. Crock HV, Yoshizawa H, Kame SK. Observations on the venous drainage of the human vertebral body. J Bone Joint Surg Br 1973; 55:528–533.

33. Louis R, Ouiminga RM, Obounou D. The azygos or vertebro-parietal venous anastomotic system. Bull Assoc Anat (Nancy) 1976; 60:381–397.

33a. Groen RJ, du Toit DF, Phillips FM, et al. Anatomical and pathological considerations in percutaneous vertebroplasty and kyphoplasty: a reappraisal of the vertebral venous system. Spine 2004; 29:1465–1471.

34. Batson OV. The function of the vertebral veins and their role in the spread of metastases. Ann Surg 1940; 112:138–149.

35. Batson OV. The role of the vertebral veins in metastatic processes. Ann Intern Med 1942; 16:38–45.

36. Coman DR, deLong RP. The role of the vertebral venous system in the metastasis of cancer to the spinal column; experiments with tumor-cell suspensions in rats and rabbits. Cancer 1951; 4:610–618.

37. Nagasaka A, Miyamoto T, Yoshizaki H, et al. Vertebral bone metastasis of small cell carcinoma of lung in a diabetic patient, initially diagnosed as pyogenic vertebral osteomyelitis. Diabetes Res 1993; 22:135–144.

38. Coman DR, deLong RP, Mccutcheon M. Studies on the mechanisms of metastasis; the distribution of tumors in various organs in relation to the distribution of arterial emboli. Cancer Res 1951; 11:648–651.

39. Jaffee WF. Tumors and tumorous conditions of the bones and joints. Philadelphia, PA: Lea and Febiger; 1958.

40. Galasko CS. Mechanisms of bone destruction in the development of skeletal metastases. Nature 1976; 263:507–508.

41. Wright RL. Malignant tumors in the spinal extradural space: results of surgical treatment. Ann Surg 1963; 157:227–231.

42. Fornasier VL, Horne JG. Metastases to the vertebral column. Cancer 1975; 36:590–594.

43. Fornasier VL, Czitrom AA. Collapsed vertebrae: a review of 659 autopsies. Clin Orthop 1978; 131:261–265.

44. Wong DA, Fornasier VL, MacNab I. Spinal metastases: the obvious, the occult, and the impostors. Spine 1990; 15:1–4.

45. Gilbert RW, Kim JH, Posner JB. Epidural spinal cord compression from metastatic tumor: diagnosis and treatment. Ann Neurol 1978; 3:40–51.

46. Stener B, Henriksson C, Johansson S, Gunterberg B, Pettersson S. Surgical removal of bone and muscle metastases of renal cancer. Acta Orthop Scand 1984; 55:491–500.

47. Weinstein JN, Collalto P, Lehmann TR. Long-term follow-up of nonoperatively treated thoracolumbar spine fractures. J Orthop Trauma 1987; 1:152–159.

48. Weinstein JN, McLain RF. Primary tumors of the spine. Spine 1987; 12:843–851.

49. Mareel M, Vermeulen S, Bracke M. [Molecular mechanism of cancer seeding: adhesion molecules and signal transduction networks]. Verh K Acad Geneeskd Belg 1997; 59:327–351.

50. Chishima T, Miyagi Y, Wang X, et al. Visualization of the metastatic process by green fluorescent protein expression. Anticancer Res 1997; 17:2377–2384.

51. Sastre-Garau X. [How to understand mechanisms of metastases]. Rev Med Interne 1992; 13:115–119.

52. Fidler IJ, Gersten DM, Hart IR. The biology of cancer invasion and metastasis. Adv Cancer Res 1978; 28:149–250.

53. Kinsey DL. An experimental study of preferential metastasis. Cancer 1960; 13:674–676.

54. Spar IL, Bale WF, Marrack D, et al. 131-I-labeled antibodies to human fibrinogen. Diagnostic studies and therapeutic trials. Cancer 1967; 20:865–870.

55. Wood S, Jr. Experimental studies on the spread of cancer, with special reference to fibrinolytic agents and anticoagulants. J Med 1974; 5:7–22.

56. Clark RL. Systemic cancer and the metastatic process. Cancer 1979; 43:790–797.

57. Springfield DS. Mechanisms of metastasis. Clin Orthop 1982; 169:15–19.

58. Galasko CS. Skeletal metastases and mammary cancer. Ann R Coll Surg Engl 1972; 50:3–28.

59. Powles TJ, Dowsett M, Easty GC, Easty DM, Neville AM. Breast-cancer osteolysis, bone metastases, and anti-osteolytic effect of aspirin. Lancet 1976; 1:608–610.

60. Faccini JM. The mode of growth of experimental metastases in rabbit femora. Virchows Arch A Pathol Anat Histol 1974; 364:249–263.

61. Chikazu D, Li X, Kawaguchi H, et al. Bone morphogenetic protein 2 induces cyclo-oxygenase 2 in osteoblasts via a Cbfa1 binding site: role in effects of bone morphogenetic protein 2 in vitro and in vivo. J Bone Miner Res 2002; 17:1430–1440.

62. Nauman EA, Satcher RL, Keaveny TM, Halloran BP, Bikle DD. Osteoblasts respond to pulsatile fluid flow with short-term increases in PGE(2) but no change in mineralization. J Appl Physiol 2001; 90:1849–1854.

63. Higashi S, Ohishi H, Kudo I. Augmented prostaglandin E2 generation resulting from increased activities of cytosolic and secretory phospholipase A2 and induction of cyclooxygenase-2 in interleukin-1 beta-stimulated rat calvarial cells during the mineralizing phase. Inflamm Res 2000; 49:102–111.

64. Ho ML, Chang JK, Chuang LY, Hsu HK, Wang GJ. Effects of nonsteroidal anti-inflammatory drugs and prostaglandins on osteoblastic functions. Biochem Pharmacol 1999; 58:983–990.

65. Kajii T, Suzuki K, Yoshikawa M, et al. Long-term effects of prostaglandin E2 on the mineralization of a clonal osteoblastic cell line (MC3T3-E1). Arch Oral Biol 1999; 44:233–241.

66. Yokozeki M, Afanador E, Nishi M, et al. Smad3 is required for enamel biomineralization. Biochem Biophys Res Commun 2003; 305:684–690.

67. Zhang H, Ahmad M, Gronowicz G. Effects of transforming growth factor-beta 1 (TGF-beta1) on in vitro mineralization of human osteoblasts on implant materials. Biomaterials 2003; 24:2013–2020.

68. Attia P, Phan GQ, Duray PH, Rosenberg SA. Parathyroid hormone-related protein and hypercalcemia in patients with metastatic melanoma: case report and review. Am J Clin Oncol 2003; 26:42–45.

69. Sowa H, Kaji H, Yamaguchi T, Sugimoto T, Chihara K. Smad3 promotes alkaline phosphatase activity and mineralization of osteoblastic MC3T3-E1 cells. J Bone Miner Res 2002; 17:1190–1199.

70. Saygin NE, Tokiyasu Y, Giannobile WV, Somerman MJ. Growth factors regulate expression of mineral associated genes in cementoblasts. J Periodontol 2000; 71:1591–1600.

71. Fielding JW, Pyle RN, Jr., Fietti VG, Jr. Anterior cervical vertebral body resection and bone-grafting for benign and malignant tumors. A survey under the auspices of the Cervical Spine Research Society. J Bone Joint Surg Am 1979; 61:251–253.

72. Mundy GR, Raisz LG, Cooper RA, Schechter GP, Salmon SE. Evidence for the secretion of an osteoclast stimulating factor in myeloma. N Engl J Med 1974; 291:1041–1046.

73. Mohammad KS, Guise TA. Mechanisms of osteoblastic metastases: role of endothelin-1. Clin Orthop 2003; (415):S67–S74.

74. Bennett A, McDonald AM, Simpson JS, Stamford IF. Breast cancer, prostaglandins, and bone metastases. Lancet 1975; 1:1218–1220.

75. Greaves M, Ibbotson KJ, Atkins D, Martin TJ. Prostaglandins as mediators of bone resorption in renal and breast tumours. Clin Sci (Lond) 1980; 58:201–210.

76. Nimberg RB, Humphries DE, Lloyd WS, et al. Isolation of a bone-resorptive factor from human cancer ascites fluid. Cancer Res 1978; 38:1983–1989.

77. Galasko CS, Bennett A. Relationship of bone destruction in skeletal metastases to osteoclast activation and prostaglandins. Nature 1976; 263:508–510.

78. Asdourian PL, Weidenbaum M, DeWald RL, Hammerberg KW, Ramsey RG. The pattern of vertebral involvement in metastatic vertebral breast cancer. Clin Orthop 1990; 250:164–170.

79. Braunstein EM, Kuhns LR. Computed tomographic demonstration of spinal metastases. Spine 1983; 8:912–915.

80. Thompson JE, Keiller VH. Multiple skeletal metastases from cancer of the breast. Surg Gynecol Obstet 1924; 38:367–375.

81. Fujita T, Ueda Y, Kawahara N, Baba H, Tomita K. Local spread of metastatic vertebral tumors. A histologic study. Spine 1997; 22:1905–1912.

82. Tomita K, Kawahara N, Kobayashi T, et al. Surgical strategy for spinal metastases. Spine 2001; 26:298–306.

83. Tokuhashi Y, Matsuzaki H, Toriyama S, Kawano H, Ohsaka S. Scoring system for the preoperative evaluation of metastatic spine tumor prognosis. Spine 1990; 15:1110–1113.

84. Tomita K, Kawahara N, Baba H, et al. Total en bloc spondylectomy. A new surgical technique for primary malignant vertebral tumors. Spine 1997; 22:324–333.

85. Tomita K, Kawahara N, Baba H, et al. Total en bloc spondylectomy for solitary spinal metastases. Int Orthop 1994; 18:291–298.

86. Findlay GF. The role of vertebral body collapse in the management of malignant spinal cord compression. J Neurol Neurosurg Psychiatry 1987; 50:151–154.

87. Fessler RG, Dietze DD, Jr., Millan MM, Peace D. Lateral parascapular extrapleural approach to the upper thoracic spine. J Neurosurg 1991; 75:349–355.

88. Rompe JD, Eysel P, Hopf C, Heine J. Decompression/stabilization of the metastatic spine. Cotrel-Dubousset-Instrumentation in 50 patients. Acta Orthop Scand 1993; 64:3–8.

89. Sundaresan N, Choi IS, Hughes JE, Sachdev VP, Berenstein A. Treatment of spinal metastases from kidney cancer by presurgical embolization and resection. J Neurosurg 1990; 73:548–554.

90. Sundaresan N, DiGiacinto GV, Krol G, Hughes JE. Spondylectomy for malignant tumors of the spine. J Clin Oncol 1989; 7:1485–1491.

91. Sundaresan N, Galicich JH, Lane JM, Bains MS, McCormack P. Treatment of neoplastic epidural cord compression by vertebral body resection and stabilization. J Neurosurg 1985; 63:676–684.

92. Siegal T. Surgical Management of malignant epidural tumors compressing the spinal cord. In: Schmidek, ed. Operative Neurosurgical Techniques: Indications, Methods and Results. 3 ed. Philadelphia, PA: WB Saunders; 1995:1997–2005.

4 Tumor Behavior

Barriers to Growth and Spread

ROBERT F. MCLAIN, MD

CONTENTS

INTRODUCTION
LOCAL GROWTH
SYSTEMIC SPREAD
CONCLUSION
REFERENCES

1. INTRODUCTION

Tumors arising in the vertebral body itself pose little danger to health and survival until they find a way into the larger system and either successfully metastasize or grow to a large enough size to threaten local vital organs. The barriers that must be overcome start with the basement membrane in either circumstance. Thereafter, the tumor must either demonstrate the ability to cross the vascular wall of the local capillary bed, survive in the circulation, and successfully implant elsewhere or the tumor must be able to overcome the local, physical barriers of the trabecular bone and cortical shell of the vertebra itself, the periosteum and overlying ligaments of the spinal column, and, finally, the muscular sheath with its many fascial layers and apposed parietal pleura.

The invasion of normal tissues by cancer cells occurs by two mechanisms: (1) growth-related tumor expansion, forcing tumor cells through planes of adjacent tissue along the path of least resistance, or (2) active locomotion, invasion, and then circulation of cancer cells.

Tumor growth generates intrinsic pressure and expansive forces, which tend to push the tumor along fascial planes and into potential spaces. Areas of dense and impenetrable tissue form barriers that either halt expansion or force the tumor in a new direction. Vascular channels and foramen often prove a portal of extension from one compartment to another, allowing a tumor to extend into a space with more room for growth and less resistance to expansile pressure. Over time, however, even rigid and impenetrable tissues will bow to pressure—bone remodels, thins, and expands or fractures, ligamentous tissues and fascia distend, and periosteum is lifted away from bone.

Tumors that will be successful in metastasis also begin with the process of direct expansion within their local environment,

but are more successful in crossing barrier membranes and tissues, gaining access to the circulation and lymphatics through combined behaviors of locomotion, invasion, and tissue degradation.

2. LOCAL GROWTH

2.1. DIRECT EXTENSION AND EXPANSION

As the growing neoplasm extends eccentrically from its initial focus, it must either displace these tissues or penetrate them. Slow-growing lesions will displace bone in such a way that the cortical shell will continually remodel, maintaining the mass within. These expansile lesions are usually benign or at least low grade. High-grade malignancies grow too rapidly for the damaged tissues to respond, pushing through vascular channels in the cortex to escape the bone barrier before it can react. As the tumor expands it builds up mass under the next barrier layer, periosteum and longitudinal ligaments, and elevates these away from the cortical bone. The progressively expanding periosteum may lay down a series of thin ossified shells in an attempt to respond to this injury, resulting in soft tissue calcifications. These tumors may also locate portals of egress unprotected by periosteum. When a tumor extends through the primary nutrient foramen at the midpoint of the dorsal vertebral cortex, the thin posterior longitudinal ligament is the only structure to retard its expansion. Once this structure is displaced tumor growth competes for space with the spinal cord or cauda equina, and the dural sheath is the only barrier to direct extension into the central nervous system. Breach of the dura is extremely rare, but adhesions to the dura are common and represent a contaminated margin.

Tumor extending anteriorly or laterally away from the vertebral body may continue to distend and stretch the periosteal layer until it becomes incompetent, or may degrade the collagen sheet and penetrate directly into the muscular layer. By this time many high-grade lesions will have successfully seeded distant tissues, but some intermediate and many low-

From: *Current Clinical Oncology: Cancer in the Spine: Comprehensive Care.*
Edited by: R.F. McLain, K-U. Lewandrowski, M. Markman, R.M. Bukowski,
R. Macklis, and E.C. Benzel © Humana Press, Inc., Totowa, NJ

grade lesions will continue to expand locally for some time before metastasizing (or at least before metastases can be detected). In these tumors the expanding front of the neoplasm continues to stretch and compress the surrounding soft tissue and muscle layers into a dense and fibrous pseudocapsule, the last barrier between the tumor and the visceral cavities. The pseudocapsule appears tough and resistant to penetration on a gross level, but is really only a distortion of much looser and more easily transgressed tissues. The pseudocapsule is often extensively contaminated with neoplastic foci, and is not a reliable barrier to invasion.

There is one other, more traumatic, means for tumor to escape its local barriers: pathological fracture. Even if the tumor has not been able to successfully metastasize or penetrate the shell of cortex and periosteum, it can, by destroying enough vertebral bone, escape through fracture and collapse of the diseased vertebra. Low-grade lesions will continue to expand and disrupt bone to the point that mechanical integrity is lost, or that minor trauma precipitates fracture. Higher-grade lesions may outstrip blood supply leading to bone necrosis. Once fracture occurs, all barriers may be breached at once, allowing tumor to spill into the surrounding musculature or the abdominal or thoracic cavity (Fig. 1). Hematoma may extend the contamination far beyond the local fracture site.

More often collapse is progressive and less acute. Tumor extends beyond the cortical shell and into the periosteal barrier, but extensive spread is not certain. Still, resection of a primary sarcoma associated with vertebral fracture must include a wide cuff of muscle and pseudocapsule if *en-bloc* excision is to be successful.

Once the tumor escapes the confines of the connective tissue sheath that surrounds the vertebral body, there is little to restrain further growth and extension. In the cervical spine, extension can occlude the vertebral artery system within the vertebral ring, and may impinge on airway or vascular structures once the vertebral barriers are breached. In the thoracic region, extension into the chest can result in diffuse metastases, or in an extensive soft tissue mass, before growth is appreciated.

The lumbar segments are encased in a more dense and extensive soft tissue envelope, but once these barriers are exceeded, extension into the abdominal cavity can occur. Locally aggressive tumors may push cranially and caudally under the longitudinal ligament and psoas muscle to directly involve adjacent vertebrae. Local invasion into the lymphatics and the great vessels, and neovascular recruitment lead to local extension and distant spread that can impair treatment.

The sacropelvic region is particularly problematic. The anterior soft tissue envelope is thin, with no muscular layer over the anterior cortex of the sacrum. Distension and rupture of the anterior cortex allows the tumor to extend into a large-volume potential space, with few structures to immediately signal the mass effect. The pelvis, anthropomorphically designed to accommodate pregnancy and a large displacement volume, can conceal a very large tumor mass before symptoms develop (Fig. 2). Tumors escaping the margins of the sacrum can extend directly into the peritoneum, colon, rectum, or bladder, where invasion can result in serious complications and morbidity. At the same time, tumors arising in the colorectum, bladder, kid-

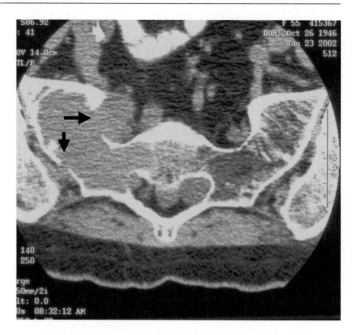

Fig. 1. An insufficiency fracture through the sacral ala allows this solitary plasmacytoma to escape the barriers of the sacral cortex and contaminate both the sacroiliac joint and the retroperitoneal space (arrows). Fortunately, the prognosis for local control is not seriously altered in this radio-sensitive tumor.

ney, and adrenals can gain access to the vertebral body through direct extension as well as vascular spread. Adherence of recurrent colorectal carcinomas can necessitate sacrectomy as part of the local control of the tumor.

2.2. PHYSICAL BARRIERS WITHIN THE SPINAL COLUMN

The spine is an extensive organ, constructed of multiple segments traversing the length of the neck, torso, abdomen, and pelvis. Vertebral segments find themselves in direct continuity with all of the visceral organs likely to develop neoplastic disease, and share venous drainage with many of these organs. The spine itself is a potential source of many types of primary tumors, and the cancellous marrow is a rich environment for tumor metastasis. The ability to treat many of these tumor types for long-term local control or cure depends on how far the tumor has spread at diagnosis and to what tissues.

2.3. CORTICAL BONE

Once the tumor has arisen in the cancellous bone of the vertebral body, it begins to extend along the planes of least resistance—through the vascular sinusoids of the vertebral marrow. After extending through the vertebral body, the tumor encounters the cortical shell of the vertebral body and pedicle. This is the first physical barrier to tumor extension. Although slow-growing and locally aggressive tumors will tend to distend and disrupt the cortical shell, over time, more aggressive tumors may escape the cortical barrier through the numerous perforations intended to provide egress of the nutrient vessels. Either tumor type may disrupt the trabecular architecture to the point that the bone fails and fractures. Once the cortical shell is fractured, the tumor is able to extend outward to the surrounding soft tissues, anteriorly into the chest or abdomen, or posteriorly into the spinal canal.

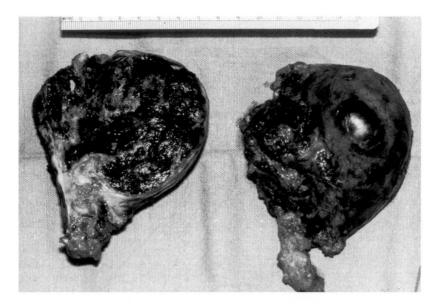

Fig. 2. Direct extension into the pelvis by a sacral chordoma may reach great dimensions before significant symptoms arise.

2.4. INTERVERTEBRAL DISCS

The intervertebral discs are, for all practical purposes, impenetrable to tumor tissue. The disc is dense, highly organized, and crosslinked with collagen fibers, and essentially avascular. Even if tumor cells have the mechanism to breakdown and invade the disc margins, the structure is several millimeters thick at any level, and crossing the disc would take an impossibly long time. In patients with severe disc disease, the disc space may be narrowed and devoid of disc material in some areas, making extension possible. Even then, direct extension of tumor from one vertebral body to the next is rare. When two adjacent vertebrae are consumed by a destructive process crossing the disc space, the diagnosis is always more likely to be infection.

When tumor extends from one vertebral body to the next, the most common route is around the disc, extending longitudinally within the spinal canal, or pushing proximally or distally underneath the anterior longitudinal ligament or periostium to reach the adjacent vertebra (Fig. 3). A bridge of tumor may be seen anterior to the disc, connecting the involved vertebrae. Even this process is time consuming, and adjacent vertebrae are still more likely to be individually seeded by multiple hematogenous metastases.

2.5. PERIOSTEUM

The periosteum of the vertebral body is relatively thin by comparison to the covering found in the long bones of the upper and lower extremities. This barrier to immediate extension into the paraspinous soft tissues can respond to slow, progressive tumor extension by ossifying and thickening, but may rapidly give way to aggressive lesions. The anterior and posterior thickenings of the periosteum, the longitudinal ligaments, provide a considerably more substantial barrier to extension, but they are incomplete, covering only a portion of the circumference of the body in either case.

Tumors extending through nutrient foramenae or defects in the cortex will tend to elevate the periosteum away from the cortical surface, disrupting adhesions and nutrient vessels as

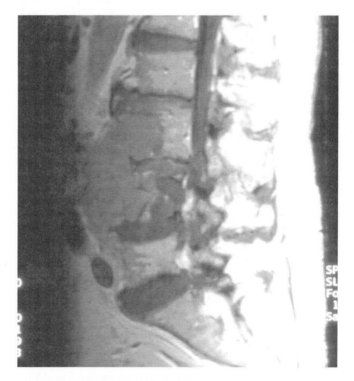

Fig. 3. An isolated renal cell metastasis of the L4 body, extending anteriorly and superiorly under the anterior longitudinal ligament to invade the L3 vertebra. Two-level corpectomy provided local control, pain relief, and 4 yr of "disease-free" survival.

the space is extended. This injury stimulates a reactive ossification of the periosteum in an attempt to repair the bone and combat the distortion. Rapidly growing tumors will repeatedly extend the periosteum away from this line of ossification, creating a distinctive "onion-peel" appearance on radiographs, created by repeated layers of ossification, one on top of the other as the tumor expands.

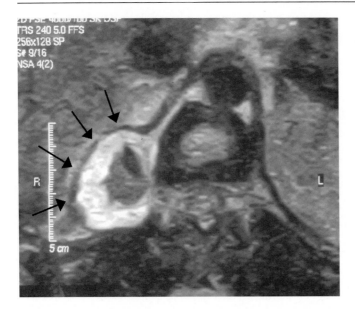

Fig. 4. Extension from the lateral aspect of the thoracic vertebra results in a large intrathoracic mass. This chondrosarcoma was still contained within a pseudocapsule of periosteum and muscle, further covered by the parietal pleura (arrows). Resection of these tissues with the tumor provided a disease-free margin.

2.6. DURA MATER

Extension of tumor tissue through the dura into the central nervous system is unusual, but can occur. More often intradural/extradural tumors begin within the thecal sack as neural tumors, extending outward as they expand.

Adhesions to the thecal sack are not uncommon, however, and represent a compromised margin when encountered. For primary sarcomas and locally aggressive tumors, dural excision is occasionally warranted to obtain a complete excision and the highest likelihood of local control and cure.

2.7. PLEURA AND PERITONEUM

The visceral and parietal reflections of these tissues form two more barriers to tumor extension within the chest and abdomen. They also create a potential space within which the tumor can extend and disseminate. Tumor cells escaping the periosteal barrier may either invade and cross the parietal and pleural membranes or distend and mechanically force tissue across the barrier (Fig. 4).

Tumor cells crossing these structures may implant there and create a focal extension of tumor mass that extends physically across either side of the membrane. These tumor foci may shed cells into the potential space between the layers, which is made a real space when tissue reaction creates an effusion. This malignant effusion may disseminate tumor metastases throughout the hemithorax or abdomen.

3. SYSTEMIC SPREAD

In addition to direct spread through expansion, tumor cells are able to migrate from their local address to new tissues, either immediately adjacent to the tumor margin, or into the circulation or lymphatic system where they can disperse widely throughout the body. Active locomotion of cells has been observed for decades, and locomotion of cancer cells was

reported as early as 1911 (1). At the present, many aspects of cellular locomotion remain speculative, but principle mechanisms are known. Signals within the surrounding stroma, either electric or soluable, trigger cell responses through action on membrane bound surface receptors. The signal drives an interaction of actin and myosin within the ceoll, in conjunction with two families of proteins, the dyneins and kinesins. Cellular motion occurs as the cell extends its leading edge outward into the surrounding substrate, and detaches itself from its original colony of tumor cells (2).

3.1. VASCULAR INVASION

Tumor cells within the spine may reach the vascular circulation by invading the sinusoids that drain the vertebral cancellous bone, the reverse of the way most metastases reach the vertebral body. The same paravertebral plexus that allows communication between the spinal venous drainage and the azygos veins draining the breast, allows cells from the vertebral levels to drain back into the pulmonary flow and metastasize into the lungs (3). Similarly, the pelvic drainage that may direct colon carcinoma or prostate carcinoma into the spinal column, may drain spinal lesions into the liver (4).

Direct extension through vessel walls can occur, and adherence to and invasion of the great vessels can render some primary tumors essentially unresectable. Tumor extending through the vascular wall may generate bulk emboli that may seed the pulmonary or hepatic beds or produce local thrombosis. In the cervical spine direct extension may occlude or encompass the vertebral arteries, complicating excising or producing neurological symptoms in patients with inadequate perfusion from the contralateral vessel.

3.2. LOCOMOTION AND INVASION

Invasion is the first morphologically identifiable act of cancer dissemination beyond the local environment. The process begins when the cell breaches the basal lamina. Hematogenous metastasis is usually attributed to invasion of the veins draining the primary tumor bed. In some sarcomas, however, metastases can enter the bloodstream through clefts in the tissue structure that drain into the vascular supply, or through the imperfect membranes formed by neovascular elements derived through angiogenesis. Further, there is some evidence that direct extension of growing tumors into disrupted tissues can seed the blood supply through shedding of cells into the ruptured vasculature.

Progression from a focal primary tumor to an invasive lesion is characterized by penetration of the basement membrane by migrating tumor cells. Fragmentation of the basement membrane occurs in both *in situ* and invasive lesions, suggesting that cells within the *in situ* lesion may prepare the surrounding stroma for later invasion (5).

The basement membrane is a three-layered structure of varying thickness, which form the stroma to the parenchyma. The structural components of the basement membrane include type IV collagen, confined to the lamina densa, the basal lamina; and type V collagen in the surrounding two layers the lamina lucida externa and the lamina lucida interna. Other components include the glycoproteins laminin and fibronectin, proteoglycans and entactin. Outside the basement membrane, the interstitial tissues are organized by fibers of types I, III, and V collagen and elastin, which—together with fibronectin—stabilize additional proteoglycans and glycoproteins in the matrix. The density of collagen and proteoglycan elements is similar to that seen in cartilage, a tissue of type I and II collagen, proteoglycan, glycosaminoglycans, and elastin, which is virtually impenetrable to tumor cells and neovasculature (6). The resistance of cartilage to invasion can be attributed to three characteristics: density, non-degradable matrix elements, and substances inhibiting the invasive apparatus of endothelial and neoplastic cells. These same characteristics confer barrier characteristics to other musculoskeletal and parenchymal tissues. "Successful" neoplasms use a variety of mechanisms to overcome these barriers to invasion and metastasis.

3.3. TISSUE DEGRADATION

The ability of rare tumors (e.g., some osteosarcomas) to invade and break down cartilage tissues depends on the ability find a cleft or vascular channel to invade, and on the subsequent ability of the neoplastic cells to degrade the cartilage matrix through protease and collagenase-driven proteolysis. The fact that proteases are also involved in the cycle of cell division and in cellular locomotion points strongly to this family of proteins as primary determinants in cancer expansion and spread. The process by which cells use these elements to invade cartilage is representative of the methods by which many tumor types cross the other barriers previously listed, gaining access to the visceral spaces or venous and lymphatic drainage.

Proteolysis is an important aspect of regulation of transmembrane signals generated by activation, inactivation, or transformation of cell surface molecules. These signals regulate various cellular functions, such as proliferation, apoptosis, differentiation, and invasion and derangements of extracellular protease activity may be critically reflected in the behavior of malignant cancer cells (7).

Whether directly extending into surrounding stroma, or invading and extending into the vascular elements in the process of metastasizing, tumor cells must cross the basement membrane, penetrate the endothelial cell barriers, and establish a successful neovascular supply before they can begin to proliferate. This complex process results in a low rate of successful metastasis, and determines that only specifically adapted cells can complete the process of invasion and metastasis. During the process of invasion, continuous degradation of the extracellular matrix must occur along the advancing front of the migrating cells, in combination with active cell locomotion. Although a number of proteases have been implicated in this process, matrix metalloproteinases (MMPs) have emerged as principle agents in cellular invasion (8). MMPs play a major role in the degradation of extracellular matrix molecules, and matrix metalloproteinase inhibitors (TIMPs) may play a role in controlling invasion and tumor extension (9–12). Both are involved in normal physiological maintenance of the basement membrane. The process of extracellular matrix degradation is carefully balanced, even in neoplastic invasion, because unregulated proteolysis would leave an unsuitable environment for tumor cell survival. It appears that the production of both MMPs and TIMPs may be carefully balanced in successful tumor phenotypes to allow invasion without dissolution of the matrix (13). Even more interesting, MMP action appears to specifically expose chemotactic sites on laminin molecules, potentially signaling breaks in the basement membrane to other tumor cells (14,15). An important host-contribution to invasion and tumor cell survival is the frequent association of local MMP production by stimulated stromal fibroblasts encountered by invading tumor cells (16).

3.4. LOCOMOTION

Even with the capacity to create a defect in the basement membrane and digest elements of the extracellular matrix that would otherwise block transit, tumor cells must physically migrate from their initial focus into new territory to accomplish invasion or metastasis.

Cell migration requires transmission of propulsive forces from the cell to the elements of the extracellular matrix through the repeated assembly and contraction of cytoskeletal elements forming lamellipodia (broad ruffles), filopodia (thin, cylindrical projections), and pseudopodia (thicker projections) (17,18). Migration starts with formation and then protrusion of a filopod or lamellipod, formed by the polymerization of actin filaments to form elongated central rods within the filapod or a meshwork within the lamellopod. At the leading edge of the protruding element integrins concentrate and anchor the cell to elements of the extracellular membrane (19). With this anchor in place, contraction of the actin filaments draws the cell body forward into the matrix. As the cell moves forward, the integrin anchors appear to move in a retrograde fashion along the cell surface (20,21). As the anchor points reach the trailing edge of the migrating cell, they release and the cell continues forward.

Tumor cell motility reflects the invasive and metastatic potential of the individual tumor type. Measurable parameters, such as pseudopod extension, membrane ruffling, and vectoral translation, are quantitatively increased among highly invasive tumor cells, and are further exaggerated by chemotactic and motility factors elicited by some tumor cells themselves (22).

4. CONCLUSION

Aggressive high-grade sarcomas and carcinomas can gain access to the vascular system or penetrate the surrounding periosteum to escape the spinal column early in their development. More slow-growing lesions will tend to be bound by the margins of vertebral cortices, periosteum, pleura, and intervertebral disc. If the tumor remains contained within the cortical shell, excision with a cuff of overlying periosteum and muscle offers a reasonable chance for a clear margin. If the tumor has penetrated the cortex, the surrounding musculature and the overlying fascia or pleura should be excised *en-bloc* with the tumor to provide the best chance for local control.

REFERENCES

1. Carrel A, Burrows MT. Cultivation in vitro of malignant tumors. J Exp Med 1911; 13:571–575.
2. Stossel TP. On the crawling of animal cells. Science 1993; 260:1086–1094.
3. Batson OV. The role of the vertebral veins in metastatic processes. Ann Intern Med 1942; 16:38–58.
4. Harrington KD. Metastatic disease of the spine. In: KD Harrington ed. Orthopaedic Management of Metastatic Bone Disease. St. Louis, MO: CV Moseby; 1988.

5. Weiss L. Metastasis of cancer: a conceptual history from antiquity to the 1990s. Cancer and Metastasis Rev 2000; 19:257–279.

6. Kuettner KE, Pauli BU. Resistance of cartilage to invasion. In: L Weiss L, Gilbert HA, eds. Bone Metastasis. Boston MA: GK Hall; 1981.

7. Seiki M, Koshikawa N, Yana I. Role of pericellular proteolysis by membrane-type 1 matrix metalloproteinase in cancer invasion and angiogenesis. Cancer and Metastasis Rev 2003; 22:129–143.

8. Kleiner DE, Stetler-Stevenson WG. Matrix metalloproteinases and metastasis. Cancer Chemother Pharmacol 1999; 43:S42.

9. Kajita M, Itoh Y, Chiba T, et al. Membrane type-1 matrix metalloproteinase cleaves CD44 and promotes cell migration. J Cell Biol 2001; 153:893–904.

10. Mignatti P, Rifkin DB. Biology and biochemistry of proteinases in tumor invasion. Physiol Rev 1993; 73:161–195.

11. Sato H, Takino T, Okada Y, et al. A matrix metalloproteinase expressed on the surface of invasive tumor cells. Nature 1994; 370:61–65.

12. Zucker S, Vacirca J. Role of matrix metalloproteinases (MMPs) in colorectal cancer. Cancer and Metastasis Rev 2003; 23:101–117.

13. Nagase H, Woessner JF. Matrix metalloproteinases. J Biol Chem 1999; 274:21,491–21,494.

14. Gianelli G, Falk-Marzillier J, Schiraldi O, Stetler-Stevenson WG, Quaranta V. Induction of cell migration by matrix metalloproteinase-2 cleavage of laminin-5. Science 1997; 277:225–228.

15. Koshikawa N, Gianelli G, Cirulli V, Miyazaki K, Quaranta V. Role of cell surface metalloproteinase MTI-MMP in epithelial cell migration over laminin-5. J Cell Biol 2000; 148:615.

16. Chambers AF, Matrisian LM. Changing views of the role of matrix metalloproteinases in metastasis. J Natl Cancer Inst 1997; 89: 1260–1270.

17. Gumbiner BM. Cell adhesion: the molecular basis of tissue architecture and morphogenesis. Cell 1996; 84:345–358.

18. Lauffenburger DA, Horwitz AF. Cell migration: a physically integrated molecular process. Cell 1996; 84:359–369.

19. Mitchson TJ, Cramer LP. Actin-based cell motility and cell locomotion. Cell 1996; 84:371–379.

20. Choquet D, Felsenfeld DP, Sheetz MP. Extracellular matrix rigidity causes strengthening of integrin-cytoskeleton linkages. Cell 1997; 88:39–48.

21. Sheetz MP, Felsenfeld DP, Galbraith CG. Cell migration: regulation of force on extracellular-matrix-integrin complexes. Trends Cell Biol 1998; 8:51–54.

22. Niinaka Y, Paku S, Haga A, Watanabe H, Raz A. Expression and secretion of neuroleukin/phosphohexose isomerase/maturation factor as autocrine motility factor by tumor cells. Cancer Res 1998; 58:2667–2674.

5 Fundamentals of Cancer Treatment

Effects of Chemotherapy on Neoplastic Cells

SUJITH KALMADI, MD AND DEREK RAGHAVAN, MD

CONTENTS

1. INTRODUCTION

Cytotoxic chemotherapy evolved from the concepts of Lissauer and Ehrlich over the last century. The initial chemotherapy protocols they devised were characterized by a lack of specificity, and walking a fine line balancing the toxicities experienced by the host and the tumor. This has been subsequently improved owing to a better understanding of tumor biology and the biochemical basis of action of the chemotherapy regimens. Radiation therapy started after the discovery of X-rays by Roentgen in 1895. Refinement of these modalities has resulted in therapeutic options for patients with several types of malignancies. Innovative modern techniques in the 1990s have provided insight into the intracellular pathways that result in sensitivity and resistance of the neoplastic cells to drug treatment.

2. CYTOKINETICS

The biological behavior and heterogeneity of tumors is explained by several factors including variation of constituent cell populations, cell regulatory functions, nutritional factors, and cytokinetics (1). This can lead to wide variations in the cell cycles of different tumors. Extensive research has given more insight into the growth cycle of cells (2). Cells grow through an orderly sequence of steps:

1. Resting phase (G0).
2. Cells with the biological intention to multiply enter the interphase (G1) that is characterized by synthetic processes involving RNA and proteins, which prepares the cell to enter the next phase.
3. DNA synthetic phase (S) where the DNA content is doubled.
4. Second resting (G2) phase before undergoing mitosis.
5. Mitotic phase (M) in which the chromosomes separate, causing cell division and two daughter cells.

Mitosis of cells results in daughter cells, which consist of (1) nondividing, terminally differentiated cells; (2) resting cells (G0), which can be recruited into the cell cycle; and (3) continually dividing cells that enter into G1 phase again. Major checkpoints in the cell proliferation occur in G1 when cells must commit themselves to division and in G2 before undergoing mitosis. Cells capable of replicating do so in response to various stimuli that affect the cell surface receptors. The cell cycle is under the control of numerous regulatory mechanisms, including cyclins and cyclin-dependent kinases (CDK). Cyclins are proteins that act as positive regulators of the activity of CDKs. CDKs are kinases, which are present in all phases of the cell cycle and control the cascade of proliferative signals. Regulation of these CDKs by the cyclin molecules cause their levels to fluctuate, synchronizing the progression of cell division.

Chemotherapy/radiation therapy works best when cells are in the cell cycle (Fig. 1). Categorization of chemotherapeutic drugs can be done by their activities relative to the cell cycle as phase specific and phase nonspecific.

1. Phase-specific drugs are effective only if present in the tumor cell during a specific phase of the cell division. Increasing drug levels will not result in more tumor kill. However, if the concentration is maintained over a longer period of time, more cells will enter the specific lethal

From: *Current Clinical Oncology: Cancer in the Spine: Comprehensive Care.*
Edited by: R. F. McLain, K-U. Lewandrowski, M. Markman, R. M. Bukowski,
R. Macklis, and E. C. Benzel © Humana Press, Inc., Totowa, NJ

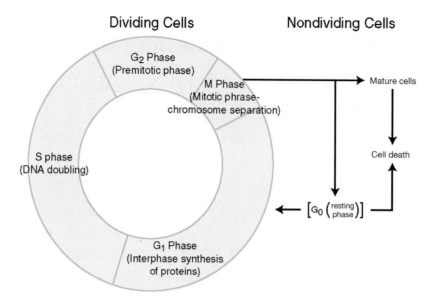

Fig. 1. Cell cycle.

phase of the cycle and get killed, (e.g., L-asparaginase, antisense therapies during G1 phase, antimetabolites during S phase, taxanes and alkaloids during G2 and M phase).

2. Phase-nonspecific agents can be further divided into cycle-nonspecific drugs, which can kill nondividing cells (e.g., steroids, some antitumor antibiotics) and cycle-specific, which can kill cells, which enter into the cell cycle (e.g., alkylating agents). Phase-nonspecific agents have a linear dose–response curve: the higher the dose administered, the greater the fraction of cells killed.

2.1. TUMOR KINETICS

The growth of a tumor can be simplistically visualized as being dependent on several variables, which include rate of cell loss, growth fraction (proportion of cells in proliferative phase), and cell doubling time. Numerous models have been devised that explain the impact of therapeutic regimens on the tumor cell cycle (3). We review these proposed models and our understanding of current chemotherapy/radiotherapy models in a historical fashion, sketching out their evolution.

The Skipper-Schabel-Wilcox model (Log Kill model), originally proposed at the Southern Research Institute in 1964, was based on the L1210 leukemia cell lines in rodents (4,5). They postulated that the increase in life-span of the host after chemotherapy was because of the cytocidal effects on the cancer cells. It also conceptualized that both tumor growth and tumor regression in response to chemotherapy were exponential in nature. Thus, a drug that would cause the tumor burden to decrease from 10^{10} to 10^9; if given in the same dose, the drug would decrease the burden from 10^5 to 10^4. These are both examples of a 90% tumor cell kill. This formed the basis for repetitive cycles of chemotherapy to achieve maximal tumor eradication. Over time, we have, however, realized that exposure to the same regimen for more than four to six times has not resulted in improved efficacy. We now understand the growth models of tumor have also a mixed nature with respect to different cancer cells in vivo (6). The Gompertzian sigmoid-shaped

growth is characteristic of many solid tumors. Tumors grow most rapidly at smaller sizes and then slow down, as they become larger secondary to problems with vascularity, hypoxia, and interaction with the other cells in their microenvironment (7–10) (Fig. 2).

There were attempts made to address the pattern of resistance to chemotherapy. Luria and Delbruck in their work with microbes, realized that bacteria develop resistance at random phases of their growth. This concept was then applied to the study of antimetabolites in L1210 cells and resistance was found to be acquired at various times of growth. Goldie and Coldman (11) then extended these concepts to human tumor cells. They concluded that larger tumors have more cells, which in turn have a cumulatively greater chance of developing spontaneous mutations. These mutations were believed to confer resistance to chemotherapy and also foster metastasis. This also led to the belief that tumors are better treated at a smaller size, before they have the ability to develop mutations and metastasis. Out of this was born the concept of multiagent noncross resistant chemotherapy, which would have a greater tumor kill and prevent development of resistance.

The Norton-Simon regression hypothesis, proposed 25 yr ago, included two different concepts (12). The first concept is that delivering chemotherapy at reduced intervals (dose-intense chemotherapy) will maximize the chances of obliterating the tumor. As known from previous experience, tumors do not grow in a simple exponential manner, but follow a Gompterzian growth pattern with faster growth in the beginning and slower growth as the tumor gets larger (13). So they concluded that if tumors were given less time to regrow between treatments, the likelihood of cure is improved. The second concept involves the use of sequential dose-dense, noncross resistant regimens to minimize drug resistance by obliterating a dominant tumor population initially and then using different agents to deal with the residual resistant cells. These two concepts brought into context, adjuvant chemotherapy after surgery/radiation result-

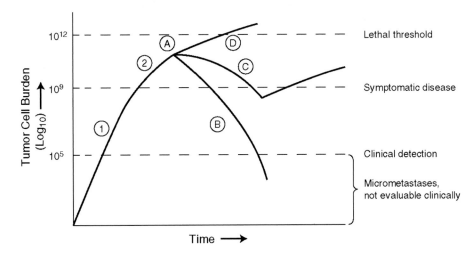

Fig. 2. Gompertizan model of tumor growth: relation between tumor mass, diagnosis, and treatment regimens. Growth phases: (1) high growth phase and (2) plateau phase with slower growth. Treatment responses: (A) initiation of treatment with surgery, radiation, and/or chemotherapy; (B) curative therapy; (C) initially sensitive tumor with secondary resistance; and (D) resistant tumor with primary resistance.

ing in less regrowth between therapies causing increased overall regression and minimized drug resistance *(14,15)*. From all these models numerous chemotherapy/radiotherapy combinations with noncross resistant drugs, concurrent chemoradiation, induction-intensification, and adjuvant approaches have been developed in a variety of different fashions.

3. CHEMORADIATION IN CANCER THERAPY

Sole modality surgical treatment in cancer often fails because of the presence of micrometastatic disease or malignant cells beyond the surgical margins at the time of resection. Combined chemotherapy and radiation can address both these mechanisms of failure. Steel and Peckham *(16)* have developed principles guiding the integration of these modalities.

1. Spatial cooperation is used to describe the action of one modality to treat disease missed by another. This can be seen in small cell lung cancer, childhood leukemia where radiation is used to treat a potential sanctuary site, such as the central nervous system. Here the dose and timing of these modalities are adjusted to minimize central nervous system effects.
2. Toxicity independence has been widely used in the designing of combination chemotherapy regimens, with improved therapeutic results seen by combining drugs with non-overlapping toxicities. When combining chemotherapy with radiation, drugs that enhance radiation-induced normal tissue damage may need to be avoided or timed sequentially (e.g., anthracyclines in adjuvant breast cancer treatment).
3. Enhancement of tumor response secondary to an additive or synergistic effect is the focus of most concurrent chemoradiation regimens. This has resulted in organ preservation (larynx cancer, sarcoma of the extremities) without compromise of overall survival. Enhanced understanding of the radio-sensitization of chemotherapeutic agents implicate pathways involving increased initial damage (e.g., antimetabolites), repair inhibition of damage inflicted by ionizing radiation (e.g., platinum compounds), and redistribution of cell cycle phase, which will make

cells more susceptible to damage by radiation (e.g., taxanes causing G2M arrest).

3.1. PHARMACOLOGY OF ANTINEOPLASTIC AGENTS

The clinical pharmacology of antineoplastic agents is being clarified through the advent of analytical tools, such as liquid chromatography and mass spectroscopy. Most of these drugs are designed with the narrowest therapeutic index compared with other branches of medicine. Study of the drugs can be simplistically classified into pharmacokinetics ("what the body does to the drug") and pharmacodynamics ("what the drug does to the body").

3.1.1. Pharmacokinetics

Pharmacokinetics involves the study of absorption, distribution, metabolism, and excretion of the drugs. Absorption has historically not been a major issue for oncologists because most drugs were administered intravenously. However, with the advances in drug delivery involving orally administered molecular agents and prodrugs, this has become an issue with oral and cutaneously absorbed drugs. Bioavailability (degree of absorption) is calculated by comparing the area under the curve (AUC) of an oral drug to the same given intravenously.

Clearance of the drug is the most critical aspect and can be conceptualized as being a function of drug distribution, metabolism, and elimination. Drug distribution can be simplistically visualized as being extracellular and intracellular. However, in reality this is more complex and has to be understood as a multicompartment model with frequent redistribution within. The presence of sanctuary sites with poor penetration of the drug results in relapse of tumors otherwise responsive to chemotherapy. Distribution can also be affected by disease states, such as cardiac failure resulting in pleural effusions and ascites creating pathological compartments (e.g., congestive heart failure can result in pleural effusions, and administration of methotrexate in this setting can result in toxicity owing to prolonged exposure of methotrexate that accumulates in the pleural effusion). Elimination is studied along two different models: linear vs nonlinear. Linear kinetics assume that the half-life of the drug will be constant. Nonlinear kinetics assumes that the elimination of the drug is saturable resulting in different rates of excretion at different concentrations resulting in variable half-lives.

The metabolism of these agents is determined by the amount of resemblance that they show to physiologic substrate. Drugs (e.g., purine and pyrimidine analogs) that show a resemblance to normal metabolites are processed by the same mechanism intracellularly as the normal metabolites. Those without resemblance to normal substrates, are degraded in the liver, in reactions involving oxidation (controlled by the cytochrome P450 enzymes) and conjugation. Knowledge of these pathways helps in the design of regimens and also in predicting toxicity. The ultimate excretion of the drug from the body is via the hepatobiliary system and/or the kidney. Reduced function of either of these organ systems may lead to dose modification or reduces the possibility of using certain chemotherapy agents. Creatinine clearance is often used as a surrogate marker of renal function. Creatinine clearance does assess the glomerular function rate, however, tubular secretion and reabsorption plays a role in the excretion of some drugs. These changes in the renal excretion of the drugs can alter their efficacy and toxicity profile. Hepatic excretion involves a number of transport systems including P-glycoprotein, cMOAT (Canalicular multispecific organic anion transporter). Enterohepatic recirculation also plays a major role, especially in the drugs metabolized by the glucuronide pathway. The cytochrome P450 system of enzymes is extremely important in the metabolism of certain drugs. Up- or downregulation of the cytochrome system by other medications being used by the patient will cause changes in the levels of chemotherapeutic agents metabolised by this system. Utilizing the liver function tests to modify the dosage of the drugs metabolised is fraught by numerous pitfalls because it does not always accurately predict the toxicity risk because they do not accurately estimate the level of dysfunction in the systems previously mentioned (17).

Understanding the pharmacokinetics is further complicated by interpatient pharmacokinetic variability (18). Pharmacogenetic variation explains some of the variability in the response and toxicity of patient groups to agents like 5-FU and irinotecan (19). Deficiency of dihydropyrimidine dehydrogenase (owing to different polymorphisms of the DPD gene), which inactivates 5-FU, will lead to increased toxicity from 5-FU. The active form of irinotecan, SN38, is inactivated via glucuronidation. Reduced activity of UGT1A1 involved in this glucuronidation leads to dose-limiting diarrhea and neutropenia. Patients with Gilbert's syndrome phenotype commonly have this abnormality. The variability in absorption of oral drugs secondary to chemotherapy insults to the mucosa can have drastic consequences both in terms of efficacy and toxicity of these agents. Most chemotherapy regimens are dosed based on body surface area, which is calculated by using body weight and height. Obesity, which causes increase in the lipophilic compartment, is not well factored into this methodology of drug dosing. The amount of lipid penetrance of a drug can cause changes in the drug levels in the obese. Hypoalbuminemia causing decreased binding and increased free concentration of the drug can increase side effects. Interdrug interactions need to be taken into account when devising combination chemotherapy regimens.

3.1.2. Pharmacodynamics

The fundamental objective of pharmacodynamics is to understand dose-response relationships (20). Phase I clinical studies attempt to define the maximally tolerated dose and the dose-limiting toxicities as a function of dose. Initial pharmacodynamic principles were based on Wagner's proposal that all drugs will have a sigmoidal shape in their drug effect based on the theory that drugs require a receptor interaction for their effect (21). However, this rule is not valid for phase-specific antineoplastic agents. When cells are not in the specific phase, increasing the dose will not increase the sensitivity, but increasing the exposure duration could achieve the desired effect.

Predicting toxicity and response in an individual patient has to be based on both pharmacokinetic and pharmacodynamic principles. Reducing drug dose for excessive toxicities is a logical practice. Changes in the patients pharmacokinetics (secondary to altered renal or hepatic function) or pharmacodynamics (increased sensitivity owing to prior exposure to the drug resulting in lower reserve, usually hematologic) can be the basis of this increase in toxicity. Whereas decreasing the drug in the first instance results in an appropriate drug exposure in vivo, the latter instance will potentially result in a subtherapeutic exposure. This type of patient may be better served by switching to an alternative chemotherapy regimen.

In most other areas of medicine, monitoring of drugs with a narrow therapeutic index (e.g., digoxin, aminoglycosides) is usually preformed by monitoring drug levels in the body. This has certain limitations in antineoplastic agents because of the use of combination chemotherapy. As mentioned earlier, investigators in pharmacodynamic studies used to correlate the total exposure (AUC) with toxicity. However, with the realization that threshold concentration over time is important in predicting response, newer work has focused on using the same concept in predicting toxicity (e.g., taxanes/topoisomerase inhibitors). Dosing techniques, such as weekly dosing (e.g., taxane) and using the AUC with creatinine clearance (carboplatin), are being used to limit toxicity without compromising efficacy.

3.1.3. Drug Resistance Mechanisms

Responses of tumors can be divided simplistically into three groups. Drug-sensitive tumors with cure, highly responsive tumors with eventual refractoriness, and tumors with some responsiveness to chemotherapy. Drug resistance has been studied in both in vivo and in vitro models. Multiple reasons involving anatomical, pharmacological, and biochemical reasons exist for tumor resistance. There are several mechanisms of drug resistance.

1. Reduced intracellular levels secondary to transport system inhibition (e.g., folate transport mechanism leading to methotrexate resistance), reduced diffusion across the cell membrane or increased efflux (P-glycoprotein MDR1 drug efflux pump). Classic multidrug resistance (MDR) is secondary to overexpression of P-glycoprotein (MDR1, P-170) (22,23). This causes increased efflux of various antineoplastic agents from the cell leading to decreased accumulation intracellularly. This has been implicated in the cross-resistance pattern to anthracyclines (e.g., doxoru-

bicin), taxanes (e.g., paclitaxel), vinca alkaloids (e.g., vincristine), and the topoisomerase inhibitors (e.g., etoposide). Tumors that express this gene, have sometimes demonstrated increased resistance and poor response to chemotherapy.

2. Alteration of drug targets including receptors (e.g., Thymidylate synthetase in 5-FU resistance). Increased levels of cell protective agents (e.g., glutathione in cisplatin resistance), which prevent oxidative damage and death of the cell, have been implicated.

3. Defects in cellular death mechanisms. Alkylating agents cause cell death by intrastrand DNA linkages. This results in cell repair systems to lead to cell death. However, if this system does not recognize the DNA defects, this will prevent tumor cell death, resulting in resistance (24). Defects in the apoptotic pathway can also involve Bcl-2 family of proteins and other regulatory mechanisms like p53. Bcl-2 family proteins comprise both up- and downregulators of apoptosis. Chemotherapy induced damage to cells is perceived by p53, which can then initiate either apoptosis or cell repair. Altered p53 is the most common genetic abnormality seen in solid tumors. Expression of wild type p53, changes in Bcl-2 family members can result in altered sensitivity of the tumor cell to chemotherapy agents (25).

4. Modification of drug metabolism can be catastrophic to antineoplastics that are designed as prodrugs (e.g., cyclophosphamide, irinotecan, which needs to be converted to SN-38).

5. Tumor cell heterogeneity with spontaneous genetic mutations occurs even before exposure to treatment (26,27). After chemotherapy eliminates the sensitive cells, these resistant cells may grow to become the predominant cell population.

Approaches to circumvent drug resistance have involved multidrug combinations, dose escalation (e.g., high-dose methotrexate, cytosine arabinoside), agents that reverse increased efflux (e.g., PSC-833 and verapamil on MDR1 reversal), cofactors that amplify drug efficacy (e.g., leucovorin with 5-FU), and inhibition of drug inactivation. Recently, liposomal (e.g., liposomal formulations of doxorubicin, cytarabine, vincristine) and nanoparticle, albumin-stabilized formulations (e.g., nanoparticle paclitaxel) have started coming into the forefront to overcome drug resistance (28). These increase the delivery of chemotherapy to the tumor cell while minimizing toxicity. Advantages of this include passive targeting to tumor, improved delivery of hydrophobic molecules, increased stability, and improved pharmacokinetics.

3.2. COMBINATION CHEMOTHERAPY PRINCIPLES

Single agents with few exceptions (e.g., choriocarcinoma) are unable to achieve cure. In view of this, combination chemotherapy regimens have been devised to accomplish the major objectives of attaining maximum tumor kill with minimal toxicity and to prevent drug resistance (29). The era began when numerous active drugs became available simultaneously and was used in leukemias and lymphomas. Fundamental principles used in the selection of these drugs in combination include:

1. Drugs with activity against the tumor.
2. Different patterns of resistance.

3. Varying mechanism of action with potential synergy.
4. Non-overlapping dose-limiting toxicities.
5. Optimal dosing and timing in combination to make the treatment free interval be the shortest.

The pragmatic view is that all curative regimens have been of a combination nature. The relation between doses and combination of these agents is complex (30). The maintenance of dose intensity has proved to be important in the success of many of these regimens. Reduction of dose can result in significantly decreased cure rates, especially in the more responsive tumors such as lymphoma, leukemia, and testicular cancer. Thus, although responses continue to be observed with dose reduction, residual tumor cells often persist leading to eventual relapse and decreased survival. The concept of relative dose intensity (amount of drug delivered in a given time frame) has evolved through the studies of Hyrniuk (31). Drugs should be used in their optimal schedule and dosage even when being combined with other agents. Interval also needs to be consistent, keeping the treatment-free interval to be the shortest time necessary for resolution of the dose limiting toxicity (usually bone marrow toxicity) to maintain dose intensity (32).

The selection of patients to receive combination chemotherapy has also undergone refinement. It may not be appropriate for a patient with an Eastern Cooperative Oncology Group (ECOG) performance score of 3 or less (Table 1) to be given a toxic regimen, unless there is substantial evidence that his disease is likely to be highly treatment sensitive and he is extremely motivated in getting treatment.

Tumor response evaluation after these chemotherapy regimens has also been standardized (33). The World Health Organization (WHO) criteria utilizes bidimensional measurement whereas the Response Evaluation Criteria In Solid Tumors (RECIST) criteria uses unidimensional measurement (Table 2).

4. TUMOR RESPONSIVENESS

It is important to understand the responsiveness of various tumor types before devising chemotherapeutic regimens (34). Tumors can be classified broadly into the following categories (35).

4.1. HIGHLY SENSITIVE

1. Childhood cancers like acute lymphocytic leukemia, Wilms tumor, Ewing's tumor, retinoblastoma, and rhabdomyosarcoma.
2. Hodgkin's lymphoma.
3. Carcinoma of the testis.
4. Choriocarcinoma.
5. Burkitts tumor.
6. Acute promyelocytic leukemia.

4.2. MODERATELY SENSITIVE

1. Adenocarcinoma of breast.
2. Non-Hodgkin's lymphoma.
3. Lung cancer.
4. Osteosarcoma.
5. Adult myeloid and lymphocytic leukemia.
6. Carcinoma of the prostate.
7. Colorectal carcinoma.
8. Female cancers of the ovary, endometrium, and cervix.

Table 1
ECOG Performance Status Scale

Status	Definition
0	Normal activity
1	Some symptoms, but ambulatory
2	In bed <50% of the time
3	In bed >50% of the time
4	100% bedridden

Table 2
World Health Organization (WHO) and Response Evaluation Criteria In Solid Tumors (RECIST) Criteria for Tumor Response

Measurability	WHO bidimensional measurement	RECIST unidimensional measurement
Number of lesions measured	5/organ; total of 10	No maximum number specified
Objective responses		
Complete response (CR)	Disappearance of all known lesion(s); confirmed at 4 wk	Disappearance of all known lesion(s); confirmed at 4 wk
Partial response (PR)	More than 50% decrease; confirmed at 4 wk	More than 30% decrease; confirmed at 4 wk
Stable disease (SD)	Neither PR nor PD criteria met	Neither PR nor PD criteria met
Progressive disease (PD)	25% increase; no CR, PR, or SD documented before increased disease, or new lesion(s)	20% increase; no CR, PR, or SD documented before increased disease, or new lesion(s)

4.3. MINIMALLY SENSITIVE

1. Endocrine gland cancers.
2. Malignant melanoma.
3. Hepatocellular carcinoma.
4. Renal carcinoma.
5. Pancreatic carcinoma.

5. TIMING OF CHEMOTHERAPY

The role of chemotherapy can be divided into several different clinical settings (36).

5.1. INDUCTION CHEMOTHERAPY

Induction chemotherapy is the use of drugs given as primary treatment when no alternative viable treatment modalities exist. An example would be the use of anthracyclines and cytosine arabinoside in the treatment of acute myeloid leukemia to induce a complete remission.

5.2. NEOADJUVANT (PRIMARY) CHEMOTHERAPY

Neoadjuvant (primary) chemotherapy is the use of chemotherapy as the initial treatment and is given in the hope of reducing the extent of local treatment needed or to increase its effectiveness. This would also address micrometastases and be an effective bioassay to assess responsiveness of the tumor to chemotherapy. An example would be the use of chemotherapy to decrease the extent of surgical resection in breast cancer or along with radiation in other malignancies to deem a tumor surgically resectable.

5.3. ADJUVANT CHEMOTHERAPY

Adjuvant chemotherapy is used after eradication of all measurable disease with local treatment (surgery and/or radiation). The rationale is to treat microscopic disease to prohibit local or distant relapse (37). This is used after optimal local treatment so that tumor mass would be at a minimum, enhancing the efficacy of antineoplastic agents. This is used commonly in numerous different malignancies including breast cancer (38) and ovarian cancer.

5.4. MAINTENANCE CHEMOTHERAPY

Maintenance chemotherapy is used usually at lower doses to prolong the duration of remission achieved with more aggressive treatment. This is used in acute lymphocytic leukemia and is being tested in clinical trials in other diseases like ovarian cancer, lymphoma, and others.

5.5. PALLIATIVE CHEMOTHERAPY

Palliative chemotherapy is used solely in the hope of palliating symptoms of the patient when the cancer is deemed incurable by any modality or combination. It does not require symptoms to be present; it is used with the hope of preventing symptoms from appearing or reoccurring or to prolong life if possible. This has been used in varying combinations with radiation, surgery, or as a single modality in cancers such as lung, prostate, and several others.

6. HIGH-DOSE CHEMOTHERAPY AND STEM CELL TRANSPLANTATION

High-dose chemotherapy involves the use of dose-intensive chemotherapy with or without radiation followed by rescue with hematopoietic stem cells and is predicated on the concept that there is a dose-response relationship for a specific regimen in certain tumors. This modality is used in hematologic malignancies (e.g., leukemia, lymphoma, myeloma), and also where high-dose chemotherapy has proven helpful in some solid malignancies (e.g., relapsed germ cell cancer) where hematologic toxicity would prevent curative doses to be administered. Stem cell source can be peripheral blood or directly from the bone marrow. Different sources of donor stem cells can be used and we have briefly described the salient features of each in Sections 6.1. and 6.2.

6.1. ALLOGENEIC BONE MARROW TRANSPLANTATION

Allogeneic bone marrow transplantation involves obtaining the stem cells from a donor who has some human leukocyte antigen (HLA)-match with the patient. This can include matched related donor (e.g., sibling), matched unrelated donor (e.g., HLA-matched donor from the bone marrow registry), stored cord blood, syngeneic (e.g., twin sibling), and haploidentical transplantation (e.g., sibling/parent who is half-matched to the patient). Complexities of allogeneic bone marrow transplantation involve immunosuppression after the transplant to prevent rejection of the donor cells by the host. This milieu of intense cytotoxic damage to the bone marrow and immunosuppression allows the donor graft cells to launch a response against the recipient termed as graft-vs-host disease (GVHD). GVHD can also have a positive effect on the tumor by having a graft vs tumor effect, which can be curative in some malignancies like chronic myelogenous leukemia. Advantages of allogeneic bone marrow transplantation include the graft-vs-tumor effect, curative option in patients with tumor involvement of the bone marrow, and no tumor contamination of the graft cells. Disadvantages include GVHD, higher treatment-related mortality, higher infectious complications secondary to immunosuppression needed after transplant, and the need to locate a suitable donor.

6.2. AUTOLOGOUS BONE MARROW TRANSPLANTATION

Autologous bone marrow transplantation uses the patient's own hematopoietic stem cells, which are harvested and cryopreserved before treatment initiation. After the completion of high-dose chemotherapy and/or radiation, this is then reinfused. Advantages include no immunosuppressive therapy needed after infusion of stem cells, no GVHD, can be used for older patients, no donor needed, and lower treatment related mortality of about 2 to 5%. Disadvantages are that there is no graft vs tumor effect, and it also cannot be used effectively if there is involvement of the stem cells with the malignancy.

7. REGIONAL CHEMOTHERAPY

Regional chemotherapy is used to deliver a higher concentration of the drugs by direct instillation into the specific regions affected by the tumor. This exposes the tumor to a higher concentration of the drug for a longer period of time than can be done safely by systemic administration avoiding systemic toxicities. This also prevents the removal of the agent by first-pass metabolism through the liver. Advances in interventional radiology-guided procedures over the last decade has allowed the evolution of this from a theoretical dream to a practical possibility. The extreme pharmacokinetic advantage from this technology is however limited by several practical issues *(39)*. Indications and clinical trials in this technology are being explored. Current examples include intrathecal therapy in the treatment and prevention of meningeal leukemia, intravesical therapy for bladder cancer, intraperitoneal chemotherapy in ovarian cancer, and intrahepatic therapy for cancer in the liver.

8. CHEMOTHERAPEUTIC AGENTS *(40)*

8.1. ALKYLATING AGENTS

These agents form the backbone of numerous regimens. They were initially discovered during World War II and then initiated the era of modern chemotherapy in combination regimens. They impair cell function by transferring alkyl groups to amino, carboxyl, phosphate, or sulfhydryl groups of nucleic acids (DNA and RNA). The most actively alkylated site is the N-7 position of guanine. This results in crosslinked DNA strands that cannot replicate, impaired transcription of RNA, and other damage to the genetic material. They are cell cycle specific, however, not phase specific. They have traditionally been divided into five classes, however, the platinum compounds because of a similar mechanism of action have been included as a sixth class. Nausea, vomiting, alopecia, and myelosuppression are fairly common acute side effects of this class of agents. They can also cause secondary acute leukemia several years after the onset of therapy, typically preceded by

a myelodysplastic phase of variable duration. This is associated with abnormalities of chromosome 5, 7, or 8 (Table 3).

8.2. ANTIMETABOLITES

Antimetabolites have been used since 1948, when they first produced temporary remission in children with acute lymphoblastic leukemia. Subsequently, methotrexate proved that chemotherapy could cure cancer as a single agent in gestational trophoblastic neoplasia. These constitute a large group of drugs, which interfere with the building blocks of DNA/RNA synthesis. They can be structural analogs of normal molecules needed for cell growth or inhibit enzymes needed for the synthesis of essential compounds. Therefore, their activity is greatest in the S phase of the cell cycle. Pharmacokinetics is characterized by their nonlinear dose–response curve (exception being 5-FU). After a certain dose, there is no more cell death, however, increasing the length of time that the cells are exposed will increase the cell killing potential (Table 4).

8.3. ANTITUMOR ANTIBIOTICS

They are generally derived from micro-organisms. They interfere with DNA by intercalation, wherein the drug inserts between DNA basepairs. This interferes with DNA replication and messenger RNA production. They also interfere with topoisomerase function. They are cell cycle-nonspecific drugs. This increases their importance in combination chemotherapy regimens where they are an extremely important component against slow-growing tumors with a low growth fraction. As a class they tend to be vesicants, and need to be given with extreme precaution to prevent extravasation causing skin necrosis and ulceration. Common side effects include nausea, vomiting, alopecia, and myelosuppression. Several of these agents synergize with the effect of radiotherapy, and caution should be exercised if both modalities are to be used (Table 5).

8.4. TUBULIN-TARGETING AGENTS

Early studies on anti-tubule drugs were done on colchicine, which was developed by the ancient Egyptians to treat gout. This class now includes the vinca alkaloids and taxanes. The primary target of these drugs is the mitotic spindle, which has led to the broad terminology of mitotic spindle poisons. The vinca alkaloids bind to microtubular proteins inhibiting their assembly (M phase), leading to mitotic spindle dysfunction, mitotic arrest, and eventually cell death from apoptosis. The taxanes bind to tubulin polymers, promoting their assembly, but make them resistant to depolymerization resulting in nonfunctional microtubules (Table 6).

8.5. TOPOISOMERASE INHIBITORS

Podophyllotoxins were used as a folk remedy by the Native Americans for its gastrointestinal effects of catharsis, emesis, and antihelminthic properties. In Russia, peasants use them as simple anti-cancer agents. Semisynthetic glycosides of this called the epipodophyllotoxins (etoposide and tenoposide) have been in clinical use for a long period of time. Recently we have seen the development of camptothecin derivatives (irinotecan and yopotecan). DNA attachment to the nuclear matrix occurs at areas called "domains." Topoisomerases bind to these areas, forming a complex allowing DNA to unwind for cell division. Topoisomerase I helps in the relaxation of supercoiled DNA, whereas topoisomerase II catalyzes the breaking and resealing of DNA. These enzymes are crucial in several critical steps of the cell cycle. Epipodophyllotoxins inhibit topoisomerase I and

Table 3
Major Alkylating Agents in Clinical Practice

Drug	Pharmacology	Uses	Toxicity
Busulfan (Myleran™, Busulfex)	Clinical response seen in 2 wk. Catabolized in the liver to inactive products, which are renally excreted.	Chronic myelogenous leukemia (CML), polycythemia vera, bone marrow transplantation (BMT)	Dose-limiting toxicity (DLT) = reversible and irreversible myelosuppression, with slow recovery. High doses for BMT can result in seizures and is given with anti-epileptics.
Carboplatin (Paraplatin™)	Second generation platinum compound similar to cisplatin with different toxicity. Half-life is shorter than cisplatin.	Ovarian, endometrial, lung.	DLT = Myelosuppression especially thrombocytopenia. Dosage typically done by area under the curve (AUC) with Calvert's formula.
Cisplatin (Platinol™)	First heavy metal anti-neoplastic. Long half-life, may remain in tissues for months. Poor central nervous system (CNS) penetration. Primarily excreted in the urine. Clinical cross-resistance with carboplatin.	Widely used. Testicular, bladder, cervical, head, and neck cancer.	DLT = Cumulative nephropathy, which can be reduced to <5% with vigorous hydration. Cumulative peripheral sensory neuropathy. Ototoxicity with tinnitus and high-frequency hearing loss.
Cyclophosphamide (Cytoxan™)	Both oral and intravenous forms. Requires activation in the liver to form acrolein and an alkylating metabolite. Drugs affecting microsomal enzymes will affect efficacy.	Used widely. Leukemia, lymphoma, breast, myeloma, BMT.	DLT = myelosuppression. High dose as preparation for BMT can cause cardiac necrosis. Hemorrhagic cystitis is secondary to a metabolite and can be prevented by hydration and mesna.
Dacarbazine (DTIC™)	Requires activation by the microsomal enzymes in the liver.	Melanoma, Hodgkin's lymphoma.	DLT = myelosuppression.
Ifosfamide (Ifex)	Intravenous formulation. Requires activation in the liver similar to cyclophosphamide	Non-Hodgkin's lymphoma, sarcoma.	DLT = myelosuppression. Hemorrhagic cystitis. High doses can lead to encephalopathy.
Melphalan (Alkeran)	Oral and iv forms. Acts directly.	Multiple myeloma, ovarian.	DLT = myelosuppression, can be cumulative and recovery prolonged.
Nitrosureas lomustine (CCNU™), and carmustine (BCNU™)	Highly lipid soluble. Rapidly biotransformed.	Brain cancer, melanoma.	DLT = myelosuppression, can be prolonged and cumulative. Nausea and vomiting can last up to 24 h.
Streptozocin (Zanosar™)	Nitrosurea compound. Short plasma half-life.	Endocrine tumors.	DLT = Nephrotoxicity initially as proteinuria and progresses to renal failure if drug is continued. Gastrointestinal (GI) toxicity.
Temozolamide (Temodar™)	Oral medication, which is activated spontaneously to the same active metabolite as DTIC.	Anaplastic astrocytoma, melanoma, glioma.	DLT = Myelosuppression especially thrombocytopenia. Moderate gastrointestinal side effects.

Table 4
Antimetabolites in Clinical Practice

Drug	Pharmacology	Uses	Toxicity
Azacitidine (Vidaza™)	Requires phosphorylation to be activated. Interferes with nucleic acid metabolism.	Myelodysplastic syndrome.	Dose limiting toxicity (DLT) = myelosuppression.
Capecitabine (Xeloda™)	Prodrug of 5-FU, which can be given orally.	Breast, colon cancer.	DLT = diarrhea. Hand-foot syndrome is common and can be dose limiting.
Cytarabine (Ara-c, Cytosar™)	Phosphorylated metabolite competitively inhibits enzymes of DNA synthesis and repair.	Acute leukemia, CML, meningeal leukemia.	DLT = myelosuppression. High doses can lead to cerebellar toxicity. Conjunctivitis occurs with high dose, which can be reduced with prophylactic steroid eye drops.
Fludarabine (Fludara™)	After activation inhibits DNA synthesis enzymes.	Chronic lymphocytic leukemia, indolent lymphomas.	DLT = cumulative myelosuppression. Increased frequency of opportunistic infections (e.g., pneumocystis, listeria, and cryptococcus).
Fluorouracil (5-FU™)	Inhibition of thymidylate synthetase by inhibits DNA synthesis. Other metabolites may interfere with RNA function. Differs from other antimetabolites in having a log linear cell kill. Leucovorin enhances the action by acting at thymidylate synthetase.	Carcinoma of colon, breast, rectum, stomach, pancreas, esophageal, head, and neck.	DLT = myelosuppression (more common with bolus regimens), mucositis, and diarrhea (more common with infusion regimens). Other toxicities include cardiac, excessive lacrimation, nasal discharge, and cerebellar toxicity.
Hydroxyurea (Hydrea™)	Inhibits nucleotide reductase inhibiting DNA synthesis. Oral drug.	CML, myeloproliferative disorders.	DLT = Myelosuppression, which recovers rapidly. Long term use possibly implicated in acute leukemia.
Methotrexate (MTX™)	Synthetic analog of folic acid, which blocks the enzyme Dihydrofolate reductase preventing formation of reduced folic acid that interferes with vital cellular enzymes.	Choriocarcinoma, ALL, meningeal leukemia, sarcoma, and bladder cancer.	DLT = Myelosuppression, stomatitis, renal dysfunction, and neurotoxicity, depending on dose and duration of use. Leucovorin rescues normal tissues from toxicity and is used in high dose regimens.

Table 5
Antitumor Antibiotics

Drug	Pharmacology	Uses	Toxicity
Actinomycin D (Dactinomycin™)	Extensively tissue bound with long half-life (36 h).	Wilms tumor, sarcoma.	DLT = myelosuppression.
Bleomycin (Blenoxane™)	Activated by microsomal reduction. Radiation sensitizer.	Lymphoma, testicular cancer.	Chills and febrile reactions that are infusion related. Pneumonitis can occur 4–10 wk after initiation.
Doxorubicin (Adriamycin™), epirubicin (Ellence™) is an epimer of doxorubicin	Extensively plasma protein bound with long half-life. Liposomal formulation (Doxil) is used in Kaposi's sarcoma, ovarian carcinoma. Idarubicin (Idamycin) is another anthracycline with a better cellular uptake.	Extensively used. breast, bladder, lymphoma, leukemia, and gastric cancer.	DLT = myelosuppression, commonly leukopenia. Cardiomyopathy with CHF is more frequent after a cumulative dose of 550 mg/m^2 (400 mg/m^2 with previous mediastinal irradiation). Dexrazoxane may have cardioprotective effects.
Mitomycin	Also functions as an alkylating agent	Gastric, pancreatic carcinoma.	DLT = myelosuppression, which can be cumulative and prolonged. Thrombocytopenia may occur up to 8 wk.

Table 6
Tubulin Targeting Agents

Drugs	Uses	Toxicity
Docetaxel (Taxotere™)	Breast, non-small cell lung, ovarian, and prostate.	DLT = myelosuppression. Fluid retention is dose dependent, secondary to increased capillary permeability and is reversible. Hypersensitivity reactions similar to paclitaxel (despite not being formulated in cremophor) can occur.
Paclitaxel (Taxol™)	Breast, non-small cell lung, and ovarian carcinoma.	DLT = myelosuppression. Hypersensitivity (3%) to cremophor (carrier vehicle) occurs usually within 20 min of initiating treatment, 90% of which happen within the first two doses. Premedication with steroids and histamine blockers is routinely recommended. Peripheral neuropathy is dose dependent.
Vincristine (Oncovin™)	Widely used in combination regimens secondary to minimal myelosuppression.	DLT = dose-dependent peripheral neuropathy universally develops. It is reversible, however, can take several months. This can result in cranial nerve palsies, abdominal pain, obstipation, ataxia, foot-drop, cortical blindness, and seizures.
Vinorelbine (Navelbine™)	Non-small cell lung cancer and breast cancer.	DLT = myelosuppression.

Table 7
Topoisomerase Inhibitors

Drugs	Pharmacology	Uses	Toxicities
Etoposide (VP-16™)	Can be used orally and intravenously. Bioavailability is 50%, however, it is non-linear and decreases with doses higher than 200 mg.	Germ cell tumor, lung cancer, lymphoma, and bone marrow transplantation (BMT).	Dose-limiting toxicity (DLT) = neutropenia. Gastrointestinal toxicities common with oral drug.
Irinotecan (CPT-11™, Camptosar™)	Needs to be activated to SN-38. This conversion occurs primarily in the liver, but can also occur in the plasma and in the intestinal mucosa.	Colorectal and lung cancer.	Early diarrhea within 24 h of the infusion is cholinergic and is controlled with atropine. Late diarrhea is owing to SN-38 and needs to be controlled with antibiotics and loperamide.
Topotecan (Hycamtin™)	Lactone ring form is the active ingredient.	Ovarian and small cell lung cancer.	DLT = Myelosuppression. Gastrointestinal side effects are common too.

camptothecins inhibit topoisomerase II. Anthracyclines also exhibit topoisomerase inhibition. Topoisomerase II inhibitors can cause secondary leukemia with a shorter latency period than with alkylating agents (2–4 yr) and not typically preceded by a myelodysplastic phase. They are associated with a balanced translocation involving chromosome 11 (11q23) or 21 (21q22) (Table 7).

8.6. HORMONAL AGENTS

Hormones are pivotal in the development and growth of several organs. Numerous hormonal manipulations have been tried in cancers originating from organs where hormones are regulatory in the function or development of the tumor akin to the target organ.

8.6.1. Tamoxifen (Nolvadex™)

Arguably, the most famous of the hormonal agents, has been the focus of trials involving thousands of patients. It is a non-steroidal agent that exerts its effect by binding to estrogen receptors and may exert antiestrogenic, weak estrogenic, or both effects. Is being used in breast cancer in both the adjuvant and metastatic settings. Side effects include hot flashes, menstrual changes, "flare response" in the first month of therapy, thrombosis, and increased occurrence of endometrial cancer when used long term.

8.6.2. Aromatase Inhibitors

These include steroidal (exemestane/Aromasin®) and non-steroidal (anastrozole/Arimidex®, letrozole/Femara®) agents with minor differences in their pharmacokinetic and pharmacodynamic profiles. They act by inhibiting aromatase, which converts adrenal androgens to estrogens in peripheral tissues and the tumor cells. It is used primarily in postmenopausal women with breast cancer in the adjuvant and metastatic setting. Toxicities include antiestrogen effects related to osteoporosis, vaginal bleeding, and musculoskeletal side effects.

8.6.3. Adrenocorticosteroids (Dexamethasone, Prednisone)

These are used in a wide variety of tumor conditions both for treatment and for symptom control. Prominent among its uses include symptomatic brain metastases, spinal cord compression, combination chemotherapy regimens to enhance cytotoxicity, immune cytopenias in chronic lyphocytic leukemia, and prophylaxis against chemotherapy induced nausea/vomiting.

Side effects are numerous, which are also enhanced by long term use. Peptic ulcer disease, myopathy, hypertension, osteoporosis, psychosis, and susceptibility to infection are among the most dreaded complications.

8.6.4. Luteinizing Hormone-Releasing Hormone (LHRH) Agonists (Leuprolide/Lupron™, Goserelin/Zoladex™)

It desensitizes the LHRH receptor resulting in castrate levels of testosterone in men and estradiol in women within a fortnight of administration. Uses include breast and prostate cancer. Usually administered in injection form once every 1 to 3 mo. Side effects are related to hormone depletion and include hot flashes, decreased libido, impotence, gynecomastia, and amenorrhea.

8.6.5. Progestins (Medroxyprogesterone/Depo-Provera™, Megestrol/Megace™)

Works at the progesterone receptor level. Has been used in breast carcinoma, prostate carcinoma, endometrial carcinoma, and as an appetite stimulant. Side effects include menstrual changes and fluid retention.

8.6.6. Antiandrogens (Bicalutamide, Flutamide, Nilutamide)

Nonsteroidal agents, which inhibit androgen binding at receptor level competitively. Its use complements medical (LHRH agonists) or surgical (orchiectomy) treatments for prostate cancer, which by themselves would result in reduction of testicular but not adrenal androgen production. Side effects are related to androgen depletion.

8.7. BIOLOGICAL AGENTS

These agents evoke immune responses, which target receptors, signaling pathways, or tumor stroma, to induce tumor regression.

8.7.1. Interleukin (IL)-2 (Aldesleukin™)

It is a highly purified lymphokine, which possesses immunomodulatory capacity related to T-cell and NK-cell activation, generation of lymphokine-activated killer cell activity, and production of γ-interferon by macrophages. It has induced tumor regression in renal cell carcinoma and melanoma. High-dose therapy is toxic and can cause capillary leak syndrome leading to hypotension, cardiac arrhythmias, and several other organ system toxicities.

8.7.2. Interferons

This family consists of more than 20 related, antigenically discrete proteins with immunomodulatory function. In this group, interferon-α has been most studied in malignancies. They are believed to work by immunomodulation involving cytotoxic T-lymphocytes, NK-cell activation, and induction of major histocompatibility complex. It is being used in melanoma, chronic myelogenous leukemia, hairy cell leukemia, renal cell carcinoma, Kaposi sarcoma, low-grade lymphoma, and multiple myeloma. Toxicities include flu-like syndrome, which is almost universal, myelosuppression, and elevated liver function tests.

8.7.3. Octreotide (Sandostatin)

Octreotide (sandostatin) is a long acting-somatostatin analog, which inhibits the secretion of various gastrointestinal enzymes. Antitumor efficacy is still investigational, however, it has demonstrated activity in the control of symptoms in carcinoid syndrome, VIP-secreting tumors, or secretory diarrhea caused by chemotherapeutic agents. Toxicities are mostly gastrointestinal causing abdominal pain, vomiting, and loose stools.

8.8. TARGETED THERAPY

Ever since Paul Ehrlich proposed the concept of the "magic bullet" to cure each disease with a specific targeted drug in his work with microbes, there has been a constant optimism that this will be true for cancer. Although some of the antineoplastic agents previously discussed do represent targeted therapy, they truly have widespread effects as reflected by their toxicity profile. Discovery of drugs with targets that are differentially expressed (quantitatively or qualitatively) in neoplastic cells would result in higher efficacy with minimal toxicity. Recently, with better understanding of the molecular pathways, more of these targeted therapies are coming into the forefront.

8.8.1. Imatinib Mesylate (Gleevec™, STI-571)

Imatinib mesylate (Gleevec, STI-571) has been the dream drug of the last decade and has generated a large amount of enthusiasm among cancer researchers to devise more of the targeted agents. It is a signal transduction inhibitor that inhibits the BCR-ABL protein and related tyrosine kinases, which is the constitutive abnormality created by the Philadelphia chromosome (reciprocal translocation between the long arms of chromosome 9 and 22) in chronic myeloid leukemia. This inhibits differentiation, proliferation, and induces apoptosis in Bcr-Abl positive cells. Gastrointestinal stromal tumors (GIST) with c-kit protooncogene overexpression have also expressed responsiveness to imatinib believed to be secondary to tyrosine kinase inhibition. Toxicities are fluid retention, nausea/vomiting, and myelosuppression.

8.8.2. HER Family of Membrane Receptors

This is composed of four members HER1 (also termed as epidermal growth factor receptor [EGFR]), HER 2 (ErbB2 or HER2/Neu), HER3, and HER4. They have a similar structure with an extracellular ligand binding domain, a transmembrane domain, and an intracellular domain with tyrosine kinase activity. Binding of ligands to the receptor can initiate signal transduction cascades, which influence numerous pathways in the cell cycle. These receptors are overexpressed in many malignancies.

- HER1 (EGFR) receptor has been targeted using monoclonal antibodies (MAbs) against the external domain and tyrosine kinase (TK) inhibitors which compete with adenosine triphosphate to bind to the receptor's kinase pocket. Cetuximab (IMC-C225) is a chimeric human-mouse MAb, which has recently been approved for use in metastatic colon cancer. Gefitinib (Iressa) is an oral TKI, which is being used in non-small cell lung cancer. This has proven higher efficacy in female nonsmokers who developed lung cancer and also in bronchoalveolar carcinoma of the lung. Side effects of these agents include diarrhea, skin rash, and acne.

- HER2 has been shown to be dramatically overamplified in breast cancer tumors (30%). Trastuzumab (Herceptin) is a MAb, which targets the extracellular domain of HER2. This combined with chemotherapy has improved progression and overall survival in metastatic breast cancer, which overexpress HER2. This represents the first successful HER targeted therapy. Cardiotoxicity leading to congestive heart failure can occur with this agent. In view of this, it is not being used concurrently with anthracyclines. Infusion related hypersensitivity reactions also occur in half of the patients, usually with the first infusion.

8.8.3. Vascular Endothelial Growth Factor (VEGF) Pathway

Angiogenesis is crucial for tumor growth, and this is promoted by oncogene-driven expression of VEGF, interleukins, and other growth factors. In tumors, VEGF is constitutively overexpressed as compared to normal tissue, and is further increased by hypoxia. This has been targeted with MAbs and TKI similar to the approach in the HER family. Bevacizumab (Avastin™) is a recombinant humanized MAb against VEGF that has been recently approved in metastatic colorectal cancer. This is now being actively studied in combination with chemotherapy and other targeted therapies in other different cancers. Toxicities include GI perforation, poor wound healing, hypertension, and nephrotic syndrome.

8.8.4. Rituximab

MAbs in hematological malignancies began with the use of Rituximab (Rituxan™), which is a chimeric human/murine MAb directed against the CD 20 antigen found on normal and malignant B lymphocytes. Attachment to this antigen leads to B-cell lysis. This has proven to be extremely effective as single agent or in combination with chemotherapy, resulting in effective treatment options for CD20 positive non-Hodgkin's lymphoma and chronic lymphocytic leukemia. Side effects are mainly infusion related and hypersensitivity reactions. Alemtuzumab (Campath™) is a recombinant humanized MAb directed against the CD 52 expressed on most normal and malignant B and T lymphocytes, NK cells, monocytes, and macrophages, but not on hematopoietic stem cells or mature plasma cells. It is used mainly in chronic lymphocytic leukemia. Toxicities include infusion related reactions and immunosuppression, which can lead to opportunistic infections. Gemtuzumab Ozogamicin (Mylotarg) is a MAb against CD 33 linked to an antibiotic calicheamicin. CD 33 is expressed on myeloid leukemia cells and this results in cytotoxicity from this compound. Side effects are infusional and hepatoxicity. Radioimmunoconjugates (Ibritumomab [Zevalin®] and Tositumomab [Bexxar®]) have been developed combining MAb with radioactive molecules. These have been approved in the treatment of non-Hodgkin's lymphoma. Side effects include infusion-related toxicities and myelosuppression.

REFERENCES

1. Tannock IF. Cell kinetics and chemotherapy. A critical review. Cancer Treat Rep 1978; 62:1117–1133.
2. Young RC, De Vita VT. Cell cycle characteristics of human solid tumors in vivo. Cell Tissue Kinet 1970; 3:285–290.
3. Alberts DS. A unifying vision of cancer therapy for the 21st century. J Clin Oncol 1999; 17:13–21.
4. Yankee RA, De Vita VT, Perry S. The cell cycle of leukemia L 1210 cells in vivo. Cancer Res 1968; 27:2381–2385.
5. Skipper HE, Schabel FM, Wilcox WS. Experimental evaluation of potential anticancer agents XII: on the criteria and kinetics associated with "curability of leukemia". Cancer Chemother Rep 1964; 35:1–111.
6. Schnipper L. Clinical implications of tumor-cell heterogeneity. N Engl J Med 1986; 314:1423–1431.
7. Hanahan D, Weinberg RA. The hallmarks of cancer. Cell 2000; 100:57–70.
8. Tubiana M. Tumor cell proliferation kinetics and tumor growth rate. Acta Oncol 1989; 28:113–121.
9. Brown JM, Giaccia AJ. The unique physiology of solid tumors: opportunities (and problems) for cancer therapy. Cancer Res 1998; 58:1408–1416.
10. Nowell PC. The clonal evolution of tumor progression. Science 1976; 194:23–28.
11. Nowell P: Mechanisms of tumor progression. Cancer Res 1986; 46:2203–2207.
12. Steel GG. The growth kinetics of tumors in relation to their therapeutic response. Laryngoscope 1975; 85:359–370.
13. Coldman AJ, Goldie JH. Impact of dose-intense chemotherapy on the development of permanent drug resistance. Semin Oncol 1987; 14:29–33.
14. Norton L, Simon R. The Norton-Simon hypothesis revisited. Cancer Treat Rep 1986; 70:163–169.
15. Norton LA. A gompertzian model of human breast cancer growth. Cancer Res 1988; 48:7067–7071.
16. Steel GG, Adams GE, Peckham MJ, eds. The Biologic Basis of Radiotherapy. The Netherlands: Elsevier; 1983:239–248.
17. Gurney H. Dose calculation of anticancer drugs: a review of the current practice and introduction of an alternative. J Clin Oncol 1996; 14: 2590–2611.
18. Canal P, Chatelut E, Guichard S. Practical treatment guide for dose individualization in cancer chemotherapy. Drugs 1998; 56: 1019–1038.
19. Iyer L, Ratain MJ. Pharmacogenetics and cancer chemotherapy. Eur J Cancer 1998; 34:1493–1499.
20. Ratain MJ, Schilsky RL, Conley BA, Egorin MJ. Pharmacodynamics in cancer therapy. J Clin Oncol 1990; 8:1739–1753.
21. Wagner JG. Kinetics of Pharmacologic Response. I. Proposed relationships between response and drug concentration in the intact animal and man. J Theor Biol 1968; 20:173–201.
22. Endicott JA, Ling V. The biochemistry of P-glycoprotein mediated multidrug resistance. Annu Rev Biochem 1989; 58:137–171.
23. Goldstein LJ, Galski H, Fojo A, et al. Expression of multidrug resistance gene in human tumors. J Natl Cancer Inst 1989; 81:116–124.
24. Hickman JA. Apoptosis and chemotherapy resistance. Eur J Cancer 1996; 32A:921–926.
25. Schmitt CA, Lowe SW. Apoptosis and therapy. J Pathol 1999; 187:127–137.
26. Moolgavkar SH, Knudsen AG. Mutation and cancer: a model for human carcinogenesis. J Natl Cancer Inst 1981; 66:1037–1052.
27. Fearon EC. Human cancer syndromes: clues to the origin and nature of cancer. Science 1997; 278:1043–1058.
28. Sikic BL. Modulation of multidrug resistance: at the threshold. J Clin Oncol 1993; 11:1629–1635.
29. DeVita VT, Schein PS. The use of drugs in combination for the treatment of cancer: rationale and results. N Engl J Med 1973; 228:998–1006.
30. Skipper HE. Critical variables in the design of combination chemotherapy regimens to be used alone or in adjuvant settings. Colloque INSERM 1986; 137:11.
31. Hyrniuk WM. Average relative dose intensity and the impact on design of clinical trials. Semin Oncol 1987: 14:65–74.
32. Day RS. Treatment sequencing, asymmetry, and uncertainty: protocol strategies for combination chemotherapy. Cancer Res 1986; 46:3876–3885.
33. Therasse P, Arbuck S, Eisenhauer E, et al. New guidelines to evaluate the response to treatment of solid tumors. J Natl Cancer Inst 2000; 92:205–216.
34. Frei E III. Curative cancer chemotherapy. Cancer Res 1985; 45:6523–6537.
35. Krakoff IH. Systemic treatment of cancer. CA Cancer J Clin 1996; 46:137–141.
36. Rideout DC, Chou TC. Synergism, potentiation and antagonism in chemotherapy. An overview. In: Chou TC, Rideout DC, eds. Synergism and Antagonism in Chemotherapy. San Diego, CA: Academic Press; 1991:3.
37. Henderson IC, Gelman RS, Harris JR, Canellos GP. Duration of therapy in adjuvant chemotherapy trials. NCI Monogr 1986; 1:95–98.
38. Hellman S. Stopping metastases at their source. N Engl J Med 1997; 337:996–997.
39. Collins JM. Pharmacokinetic rationale for regional drug delivery. J Clin Oncol. 1984; 2:498–504.
40. Perry MC, ed. The Chemotherapy Sourcebook. 3rd ed. Philadelphia, PA: Lippincott, Williams and Wilkins; 2001.

6 The Role of Surgical Therapy

Principles of Effective Surgical Treatment

Robert F. McLain, MD

Contents

1. INTRODUCTION

The correct treatment of any spinal column tumor depends on a number of characteristics or factors unique to the individual patient and their individual tumor. There is a broad spectrum of therapies available to treat spinal tumors, ranging from observation to total vertebrectomy. Both undertreatment and overtreatment can lead to trouble. A successful surgical plan follows from a concise, step-wise investigational algorithm:

1. Identify and characterize the tumor.
2. Classify the tumor as stage and extension.
3. Identify an indication for surgery—relative or absolute.
4. Review the non-operative options.
5. Review the options for resection and reconstruction.
6. Determine the role of adjuvant therapy.
7. Formulate a treatment plan that takes all steps into consideration.

The physician evaluating a patient with a suspect spinal lesion for the first time is faced with a hierarchy of clinical questions that must be answered before a definitive plan can be proposed. Is this tumor benign or malignant? If malignant, is it primary or metastatic? Is the patient systemically ill or fit? Is the tumor slow-growing, locally aggressive, or widely disseminated? Is there any neurological compromise? Is there a fracture or instability?

The spectrum of potential therapies runs the gamut from simple diagnosis and observation to radical resection and reconstruction depending on the tumor and its stage (Table 1). The physician cannot reliably offer the patient the best treatment until all of the previous questions have been adequately addressed.

In any event, tumors arising in the spinal column present special problems compared to tumors in other areas of the musculoskeletal system. A true *radical excision* cannot be

Table 1
The Role of Surgery With Respect to Tumor Type

Treatment option	Tumor types
Observation	Indolent and clearly benign tumors—hemangioma, osteochondroma, bone island or infarct.
Radiotherapy	Metastatic lesions from a radio-sensitive primary—disseminated myeloma, breast carcinoma.
Chemotherapy	Metastatic lesions from a chemosensitive primary tumor—thyroid (usually with radiotherapy).
Intralesional excision-curettage	Benign tumors with limited potential for local recurrence—aneurysmal bone cyst, osteoblastoma, and metastatic lesions in which local control will be obtained through radiotherapy.
Marginal excision (with or without adjuvant cryotherapy or radiotherapy)	Locally aggressive benign lesions—giant cell tumor; primary and metastatic lesions. sensitive to radiotherapy—solitary plasmacytoma, breast/prostate metastases; and low-grade malignancies—soft-tissue chondrosarcoma.
Wide excision (modified)	All primary malignancies without known metastases—osteosarcoma, chondrosarcoma, chordoma; solitary metastases with likelihood of prolonged survival—breast, prostate, renal cancer; locally aggressive benign tumors—giant cell tumor.

achieved in the spinal column, because any break in the vertebral ring violates the osseous "compartment." The necessary cuts through the bony ring of the vertebra may expose normal tissues to contamination even in well-circumscribed tumors. Hemorrhage from the cut bone surfaces can spread tumor cells throughout the surgical field, reducing the chance for local control. If the tumor has extended beyond the vertebral cortex, even a marginal excision may be hard to obtain. A tumor that

From: *Current Clinical Oncology: Cancer in the Spine: Comprehensive Care.*
Edited by: R. F. McLain, K-U. Lewandrowski, M. Markman, R. M. Bukowski,
R. Macklis, and E. C. Benzel © Humana Press, Inc., Totowa, NJ

adheres to or invades the dura mater or aorta may prove difficult or impossible to resect, and tumor that involves the vena cava is usually unresectable. In these cases the risks of attempting a wide resection with vascular or dural grafting must be weighed against those of following up a marginal excision with adjuvant radiation.

2. GOALS OF SURGICAL TREATMENT

2.1. TREATMENT OF METASTATIC SPINAL TUMORS

When conservative therapy fails to control metastatic disease, the physician must determine whether surgery is likely to improve the patient's function, quality of life, or longevity. Patients with an asymptomatic or minimally symptomatic spinal metastasis often do not require surgery. In cases of severe pain, segmental instability, or neurological compromise, however, operative intervention may provide great benefit.

2.2. TREATMENT OF PRIMARY BENIGN TUMORS

The principle reasons for operating on benign tumors are to establish the diagnosis, treat pain, and to prevent local tumor expansion. Intralesional excisions are adequate in many tumor types (aneurysmal bone cyst, osteoblastoma) and should be carried out through the most direct approach with the least disruption of normal vertebral elements.

2.3. TREATMENT OF PRIMARY MALIGNANT TUMORS

In primary malignancies, the principle goal of surgical treatment is local control of the disease. Plan the approach and resection to give the best chance of an adequate resection margin with the least disruption of vertebral stability.

3. INDICATIONS FOR SURGERY

Patients with spinal malignancies are often compromised and at higher risk for surgical and medical complications after aggressive treatment. If surgery is offered as part of the treatment plan, there must be a clear rationale with well-defined goals and benefits. Patients with metastases from a known primary, or with a peripheral metastasis that can be biopsied easily, may not require any spinal procedure. Unless there is neurological impingement or mechanical instability, radiation or chemotherapy can often retard tumor progression and control the spinal lesion from radio-sensitive primaries. The broadly accepted indications for surgical treatment of a spinal tumor include:

1. Inability to establish a tissue diagnosis by other methods.
2. Neurological compression owing to pathological fracture with bony impingement.
3. Mechanical instability with severe pain or impending neurological injury.
4. Tumor progression in face of, or following radiotherapy.
5. Known radio-resistant tumor.
6. Primary malignant tumor without known metastases.
. Resectable solitary metastasis in patient with potential long-term survival.

3.1. DIAGNOSIS AND BIOPSY

Biopsy is necessary in undiagnosed metastatic disease and all but a few primary lesions.

When the differential diagnosis is limited to lesions that are easily distinguished histologically, needle biopsy is ideal. Fine-needle aspiration or biopsy can be carried out with computed tomography (CT) guidance and minimal risk to the patient. The sample obtained is small, and there is a possibility of sampling nondiagnostic regions of the tumor. Needle biopsy is not adequate to differentiate cartilage tumors, osteoblastic tumors, or most spindle cell tumors, but can distinguish between infection, adenocarcinoma, and sarcoma. Craig-needle biopsy is more likely to obtain diagnostic material, but is also more invasive. More subtle differentials usually require an open biopsy.

Incisional biopsy is carried out as the last step in tumor staging, just before or at the time of definitive resection. A section of tissue large enough for histological and ultrastructural analysis, as well as immunological staining, should be cut from the margin of the lesion using a sharp scalpel. Central sections of an aggressive tumor may be necrotic. Occasionally, circumscribed lesions may present an opportunity for *en-bloc* excision at the first procedure. There are only a few tumors (i.e., chondrosarcoma) that present so classic an image that vertebrectomy may be planned without first obtaining a biopsy specimen.

3.2. DECOMPRESSION

Acute spinal cord compression typically results from rapid tumor growth or bony destruction leading to an acute pathological fracture *(1,2)*. Patients with rapidly progressive paralysis owing to compression have a poor prognosis for recovery. Although between 60 and 95% of ambulatory patients will retain that ability after treatment, only 35 to 65% of paraparetic patients and less than 30% of paraplegic patients will regain the ability to stand and walk after either surgical or medical treatment *(3,4)*.

Compression may be caused by the tumor's enlarging soft tissue mass, a pathological fracture forcing bone fragments into the canal, vertebral collapse and kyphosis, or direct metastasis or extension into the meninges or epidural space *(5,6)*. Surgical decompression is absolutely indicated in cases of bony compression or rapidly progressive paraplegia from any other cause. Early recognition and treatment of spinal cord compression is necessary to prevent permanent neurological injury.

3.3. STABILIZATION

Modern spinal instrumentation is rigid, attaches to the spine at multiple points, and is able to function even in segments that have no laminae or suffer from poor bone quality. Used correctly, instrumentation prevents early progressive deformity owing to bone destruction, limits pain because of segmental instability, and improves spinal fusion. Most contemporary instrumentation systems permit postoperative imaging with CT and magnetic resonance imaging (MRI).

Segmental instrumentation systems provide the surgeon with a highly versatile tool for stabilizing the spine. Hooks and screws placed at multiple levels distribute fixation forces and improve construct strength, whereas pedicle screws allow fixation of levels with no intact laminae. Screw and plate constructs can be used in the upper thoracic spine to stabilize the cervicothoracic junction, to treat laminectomized segments, and to limit the bulk of instrumentation placed under thin, irradiated soft tissues.

Combined with an anterior strut, screw/rod and screw/plate constructs provide superior axial, torsional, and sagittal rigid-

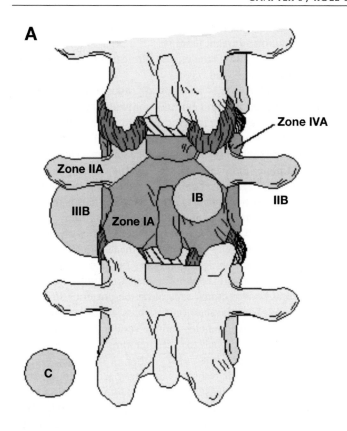

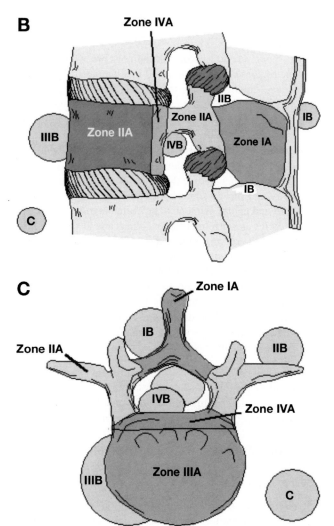

ity, allowing the patient to get out of bed immediately, and begin ambulation or mobilization within 24 to 48 h of surgery.

3.4. RADIO-RESISTENT TUMOR

Progression of the spinal tumor, heralded by neurological symptoms or bony collapse, may occur after or even in the face of radiotherapy. In some cases the tumor simply does not respond to the therapy. In others, the bony destruction may already be so severe that fracture is inevitable irrespective of tumor response. In these cases, surgical treatment may be needed to reduce the tumor burden, decompress the neurological elements, or to stabilize the spine. In other instances, the tumor type is known to be refractory to radiotherapy. Surgical resection represents the only means of local control, and is best carried out early, through nonirradiated tissue.

3.5. RESECTION

When a primary malignant lesion can be completely resected, patient survival improves significantly. The anterior and posterior longitudinal ligaments, vertebral body, adjacent discs, and even the overlying dura mater may need to be resected to obtain local control. If necessary, one or more nerve roots may be sacrificed to provide a wide margin of excision. In some metastatic lesions, a complete resection can confer improved survival and quality of life. Solitary renal cell metastases, some breast metastases, and local recurrences of colorectal carcinomas may occasionally be approached with idea of providing long-term disease free survival, if not outright cure. The decision to attempt a wide resection in these lesions must be weighed against the surgical morbidity and the risks of vascular and neurological injury. In some cases the most prudent approach may be to accept a marginal or intralesional resection, supplemented with adjuvant radio- or cryotherapy.

Fig. 1. Characterizing tumor stage. The vertebra is divided into four zones based on the anatomic structures involved, the adjacent structures at risk and the approach to resection. Large tumors frequently involve more than one zone, and extension from zone 4 into zone 2 commonly complicates the plan for wide marginal excision. (A) Intraosseous lesions offer the best chance of successful excision, but (B) extraosseous extension does not exclude the possibility. (C) Distant metastases indicate that the best outcome for the spine surgery will be local control, with systemic control dependent on medical therapy. (A) Anterior–posterior view, (B) lateral view, (C) axial cross-sectional view.

3.6. CLASSIFYING TUMOR STAGE AND EXTENSION

The surgical plan and potential resection margins can be developed from a simple staging system, based on the anatomic structures of the vertebral column and the surgical approach needed to reach them. The vertebra is divided into four anatomic zones of involvement, and the degree of tumor extension is defined by three degrees of tumor spread: intraosseous containment, extraosseous extension, and metastatic spread (Fig. 1). More extensive classification systems have been proposed, and offer greater specificity in terms of database and research descriptions, but these are cumbersome and hard to apply in clinical situations.

Weinstein's staging system *(7)* divides the vertebral elements into four zones:

1. Tumors in zone 1 involve the spinous process or laminae, the regions routinely removed in a laminectomy.
2. Zone 2 tumors involve the pedicle, transverse processes, and/or facets. These tumors can still be removed from a posterior approach, though the spinal canal must be opened widely to get to the base of the pedicle.
3. Zone 3 lesions involve the anterior vertebral body, and must be approached anteriorly.
4. Zone 4 lesions involve the posterior-third of the vertebral body and the vertebral cortex just anterior to the spinal cord and neural elements. They often involve one or both pedicles as well. In order to address any lesion involving zone 4, the surgeon must remove most of zone 3, and must separate the vertebral body, anteriorly, from the pedicles, posteriorly, resecting vertebral zones 1 and 2 in the process. In order to obtain a clear resection margin, zone 4 lesions require a total or near-total vertebrectomy. This is most feasible if the tumor is still intraosseous (grade A), without extraosseous spread (grade B). Distant metastases (grade C) usually contraindicate such an aggressive approach.

CT and MRI provide most of the information needed to stage the tumor, and bone scan, chest and abdominal CT, and serologies aid in determining metastatic status. Grade B lesions may prove unresectable if vital structures are directly invaded by tumor.

3.7. PRINCIPLES OF SURGICAL TREATMENT

Three principle issues must be considered in developing a surgical plan for any patient:

1. What is the proper margin of resection for this tumor (of primary concern in locally aggressive and malignant primary tumors)?
2. Is there a need for neurological decompression?
3. What extent and means of reconstruction will be needed?

3.8. RESECTION

Musculoskeletal tumor surgery recognizes that, although not every tumor can be removed *en bloc*, without leaving any residual disease, the quality of the resection margin has great prognostic importance. Extremity resections are usually discussed in terms of intralesional, marginal, wide, and radical margins. True radical margins cannot be obtained in the spine, so the best that we can hope for is clean, wide margin of resection.

Numerous studies show that the ability to completely resect the primary lesion significantly improves patient survival *(8–11)*. Even in metastatic lesions, a *wide* resection can confer improved survival and quality of life *(12)*. In locally aggressive tumors, the surgeon must resect the anterior and posterior longitudinal ligaments, vertebral body, adjacent discs, and the overlying dura mater, if necessary, to avoid leaving residual tumor behind. In order to obtain a clean margin the surgeon must take care not to enter the soft tissue mass of the tumor either surgically or with retractors or rakes. To insure that the margins are clear, the surgeon will excise a cuff of normal muscle tissue with the tumor. It is sometimes necessary to sacrifice one or more nerve roots to provide a suitable margin of excision. Once extensive collapse has occurred, as in vertebra

plana, a wide surgical margin is not possible and local control is dependent on adjuvant therapy.

The surgeon chooses the proper surgical approach based on the tumor type and location.

Zone 1 and 2 tumors are typically approached through a posterior longitudinal, mid-line incision, centered over the level of the tumor. Transverse incisions should *never* be used in any approach to a spinal neoplasm. The extent of the incision is based on the extent of the soft tissue mass, if any. The laminectomy and bone removal necessary for tumor resection often results in some degree of segmental instability. Posterior instrumentation and fusion may be performed when this is the case.

Zone 3 lesions are often addressed through an anterior approach alone. Depending on the extent of resection a formal reconstruction may or may not be necessary.

Zone 4 lesions require a combined surgical approach if a marginal or wide margin is to be obtained. Complete resection of the vertebral body requires separating the posterior structures (zones 1 and 2) from the anterior structures (zones 3 and 4), at the junction between the pedicles and the vertebral body (Fig. 2).

The standard approach to vertebrectomy combines a midline posterior incision with either a retroperitoneal, thoracoabdominal, or transthoracic approach to the anterior vertebral body. If at least one pedicle is uninvolved, a wide margin is possible *(13)*. An alternative approach is to extend the posterior dissection around the side of the vertebral body, completing the vertebrectomy through a posterolateral resection *(14)*. Complete vertebrectomy requires both anterior and posterior stabilization, but experience has shown that this aggressive surgical approach does improve patient survival and neurological function even when cure cannot be obtained *(15)*.

For sacral lesions a high sacral amputation is the procedure of choice *(19)*. This combined anterior/posterior sacral approach provides improved outcome with surprisingly little long-term morbidity. As long as the S2 nerve roots are spared bilaterally, or S2 and S3 are spared unilaterally, bowel and bladder function are usually retained *(16,17)*. In more proximal tumors these roots must be sacrificed in order to obtain local control and a reasonable likelihood of survival.

When a wide margin is not possible, the surgeon must accept a *marginal* margin. This will not provide adequate local control in some tumors, unfortunately, and recurrence of locally aggressive, radio-resistant tumors, such as chordoma, chondrosarcoma, and giant cell tumor, can be anticipated. Intra-operative strategies to improve results in marginal excisions have included cryotherapy (applying liquid nitrogen or polymethylmethacrylate to the tumor bed), intra-operative radiotherapy, and repeated resections of compromised margins.

Considering the extraordinary morbidity of reoperating on the spinal column, particularly in the face of vascular and neural adhesions, irradiated tissues, and hypervascular tumor tissue, surgeons will want to take every opportunity to avoid tumor recurrence. For this reason, *intralesional* tumor resection is avoided in any but the most clearly benign and self-limited lesions. If the patient already has disseminated disease, or if local involvement is already so extensive as to make resection impossible, curettage and "piecemeal resection" may be adequate to provide temporary local control. The other circum-

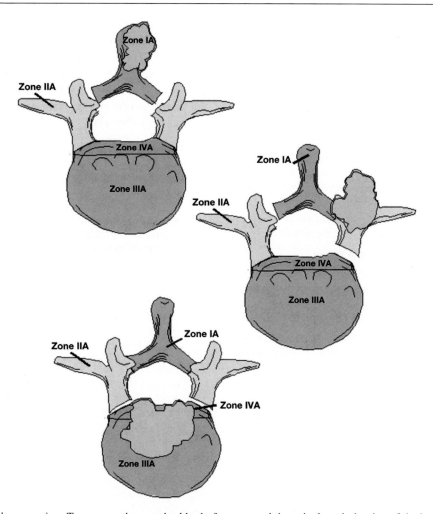

Fig. 2. Principles of *en-bloc* resection. To remove the vertebral body from around the spinal cord, the ring of the bony elements must be cut in two places. The typical point for release is at the junction of the vertebral pedicle with the posterior corner of the vertebral body. Axial and lateral views show the point at which the pedicle can be cut from a posterior approach to allow the vertebral body to be removed in one piece through an anterior approach.

stance in which an intralesional resection makes good sense is when the tumor is reliably radio-sensitive, and adjuvant therapy is sure to irradicate tumor left behind.

3.9. DECOMPRESSION

As many as 20% of all patients with disseminated carcinoma develop symptomatic spinal cord compression *(1,2)*. Patients often complain of progressive back pain, radicular symptoms or belt-like pain, lower extremity weakness, sensory loss, and bowel or bladder dysfunction.

Radiotherapy remains the appropriate treatment for most of these patients, though different tumor types exhibit different levels of radio-sensitivity. Lymphoreticular neoplasms and many adenocarcinomas are reliably radio-sensitive, and satisfactory local control can be gained through radiotherapy *(18)*. Gastrointestinal and renal neoplasms often respond incompletely to irradiation, and a number of primary tumors (i.e., chondrosarcoma, chordoma) are not at all radio-sensitive. Consequently, neurological compromise because of these tumors is best treated surgically.

Surgical decompression is most reliably effective when the approach is properly matched to focus of compressive: anterior

approaches for anterior compression and posterior approaches for posterior compression. "Surgery" is often unhelpful to patients with neurological symptoms, stemming from the historical practice of treating all compromised patients with laminectomy. Compared to radiotherapy alone, laminectomy provides no added benefit in treating anterior cord compression, the most common site of compression, and can compound problems by introducing or increasing segmental spinal instability *(6,19)*. In large series, decompressive laminectomy has provided neurological improvement in only 33% of cases, and a satisfactory outcome (maintenance of ambulation and sphincter control) in 37% *(20)*. By comparison, anterior decompression provided improvement in 79%, and a satisfactory outcome in 80%.

3.10. RECONSTRUCTION

Spinal instrumentation and fusion are often needed after tumor resection to restore stability, prevent progressive deformity, and to facilitate graft incorporation and fusion. The surgeon must choose an instrumentation construct that can meet the mechanical demands it will face following tumor resection, can compensate for loss of bony elements owing to resection or laminectomy, and permit postoperative imaging with CT and MRI. Key principles to satisfactory spinal reconstruction are to:

1. Restore the anterior weight-bearing column, preventing vertebral collapse and kyphosis.
2. Apply posterior instrumentation after laminectomy, compensating for lost muscular attachments and preventing post-laminectomy kyphosis.
3. Combine anterior and posterior constructs to restore axial, sagittal, and torsional stability after vertebrectomy.
4. Anticipate disease progression, extending fixation over longer segments, and maximizing the number of fixation points to insure construct survival.
5. Anticipate *improved patient survival*, strive for spinal fusion among patients likely to live more than 3 to 6 mo.

3.11. POSTERIOR INSTRUMENTATION

Newer segmental instrumentation systems are versatile and resilient. They allow the surgeon to neutralize the overall length of the spine while either compressing or distracting the internal spinal segments involved in the reconstruction. These systems have superior torsional and sagittal strength, and are widely available in titanium, improving postoperative imaging capabilities. These versatile systems also allow the surgeon to address multiple levels of vertebral involvement, restoring normal thoracic kyphosis and lumbar lordosis in the same construct.

Pedicle screw fixation is particularly helpful in patients who have undergone previous laminectomy. Combined with an anterior strut, pedicle screw constructs provide sufficient rigidity to allow the surgeon to instrument only two-motion segments when treating primary and metastatic lesions of the thoracolumbar spine *(21)*. Screw failure can be expected, however, if the anterior weight-bearing column is not restored *(22)*.

3.12. ANTERIOR INSTRUMENTATION

Anterior column reconstruction may be carried out in combination with posterior procedures, or as the preferred approach to instrumentation in selected patients. There is a significant incidence of wound complications associated with posterior surgery in spinal tumor patients. These patients are often systemically ill, many have undergone regional radiation therapy, and most have impaired healing potential. Because of illness, malnutrition, and inactivity, many have lost muscle mass and have little subcutaneous fat. Wound dehiscence, infection, and skin problems are common enough to prompt many surgeons to consider anterior reconstruction as their primary avenue of treatment.

Once the tumor is removed, something must fill the space left behind, both to bear the load of the upper body, and to augment the stability provided by the spinal instrumentation. Polymethylmethacrylate (PMMA) bone cement is frequently used to reconstruct the vertebral column in metastatic disease. It is resilient in compression, but it has no potential for biological incorporation. It has a tendency, therefore, to loosen and displace over time. To prevent migration of the PMMA strut, surgeons have either driven longitudinal Steinmann pins proximally and distally into the adjacent vertebrae to anchor the cement and improve its bending resistance, or alternately, inserted fixation rods into the vertebrectomy defect to restore height and anchor the PMMA mass *(23)*.

A tricortical bone graft strut or titanium cage with morselized autograft is favored in the treatment of benign or slow-growing tumors, in which survival is likely to be measured in years, and bony fusion is crucial. Similarly, in some malignant primaries, in which successful treatment will result in prolonged survival, the reconstruction must provide a solid fusion if late complications are to be avoided.

REFERENCES

1. Constans JP, Divitiis E, Donzelli R, Spaziante R, Meder JF, Haye C. Spinal metastases with neurological manifestations: review of 600 cases. J Neurosurg 1983; 59:111–118.
2. Siegal T, Siegal T. Current considerations in the management of neoplastic spinal cord compression. Spine 1988; 14:223–228.
3. Harrington KD. Anterior decompression and stabilization of the spine as a treatment for vertebral collapse and spinal cord compression from metastatic nalignancy. Clin Orthop 1988; 233:177–197.
4. Kostuik JP, Errico TJ, Gleason TF, Errico CC. Spinal stabilization of vertebral column rumors. Spine 1988; 13:250–256.
5. Boland PJ, Lane JM, Sundaresan N. Metastatic disease of the spine. Clin Orthop 1982; 169:95–102.
6. Harrington KD. Current concepts review: metastatic disease of the spine. J Bone Joint Surg 1986; 68:1110–1115.
7. Weinstein JN. Surgical approach to spine tumors. Orthopaedics 1989; 12:897–905.
8. Bohlman HH, Sachs BL, Carter JR, Riley L, Robinson RA. Primary neoplasms of the cervical spine. J Bone Joint Surg 1986; 68:483–494.
9. Shives TC, Dahlin DC, Sim FH, Pritchard DJ, Earle JD. Osteosarcoma of the dpine. J Bone Joint Surg 1986; 68:660–668.
10. Stener B. Total spondylectomy in chondrosarcoma arising from the seventh thoracic vertebra. J Bone Joint Surg 1971; 53:288–295.
11. Weinstein JN, McLain RF. Primary tumors of the apine. Spine 1987; 12:843–851.
12. Sundaresan N, Sachdev VP, Holland JF, et al. Surgical treatment of spinal cord compression from epidural metastasis. J Clin Oncol 1995; 13:2330–2335.
13. Boriani S, Biagini R, De Lure F, et al. En-bloc resections of bone tumors of the thoracolumbar spine. A preliminary report on 29 patients. Spine 1996; 21:1927–1931.
14. Fidler MW. Radical resection of vertebral body tumors: a surgical technique used in ten cases. J Bone Joint Surg 1994; 76:765–772.
15. Stener B, Gunterberg B. High amputation of the sacrum for extirpation of tumors. Spine 1978; 3:351–366.
16. Gennari L, Azzarelli A, Quagliuolo V. A posterior approach for the excision of sacral chordoma. J Bone Joint Surg 1987; 69:565–568.
17. Samson IR, Springfield DS, Suit HD, Mankin HJ. Operative treatment of sacrococcygeal chordoma. A Review of twenty-one cases. J Bone Joint Surg 1993; 75:1476–1484.
18. Tomita T, Galicich JH, Sundaresan N. Radiation therapy for spinal epidural metastases with complete block. Acta Radiol Oncol 1983; 22:135–143.
19. Gilbert RW, Kim JH, Posner JB. Epidural spinal cord compression from metastatic tumor: diagnosis and treatment. Ann Neurol 1978; 3:40–51.
20. McLain RF, Weinstein JN. Tumors of the spine. Seminars in Spine Surgery 1990; 2:157–180.
21. McLain RF, Kabins M, Weinstein JN. VSP stabilization of lumbar neoplasms: technical considerations and complications. J Spinal Disord 1991; 4:359–365.
22. McLain RF, Sparling E, Benson DR. Failure of short segment pedicle instrumentation in thoracolumbar fractures: complications of Cotrel-Dubousset instrumentation. J Bone Joint Surg 1993; 75:162–167.
23. Siegal T, Tiqva P, Siegal T. Vertebral body resection for epidural compression by malignant tumors. J Bone Joint Surg 1985; 67:375–382.

7 Presenting History and Common Symptoms of Spine Tumors

DANIEL SHEDID, MD AND EDWARD C. BENZEL, MD

CONTENTS

1. INTRODUCTION

Spinal tumors may cause a variety of symptoms depending on their type, location, and rate of growth. The symptomatology differs depending on tumor location (e.g., extradural or vertebral column vs intradural-extramedullary vs intramedullary). Vertebral column tumors are divided into primary and metastatic. Primary tumors include neoplasms of the marrow (e.g., multiple myeloma), and tumors of the bone or the cartilage of the spine *(1)*. Metastatic spinal pathology is much more common than primary neoplastic pathology. The spine is the most common site of skeletal metastasis *(2)*. A spinal metastasis is found in as many as 70 to 90% of patients dying of cancer *(3,4)*. The most common tumors that metastasize to the spine are tumors of the lung, breast, prostate, kidney, lymphoma, melanoma, and gastrointestinal tract *(5)*. In the pediatric population, spinal metastasis commonly arise from neuroblastoma, rhabdomyosarcoma, leukemia, and histiocytosis; less commonly from lymphoma, Wilms' tumor, and primitive neuroectodermal tumor *(6)*. Meningiomas and nerve sheath tumors (schwannomas and neurofibromas) comprise the overwhelming majority of the intradural-extramedullary tumors. Astrocytoma, ependymoma, and hemangioblastoma account for the majority of the intramedullary tumors.

2. METASTATIC EPIDURAL TUMORS

Pain is the most common presenting symptom of spinal metastases (85% of patients with metastasis to the spine) *(7)*. In patients already diagnosed with cancer, the onset of spinal pain

may indicate a spinal fracture caused by weakening of the vertebrae by metastatic tumor. Nocturnal bone pain suggests metastatic involvement. The pain is often difficult to distinguish from back pain owing to muscle strain or degenerative disease. However characteristics that suggest the diagnosis of neoplasm are pain that is gradual in onset but progressive, unrelenting, nonmechanical, and nocturnal *(2,7–9)*. The pain usually localizes to the site of the lesion. Radicular pain is of localizing value as well, as it tends to radiate in the dermatomal distribution of the compressed nerve root(s). This pain should be differentiated from that caused by disc degenerative disease. Pain of degenerative origin tends to affect the cervical or low lumbar area, whereas pain of metastatic epidural compression occurs at any level. Lying down often improves the pain of degenerative disease, but worsens the pain associated with metastatic compression *(9)*.

Motor dysfunction rarely occurs as an initial symptom, but is present in 76% of patients at the time of diagnosis *(5)*. Motor weakness usually follows the development of pain by weeks or months. It affects predominantly proximal muscles, creating difficulty when climbing stairs or rising from a chair *(9)*. Half of these patients have sensory dysfunction, such as numbness or paresthesia, whereas more than 50% have bowel and bladder dysfunction. Sphincter dysfunction is usually associated with sensory and motor dysfunction, except in patients with lesions at or near the conus medullaris or the sacrum. Approximately 5 to 10% of patients with cancer present with spinal cord compression as their initial symptom. Among those who present with cord compression, 50% are non-ambulatory at diagnosis and 15% are paraplegic. In paraplegic patients, a flaccid paralysis of the lower limbs with a distended bladder (neurogenic bladder) are usually observed.

From: *Current Clinical Oncology: Cancer in the Spine: Comprehensive Care.*
Edited by: R. F. McLain, K-U. Lewandrowski, M. Markman, R. M. Bukowski, R. Macklis, and E. C. Benzel © Humana Press, Inc., Totowa, NJ

Ventral spinal cord compression is associated with weakness in the extremities and loss of pain and temperature sense (spinothalamic tract) below the level of the compression, with preservation of touch, position, and vibration (dorsal column). Dorsal spinal cord compression is associated with the loss of dorsal column sensation with preservation of other sensory or motor functions *(10)*. Brown-Sequard's syndrome is characterized by ipsilateral spastic paralysis below the level of the lesion (interruption of the lateral corticospinal tract) with ipsilateral loss of tactile discrimination, vibratory, and position sensation below the level of the lesion (interruption of dorsal column) and contralateral loss of pain and temperature sensation. This usually occurs two to three segments below the level of the lesion (interruption of lateral spinothalamic tract) *(11)*.

The level of motor or sensory loss usually correlates with the site of spinal cord compression. The level of motor loss is more reliable than the level of sensory loss, except with thoracic cord involvement, where the sensory level on the chest or abdomen is of useful localizing value. Abdominal reflexes may also help in localizing because their innervation originates from segments T8 to T12 *(10)*.

Compression of the cauda equina often results in sporadic nerve root involvement, because the lumbar and sacral nerve roots are loosely arranged in the thecal sac. Therefore, such compression gives rise to patchy and asymmetrical motor and sensory loss in the lower limbs. Compression of the conus medullaris is often associated with a more complete and symmetrical distribution of neurological signs. Both conus medullaris and cauda equina compression can produce saddle anesthesia and loss of sphincter control.

Finally, symptoms of weight loss, change in appetite, fatigue, hemoptysis, hematuria, melena, rectorrhagia, and masses in the breast, neck, or axilla should be part of the review of systems whenever a systemic malignancy is suspected *(8)*.

3. INTRADURAL-EXTRAMEDULLARY TUMORS

Tumors that arise from within the confines of the dura mater are rarely metastatic and are usually slow growing. Patients with these types of tumors may have pain for years before any neurological problems occur. Because these tumors grow slowly, displacement of the spinal cord is gradual, and symptoms are often less than one would anticipate after radiographic imaging *(12)*. The symptoms may be difficult to differentiate from intramedullary and extradural lesions (e.g., syringomyelia, cervical spondylotic myelopathy, multiple sclerosis, spinal arteriovenous malformation, or spinal infection) *(12)*. Furthermore, intradural-extramedullary lesions can also be associated with subarachnoid hemorrhage, intracranial hypertension, intramedullary cyst formation, and hand atrophy, which may result in falsely localizing signs, further complicating the clinical presentation *(12–15)*.

Pain is the most common initial symptom in these patients. Unilateral radicular symptoms tend to present earlier than myelopathic symptoms because nerve sheath tumors arise primarily from the dorsal nerve roots. Occipital headaches may be caused by tumors located high in the cervical region and thoracic tumors may produce symptoms mistakenly attributed to visceral pathologies. Patients with meningioma can present with focal back or neck pain, rather than radicular pain. This symptom complex often progresses to myelopathy before the development of radiculopathy *(12,16)*. Filum terminale lesions, such as myxopapillary ependymomas, are associated with low back pain radiating into one or both legs. The pain may progress for several years before other symptoms occur, owing to the larger size of the thecal sac in this region. Sphincter dysfunction is most commonly seen in advanced cases or when the tumor involves the conus medullaris. Therefore, these lesions may mimic lumbar spondylosis *(12,17)*.

4. INTRAMEDULLARY TUMORS

The clinical features of intramedullary lesions are variable. Most tumors are benign and slow growing. This often results in a prolonged symptom duration before the establishment of the diagnosis (2–3 yr). Malignant lesions present with a much shorter course. Intratumoral hemorrhage in this latter group produces an ictal event and a precipitous presentation.

In the adult population, pain is the most common presenting symptom. It occurs in 60 to 70% of patients *(18)*. Pain is less common as a presenting symptom in the pediatric population. Motor and gait disturbances predominate in this age group *(19)*. The pain is usually poorly described, of variable intensity, localized to the general level of the lesion, rarely radicular, infrequently affected by activity or Valsalva maneuvers, and often described as a localized ache or muscle spasm. It may worsen at night or with recumbency *(18)*. In the case of an intramedullary tumor, a so-called dissociated sensory loss is common (Fig. 1). In these cases, there is loss of sensitivity to pain and temperature below the segmental spinal level of the tumor, but preserved sensitivity to light touch. Sensory or motor complaints are the initial symptom in about one-third of patients. Unilateral or asymmetric involvement is typical. Numbness is a common complaint and typically begins distally in the legs, with proximal progression. Urinary frequency is a common complaint and gait difficulties are common and related both to spasticity and to sensory dysfunction.

Tumors of the middle and lower cervical regions produce a suspended, cape-like sensory loss with pain involving the upper extremities, most often the shoulders or fingers (Fig. 2). A Horner's syndrome may be seen unilaterally or bilaterally, depending on the degree of involvement of the sympathetic system.

Involvement of the upper thoracic region produces pain in a girdle-type or belt-like distribution. If tumor expansion is asymmetric, symptoms of nerve compression may be unilateral. This is occasionally mistaken for angina pectoris, myocardial infarction, or pleurisy (Fig. 3). Lesions in the middle and lower thoracic regions may evoke pain that may erroneously suggest an abdominal lesion.

Tumors of the lumbar enlargement and conus medullaris often present with a history of back pain and leg pain, which may be radicular in origin. Urogenital and anorectal dysfunction are common. These symptoms may be mistakenly attributed to herniated nucleous pulposus or spondylosis *(18,20)*.

Intramedullary tumors in children may be associated with orthopedic deformities (kyphoscoliosis) and extremity weakness. Gait abnormalities or deformities of the feet (i.e., talipies

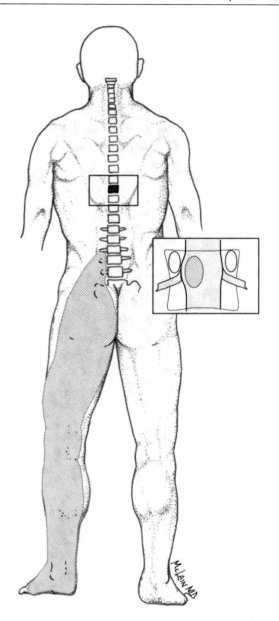

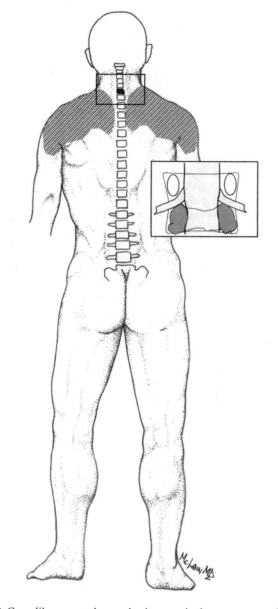

Fig. 1. Dissociative sensory loss caused by intramedullary tumors results in loss of pain and temperature sensitivity, with sparing of light touch and motor function distal to the lesion.

Fig. 2. Cape-like sensory loss and pain occur in the upper extremities when cervical level tumors compress the cord and nerve roots bilaterally.

equinovarus or pes cavus) may be observed in the young child. Enuresis in the previously toilet-trained child is another symptom of caudal tumor involvement. Sinus tract or a hairy or pigmented cutaneous lesion suggest the diagnosis of teratomas, epidermoid, and dermoid lesions *(21)*.

5. TUMORS OF THE CRANIOVERTEBRAL JUNTION

A variety of pathological lesions may occur at the level of the foramen magnum. However, meningiomas and neurofibromas predominate and constitute approx 70% of such lesions *(22)*. No definitive clinical markers for foramen magnum lesions exist, and the clinical profiles of the patients with foramen magnum tumors are varied. The latter includes neck pain, dyesthesias, cruciate hemiparesis, and pseudoathetoid movements of the upper limbs *(23)*.

These tumors may cause symptoms by compression of neighboring structures or by traction, and, thus, may have widespread effects such as hydrocephalus, syringomyelia, and vascular compromise *(24)*. The most common presentation is craniocervical pain, described as an aching sensation that is aggravated by head and neck motion and is referred to the second cervical dermatome *(25)*. Pain and temperature sensation is frequently affected, followed by loss of joint sensation. It is seen often in the upper extremities and may then march in a clockwise fashion around the limbs *(26)*. A suspended sensory loss with patches of preservation of sensation may also be seen *(27)*. Spasticity and weakness is a feature of foramen magnum tumors. The weakness usually originates in as an ipsilateral motor deficit limb and may follow a clockwise pattern (rotating paralysis) *(26,28)*.

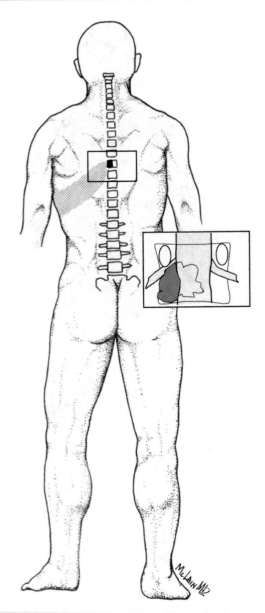

Fig. 3. Belt- or girdle-like pain and numbness occur when thoracic level tumors compress the nerve roots at the involved level. Unilateral compression produces symptoms of flank or rib pain on the involved side.

Foramen magnum tumors present as a unique syndrome, with a disproportionate loss of position and vibration sense in the upper (as compared to the lower) extremities, and with atrophy of the intrinsic muscles of the hand. These lower motor neuron findings are probably because of venous infarction at lower cervical levels (C8–T1) (29,30).

Besides sensory and motor symptoms, cranial nerves may also be affected in tumors of the foramen magnum. The most common cranial nerves affected are the vagus, glossopharyngeal, and hypoglossal. This leads to dysphagia, slurred speech, and repeated episodes of aspiration (30). Involvement of the spinal root of the accessory nerve may manifest as torticollis and weakness of the trapezius and sternocleidomastoid muscles. Involvement of the eighth cranial nerve may be associated with vertigo, tinnitus, and hearing loss. Nystagmus may be the result of involvement of the sulcomarginal fibers, which are an extension of the median longitudinal fasciculus (30).

Vascular changes as a result of compression, traction, or instability in the region of the foramen magnum may result in transient and episodic symptoms such as drop attack, migraine, paralysis, and visual loss (24,31).

6. SUMMARY

Spine tumors may have a wide variety of neurological symptoms. Some symptoms can correlate with the localization of the lesion. Neurological examination and radiological imaging remain important adjunct in the localization and the nature of the pathology.

REFERENCES

1. Swenson R. Differential diagnosis: a reasonable clinical approach. Neurol Clin 1999; 17:43–63.
2. Walker MP, Yaszemski MJ, Kim CW, Talac R, Currier BL. Metastatic disease of the spine: evaluation and treatment. Clin Orthop 2003; 415:S165–S175.
3. Black P. Spinal metastasis: current status and recommended guidelines for management. Neurosurgery 1979; 5:726–746.
4. Fornasier VL, Horne JG. Metastases to the vertebral column. Cancer 1975; 36:590–594.
5. Gilbert RW, Kim JH, Posner JB. Epidural spinal cord compression from metastatic tumor: diagnosis and treatment. Ann Neurol 1978; 3:40–51.
6. Faerber EN, Roman NV. Central nervous system tumors of childhood. Radiol Clin North Am 1997; 35:1301–1328.
7. Riley LH, Frassica DA, Kostuik JP, Frassica FJ. Metastatic disease to the spine: diagnosis and treatment. Instr Course Lect 2000; 49:471–477.
8. Daw HA, Markman M. Epidural spinal cord compression in cancer patients: diagnosis and management. Cleve Clin J Med 2000; 67:497, 501–544.
9. Sharma BS, Gupta SK, Khosla VK, et al. Midline and far lateral approaches to foramen magnum lesions. Neurol India 1999; 47:268–271.
10. Finelli PF, Leopold N, Tarras S. Brown-Sequard syndrome and herniated cervical disc. Spine 1992; 17:598–600.
11. McCormick PC, Torres R, Post KD, Stein BM. Intramedullary ependymoma of the spinal cord. J Neurosurg 1990; 72:523–532.
12. McCormick PC, Post KD, Stein BM. Intradural extramedullary tumors in adults. Neurosurg Clin N Am 1990; 1:591–608.
13. Blaylock RL. Hydrosyringomyelia of the conus medullaris associated with a thoracic meningioma: case report. J Neurosurg 1981; 54:833–835.
14. De Divitiis E, Maiuri F, Corriero G, Donzelli R. Subarachnoid hemorrhage due to a spinal neurinoma. Surg Neurol 1985; 24:187–190.
15. Feldmann E, Bromfield E, Navia B, Pasternak GW, Posner JB. Hydrocephalic dementia and spinal cord tumor. Report of a case and review of the literature. Arch Neurol 1986; 43:714–418.
16. Davis RA, Washburn PL. Spinal cord meningiomas. Surg Gynecol Obstet 1970; 131:15–21.
17. Fearnside MR, Adams CB. Tumours of the cauda equina. J Neurol Neurosurg Psychiatry 1978; 41:24–31.
18. Black P. Injuries of the vertebral column and spinal cord: mechanisms and management in the acute phase. In: Zuidema GD, Rutherford RB, Ballinger WF (eds). The Management of Trauma. 3rd ed. Philadelphia, PA: Saunders; 1979:226–253.
19. Epstein FJ, Farmer JP. Pediatric spinal cord tumor surgery. Neurosurg Clin N Am 1990; 1:569–590.

20. DeSousa AL, Kalsbeck JE, Mealey J, Campbell RL, Hockey A. Intraspinal tumors in children. A review of 81 cases. J Neurosurg 1979; 51:437–445.
21. Riley LH, Frassica DA, Kostuik JP, Frassica FJ. Metastatic disease to the spine: diagnosis and treatment. Instr Course Lect 2000; 49:471–477.
22. Stein BM, McCormick PC. Intramedullary neoplasm and vascular malformations. Clin Neurosurg 1992; 39:361–387.
23. Bull J. Letter: missed foramen-magnum tumours. Lancet 1974; 1:91.
24. VanGilder JC, Menezes AH, Dolan KD. The Craniovertebral Junction and its Abnormalities. Mount Kisco, NY: Futura; 1987.
25. Meyer FB, Ebersold MJ, Reese DF. Benign tumors of the foramen magnum. J Neurosurg 1984; 61:136–142.
26. Beatty RA. Cold dysesthesia: a symptom of extramedullary tumors of the spinal cord. J Neurosurg 1970; 33:75–78.
27. Endtz LJ, Frenay JJ. Studies on asterognosis and amyotrophy of the hand in brainstem syndromes. Relation to the symptomatology of tumours at the spinocranial junction. J Neurol Sci 1980; 44:241–246.
28. Taylor AR, Byrnes DP. Foramen magnum and high cervical cord compression. Brain 1974; 97:473–480.
29. Stein BM, McCormick PC. Spinal intradural tumors. In Wilkins RE, Rengachary S, eds. Neurosurgery. New York, NY: McGraw-Hill; 1996:1769–1781.
30. Menezes AH, VanGilder JC. Transoral-transpharyngeal approach to the anterior craniocervical junction. Ten-year experience with 72 patients. J Neurosurg 1988; 69:895–903.
31. Benzel EC. Biomechanics of Spine Stabilization. Rolling Meadows, IL: American Association of Neurological Surgeons Publications; 2001.

8 Physical Examination

Signs of Pathology and the Spine Examination

EERIC TRUUMEES, MD

CONTENTS

"More mistakes are made from want of a proper examination than for any other reason," Russell Howard (1)

"A cursory exam is worse than no exam at all because it may give the false hope that the lesion is minor," (1)

1. INTRODUCTION

Each year, 1.3 million new cancers are diagnosed in the United States *(2)*. Carcinomas of the lung, breast, prostate, and kidney are the most common *(3–5)*. More than 70% of these patients will develop skeletal metastases, most commonly in the spine *(6)*. Primary malignancies of the spine are not rare, but in adults, the vast majority of spine lesions represent lymphatic or hematogenous metastasis *(7)*.

Spinal tumors are also seen in children. Although the majority are benign, up to 30% are malignant *(8,9)*. Unlike adults, primary tumors and multicentric malignancies are more common than metastases in children *(10,11)*. Metastatic disease is seen in younger children (<8 yr old) and occurs with dissemination of neuroblastoma, retinoblastoma, and rhabdomyosarcoma *(9,10,12)*. The most common cancer in children is leukemia. Although leukemia affects all organ systems, back pain and vertebral collapse are the initial findings in 6% of children *(13)*.

In patients with suspected cancer of the spine, physical examination takes place in three settings. First, undiagnosed patients present with spinal pain. Distant findings, such as spine pain, predate symptoms from the primary lesion in up to one-third of patients *(14)*. Up to 24% of patients with metastatic disease will present with a pathological fracture *(15)*. In this setting, use the physical examination to search for the primary lesion. Second, there is a search for distant spread in patients with primary spine tumors. Other patients present with a known active malignancy and suspected spine involvement. Here, spinal findings may be more obscure. Perform a detailed evaluation to discriminate between spinal and extra-spinal causes of symptoms. Finally, patients with a remote history of cancer present with new onset spinal pain. Focus the spine examination on the strong possibility of cancer recurrence *(16)*.

2. CLINICAL SYNDROMES

Cancer in the spine has many sources and manifestations. It affects any age and either gender. Spinal malignancy can attack the bone or soft tissue structures of any vertebral level. Lesions may be contained by the spinal column or may extend into the paraspinal tissues. This wide variety of underlying disease states and patient types ensures a great diversity of physical findings. Four common clinical syndromes predominate:

1. Detection of spinal cancer in an asymptomatic individual.
2. Spinal cancer presenting with mild pain and stiffness.

From: *Current Clinical Oncology: Cancer in the Spine: Comprehensive Care.*
Edited by: R. F. McLain, K-U. Lewandrowski, M. Markman, R. M. Bukowski,
R. Macklis, and E. C. Benzel © Humana Press, Inc., Totowa, NJ

3. Spinal cancer causing severe pain and major neurological deficit.
4. Referred back pain from anatomic sites outside the spine.

In Burger and Lindeque's series *(17)*, in 17 of 78 patients with malignancy, back pain arose from shoulder, hip, or other extraspinal involvement. Other patients will have multiple bone metastases. To guide appropriate therapy, use the physical exam to identify the symptomatic lesion *(18)*.

3. IMPORTANCE OF THE EXAM

No physical findings point unequivocally toward spinal tumor. Many patients will have no prominent physical findings *(3)*. In Bohlman's series *(19)* of cervical spine tumors, no physical exam finding conclusively led to the diagnosis of neoplasm. Radiological imaging was required for further delineation of the lesion. In Ruff and Lanska's series, no single sign was both highly specific and sensitive *(20)*. In these patients, radicular pain and vertebral percussion tenderness were both sensitive, but not specific. Interobserver variability and reproducibility of physical signs is dependant on methods and care employed *(21)*. Rougraff et al. *(22)* assessed the diagnostic strategy they used to identify the source of skeletal metastases. Physical findings revealed the occult primary in the 8% of patients with masses and was non-diagnostic in 90% *(22)*.

The lack of specific findings accounts for the limited discussion of examination findings in the literature. Historically, close physical examination was underemphasized because of the perceived hopelessness of the disease. With improved treatment and prolonged survival, close physical evaluation is mandatory *(23)*. A careful physical examination will:

1. Aid in the diagnosis.
2. Allow earlier detection of spinal cancer, giving the best opportunity for cure *(8)*.
3. Highlight areas of concern (such as nutritional problems).
4. Direct treatment (urgent surgical intervention for progressive neurological decline).
5. Have prognostic significance *(24)*.

In patients with neurological dysfunction, the extent and the rapidity of decline have strong implications for the prognosis of both neurological recovery and patient survival *(6,25)*.

4. CLINICAL PRESENTATION

More than 85% of spine cancer patients present with back pain *(6)*. Back pain is the only symptom in 30%. The degree of spinal involvement and the severity of the presenting signs are not directly related *(26)*. However, a typical progression of signs and symptoms was described in 153 patients with metastatic spinal column involvement *(27)*. These patients presented with, in decreasing order of occurrence:

1. Radicular pain, which predominated in the lumbar area.
2. Motor weakness, which was associated with thoracic involvement.
3. Sensory changes.
4. Bladder dysfunction.

Leg pain is the only symptom in 10% of patients. Twenty-eight percent present with a combination of pain and neurologi-

Table 1
Signs of Metastatic Epidural Cord Compression in Adult Veterans[a]

Radicular pain	93%
Vertebral percussion tenderness	33%
Radicular sensory loss	17%
Radicular motor loss	16%
Leg weakness	29%
Spastic paraparesis	17%
Spinal sensory level	18%
Urinary retention or incontinence	20%

[a]From ref. *20*.

cal deficit. Spinal cancer is an incidental finding in 2% of patients *(6)*.

In a series of 130 patients with spinal cord compression, only 10 (8%) presented with neurological involvement as their first symptom of cancer *(28)*. Siegal and Siegal *(25)* reported that 16 of 113 patients (14%) with cord compression presented with primary neurological involvement. Objective neurological deficit is significantly more likely to be caused by a malignant than benign tumor. In Weinstein and McLain's series, an objective neurological deficit could be identified in 55% of patients with malignant primary tumors of the spine, but only 35% of patients with benign lesions *(8)*. Similar findings were noted in the series of Shives et al. *(29)*, Thommeson and Poulsen *(30)*, and Sim et al. *(31)*. Sixteen percent of patients have a mass or deformity *(8)*. In most cases, pain will localize to the metastatic deposit, occasionally the pain will be referred *(32)*. Ruff and Lanska *(20)* delineated the presenting signs in veterans subsequently demonstrated to have epidural metastases (*see* Table 1).

The presentation of cancer of the spine in children is also nonspecific. However, although more than 80% of adult back pain is self-limited, less than 30% of back pain in children is self-limited. In most cases there is a skeletal cause *(33)*. Back pain is reported in 93%, whereas severe neurological deficits are seen in only 7.5%. Palpable masses are noted in 5.5%, but these usually stem from benign tumors of the posterior elements *(33)*. In Freiberg and coworker's *(34)* report of 19 children with metastatic vertebral disease, 12 demonstrated vertebral tenderness, 8 had neurological findings, 1 was hypertensive, and 2 were discovered incidentally. In Leeson's *(9)* autopsy study, each child had complained of pain, 11 of 39 had had pathological fractures, and 3 had presented with acute spinal cord injury syndrome. In children with leukemia, 5.6% had back pain and 50% had systemic findings *(35)*. The presenting signs in Fraser's series are depicted in Table 2 *(12)*.

Cervical vertebral bodies are smaller and the spinal canal has relatively more space for the cord. In Bohlman's series *(19)*, neck pain was the most common presenting complaint, but neck mass, persistent headaches, stiff neck, radiating arm pain without neck pain, long tract signs, and myelopathy were also noted. There was only one case of quadriparesis in 23 patients. In Marchesi's series *(36)*, 42% had radicular pain, and 31% had objective neurological findings.

Table 2
Signs of Spinal Malignancy in Children[a]

Muscle weakness	67%
Pathological reflexes	60%
Sensory loss	30%
Mass	20%
Paravertebral muscle spasm	15%
Sphincter laxity	occ
Palpable bladder	occ
Muscle atrophy	occ
Pain with straight leg raise	occ
Scoliosis	occ
Local tenderness	occ
Torticollis	occ
Ataxia	occ
Cutaneous sinus	occ
Sagittal plane change	occ

[a]From ref. *12*.

5. PARANEOPLASTIC SYNDROMES AND SIGNS OF DISSEMINATED NEOPLASIA

Patients with metastatic cancer are systemically ill. Paraneoplastic syndromes are systemic manifestations of metastatic cancer and fall into three categories:

1. Clinical syndromes.
2. Neurological syndromes.
3. Hematological syndromes.

Suspected causes of these syndromes include:

1. Hormones synthesized by a tumor.
2. Immune complex formation.
3. Ectopic hormone receptor production.
4. Release of physiologically active compounds by a tumor.
5. Unknown causes.

The paraneoplastic syndromes may mimic spinal pathologies. A previously undiagnosed patient may present with a paraneoplastic syndrome symptom complex and therefore they must be recognized *(37)*.

Tumors may cause endocrine imbalance. For example, fasting hypoglycemia may be derived from insulin secretion from an insulinoma. Diarrhea may result from vasoactive intestinal polypeptide release from an islet cell tumor. Epinephrine and norepinephrine secretion from a pheochromacytoma often produces hypertension. Ectopic adrenocorticotropic hormone and antidiuretic hormone are produced by some lung cancers. Parathyroid hormone is produced by squamous cell lung cancer, head and neck cancers, and bladder cancer. Some breast cancers, small cell lung cancer, and medullary thyroid carcinomas release calcitonin *(38)*.

Dermatomyositis and, to a lesser degree, polymyositis are common in cancer patients. A progressive, proximal muscle weakness, a dusky, erythematous butterfly rash on the cheeks, and periorbital edema are seen *(39)*.

Pigmented skin lesions or keratoses are common in patients with disseminated cancer. These include acanthosis nigricans in patients with a gastrointestinal malignancy, generalized melanosis in patients with lymphoma, melanoma, and hepatocellular carcinoma, and Bowen's disease in patients with lung, gastrointestinal (GI), and genitourinary malignancies *(40)*. Patients with lymphoma and GI malignancy may also bear multiple, large seborrheic keratoses, i.e., the sign of Leser-Trélat *(41)*.

The neurological paraneoplastic syndromes occur in less than 1% of cancer patients and are more frequent with oat cell carcinoma of the lung, breast, and ovarian cancer. These syndromes are not limited to the nervous system but frequently affect it. Their etiology is unknown, but autoimmune mechanisms have been proposed and circulating antibodies against nervous system tissues are often found *(42,43)*.

These neurological syndromes are classified by location and often have central effects such as progressive dementia, alteration of mood, and seizures. They may also present with focal motor or sensory signs, which makes their identification in patients with presumed malignancy of the spine especially important. Unless characteristic autoantibodies are detected, the diagnosis of neurological paraneoplastic syndrome is one of exclusion *(44)*.

Subacute cerebellar degeneration leads to progressive bilateral leg and arm ataxia and dysarthria. Neurological signs include dementia, nystagmus, and extensor plantar signs. The syndrome progresses over weeks to months, often causing profound disability. It may precede discovery of the causative cancer by weeks to years. Anti-Yo, a circulating autoantibody, may be detected in the serum or CSF *(42,43)*.

Paraneoplastic sensory neuropathy may occur with or without encephalomyelitis. It usually accompanies small cell lung carcinoma and presents with painful neuropathy and loss of all sensory modalities. An associated limbic encephalitis may progress from anxiety and depression, to memory loss, agitation, confusion, hallucinations, and behavioral abnormalities. Some patients will have anti-Hu, a circulating autoantibody, in the serum and spinal fluid.

Spontaneous chaotic eye movements, opsoclonus, represents a rare cerebellar syndrome accompanying childhood neuroblastoma. Opsoclonus is also associated with cerebellar ataxia and myoclonus of the trunk and extremities. The circulating antibody, Anti-Ri, may be present *(45)*.

Subacute motor neuropathy is a rare disorder of painless weakness of both upper and lower extremities. It is seen in patients with Hodgkin's disease or other lymphomas and is thought to represent degeneration of the anterior horn cells. Subacute necrotic myelopathy is a rare, rapidly ascending destruction of the gray and white matter of the spinal cord, leading to paraplegia *(46)*.

Peripheral neuropathy is the most common neurological paraneoplastic syndrome. This distal sensorimotor polyneuropathy produces mild motor weakness, sensory loss, and absent distal reflexes and is indistinguishable from similar changes that accompany many chronic illnesses.

Guillain-Barré and Eaton-Lambert syndromes are immune-mediated neurological conditions more common in patients with cancer than in the general population. Eaton-Lambert syndrome, an immune-mediated, myasthenia-like syndrome, weakens the limbs, but spares the ocular and bulbar muscles. An immunoglobin G antibody impairs release of acetylcholine from nerve terminals. Eaton-Lambert can precede, occur with, or develop after the diagnosis of cancer, particularly in men with intrathoracic tumors (47).

Hematologic paraneoplastic syndromes include: pure red blood cells aplasia, anemia of chronic disease, leukocytosis (the leukemoid reaction), thrombocytosis, eosinophilia, and basophilia. These conditions are seen particularly in lymphoid malignancies and Hodgkin's disease. For surgical patients, recognition of potential paraneoplastic disseminated intravascular coagulation, idiopathic thrombocytopenic purpura, and a Coombs-positive hemolytic anemia is critical to safe intra- and postoperative management.

Other paraneoplastic complications represent contiguous extension of tumor into surrounding neurovascular structures. Horner's syndrome reflects tumor invasion into the cervical sympathetic chain and presents with enophthalmos, miosis, ptosis, and ipsilateral facial anhidrosis. Pancoast syndrome, owing to infiltration of the brachial plexus and neighboring ribs and vertebrae, consists of pain, numbness, and weakness of the affected arm. Pancoast syndrome may coexist with Horner's Syndrome. Superior vena cava syndrome occurs when tumor constricts the superior vena cava and obstructs of venous drainage. Patients present with dilation of collateral veins in the upper part of the chest and neck and edema and plethoric facies, neck, and torso. Lymphangitic carcinomatosis results from the intrapulmonary spread of a primary or secondary cancer and causes cor pulmonale, worsening hypoxemia, and severe dyspnea.

Direct bone destruction or endocrine dysfunction may produce hypercalcemia. Although many patients are asymptomatic, clinical manifestations include constipation, anorexia, nausea and vomiting, abdominal pain, and ileus. Increased free calcium is also associated with emotional lability, confusion, delirium, psychosis, stupor, and coma. Neuromuscular involvement may cause prominent skeletal muscle weakness (48). Endocrine-mediated bone loss may be massive. In many patients with metastatic carcinoma, bone loss leads to non-neoplastic osteoporotic compression fractures (49).

Hypertrophic pulmonary osteoarthropathy occurs in 5% of those with lung cancer, lung metastases, thymoma, sarcoma, Hodgkin's disease, or mesothelioma. Clubbing, periosteal thickening, and pain in the long and short tubular bones are accompanied by swollen joints in 30 to 40% (50).

6. PHYSICAL EXAMINATION STRATEGY

Examine the gowned and otherwise unclothed patient in a warm, well-lit room. Shoes and socks should be removed. Start with a general survey of the patient's appearance and movement. Then, perform the spine examination itself. Include elements of the shoulder, pelvis, and hip exam. In cancer patients, an examination of commonly involved organ systems includes an abdominal and thoracic exam. Finally, perform a complete neurological examination. The key is to develop a thorough, efficient routine that avoids missed or duplicated steps (see Table 3).

Table 3
Suggested Physical Exam Sequence[a]

Position	Exam
On arrival	Vitals: height/weight, temperature
Standing	Inspection: general inspection, skin, deformity, spasm
	ROM: neck, shoulders, back
	Thyroid, SCM, posterior neck tenderness
	Gait and walking posture
	Functional motor eval: toe raises, heel-walking, squats
Sitting	Posture
	Motor: hip flexors, hip abductors and adductors, toe, and ankle
	Dorsiflexion, plantarflexion, inversion/eversion
	Knee flexion and extension
	Deep tendon reflexes, arms/legs
	Abnormal reflexes: Hoffman, Babinski, Oppenheim
	Sensation
	SLR
Supine	Motor: miscellaneous
	Measurements: extremity circumference for atrophy
	SLR
	Clonus
	Pulses and capillary refill, hair pattern, edema
	Hip ROM, Patrick test
	Abdominal/breast exam
Prone	Femoral nerve stretch, prone knee bend
	Thoracic and lumbar spine palpation
	Costovertebral angle tenderness
	Gluteal and hamstring strength
Lateral Decubitus	Rectal and prostate exam
	Perineal sensation
	Gaenslen's test

[a]Modified from ref. 71.
ROM, range of motion; SCM, sternocleidomastoid muscle; SLR, straight leg raise.

7. GENERAL SURVEY

Patients with metastatic disease are by definition systemically ill (16). The extent of illness is variable, and may not be apparent until a detailed exam has been performed. Manifestations apparent on first observation may include cachexia, lethargy, nausea, dehydration, and confusion (50). Document vital signs looking especially for weight fluctuations, hypertension, and fever. Also search for signs of venous thromboembolism, lymphadenopathy, skin change, and edema.

Palpate the axillary, cervical, and inguinal node-bearing areas carefully (51). Many carcinomas, synovial and epithelioid sarcomas, and rhabdomyosarcomas spread to regional lymph nodes. Lymphadenopathy is also a feature of lymphoma. Lymphatic or venous obstruction may lead to extremity edema. At each phase of the exam, inspect the skin. Local and systemic cutaneous manifestations of malignancy include acanthosis nigricans, jaundice, cyanosis, and easy bruisability (40,50). Neurofibromata may undergo malignant degeneration (40).

Table 4
Common Sources of Metastatic Lesions to the Spine

Lung
Breast
Prostate
Kidney
Gastrointestinal tract: colon, rectal
Thyroid

8. SOURCE SYSTEMS EXAMS

Most lesions to the spine originate from major thoracoabdominal organ systems. Primary spinal malignancies may metastasize to the lungs or elsewhere. A complete physical examination therefore requires assessment of potentially involved organs (*see* Table 4).

The thyroid gland lies over the thyroid cartilage at the C4–C5 vertebral level. Most patients with thyroid cancer will have a palpable mass at presentation. This nodule is asymptomatic, but rock hard on palpation *(52,53)*.

Pancreatic cancer is typically silent until late in the course of disease. Weight loss and abdominal pain occur with advanced disease. Obstructive jaundice, splenomegaly, gastric and esophageal varices, and GI hemorrhage may develop. Patients report increasingly severe upper abdominal pain radiating to the back. In these patients, pain may be relieved by bending forward or assuming the fetal position *(54)*.

Hepatocellular carcinoma or liver metastases harden and enlarge the liver. The liver may also be tender with palpable lumps. Hepatic bruits and pleuritic-type pain with an overlying friction rub are uncommon, but characteristic, signs. Without biliary obstruction by tumor, jaundice is usually absent or mild. Ascites from peritoneal seeding, on the other hand, is common *(55)*.

Renal cell carcinoma most commonly presents with gross or microscopic hematuria. Later, flank pain is reported. On exam, look for a palpable, often pulsatile, mass and costovertebral angle tenderness. On the left, this mass may be misinterpreted as splenomegaly. Vital signs may reveal fever or hypertension *(56)*.

Begin the abdominal exam with inspection. Distension, especially asymmetric distention of the superior or inferior halves may reflect a mass. Subcutaneous bleeding may be indicated by a dissecting bluish discoloration or frank ecchymoses of the costovertebral angles (Grey Turner's sign) or around the umbilicus (Cullen's sign). Abdominal tumors or ascites that stretch the skin produce striae. Further, look for limited abdominal motion with breathing. On the other hand, visible peristalsis is abnormal.

Next, auscultate all four quadrants of the abdomen with the diaphragm of stethoscope to listen for active peristalsis. The pitch and frequency of the peristalsis signal the nature of the underlying disease. High-pitched peristalsis or borborygmi in rushes suggest intestinal obstruction. Absence of sounds after 5 min of continuous listening suggests peritonitis and paralytic ileus. Severe pain with a silent abdomen warrants immediate exploration. Then, with the bell of the stethoscope listen in the epigastric region and peri-umbilical regions for bruits *(57)*.

Percuss the size and density of the abdominal organs to detect fluid (ascites), air (distention), or solid masses. Palpate all four quadrants for tenderness, rebound tenderness, and masses. Assess for costovertebral angle tenderness. Rectal and pelvic examinations are essential parts of the complete abdominal exam. Although a complete pelvic examination may be deferred to the patient's gynecologist, it should not be ignored. During the rectal exam, assess sphincter tone, palpate the prostate, and check the stool guiac.

Prostate cancer is slowly progressive and asymptomatic until late in the disease. In late disease, symptoms of bladder outlet obstruction, ureteral obstruction, and hematuria are present. Because prostrate metastases are often blastic, fractures are less frequent *(58)*. A trans-rectal prostate examination is required. In patients with locally advanced disease, induration to the seminal vesicles and fixation of the gland laterally may be appreciated.

Breast carcinoma is the principle source of spinal metastases in women *(59)*. More than 80% of breast cancers are discovered as a lump by the patient. Less commonly, a history of pain without mass is described. In these patients, breast enlargement or a nondescript, firm, asymmetrical thickening is reported. A complete breast exam is performed in stages. First, with the patient sitting and arms hanging loosely, examine the breasts for size, symmetry, contour, skin color, texture, and venous pattern. Then, ask the patient to elevate her hands to accentuate dimpling. Systematically palpate the breasts, axillae, and supraclavicular regions. Examine the axillae with the patient's arms at her side and elbows flexed to 90°. Lymph nodes should not be palpable in an adult *(57)*. Advanced breast cancers are fixed to the chest wall or to the overlying skin. These lesions also demonstrate skin dimpling, satellite nodules or skin ulcers, and the lymphedematous exaggeration of skin markings (peau d'orange). Inflammatory breast cancer is a particularly virulent variant, characterized by diffuse inflammation and enlargement of the breast, often without a mass.

Lung cancer manifestations depend on tumor location and type of spread. Most bronchogenic carcinomas are endobronchial and present with a cough, with or without hemoptysis. Bronchial narrowing may trap air leading to localized wheezing, atelectasis, ipsilateral mediastinal shift, diminished expansion, dullness to percussion, or loss of breath sounds. Infection of an obstructed lung produces fever, chest pain, and weight loss. Persistent localized chest pain suggests neoplastic invasion of the chest wall. Peripheral nodular tumors are asymptomatic until they invade the pleura or chest wall and cause pain or until they metastasize to distant organs. Late symptoms include fatigue, weakness, decreased activity, worsening cough, dyspnea, decreased appetite, weight loss, and pain. Large, malignant serosanguineous pleural effusions are common. Begin the lung examination with an inspection of the shape of the chest and the rate and rhythm of respiration. Asymmetry of chest wall expansion suggests respiratory compromise from a collapse lung or limitation of expansion by extrapleural air, fluid, or a mass. Note the midline position of the trachea. Percuss and auscultate each lung field. Palpate for crepitus, tactile fremitus, or a pleural friction rub *(57)*.

In children, the findings of disseminated malignancy are the same. Look for signs of easy bruisability, cachexia, and failure to meet growth expectations. Metastatic diseases are less common. Neuroblastoma metastases are rarely limited to one site *(9)*. Rhabdomosarcoma will often have soft tissue masses. Spinal metastases are uncommon with Wilm's tumor and have a poor prognosis *(9)*.

9. THE SPINE EXAM

9.1. INSPECTION, CONTOUR, AND PALPATION

Begin the spine examination immediately after entering the room. Note the position of the patient in the room; are they more comfortable pacing, standing, sitting, or lying down? Mechanical disorders rarely leave a patient writhing in pain, and in such a case consider a serious visceral disorder or psychological overlay *(60)*. Assess the patient's movement and gait for splinting, antalgia, ataxia (wide-based gait), circumduction, a steppage, or drop foot patterns.

Next, inspect the spinal contour from the front, sides, and back both standing and seated. Look for coronal imbalance, pelvic obliquity, or shoulder imbalance. Pass a plumb line from the C7 spinal process; it should pass through the gluteal cleft. Normal sagittal balance includes a thoracic kyphosis of 20 to 45° and a lumbar lordosis of 40 to 60°.

Gross deformity is an unusual feature of spinal neoplasia. Changes are typically subtle, such as the kyphosis engendered by pathological compression fractures. Asymmetric vertebral collapse in the anteroposterior plane may cause a sharp scoliosis. Benign bone tumors of the posterior elements, such as osteoid osteoma and osteoblastoma, are occasionally associated with scoliosis. Idiopathic scoliosis is rarely painful, whereas painful curves, with localized tenderness, muscle spasm, and limited motion more often have underlying neoplastic or inflammatory causes. Investigate unusual patterns such as left thoracic, cervical and "C"-shaped curves closely *(61,62)*. These curves come on suddenly and progress rapidly *(62)*. A sciatic list, secondary to muscle spasm, is present when standing but disappears with recumbency *(see* Fig. 1 *[63])*.

Note the patient's head position. Torticollis, from inflammation of the sternocleidomastoid muscle, causes the head to tilt toward the ipsilateral shoulder and rotates toward the contralateral side. Head tilt may also represent cerebellar or ophthalmologic disorders *(64)*. Angular deformities from cervical metastases are infrequent *(65)*.

Next, meticulously palpate the spine. Back pain is nonspecific and ubiquitous in the age groups at risk for spinal tumors. But, idiopathic back pain is typically mechanical, activity related, and self-limited. Neoplastic pain is typically progressive and unrelenting. Although it may be exacerbated by activity, it is not responsive to rest *(66)*. Neoplastic pain is well localized and readily reproduced by palpation or percussion over the involved area *(62)*.

Palpate the cervical spine while inspecting for atrophy or swelling. Separately assess the spinous process and interspinous ligaments for both pain and step-off. Put a lateral or rotatory moment on the spinous process to differentiate local, mechanical spinal pain from referred tenderness *(1)*. Next,

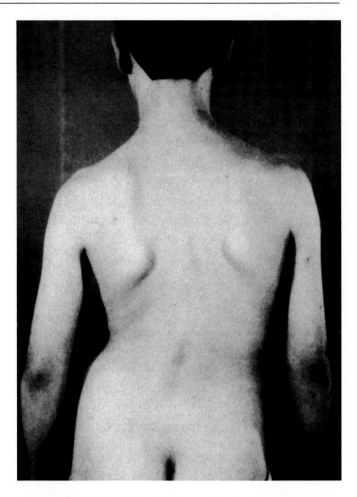

Fig. 1. Sharp left-sided scoliosis associated with a T10 tumor.

palpate the posterior superior iliac spine, scapula and ribs, iliac crests, sacrum and coccyx, and trochanters and ischial tuberosities. Undertake soft tissue palpation for spasm, fluctuance, or masses. Include the paraspinal muscles, gluteus, piriformis, and sciatic notch.

9.2. RANGE OF MOTION AND TENSION SIGNS

Next, assess spinal range of motion (ROM). In patients with spinal cancer, pain increases with ROM, but to a lesser degree than typical, mechanical spine pain *(66)*. The normal cervical spine flexes 45° to allow the chin to touch the chest. The neck extends 75° and exhibits 40° of lateral bending and 75° of rotation *(67)*.

The normal thoracolumbosacral spine exhibits 80° of forward flexion. Measure the distance of fingertips to the floor. Watch the patient return to an erect posture. This should be a smooth motion. A catch suggests instability. The normal thoracolumbosacral spine spine exhibits 20–40° of extension, 45° of rotation, and 20–40° of lateral bending *(67)*. These motions may increase radicular symptoms.

Several provocative tests are useful. To perform an Adson's test, palpate the radial pulse both before and after passively abducting, extending and externally rotating the arm. Then, turn the head toward arm in question. A decrease or loss of pulse suggests thoracic outlet syndrome, which may be caused

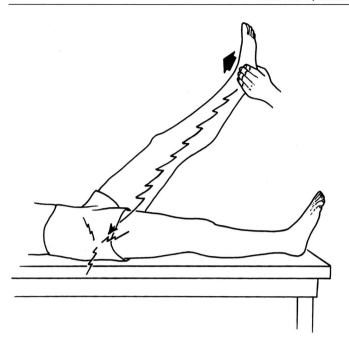

Fig. 2. The straight leg test.

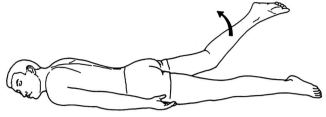

Fig. 3. The femoral nerve stretch sign.

by a mass or supraclavicular lymphadenopathy. If cervical radicular involvement is suspected, perform a cervical compression test by applying axial pressure on top of head. Increased arm pain reflects a positive test. Perform Spurling's test by compressing the head with the neck extended and turned to the painful side. Reproduction of radiating arm pain suggests nerve root entrapment in the neuroforamen (68). L'Hermitte's phenomenon refers to a shock-like sensation noted through the trunk and extremities with passive flexion and compression of head

A positive distraction test implies relief of arm pain with gentle axial traction on the head. Tension on the cervical nerve roots can also be decreased by passively abducting the shoulder. Decreased pain, a positive shoulder abduction test, is reported in 68% of those with cervical radiculopathy owing to extradural compression (69).

Seek lumbar tension signs with both a supine and sitting straight leg raise (see Fig. 2). This test is moderately sensitive, but relatively nonspecific. A negative test, therefore, does not exclude radiculopathy. The patient's response depends on exact location of compressing material (70). Perform the ankle dorsiflexion test by raising the supine patient's leg to the point of pain. Then, flex the knee slightly to relief hamstring tightness. Next, dorsiflex the foot. If the pain recurs, the source is likely radicular and not from muscle tightness. Laseque's Maneuver is undertaken with the patient supine and the hips and knees flexed to 90°. Then, extend the knee until sciatica is produced (71).

Further evidence of compression of the L4–S2 roots is confirmed with a bowstring test. With the supine patient's knee flexed to 70°, press on the tibial nerve in the popliteal fossa. Reproduction of pain in thigh or calf is a positive test (71). Compression on the upper lumber roots L2–L4 may be assessed with a femoral stretch test (see Fig. 3). Extend the thigh at the hip with the leg flexed in a prone patient. Reproduction

of leg pain is a positive test. However, this test also causes pelvic rotation, increased lumbar lordosis, and hip extension. Therefore, groin pain may reflect hip joint disease and back pain may reflect sacroiliac (SI) joint or facet joint pathology (71).

The prone knee bend also assesses upper lumbar nerve root compression. Place one hand on the patient's buttock allowing the hip to remain in extension while the knee is flexed. Compare left and right production of anterior thigh pain. Similar pain reflects quadriceps tightness, differences suggest root compression (72).

10. ASSOCIATED MUSCULOSKELETAL EXAM

The assessment of back and extremity pain is complicated by radiating pain patterns from the spine into the extremities and vice versa. Therefore, no spinal examination is complete without an assessment of at least the shoulder, hip, and pelvis.

Shoulder and cervical spine pathology often coexist. Shoulder pain may radiate medially to neck and neck pain routinely radiates laterally into shoulder. Other sources of referred pain to the shoulder include: mediastinal lesions, cardiac ischemia, and diaphragmatic irritation (5). Glenohumeral joint pain is typically felt at the deltoid insertion and radiates down the lateral arm.

Begin the shoulder examination by inspecting the shoulder contour from the front and behind, specifically comparing shoulder elevation. Look for scapular winging, which reflects injury to the long thoracic nerve. Assess the deltoid, supraspinatus, and infraspinatus contours for atrophy.

Palpate the bony shoulder girdle including the subcutaneous clavicle, scapular borders and spine, and the acromioclavicular joint. Palpate the associated soft tissue structures including the subacromial space, biceps tendon and posterior triangle. The normal shoulder has a wide arc of motion: 160° forward flexion and 50° of extension; 170° abduction (or side elevation) and 50° adduction. Internal and external rotation should be above 65° in all planes (67).

Provocative testing of the shoulder begins with the impingement test. Subacromial impingement may mimic radicular pain and is reproduced by internally rotating the elevated arm. External rotation causes apprehension in the patient with shoulder instability. Exacerbate acromioclavicular joint pain with cross body adduction. Shoulder weakness may be owing to a C5 root palsy or to a rotator cuff tear. Test each rotator cuff muscle in isolation. The subscapularis is best assessed by a lift-off test from the back. Place the arm in the impingement position and ask the patient to resist caudal pressure to test the supraspina-

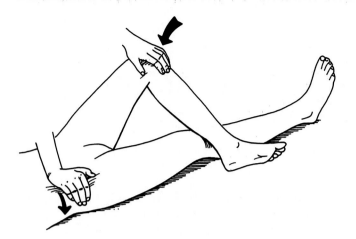

Fig. 4. The Patrick flexion, abduction, external rotation (FABER) test.

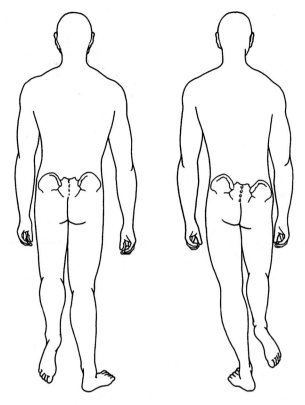

Fig. 5. The Trendelenburg test. The left-sided figure is normal. The right-sided figure demonstrates a droop of the right side signifying weakness of the left gluteus medius.

tus. Test infraspinatus function by comparing the strength of external rotation with the adducted arms.

SI joint pathology manifests as low back or buttock pain but may also refer to posterior thigh and leg. Hip joint disorders classically manifest as groin pain radiating to the anterolateral thigh and medial knee. But hip pathology can also refer pain to the back. Metastatic disease patients may have coexistent hip and spine involvement.

Begin the hip and pelvis exam with inspection of the muscular contour and overlying skin. Next, palpate the SI joints, pubic symphysis, and femoral triangle. Extraspinal sciatic nerve compression from malignancy may simulate radiculopathy. In patients with disseminated disease and radicular complaints, palpate the entire course of the sciatic nerve from its sciatic notch to the foot (73). The straight leg raise (SLR) test may localize pain to a specific point along the course of the nerve.

Normal hip ROM includes 110° of flexion and 30° of extension and approx 45° of abduction, adduction, and internal and external rotation (67).

Perform provocative tests to further delineate the origin of pain. Perform a Patrick test on the supine patient by holding the contralateral iliac crest. Then, flex, abduct, and external rotate the hip (see Fig. 4). A positive test causes increased SI joint area pain. Increased groin pain reflects hip joint pathology. Perform Gainslen's test with the patient supine at the edge of the table with both legs drawn up into the knee chest position. Allow the unsupported leg to slowly drop off the edge of the table while the supported leg remains with the hip flexed. This maneuver places strain on SI joint and is positive if it generates concordant pain (74).

Perform Maitland's Test in the lateral decubitus position with the upper hip flexed to 90° and the lower hip extended. Face the patient and put one hand on the anterior superior iliac spine (ASIS) and the heel of the other hand on the ischial tuberosity. Push your hands in opposite directions to cause rotation of the hemipelvis. A positive test produces of concordant pain in the SI joint (74). Perform a pelvic rock test on the supine patient by compressing the iliac crests. The posterior stress test

also provokes SI joint pain. Flex the hip and knee and place an axial load on the hemipelvis.

The Trendelenburg test assesses L5 nerve root function, hip abductor weakness, or primary hip joint pathology. Stand behind patient with one hand on each iliac crest. Instruct the patient to stand on one leg, then the other. A drop of the opposite side of the pelvis implies weakness of hip abductors on weightbearing side (see Fig. 5 [74]).

11. NEUROLOGICAL EXAM

Neurological deficit is more common in patients with primary spinal malignancy (55%) than in those with metastatic disease (8–14%). Although weakness is the presenting symptom in only 5% of children with malignancy, more than 65% of these children will eventually develop weakness. In this patient population, weakness progresses rapidly: 30% reach maximal deficit in less than 48 h and 90% reach maximal deficit in less than 10 d. Only 10% have more gradual progression (66).

Motor weakness may be difficult to differentiate from lethargy (6). Differentiate radiculitis (pain in radicular distribution) from radiculopathy (dermatomal sensory loss, paresthesias, and motor loss). Pay special attention to signs of cauda equina compression including bowel and bladder dysfunction, saddle anesthesia, and lower extremity sensorimotor dysfunction. Cord compression from epidural extension of tumors above the L2 level can cause myelopathy. Symptoms of cervical myelopathy include numb, cold, painful hands, and decreased fine motor skills. Myelopathy hand includes weak intrinsics with the loss of adduction and extension of ulnar two to three digits. Demonstrate the finger escape sign by asking the patient to keep his fingers in full extension. If the ulnar digits abduct, a myelopathy above the C6–C7 level is suggested *(76)*.

In patients with metastatic disease and neurological dysfunction, consider brain and paraneoplastic involvement. Assess the cranial nerves and cognitive and cerebellar function. Brain, spinal cord, nerve roots, and muscle lesions may affect motor power. Flaccid paralysis suggests nerve root compression, whereas upper motor neuron injury causes spastic paralysis. Power is graded:

5	Normal	Complete ROM against gravity with full resistance.
4	Good	Complete ROM against gravity with some resistance.
3	Fair	Complete ROM against gravity.
2	Poor	Complete ROM with gravity eliminated.
1	Trace	Evidence of slight contractility, no joint motion.
0	Zero	No evidence of muscle contraction.

Assess the three categories of sensory changes. Pain and temperature sensations are relayed through the lateral spinothalamic tracts. Report changes in pain sensation as:

1. Hyperesthetic: increased sensation.
2. Hypesthetic: decreased sensation.
3. Dysesthetic: altered sensation.
4. Anesthetic: no sensation.

The ventral spinothalamic tract carries the majority of light touch sensation. Light touch is typically the last modality lost and therefore the last modality tested when recording the spinal cord level. Test proprioception and vibratory sensation loss, subtle signs of early myelopathy *(64)*. The sensory level may be several levels below the malignant lesion *(24)*.

The reflex arc is a simple sensory-motor pathway, which functions with modulation from long tract axons. Peripheral interruption of the arc leads to loss of reflex. If the level of the arc is intact, the reflex will function despite cord disruption above. Reflexes vary considerably from patient to patient; compare both sides. Spinal cord and brain lesions eventually lead to hyperreflexia. Stretch reflexes are reported as:

+2	Normal.
+3	Increased (upper motor neuron).
+1	Decreased (nerve root pressure).
0	None (arc interruption).

Seek abnormal reflexes such as the Babinski (or plantar) response. Firmly stroke the plantar surface of the foot with a sharp instrument *(see* Fig. 6). Start from the heel and proceed distally along lateral aspect of the sole and then medially across the forefoot. A positive response is seen with upgoing and fanned toes. No motion or downgoing toes are a normal or negative response *(64)*. Patients with foot problems are better assessed with the Oppenheim test. Stroke tibial crest and look for typical Babinski responses *(64)*.

Test for clonus by quick and sustained dorsiflexion of ankle. Two to three beats may be normal if symmetric and unchanged from prior exam. However, more than four beats is always abnormal. To perform Hoffman's test, hold the middle

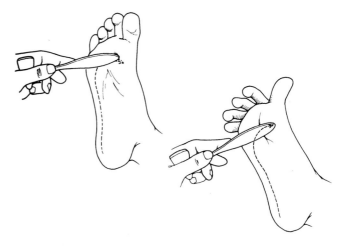

Fig. 6. Babinski's plantar response. The left-sided figure demonstrate a normal (no) response. The right-sided figure demonstrates a positive plantar response with great toe extension and fanning of the lesser toes.

finger extended, flick the distal interphalangeal joint. If the thumb and index finger flex, the test is positive. Repeated flexion and extension of the neck may accentuate this response. This test is often positive in normal patients, but may be an upper motor neuron sign, especially if asymmetric.

The cremasteric reflex tests the integrity of the T12 (efferent) and L1–L2 afferent neurological levels. When intact, a unilateral elevation of the scrotal sac is seen when the skin of ipsilateral inner thigh is stroked. Absence of elevation reflects an upper motor neuron lesion *(64)*. In patients with global hyperreflexia, pathology above the foramen magnum should be sought. Perform a jaw jerk by tapping on the patient's jaw. A brisk reflex indicates intracranial or systemic disease such as hyperthyroidism or hypercalcemia.

At presentation, autonomic dysfunctions are reported in only 2% of those with spinal malignancy *(66)*. However, subtle signs of such dysfunction can be detected in 60% at the time of diagnosis. Autonomic signs include bowel dysfunction. Constipation is typical. Incontinence signals advanced disease. Other signs include orthostatic hypotension, impotence, and decreased sweating. Order urodynamic evaluation for further assessment of bladder tone.

Test the various spinal levels individually *(see* Table 5). C1–4 are difficult to test. C2 injury may present with occipital headaches. C4 provides major innervation to the diaphragm. A brisk scapulohumeral reflex reflects compression of the upper cord (C1–3). To obtain this response, tap the tip of the scapular spine. Look for elevation of the scapula and abduction of humerus.

The C5 cord level provides sensation to the lateral arm *(see* Fig. 7). Test motor function by resisting shoulder abduction. The biceps reflex reflects mainly the C5 level, with some C6. Rest the patient's arm on medial side of your arm. Place your thumb across biceps tendon and strike your thumb with the hammer. The inverted radial reflex reflects cord and root impingement at C5. Tap the brachioradialis tendon and note a decreased brachioradialis reflex with finger flexor contrac-

Table 5
Spinal Levels

Motor levels	Muscle	Reflex	Sense
C2			GON/head
C3			Neck
C4	Diaphragm, scapular		Shoulders
C5	Biceps	Biceps	Lateral arm
C6	Wrist extensors	Brachioradialis	Radial forearm/thumb
C7	Triceps, EDC, WF	Triceps	Middle finger
C8	Finger flexors		Ulnar hand
T1	Intrinsics (spread fing)		Ulnar forearm
T2–T8	Interossei		Axilla (2), else chest
T10–T12	Abdominals		Lower abdomen
T12–L1	Cremasteric		Front upper thigh
L2	Iliopsoas (L1–L2 Adductors)		Front mid thigh
L3	Quads (with 4)		Front knee
L4	Tibialis anterior	Patellar	Medial leg, med mall
L5	EHL (with S1 hamstrings)		Front leg, dors foot, gt toe
S1	Gastrocnemius (FHL)	Ankle	Lateral foot
S2	Urethral sphincter		Back thigh
S3	Anal sphincter		Buttocks
S3–S4	Bulbocavernosus		Perineum

GON, greater occipital nerve; EDC, estensor digiti commiunis; WF, wrist flexor; EHL, extensor hallucis longus; FHL, flexor hallucis longus.

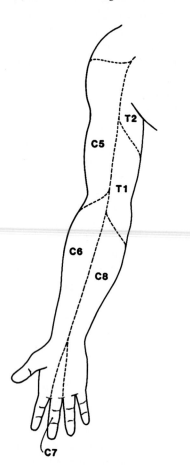

Fig. 7. The sensory dermatomes of the arm.

tion. The C6 cord level provides sensation to the lateral forearm, thumb, index, and radial half of middle fingers. There is no pure C6 level muscle, but the biceps has major C6 contribution, as do the radial wrist extensors. Assess the C6 brachioradialis reflex C6 by tapping on its tendon at distal wrist with flat part of hammer.

The C7 cord level provides sensation to the middle finger, but as C6 and C8 roots also contribute, there is no conclusive way to test C7 in isolation. Motor function is tested by elbow extension. The triceps reflex provides a C7 component through the radial nerve. Test this reflex by tapping with the point of the hammer into the olecranon fossa. C8 provides sensation to the ulnar forearm and ulnar side of the little finger. Assess grip strength. There are no reliable C8- or T1-mediated reflexes. T1 provides sensation to the medial arm. In that the intrinsics are almost pure T1 in innervation, test T1 via finger abduction and adduction.

T2 through T12 provide sensation to the thorax and abdomen. Each motor root overlaps its neighbors. Therefore, sensory changes can be subtle if only one root is involved. Motor testing is also challenging in that the intercostals, while segmentally innervated, are difficult to test individually. The rectus abdominus is segmentally innervated by anterior primary rami of T5–T12. Elicit Beevor's Sign by having the patient perform a quarter sit up with his arms crossed on his chest. During this exercise, the umbilicus should not move. If the umbilicus is drawn up or down or to one side, upper motor neuron suspect impairment.

L1 through L3 provide sensation to the anterior thigh between the inguinal ligament and the knee (see Fig. 8). There is no specific muscle for each root. Each provides some innervation to the iliopsoas and quadriceps via the lumbosacral plexus. Test these roots with hip flexion. L4 provides sensation from

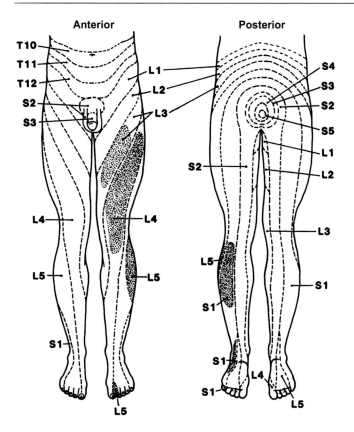

Fig. 8. The sensory dermatomes of the leg.

the medial leg to the medial foot. Test L4 motor strength by resisting ankle dorsiflexion. The patellar tendon reflex assesses predominantly L4, but has contributions from L2 and L3 as well. This reflex will decrease in the presence of knee pathology.

L5 provides sensation to the lateral leg and dorsum of the foot. Test L5 motor power by resisting toe extension and hip abduction. There is no easily obtained L5 reflex. S1 provides sensation to the lateral and plantar surface of the foot. Test S1 strength by single toe rise and resisting ankle eversion. The Achilles reflex is almost entirely S1. S2–4 provide sensation to three concentric rings around anus. While these roots provide motor innervation to the intrinsic muscles of foot, there is no efficient way to isolate them for testing. Inspect the toes for clawing or cavus deformity. The anal wink is a superficial sacral reflex.

12. CONCLUSION

Although myriad diagnostic modalities are now available to assess patient health and disease status, a careful history and physical examination remain the cornerstones of diagnosis in patients with neoplastic disease.

REFERENCES

1. McCulloch JA, Transfeldt EE. MacNab's Backache. 3d Ed.Baltimore, MD: Williams and Wilkings; 1997:257–276.
2. Landis SH, Murray T, Bolden S, Wingo PA. Cancer Statistics, 1998. CA Cancer J Clin 1998; 48:6–29.
3. Frassica FJ, Gitelis S, Sim FH. Metastatic bone disease: general principles, pathophysiology, evaluation, and biopsy. Instr Course Lect 1992; 41:293–300.
4. Frassica FJ, Sim FH. Pathogenesis and prognosis. In: Sim FH, ed. Diagnosis and Management of Metastatic Bone Disease. A Multidisciplinary Approach. New York, NY: Raven Press; 1988:1–6.
5. Frassica FJ, Sim FH. Bone Pain. In: Taylor R, ed. Difficult Diagnoses II. Philadelphia, PA: WB Saunders; 1992, pp. 52–54.
6. Harrington KD. Metastatic disease of the spine. J Bone Joint Surg Am 1986; 68:1110–1115.
7. Dahlin DC. Bone Tumors. General Aspects and Data on 6,221 Cases. 3rd ed. Springfield, IL: Thomas; 1978.
8. Weinstein JN, McLain RF. Primary tumors of the spine. Spine 1987; 12:843–851.
9. Leeson MC, Makley JT, Carter JR. Metastatic skeletal disease in the pediatric population. J Pediatr Orthop 1985; 5:261–267.
10. Young J, Miller R. Incidence of malignant tumors in U.S. children. J Pediatr 1975; 1:254–258.
11. Parham DM, Pratt CB, Parvey LS, Webber BL, Champion J. Childhood multifocal osteosarcoma. Clinicalpathologic and radiographic correlates. Cancer 1985; 55:2653–2658.
12. Fraser RD, Paterson DC, Simpson DA. Orthopaedic aspects of spinal tumours in children. J Bone Joint Surg Br 1977; 59:143–151.
13. Boriani S, Weinstein JN. Differential diagnosis and surgical treatment of primary benign and malignant neoplasms. In: Frymoyer JW, ed. The Adult Spine. Principles and Practice. 2nd ed. Philadelphia, PA: Lippincott-Raven; 1997:951–987.
14. Pedersen AG, Bach F, Melgaard B. Frequency, diagnosis, and prognosis of spinal cord compression in small cell bronchogenic carcinoma. A review of 817 consecutive patients. Cancer 1985; 55:1818–1822.
15. Koskinen EV, Nieminen RA. Surgical treatment of metastatic pathologic fracture of major long bones. Acta Orthop Scand 1973; 44:539–549.
16. Kostuik JP. Differential diagnosis and surgical treatment of metastatic spine tumors. In: Frymoyer JW, ed. The Adult Spine. Principles and Practice. 2nd ed. Philadelphia, PA: Lippincott-Raven; 1997:989–1014.
17. Burger EL, Lindeque BG. Sacral and non-spinal tumors presenting as backache. A retrospective study of 17 patients. Acta Orthop Scand 1994; 65:344–346.
18. Batson OV. The function of the vertebral veins and their role in the spread of metastases. Ann Surg 1940; 112:138–149.
19. Bohlman HH, Sachs BL, Carter JR, Riley L, Robinson RA. Primary neoplasms of the cervical spine. J Bone Joint Surg Am 1986; 68:483–494.
20. Ruff RL, Lanska DJ. Epidural metastases in prospectively evaluated veterans with cancer and back pain. Cancer 1989; 63:2234–2241.
21. Van den Hoogen HM, Koes BW, van Eijk JT, Bouter LM. On the accuracy of history, physical examination, and erythrocyte sedimentation rate in diagnosing low back pain in general practice. A criteria-based review of the literature. Spine 1995; 20:318–327.
22. Rougraff BT, Kneisl JS, Simon MA. Skeletal metastases of unknown origin: a prospective study of a diagnostic strategy. J Bone Joint Surg 1993; 75:1276–1281.
23. McLain RF. Tumors of the spine. In: Chapman MW: Chapman's Orthopaedic Surgery. 3rd ed. Philadelphia, PA: Lippincott William and Wilkins; 2001:3933–3958.
24. Boland PJ, Lane JM, Sundaresan N. Metastatic disease of the spine. Clin Orthop 1982; 169:95–102.
25. Siegal T, Siegal T. Current considerations in the management of neoplastic spinal cord compression. Spine 1988; 14:223–228.
26. Hall TC, Griffiths CT, Petranek JR. Hypercalcemia. An unusual metabolic complication of breast cancer. N Engl J Med 1966; 275:1474–1477.
27. Helweg-Larsen S, Sorenson PS. Symptoms and signs in metastatic cord compression. A study of progression from first symptom until diagnosis in 153 patients. Eur J Cancer 1994; 30A:396–398.
28. Gilbert RW, Kim JH, Posner JB. Epidural spinal cord compression from metastatic tumor. Diagnosis and treatment. Ann Neurol 1978; 3:40–51.

29. Shives TC, Dahlin DC, Sim FH, Pritchard DJ, Earle JD. Osteosarcoma of the spine. J Bone Joint Surg Am 1986; 68:660–668.

30. Thommesen P, Poulson JO. Primary tumors in the spine and pelvis in adolescents, Clinical and radiologic features. Acta Orthop Scand 1976; 47:170–174.

31. Sim FH, Dahlin DC, Stauffer RN, Laws ER. Primary bone tumors simulating lumbar disc syndrome. Spine 1977; 2:65–74.

32. Sim FH, Frassica FJ, Edmonson JH. Spine. In: Sim, FH, ed. Diagnosis and Management of Metastatic Bone Disease. A Multidisciplinary Approach. New York, NY: Raven Press; 1988, pp. 45–49.

33. Weinstein JN, Boriani S, Campanaci L. Spine neoplasms. In: Weinstein, SL ed. The Pediatric Spine. Principles and Practice. Philadelphia, PA: Lippincott Williams and Wilkins;2001:685–707.

34. Freiberg AA, Graziano GP, Loder RT, Hensinger RN. Metastatic vertebral disease in children. J Pediatr Orthop 1993; 13:148–153.

35. Rogalsky RJ, Black GB, Reed MH. Orthopaedic manifestations of leukemia in children. J Bone Joint Surg Am 1986; 68:494–501.

36. Marchesi DG, Boos N, Aebi M. Surgical treatment of tumors of the cervical spine and first two thoracic vertebrae. J Spinal Disord 1993; 6:489–496.

37. Kujawa KA, Niemi VR, Tomasi MA, Mayer NW, Cochran E, Goetz CG. Ballistic-choreic movements as the presenting feature of renal cancer. Arch Neurol 2001; 58:1133–1135.

38. Bollanti L, Riondino G, Strollo F. Endocrine paraneoplastic syndromes with special reference to the elderly. Endocrine 2001; 14:151–157.

39. Mitnick HJ. Paraneoplastic rheumatic syndromes. Curr Rheumatol Rep 2000; 2:163–170.

40. Brenner S, Tamir E, Maharshak N, Shapira J. Cutaneous manifestations of internal malignancies. Clin Dermatol 2001; 19:290–297.

41. Vielhauer V, Herzinger T, Korting HC. The sign of Leser-Trelat: a paraneoplastic cutaneous syndrome that facilitates early diagnosis of occult cancer. Eur J Med Res 2000; 5:512–516.

42. Jolobe OM. Neurological manifestations of malignant disease. Hosp Med 2000; 61:675.

43. Rudnicki SA, Dalmau J. Paraneoplastic syndromes of the spinal cord, nerve, and muscle. Muscle Nerve 2000; 23:1800–1818.

44. Bradwell AR. Paraneoplastic neurological syndromes associated with Yo, Hu, and Ri autoantibodies. Clin Rev Allergy Immunol 2000; 19:19–29.

45. Vigliani MC, Palmucci L, Polo P, et al. Paraneoplastic opsoclonus-myoclonus associated with renal cell carcinoma and responsive to tumour ablation. J Neurol Neurosurg Psychiatry 2001; 70:814–815.

46. Pranzatelli MR. Paraneoplastic syndromes: an unsolved murder. Semin Pediatr Neurol 2000; 7:118–130.

47. Carpentier AF, Delattre JY. The Lambert-Eaton myasthenic syndrome. Clin Rev Allergy Immunol 2001; 20:155–158.

48. Thompson JT, Paschold EH, Levine EA. Paraneoplastic hypercalcemia in a patient with adenosquamous cancer of the colon. Am Surg 2001; 67:585–588.

49. Wong DA, Fornasier VL, MacNab I. Spinal metastases: the obvious, the occult, and the impostors. Spine 1990; 15:1–4.

50. Mirra JM. Metastases. In: Mirra JM, ed. Bone Tumors. Philadelphia, PA: Lea and Febiger; 1986:1499–1450.

51. Enzinger FM, Weiss SW., eds. Soft Tissue Tumors. St. Louis, MO: C. V. Mosby; 1983.

52. Bell RM. Thyroid Carcinoma. Surg Clin North Am 1986; 66:13–30.

53. Leeper RD. Thyroid Cancer. Med Clin North Am 1985; 69:1079–1096.

54. Barkin JS, Goldstein JA. Diagnostic approach to pancreatic cancer. Gastroenterol Clin North Am 1999; 28:709–722, xi.

55. Perilongo G, Shafford EA. Liver tumours. Eur J Cancer 1999; 35:953–958.

56. Kiely JM. Hypernephroma. The internist's tumor. Med Clin North Am 1966; 50:1067–1083.

57. Seidel HM, Ball JW, Dains JE, Benedict GW. Mosby's Guide to Physical Examination. St. Louis, MO: CV Mosby; 1987.

58. Cumming J, Hacking N, Fairhurst J, Ackery D, Jenkins JD. Distribution of bony metastases in prostatic carcinoma. Br J Urol 1990; 66:411–414.

59. Asdourian PL, Weidenbaum M, DeWald RL, Hammerberg KW, Ramsey RG. The pattern of vertebral involvement in metastatic vertebral breast cancer. Clin Orthop 1990; (250):164–170.

60. King HA. Back pain in children. In: Weinstein, SL, ed. The Pediatric Spine. Principles and Practice. Philadelphia, PA: Lippincott Williams and Wilkins; 2001:685–707.

61. King HA. Back pain in children. Orthop Clin North Am 1999; 30:467–474, ix.

62. Keim HA, Reina EG. Osteoid-Osteoma as a cause of scoliosis. J Bone Joint Surg Am 1975; 57:159–163.

63. Khuffash B, Porter RW. Cross leg pain and trunk list. Spine 1989; 14:602–603.

64. Klein JD, Garfin SR. Clinical evaluation of patients with suspected spine problems. In: Frymoyer JW, ed. The adult spine. Principles and Practice. 2nd ed. Philadelphia, PA: Lippincott-Raven; 1997:319–340.

65. Abdu WA, Provencher M. Primary bone and metastatic tumors of the cervical spine. Spine 1998; 23:2767–2777.

66. Bos GD, Ebersold MJ, McLeod RA, et al. Lesions of the spine. In: Sim FH, ed. Diagnosis and Management of Metastatic Bone Disease. A Multidisciplinary Approach. New York, NY: Raven Press; 1988:221–236.

67. Greene WB, Heckman JD. Clinical Measurement of Joint Motion. Chicago, IL: American Academy of Orthopaedic Surgeons; 1994.

68. Spurling RG. Lesions of the Cervical Intervertebral Disc. Springfield, IL: Thomas; 1956.

69. Davidson R, Dunn E, Metzmaker J. The shoulder abduction test in the diagnosis of radicular pain in cervical extradural compressive monoradiculopathies. Spine 1981; 6:441–446.

70. Thelander U. Straight leg raising versus radiologic size, shape and position of lumbar disc hernias. Spine 1992; 17:395–398.

71. Schofferman JA. Physical examination. In: White AH, ed. Spine Care. St. Louis, MO: Mosby-Year Book; 1995:71–81.

72. Christodoulides AN. Ipsilateral sciatica on femoral nerve stretch test is pathognomonic of an L4-5 disc protrusion. J Bone Joint Surg 1989; 71B:88–89.

73. Bickels J, Kahanovitz N, Rubert CK, et al. Extraspinal bone and soft-tissue tumors as a cause of sciatica. Clinical diagnosis and recommendations: analysis of 32 cases. Spine 1999; 24:1611–1616.

74. Hoppenfeld S. Physical Examination of the Spine and Extremities. Norwalk, CT: Appleton and Lange; 1976.

75. McCombe PF. Reproducibility of physical signs in low back pain. Spine 1989; 14:909–918.

76. Ono K, Ebara S, Fuji T, Yonenobu K, Fujiwara K, Yamashita K. Myelopathy hand. J Bone Joint Surg 1987; 69:215–219.

9 Imaging

Screening for Spinal Disease

A. Jay Khanna, md, Mesfin A. Lemma, md, Bruce A. Wasserman, md, and Robert F. McLain, md

Contents

1. INTRODUCTION

Irrespective of the underlying pathology, treatment for neoplasia of the spine starts only after the disease has been identified and its extent confirmed on an objective study. Whenever there is a suspicion that cancer has involved the spine, an appropriate screening protocol should be initiated to confirm or rule out that suspicion and to provide a differential diagnosis or preliminary diagnosis that will guide initial treatment.

2. SCREENING

The presence or absence of most spinal disorders is established based on an evaluation of the patient's history, physical examination, and radiographic studies. However, it is well known that multiple acquired and degenerative findings are seen on imaging studies of asymptomatic individuals as well as on autopsy of subjects who have never had neck or back pain. These degenerative changes must be distinguished from superimposed pathology, including acute disorders such as infection and neoplasia. The accurate interpretation of radiographic and other screening studies can have significant consequences with respect to the early recognition and treatment of primary and metastatic spinal tumors.

Several authors have suggested the criteria for an effective screening program. Wilson and Junger *(1)* defined 10 requirements for a cost-effective screening program and subdivided them into four groups including knowledge of disease, feasibility, diagnosis and treatment impact, and cost. In screening for spinal malignancies, each of these factors is important to the reliability and accuracy of the process.

From: *Current Clinical Oncology: Cancer in the Spine: Comprehensive Care.*
Edited by: R. F. McLain, K-U. Lewandrowski, M. Markman, R. M. Bukowski,
R. Macklis, and E. C. Benzel © Humana Press, Inc., Totowa, NJ

A commonly referenced study performed by Boden et al. *(2)* evaluated the results of magnetic resonance imaging (MRI) studies performed on 67 patients who never had back pain, sciatica, or neurogenic claudication. Twenty percent of patients younger than 60 yr of age had a herniated nucleus pulposus and one had spinal stenosis. In the group of patients who were 60 yr of age or older, 36% of the patients had a herniated nucleus pulposus and 21% had spinal stenosis. Disc degeneration or bulging was seen in at least one lumbar level in 35% of the patients between 20 and 39 yr of age and in all but one of the patients 60 yr of age or older. Although this particular study does not involve spinal malignancies, it demonstrates that screening studies will often reveal findings of little or uncertain clinical significance. It is important to keep this in mind when ordering and interpreting a spine MRI examination or chest computed tomography (CT) scan to screen for metastatic lesions.

3. HISTORY AND PHYSICAL EXAM

Metastatic tumors are far more common than primary lesions in the spine, accounting for 97% of all recognized spinal tumors. Patients with adenocarcinoma are especially prone to spinal involvement, with primaries from lung, breast, prostate, kidney, gastrointestinal tract, and thyroid carcinoma making up the majority of clinically relevant metastases *(3)*. Certain primary tumors (chordoma, osteoblastoma) do show a predilection for the spinal column, but primary tumors of the spine still make up a very small proportion of all spinal tumors. Initial physical examination should include an examination of the breasts, thyroid, prostate, and rectum for masses, a guaiac test of the stool for blood, and a urinalysis for red blood cells.

3.1. AGE

Carcinomas and metastases demonstrate a peak incidence in ages 40–60. Myeloma and lymphoma are also most common in the ages 50–60. The middle-aged patient presenting with a painful, undiagnosed lesion of the spine deserves careful scrutiny for an underlying malignancy.

3.2. LOCATION

The majority of malignant tumors, both primary and metastatic, will arise in the anterior vertebral body and possibly one or both pedicles. Such lesions never produce a palpable mass, and may be silent until they have grown to considerable size.

3.3. SYMPTOMS

Pain is by far the most common symptom, distinguished in tumor patients by its unremitting nature and prominence at night and at rest (4). Subjective complaints of weakness, and objective neurological deficits can be identified in 35% of patients with benign tumors and 55% of patients with malignancies.

Back pain symptoms may localize to a specific spinal segment or may be more diffuse. Radicular pain in the thoracic region may result in girdle- or belt-like pain forming a band of dysesthesias circumferentially around the trunk (5).

Pathological fracture resulting from extensive vertebral body destruction may produce acute pain symptoms indistinguishable from those seen in traumatic or osteoporotic compression fractures. Fractures may also cause acute or chronic compression of the spinal cord, resulting in pain, paraparesis, or paraplegia (6).

3.4. NEUROLOGICAL DEFICITS

Cord or nerve root compression are most common in rapidly expanding malignant lesions, but any slowly progressive, expansile neoplasm may produce a deficit if left alone long enough. The clinician should maintain a high index of suspicion for patients with persistent back or radicular pain, particularly those with a known history of previous malignancies (7).

Any objective finding of cord compression or bowel and bladder dysfunction should trigger a search for the cause.

3.5. LABORATORY STUDIES

Laboratory studies important to the evaluation of spine tumor patients are discussed in detail in Chapter 11. Before establishing the diagnosis and completing the screening examination, a handful of preliminary laboratory studies should be obtained.

The erythrocyte sedimentation rate is nonspecific, but highly sensitive for systemic disease or advanced focal involvement by tumor or infection. A C-reactive protein analysis should be added to further assess the possibility of infection. These studies, along with a basic metabolic panel should be ordered at the point of initial evaluation.

Two additional laboratory studies that can be ordered at the initial visit are a prostate-specific antigen study in men, and a serum protein electophoresis/urine protein electrophoresis panel to detect immunoglobulin spikes associated with plasma cell neoplasms.

3.6. IMAGING STUDIES

3.6.1. Plain Films

Plain radiographs should be the first study ordered in any case where spinal neoplasia is suspected. Anteroposterior (AP) and lateral views of the spinal column and vertebra provide considerable information about the presence and nature of the lesion, and may be sufficient to identify diagnostic characteristic in some tumor types. The benign or malignant nature of the

lesion may be deduced from the pattern of bony destruction. Geographic patterns of bone destruction suggest a slowly expanding lesion, either benign or low-grade, whereas more rapidly growing tumors produce a moth-eaten appearance or permeative pattern of destruction (8). Radiographic evidence of bone destruction is not apparent until between 30 and 50% of the mineralized bone has been destroyed, however, such early lesions may be difficult to detect (9). Whereas 26% of patients with spinal metastases will have occult lesions undetectable on plain radiographs, careful scrutiny of plain films will reveal some evidence of disease in roughly 90% of symptomatic patients (10,11).

The classic early sign of vertebral neoplasia is the "winking owl" sign, seen on the AP view. The loss of the pedicle ring on one side results from the destruction of the pedicle cortex, usually by tumor invading from the vertebral body anteriorly. Vertebral compression fracture secondary to erosion of bone by tumor is another common radiographic finding. A pathological compression fracture may be difficult to differentiate from a traumatic or osteoporotic injury.

Acutely angled, painful scoliosis, a sclerotic region of bone or pedicle, or focal osteopenia may all suggest a neoplastic process.

Occasionally a patient presents with extensive bony destruction. In these cases, plain radiographs and active flexion and extension radiographs may define the extent of instability present and help limit the risk of cord injury through earlier surgery or radiotherapy.

High quality studies are necessary. Imaging of the cervicothoracic and thoracolumbar junctions is particularly important (Fig. 1). Radiographic films should be centered over the region of interest in order to obtain the best definition of the endplates and bony cortices.

If multiple myeloma is a concern, a skeletal survey should be ordered, as bone scan can be unreliable in these patients (12). The skeletal survey individually images the bones of the extremities, pelvis, and spine to identify areas of involvement associated with diffuse disease.

3.6.2. Bone Scan

Tecnetium bone scans (99 m) are commonly used to detect neoplastic disease of the musculoskeletal system. Highly sensitive, bone scanning is ideal for detecting lesions in patients with known visceral disease, and in undiagnosed, but symptomatic, patients with negative or equivocal radiographs (Fig. 2). Whole body scanning can determine the extent of dissemination in patients with known systemic disease and can define the most accessible lesion for biopsy in patients with an unknown primary malignancy. Bone scans have poor specificity. Nonneoplastic pathology, most often osteoarthritis, can cause focal uptake mimicking metastatic spread. The addition of single photon emission CT (SPECT), a recent technological advancement, however, improves the predictive value of planar scans by better defining the anatomical location of uptake (13,14).

If the bone scan demonstrates widely dispersed areas of skeletal involvement, the diagnosis of metastatic disease may be reliably established. If there are only a few points of involvement, the scan can guide the clinician in definitively imaging these regions with CT or MRI.

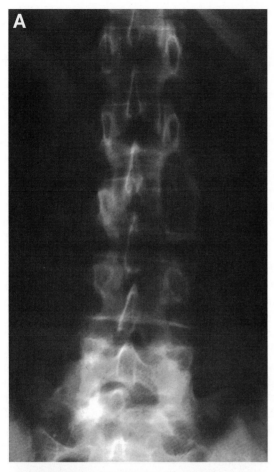

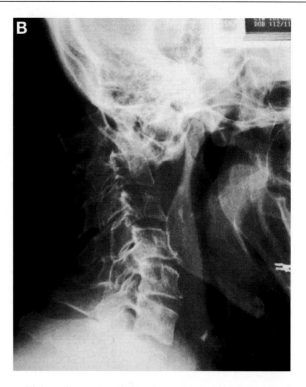

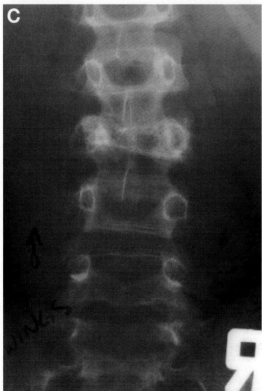

Fig. 1. Plain radiographs of spinal neoplasms. (A) Absence of the right pedicle ("winking owl" sign) and lytic destruction of the vertebral body suggest a neoplastic process. The residual integrity of the vertebral cortex (expanded but not disrupted) hints at the slower growth of a benign or low-grade malignant lesion. The patient proved to have an aneurysmal bone cyst. (B) The plain radiographs give little clue as to the type of tumor affecting this patient, but the gross instability and destruction of the C2 vertebral body suggest an aggressive and rapidly progressive malignancy, consistent with a metastasis from the patient's known breast carcinoma. (C) The vertebral collapse seen at L2 in this 13-yr-old is atypical of Ewing's sarcoma, but clearly defined the involved vertebral level, allowing more specialized radiographic analysis and biopsy, to establish the diagnosis.

3.6.3. CT Imaging

CT scanning improves the specificity in imaging of spinal neoplasms. CT is highly sensitive to alterations in bone mineral content and is able to demonstrate destructive processes far more reliably and at much higher resolution than plain radiographs can. Lesions may be visualized at an earlier time in their development, before extensive bony destruction or intramedullary extension has occurred, and before cortical erosion has progressed to the point of fracture or extension into the soft tissues. However, CT scanning is a time-consuming process that is most effective when the appropriate region is targeted. The preliminary bone scan or radiograph should identify the correct level for CT scanning, improving the yield in diagnostically difficult cases.

Newer techniques of spiral CT imaging and image analysis and manipulation make it possible to image larger fields in less time, and to create three-dimensional image products that lend value to the preoperative staging process. Stereotactic guidance systems also generate real-time data based on input from preoperative CT studies. Properly selected scanning protocols may be able to generate CT files suitable both for screening and diagnosis as well as for operative planning and stereotaxis.

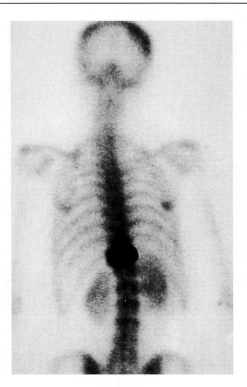

Fig. 2. Bone scan identifies T12 metastasis in a patient with colon carcinoma.

CT has two roles in the screening protocol for patients with a suspected spinal tumor: first, to establish the location, extent, and character of the spinal lesion itself; and second, to determine whether the neoplastic process has disseminated to the pulmonary or hepatic viscerae. Whereas spinal CT should include both bone and soft-tissue windows for greatest definition, a separate study should be obtained to specifically evaluate the lungs and abdominal contents. Findings of space-occupying or invasive lesions within the lung or hepatic parenchyma suggest systemic metastasis, changing the surgical perspective regarding the spinal lesions. Enlarged lymphatics and nodes, visceral masses, and evidence of unexplained infiltrates or effusions should be noted for further diagnostic testing.

3.6.4. Magnetic Resonance Imaging

MRI has become the modality of choice to evaluate the spine and its adjacent organ systems. MRI provides the best imaging of neural structures, can clearly define intramedullary, intradural, and extradural masses, and can reveal the compressive nature of the spinal lesion as well as the extent of its soft-tissue spread. The ability to generate multiplanar images and to better delineate soft tissue boundries makes MRI invaluable in diagnosis and treatment planning. Whole spine MRI is a reasonable and reliable screening method, defining the entire extent of the spinal column. It is the best method to evaluate suspected spinal cord compression in a patient with known malignancy.

MRI has the ability to detect small neoplasms within the spine because normal marrow is replaced with tumor tissue, which has an increased cellularity and extracellular water content (15). MRI is not dependent on bony disruption or reaction to provide a diagnosis. MRI can distinguish between traumatic processes and neoplastic disease, and is helpful in differentiat-

ing malignant from osteoporotic compression fractures. Characteristically, neoplasms have low signal intensity on T1 or T1-weighted images, and high signal on T2. Fat suppression techniques combined with intravenous gadolinium enhancement further increase the contrast between normal fatty marrow and tumor tissue, making MRI the imaging technique with the ability to detect neoplasms in their earliest stages (16).

Osteoporotic fractures can be distinguished from pathological fractures owing to malignancy. Malignant lesions usually have a more ill-defined margin, involvement of the pedicle, marked enhancement, and frequent paravertebral soft tissue extension, whereas benign causes of vertebral compression will usually still have fat present within the body, not involve the pedicle, demonstrate more focal edema, and not have an associated soft tissue mass (17,18). Infection can also be differentiated from neoplasm on MRI because infectious processes usually involve the disk space and end plate and incite a significant amount of edema. Neoplastic lesions are often more defined, do not involve the disk or end plates, and are associated with limited edema (Fig. 3 [15]).

3.6.5. Myelography

Myelography has now given way to MRI as the imaging study of choice in most instances. In combination with computed tomography, however, it remains a valuable tool for detecting cord compression owing to fracture and bony impingement, especially in patients who cannot undergo MRI. This includes patients with metallic implants such as heart valves, intracranial clips, or intraocular metallic bodies should be imaged via myelography.

Myelography can also provide some functional information. In a patient with multiple levels of neural compression, a myelographic block may reveal which level is critical to restoring function. Myelography can not, by itself, provide any information regarding tissues or structures outside the neural canal.

3.7. BIOPSY

Biopsy is the final step in screening and staging for spinal tumors. The importance of a carefully planned biopsy cannot be over emphasized. Once the biopsy incision has been made, there are very few choices left in planning the definitive tumor removal. When the surgeon selects an approach for biopsy they are committed to that approach from then on. The risks of inadequate or inappropriate biopsy can significantly alter a patient's prognosis for cure or prolonged survival. This risk is significantly reduced when the biopsy is performed by the *treating*, rather than the *referring*, physician.

4. EVALUATION OF SPINAL METASTASES: THE CLINICAL SCENARIO

The patient presenting for evaluation of spinal neoplasia has been separated from the rest of the back pain population based on their initial findings. Clinical symptoms and signs have prompted their primary physician to obtain either plain radiographs that have shown some lesion among the vertebrae, or an MRI study which has revealed a suspicious lesion. Occasionally, spinal involvement is identified during the staging workup of a known visceral primary, i.e., breast or prostate carcinoma. After a thorough history and physical examination and identification of the type and location of the primary malignancy if possible, the next step is to completely characterize the level

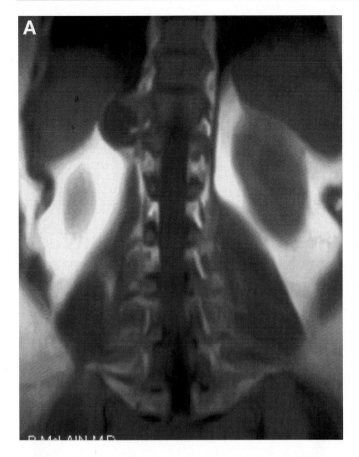

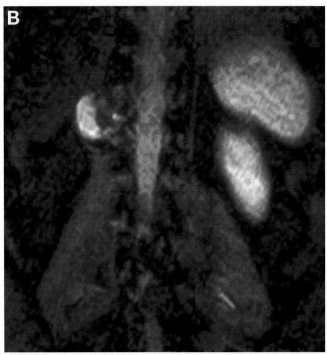

Fig. 3. Magnetic resonance imaging provides important information on the nature and extent of spinal disease. (A) T1-weighted image of a lower thoracic lesion originally identified on plain radiographs. Tumor tissue is dark in this format. (B) The T2-weighted image shows the tumor as bright or inhomogenous. This T1–T2 pattern is most consistent with neoplasm.

and degree of spinal involvement. An appreciation of those primary malignancies that have a propensity to metastasize to the spine increases the level of suspicion for a spinal metastasis and, thus, the likelihood that the diagnosis will be made. These primary sites include breast, prostate, lung, kidney, and thyroid, and physical examination should be completed at the first visit. Appropriate laboratory studies are sent at this time as well.

Conventional radiographs are the first imaging modality used to evaluate the spine, and should be obtained at the first encounter if they are not already available (Fig. 4). Even if excellent quality MRI has defined the extent of the soft tissue involvement, radiographs provide important information regarding bone destruction and stability, and should be obtained before proceeding with staging. Their additional contribution lies in their ability to provide a rapid skeletal survey and rule out other causes of back and neck pain including degenerative changes and trauma including vertebral compression fractures.

If not obtained as the initial diagnostic study, the mainstay in the evaluation of patients with suspected or known spinal tumor is MRI. Sagittal T1- and T2-weighted images of the entire spinal column should be obtained. Subsequently, axial images are obtained through regions of the spine that are felt to be symptomatic, correlate with a neurological level on physical examination or demonstrate suspicious findings on conventional radiographs, nuclear scintigraphy, or the sagittal images. The evaluation of post-Gadolinium T1-weighted images should be considered in patients with a suspicion for leptomeningeal carcinomatosis and intramedullary lesions as well as those in whom infection may be in the differential diagnosis.

At the same time, a battery of screening studies should be ordered, including bone scan, chest CT scan, and abdominal CT or ultrasound. These studies should be carefully reviewed before proceeding to biopsy, as a lytic lesion of the iliac wing will be much easier to biopsy than an anterior vertebral mass at T2. Likewise, any consideration of surgical resection and reconstruction will depend on the extent of metastatic disease identified throughout the viscerae.

Once the screening studies have been obtained and assessed, more definitive studies, including CT reconstructions, biopsy, and specific tumor antigen studies can be considered based on the most suitable differential diagnosis.

5. SUMMARY

The screening workup of a spinal tumor is intended to rapidly gather enough information to confirm the suspected diagnosis, provide an initial prognosis, and guide the definitive work-up to establish a tissue diagnosis and effective treatment. The studies included should be obtained or initiated at the first specialty visit after the possibility of spinal neoplasia has been recognized, and the important data should be in hand within the first week after the evaluation is initiated.

REFERENCES

1. Wilson JMG, Junger F. Principles and Practice of Screening for Disease (Public Health Papers No. 34). Geneva, Switzerland: World Health Organization; 1968.
2. Boden SD, McCowin PR, Davis DO, Dina TS, Mark AS, Wiesel S. Abnormal magnetic-resonance scans of the cervical spine in as-

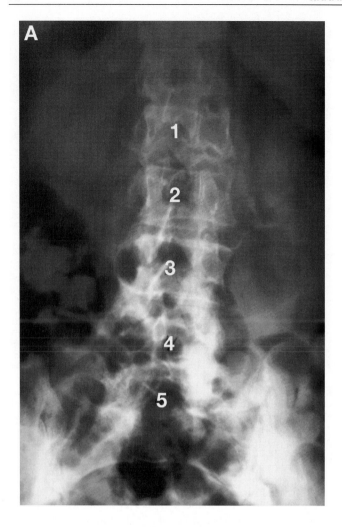

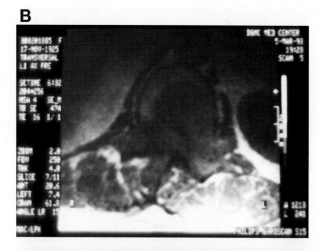

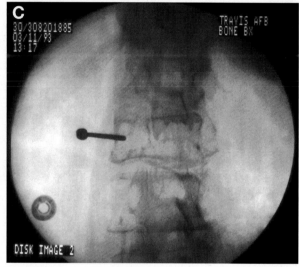

Fig. 4. Screening evaluation of a patient with thoracolumbar back pain. (A) Anteroposterior radiograph demonstrates a lytic lesion of the L1 vertebral body, with expansion or erosion of the right-sided pedicle. The process is destructive but well marginated, or geographic, suggesting a low-grade malignant process (B) Magnetic resonance imaging confirms extensive bony replacement and canal compromise by soft-tissue mass. Sedimentation rate was elevated, but not C-reactive protein. A monoclonal immunoglobulin G spike was isolated from both the urine and serum electrophoresis studies. (C) Transpedicular biopsy carried out under fluoroscopic control confirms diagnosis of plasma cell tumor. Systemic work-up confirmed a solitary lesion.

ymptomatic subjects. A prospective investigation. J Bone Joint Surg Am 1990; 72:1178–1184.

3. Jaffe, H.L. Tumors and Tumorous Conditions of the Bones and Joints. Philadelphia, PA: Lea and Febiger; 1958.

4. Weinstein JN, McLain RF. Primary tumors of the spine. Spine 1987; 12:843–851.

5. Sim FH, Dahlin DC, Stauffer RN, Laws ER. Primary bone tumors simulating lumbar disc syndrome. Spine 1977; 2:65–74.

6. Harrington KD. Current concepts review: metastatic disease of the spine. J Bone Joint Surg 1986; 68:1110–1115.

7. McLain RF. Tumors of the spine. In: Chapman's Orthopaedic Surgery. 3rd ed.Philadelphia, PA: Lippincott, Williams and Wilckins;2001:3933–3958.

8. Lodwick GS. Determining growth rates of focal lesions of bone from radiographs. Radiology 1980; 134:577–583.

9. Edelstyn GA, Gillespie PJ, Grebell ES. The radiologic demonstration of osseous metastases: experimental observations. Clin Radiol 1967; 18:158–164.

10. Wong DA, Fornasier VL, MacNab I. Spinal metastases: the obvious, the occult, and the imposters. Spine 1990; 15:1–4.

11. Weinstein JN, McLain RF. Primary tumors of the spine. Spine 1988; 12:843–851.

12. McLain RF, Weinstein JN. Solitary plasmacytomas of the spine: report of 84 cases. J Spinal Disord 1989; 2:69–74.

13. Savelli G, Chiti A, Grasselli G, Maccauro M, Rodari M, Bombardieri E. The role of bone SPET study in diagnosis of single vertebral metastases. Anticancer Res 2000; 20:1115–1120.

14. Gates, GF. SPECT bone scanning of the spine. Semin Nucl Med 1998; 28:78–94.

15. Vacarro AR, Shah SH, Schweitzer ME, Rosenfeld JF, Cotler JM. MRI description of vertebral osteomyelitis, neoplasm, and compression fracture. Orthopedics 1999; 22:67–73.

16. Yamaguchi T. Intertrabecular vertebral metastases: metastases only detectable on MR imaging. Semin Musculoskel Radiol 2001; 5:171–175.

17. Chan JH, Peh WC, Tsui EY, et al. Acute vertebral body compression fractures: Discrimination between benign and malignant causes using apparent diffusion coefficients. Br J Radiol 2002; 75:207–214.

18. Shih TT, Huang KM, Li YW: Solitary vertebral collapse: distinction between benign and malignant causes using MR patterns. J Magn Reson Imaging 1999; 9:635–642.

19. McLain RF, Weinstein JN. Tumors of the spine. Seminars in Spine Surgery, 1990; 2:157–180.

10 Imaging of the Spine

A. Jay Khanna, md, Michael K. Shindle, md, and Bruce A. Wasserman, md

Contents

1. INTRODUCTION

Multiple modalities are available for imaging the spine in patients with cancer, including conventional radiography, computed tomography (CT), radionuclide imaging, magnetic resonance imaging (MRI), functional and metabolic imaging, and interventional radiology techniques. After a careful history and physical examination, the next step in the evaluation of the patient with primary or secondary neoplastic involvement of the spine is selection of the appropriate imaging modality and its application at the appropriate region of the spine.

The purpose of this chapter is to review these techniques and their roles in the definitive diagnosis and treatment planning of the patient with cancer involving the spine.

2. CONVENTIONAL RADIOGRAPHY

Conventional radiography is often the first imaging modality used to evaluate the spine. The major advantages of this imaging modality are its wide availability and that it provides a rapid, inexpensive evaluation that covers a large extent of the spine. The major disadvantage of conventional radiography is its inability to discriminate soft tissues and its low sensitivity for the detection of osseous destruction and/or marrow replacement. It has been established that there must be approx 50% reduction in the local bone mineral density before a lesion is detectable on conventional radiographs *(1,2)*. In addition, the quality of conventional radiographic imaging is limited at the occipitocervical and cervicothoracic junctions as well as in the sacrum.

Conventional radiographs may be used to evaluate the patient with a primary malignancy or metastatic disease of the spine. Radiographs should be scrutinized for the presence of lytic or blastic lesions suggestive of a metastasis. One relatively specific finding is the "winking owl" sign often seen in the lumbar and thoracic spine on anteroposterior (AP) radiographs. This sign results from marrow replacement of the pedicle and the resultant asymmetry between the involved pedicle and adjacent pedicles. In addition, frank destruction of the osseous elements and blastic changes might be noted on AP and lateral radiographs. Metastatic carcinoma in bone has a predilection for the axial skeleton, but has a wide range of plain radiographic patterns. Bone lesions may be radiodense or radiolytic, however, certain metastatic diseases produce consistent radiographic patterns. For example, metastatic lung or renal cell carcinoma almost always produces radiolytic lesions, whereas metastatic prostate cancer usually produces radiodense lesions. Metastatic breast carcinoma is often osteoblastic, but a mixed osteolytic and osteoblastic pattern is not uncommon *(31,32)*. Another important indication for the use of conventional radiographs is preoperative planning. Although CT or MRI may often provide significantly improved evaluation of a given lesion, conventional radiographs provide the spine surgeon with a "roadmap" that allows for confirmation of the spinal level of involvement and, thus, a guide within the operating room where only conventional radiographic imaging or fluoroscopy may be available.

3. MYELOGRAPHY

Myelography is performed after the introduction of a nonionic contrast agent into the subarachnoid space via either a cervical or lumbar puncture followed by conventional radiographs and often CT to obtain indirect evidence of neural compression. Myelography augments the information obtained from conventional radiographs by allowing for assessment of the extradural compartments and occasionally the intradural-extramedullary compartment. The addition of CT increases the

From: *Current Clinical Oncology: Cancer in the Spine: Comprehensive Care.*
Edited by: R. F. McLain, K-U. Lewandrowski, M. Markman, R. M. Bukowski,
R. Macklis, and E. C. Benzel © Humana Press, Inc., Totowa, NJ

sensitivity and specificity of the diagnostic test *(3)*. The major disadvantage of myelography is that it is an invasive examination that may place the neural elements at risk. In addition to the small risk of allergic reaction, infection, bleeding, or a lowered seizure threshold, myelography can result in a decline in neurological function in patients with tumor-related spinal cord compression *(4)*. Another disadvantage is that myelography generally does not demonstrate the site of neural compression below a complete block of contrast flow *(5)*. With the relatively recent advent of MRI, which allows for excellent evaluation of all compartments of the spine as described below, the use of myelography is primarily indicated in patients for whom MRI is contraindicated. One excellent primary indication for myelography is imaging of the instrumented spine where metallic artifacts may obscure detail.

More than for other imaging modalities, a certain amount of experience is required for the successful evaluation of even routine conventional and CT myelogram studies. The requisite knowledge includes a basic understanding of the pattern of flow and distribution of cerebrospinal fluid (CSF) within the thecal sac. With this in mind, the goal in evaluating these studies is to determine whether or not the CSF distribution is normal and if it is not, determine what structure is causing a change in the contour of the contrast-filled subarachnoid space.

When reviewing a myelographic study, one should first evaluate the conventional radiographs (including AP, lateral, and oblique views) obtained after the administration of the intrathecal contrast agent. The relationship of the osseous spine to the thecal sac and nerve roots is evaluated with specific attention to regions of extrinsic compression on the thecal sac or nerve roots that may result in a deformation of the thecal sac, a suggestion of stenosis or a "cutoff" of flow below a given spinal level, or into a given nerve root sleeve. In most instances, a CT scan is also obtained after the conventional radiographs and the sagittal and coronal reconstructed images as well as the original axial images are reviewed for additional findings with the benefit of cross-sectional visualization, improved soft-tissue contrast, and osseous detail.

4. COMPUTED TOMOGRAPHY

CT allows for the acquisition of high-resolution axial images of the entire spine; its primary strength is that it affords the opportunity to evaluate the osseous elements and extradural compartment. The evaluation of now readily available sagittal and coronal reconstructed images allows for excellent depiction of the overall spinal alignment and the three-dimensional configuration of a given lesion. The more recent use of three-dimensional, volume-rendered, and surface-rendered reconstructed images are often useful for preoperative planning *(7,8)*. Newer multiple-row detector helical CT scanners have decreased imaging times to the point where the rate-limiting step is the time required to place the patient on the scanner table and vastly improving imaging quality and resolution *(9)*.

The disadvantages of CT include the use of ionizing radiation and the diminished ability to differentiate soft tissue structures as is possible with MRI. Visualization of the subarachnoid space necessitates myelographic contrast with CT, whereas this space is easily discriminated on MRI.

It is important to note that CT with bone windows is a useful study that often complements the information provided by MRI. CT allows for the determination of the nature of osseous changes seen in association with spinal tumors. If CT imaging shows sclerotic margins for a vertebral body lesion seen on MRI, the lesion is likely to be a benign or slowly growing process.

5. MAGNETIC RESONANCE IMAGING

MRI allows for high-resolution imaging of not only the osseous structures of the spine, but also the soft tissue structures, including the intervertebral discs, spinal cord, nerve roots, meninges, and paraspinal musculature in multiple orthogonal planes. MRI also provides the capability of soft tissue differentiation, including the ability to differentiate between CSF and neural tissue without the use of intrathecal myelographic contrast materials. MRI has been shown to be superior to CT in the evaluation of neoplasms of the spine *(10,11)*. CT and MRI are often complementary in the evaluation of primary extradural bone tumors. The disadvantages of MRI include its limited ability to detect calcification and small osseous fragments and the potential for image degradation from motion artifacts secondary to the longer scan times *(12)*.

Spine tumors are generally classified according to anatomic location as extradural, intradural-extramedullary, and intradural-intramedullary *(12–14)*.

5.1. IMAGING PROTOCOLS

MRI protocols for the evaluation of spinal tumors vary widely among institutions and also according to the region of the spine involved. Most protocols include sagittal and axial T1- and T2-weighted images. Coronal images are helpful for tumors with paraspinal extension; they show the extent and position of the tumor relative to the surrounding organs, i.e., the lung, liver, and aorta. Contrast enhancement is particularly useful for the evaluation of intradural-extramedullary and intramedullary tumors. Most extradural tumors enhance, however, contrast administration may be of lesser value for lesions in this space than for those in the other two compartments. Contrast-enhanced imaging may even decrease the conspicuity of the lesion because of the high signal of fat within the marrow in adults on T1-weighted images. Thus, fat suppression is useful for extradural lesion evaluation. Fat-suppression sequences are applied to T2-weighted sequences in which the lesion is often hyperintense against a hyperintense fatty background. Gradient echo sequences are generally not useful for tumor imaging unless hemorrhage is suspected (e.g., in the case of a cellular ependymoma or cavernoma). Diffusion-weighted imaging may also be useful for distinguishing between benign and pathologic compression fractures *(15)*.

5.2. CLASSIFICATION OF SPINAL CORD TUMORS

Several authors have advocated the classification of spinal cord tumors into three categories: extradural, intradural-extramedullary, and intramedullary (Table 1; Fig. 1 *[12–14]*). The MRI appearance of a spinal tumor and the careful evaluation of the tumor on axial, coronal, and sagittal images allows for the reliable assignment of the tumor into one of these three categories, leading to a differential diagnosis. Samples are provided in the next sections, however, in clinical practice, the

Table 1
Classification of Spinal Tumors

Extradural	Intradural-extramedullary	Intramedullary
Metastases	Nerve sheath tumors	Ependymoma
Myeloma	Meningiomas	Astrocytoma
Lymphoma	Lipoma	Hemangioblastoma
Hemangioma	Epidermoid	Metastases
Aneurysmal bone cyst	Dermoid	Glioblastoma
Giant cell tumor	Arachnoid cysts	
Osteoid osteoma	Paraganglioma	
Osteoblastoma	Intradural metastases	
Osteochondroma		
Eosinophilic granuloma		
Ewing's sarcoma		
Osteosarcoma		
Chordoma		
Leukemia		
Chondrosarcoma		

A

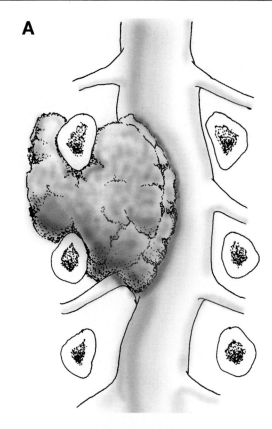

B

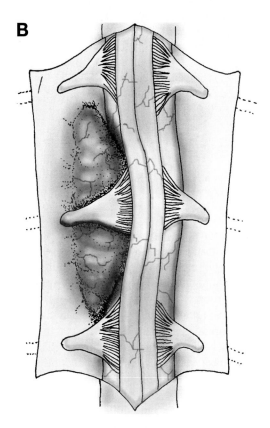

C

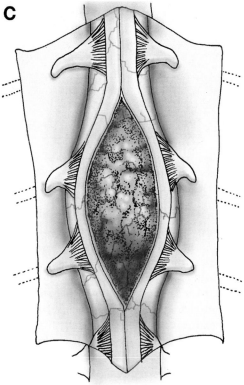

Fig. 1. These drawings illustration the typical appearance of (**A**) extradural, (**B**) intradural-extramedullary, and (**C**) intradural-intramedullary tumors.

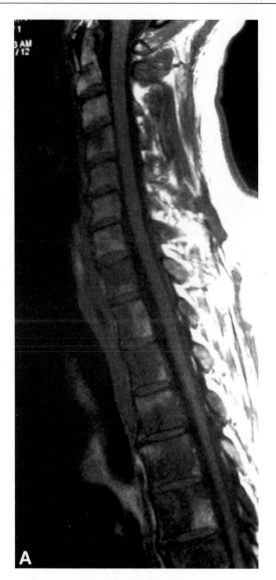

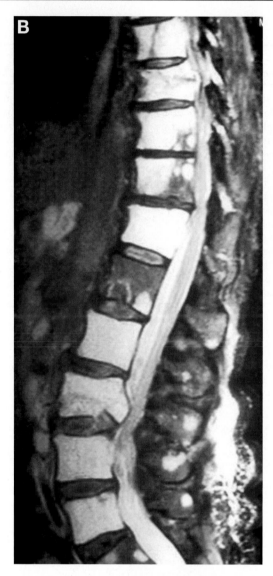

Fig. 2. Extradural lesion. (**A**) Sagittal T1-weighted cervical and (**B**) T2-weighted lumbar images show multiple extradural lesions, compatible with metastases in a patient without a known primary malignancy.

diagnoses should be modified based on patient characteristics such as age, gender, past medical history (including history of primary malignancy), and clinical symptoms.

5.2.1. Extradural Tumors

Extradural tumors account for approx 30% of all spinal cord neoplasms *(16)* and include all masses that are located peripheral to the dura mater. These lesions usually act to compress the spinal cord extrinsically and eccentrically. Extradural lesions arise from the osseous spine, disk, or adjacent soft tissue. These lesions displace the thecal sac away from the mass, resulting in compression and narrowing of the subarachnoid space above and below the mass. This narrowing of the subarachnoid space can best be seen on axial and sagittal images *(12)*.

A comprehensive differential diagnosis of extradural tumors is included in Table 1. Most extradural spinal neoplasms are metastatic and, therefore, malignant (Fig. 2). Metastases, the most common neoplasms of the spine, are usually seen in patients over 40 yr old *(12)*. Breast, lung, and prostate cancer account for most metastatic spinal disease *(12,13)*. Although

not as common, multiple myeloma and lymphoma should be placed high in the differential diagnosis because multiple myeloma is the most common primary malignant bone neoplasm and lymphoma is a frequent cause of spinal malignancy in any age group.

Extraspinal tumors extending into the spinal canal through the neural foramina are most typically seen in lymphoma and myeloma. In addition, Pancoast's tumor in the thoracic spine, renal cell cancer at the thoracolumbar junction, and neuroblastoma in children are examples of neoplasms that extend into the spinal canal from their site of origin (Fig. 3).

5.2.2. Intradural-Extramedullary Tumors

Intradural-extramedullary tumors comprise the largest group of spinal cord neoplasms and represent approx 55% of all primary spinal cord neoplasms *(17)*. Intradural-extramedullary tumors are located between the dura mater and the spinal cord. The MRI findings of intradural-extramedullary tumors are very specific. At the level of the tumor, the cord is displaced to the contralateral side, and the CSF column forms an acute angle

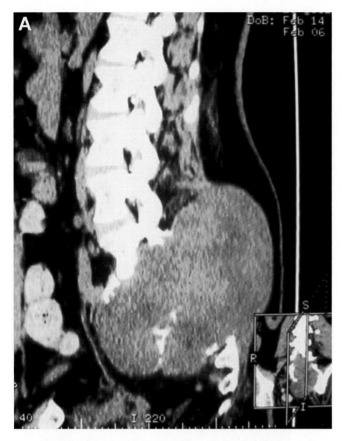
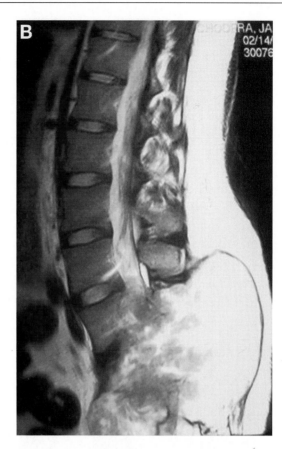

Fig. 3. Extradural lesion. **(A)** Sagittal computed tomography reconstruction and **(B)** sagittal T2-weighted images show a large sacral lesion, which was found to be a large schwanomma with extradural extension.

with the tumor at its site of attachment to the dura. The subarachnoid space is widened on the ipsilateral side and narrowed on the contralateral side. With larger tumors, the spinal cord is often flattened against the dura on the contralateral side. Myelography shows a sharp delineation of the contrast column along the surface of the mass, referred to as a "contrast meniscus."

The most common intradural-extramedullary tumors include the nerve sheath tumors (neurofibromas and schwannomas) and meningiomas, which account for approx 50% of all adult primary spinal neoplasms (Fig. 4 [13]). Meningiomas, usually located dorsal to the thoracic cord, commonly have a flat dural base. When evaluating a gadolinium enhanced MRI of the spine, sagittal, axial, and especially coronal planes should be obtained to detect "dural tails" that are very suggestive of meningioma (18). The appearance of a dural tail results from enhancement of that portion of the meningioma (the tail) that extends towards and infiltrates into the dura. Schwannomas and neurofibromas may have a dumbbell shape with both intradural and extradural components and frequently have foraminal extension. An enlarged neural foramen is highly suggestive of a nerve sheath tumor. Patients with intradural lesions commonly require imaging of the entire craniospinal axis because multiple lesions (i.e., drop metastases, neurofibromatosis, or spread from intracranial tumors) may have to be ruled out before subjecting a patient to a high-risk spinal cord operation. Multiple enhancing intradural nodules are highly suggestive of leptomeningeal disease in a patient with a history of cancer. The same

radiological findings in a patient with Von Recklinghausen's disease suggest multiple neurofibromas or schwannomas.

5.2.3. Intradural-Intramedullary Tumors

Intramedullary tumors account for 16 to 25% of spinal cord neoplasms (12,17). These tumors are located within the parenchyma of the spinal cord (Fig. 5). The characteristic MRI finding is widening of the spinal cord in all planes (sagittal, axial, and coronal), narrowing of the CSF column at the level of the lesion, and an enhancing lesion, commonly associated with a syrinx. Complete lack of enhancement, absence of spinal cord enlargement and the absence of a syrinx should alert the physician to other potential non-neoplastic conditions such as transverse myelitis. In patients who present with an ill-defined spinal cord abnormality suggestive of a plaque on MRI examination, a brain MRI can be very helpful in ruling out multiple sclerosis. The presence of multiple periventricular lesions, which are best seen on axial T2-weighted images, are highly suggestive of multiple sclerosis.

Gliomas account for approx 95% of all intramedullary neoplasms (17); approx 65% are ependymomas and 30% are astrocytomas (12,17). Children show a slight preponderance of astrocytomas relative to ependymomas, and there is a large predominance of ependymomas in and below the conus medullaris (19). Hemangioblastomas, although rare, should also be considered when evaluating a patient with an intramedullary tumor (20,21). These tumors are found most frequently at the cervicothoracic and thoracolumbar regions (13) and are

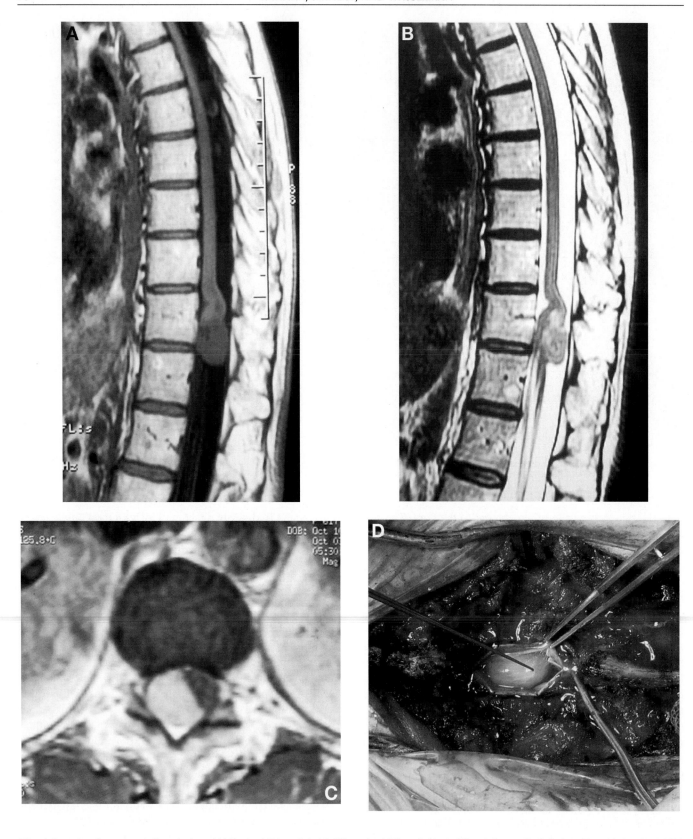

Fig. 4. Intradural-extramedullary lesion. (A) Sagittal T1-weighted, (B) sagittal T2-weighted, (C) axial post-Gadolinium T1-weighted, and (D) intra-operative images show a schwannoma in the distal thoracic spine. (Reprinted with permission from ref. *21a*.)

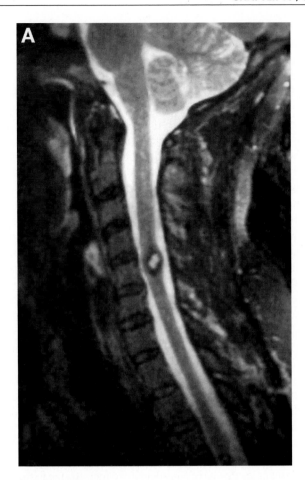

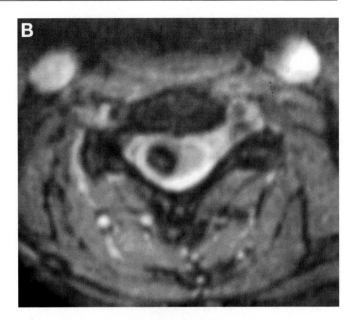

Fig. 5. Intradural-intramedullary lesion. (**A**) Sagittal T2-weighted and (**B**) axial T2-weighted images showing in intradural-intramedullary lesion compatible with a cavernoma of the cervical spinal cord at the C5 level.

typically subpial in location with a cystic component with an enhancing mural nodule and signal voids owing to their hypervascularity. Metastases can also present as intramedullary lesions. A common primary site is an intracranial neoplasm that spreads via CSF seeding to the leptomeninges, which may lead to direct invasion of the spinal cord *(13)*. Other primary sites outside of the central nervous system include lung and breast carcinoma, lymphoma, melanoma, and adenocarcinoma *(13,22)*. Intramedullary spinal cord schwannomas are rare; only 44 cases have been reported in the literature *(23)*.

Gadolinium plays an important role in the evaluation of intramedullary disease because it can aid substantially in lesion delineation and characterization *(24–26)*. With focal lesions such as hemangioblastomas and metastases, gadolinium enables accurate distinction of the solid portion of the tumors from the extensive edema *(27)*. In addition, most primary cord gliomas will show some enhancement regardless of histologic grade. This enhancement has proven useful because if an intramedullary lesion is seen, lack of enhancement makes a glioma less likely and places other processes (such as benign syrinx) higher in the differential diagnosis *(26)*. Certain tumors (i.e., intradural-extramedullary drop metastases) may be virtually invisible without the administration of gadolinium. Finally, gadolinium is useful for differentiating reactive from neoplastic cysts because reactive cysts usually do not enhance and tumor cysts are generally surrounded by enhancement and require excision. Other advantages of gadolinium include: (1) improved

biopsy yield secondary to the correlation between higher cellular activity and tumor aggression at enhancing sites *(28)*; (2) improved delineation of cord compression and differentiation of enhancing tumor from nonenhancing cord; and (3) evaluation of the response of spinal metastases to therapy. Overall, Godolinium-diethyltriamine pentaacetic acid-enhanced MRI increases MRI sensitivity and specificity and improves the reliability of spinal tumor diagnosis *(29)*.

The careful evaluation of an MRI study is critical to the treatment of spinal tumors. The clinician must focus on placing the lesion within a compartment rather than describing multiple details regarding the lesion that may not affect the final diagnosis. Determining the location (extradural vs intradural-extramedullary vs intramedullary), recognizing the characteristic signal intensity changes with various pulse sequences, and an understanding of the indications and limitations of the available imaging protocols in addition to other imaging modalities can provide a precise radiological identification of the tumor type and help guide additional evaluation, treatment, and subsequent follow-up.

5.2.4. Radionuclide Imaging

The primary indication of nuclear scintigraphy is staging and evaluation of skeletal metastases. It is important to note that nuclear scintigraphy, although quite sensitive, lacks specificity owing to the fact that multiple other processes (i.e., degenerative arthritis, trauma, and infection) also lead to an increase in radiotracer activity as is seen in patients with metastatic disease *(30,31)*. In addition, multiple myeloma and several lytic metastases can produce false-negative examinations because of their aggressive nature and the inability to allow for osseous remodeling *(32)*. Another potential use is seen in

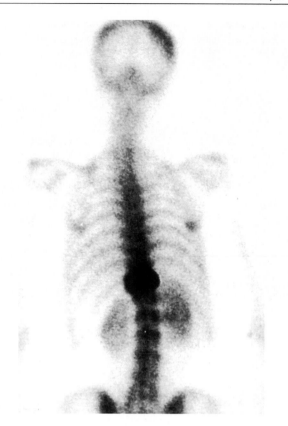

Fig 6. Radiotracer uptake in metastatic disease. Focal uptake in thoracic spine coincides with destructive lesion involving vertebral body and pedicles, not yet apparent on plain radiographs.

patients with metastatic lesions of unknown primary where nuclear scintigraphy may allow for the localization of a peripheral skeletal lesion, which is amenable to percutaneous or open biopsy *(33)*.

Most sites of metastatic tumor deposition demonstrate a focal or asymmetric increase in radiotracer activity (Fig. 6) related to an increase in osseous remodeling secondary to osteolysis resulting from the osteoclasts that have been activated by the metastatic tumor cells. When evaluating these images, it is important to have an understanding of the normal patterns of radiotracer distribution within the skeleton including increased activity in regions of rapid remodeling including the epiphyseal plates in children and in common areas of degenerative changes in older adults (i.e., knees, hips, shoulder joints, costochondral junctions of the rib cage).

5.2.5. Functional and Metabolic Imaging

Positron emission tomography (PET) images are produced after the injection of trace amounts of radionuclides that have been produced in a cyclotron and concentrate in areas of increased metabolic activity including tumors and various organs. The radiotracers are often bound to metabolites, which are specific to various tumors and may assist in evaluating their metabolic activity and response to treatment. Fluorine-18 fluorodeoxyglucose PET has been shown to have a high predictive value in differentiating spinal metastases from benign lesions when the number of foci and pattern of radiotracer activity are considered *(34)*. PET imaging is highly special-

ized and is offered at select institutions across North America and the images are best reviewed with nuclear medicine trained physicians with specialized training in PET.

5.2.6. Interventional Radiology Techniques

Interventional techniques include those that require fluoroscopic guidance to the region of interest and include vertebral biopsy, angiography, vertebroplasty, and kyphoplasty *(33)*. The latter two techniques are discussed in Chapter 34 as well as other minimally invasive surgical techniques. Vertebral biopsies are often performed to obtain a definitive diagnosis before proceeding with medical or surgical treatment. Fluoroscopic guidance can be used to navigate transpedicular and extrapedicular approaches. In addition, vertebral biopsies can be performed in conjunction with vertebroplasty and kyphoplasty procedures. Angiography is usually used to evaluate vascular lesions of the spine including hemangiomas and other vascular malformations and metastatic lesions that tend to be highly vascular, such as renal cell carcinoma and thyroid cancer. Diagnostic angiography can also be combined with endovascular embolization techniques to decrease the vascular supply to a region before proceeding with open surgical intervention.

5.2.7. Evaluation of Spinal Metastases

A common clinical scenario in the management of patients with cancer is the diagnosis and treatment of spinal metastases. After a thorough history and physical examination and identification of the type and location of the primary malignancy if possible, the next step is the identification of the level and degree of spinal involvement. An appreciation of those primary malignancies that have a propensity to metastasize to the spine increases the level of suspicion for a spinal metastasis and, thus, the likelihood that the diagnosis will be made. These primary sites include breast, prostate, lung, kidney, and thyroid *(35,36)*.

Although conventional radiographs have been shown to have a poor sensitivity for the evaluation of spinal metastases *(37)*, they are often the first imaging modality used to evaluate the spine. Their contribution lies in their ability to provide a rapid skeletal survey and rule out other causes of back and neck pain including degenerative changes and trauma including vertebral compression fractures. In addition, they assist in the localization of the level of pathology, which is useful for operative planning.

The mainstay in the evaluation of patients with suspected or known spinal metastases is MRI. Sagittal T1- and T2-weighted images of the entire spinal column should be obtained. Subsequently, axial images are obtained through regions of the spine that are felt to be symptomatic, correlate with a neurological level on physical examination or demonstrate suspicious findings on conventional radiographs, nuclear scintigraphy, or the sagittal images. The evaluation of post-Gadolinium T1-weighted images should be considered in patients with a suspicion for leptomeningeal carcinomatosis and intramedullary lesions as well as those in whom infection may be in the differential diagnosis.

6. SUMMARY

Several different imaging modalities are available for imaging the spine of a patient with cancer. It is the role of clinicians to evaluate the patient and use their basic understanding of the imaging options available along with the likely characteristics of the primary or metastatic lesion to select the appropriate imaging study, they should also consider factors such as patient risk, cost to the health care system, and the sensitivity and specificity of the study.

ACKNOWLEDGMENT

Portions of this chapter are reprinted with permission from ref. *21a*.

REFERENCES

1. Kamholz R, Sze G. Current imaging in spinal metastatic disease. Semin Oncol 1991; 18:158–169.
2. Steinbach HL. The roentgen appearance of osteoporosis. Radiol Clin North Am 1964; 50:191–207.
3. Janssen ME, Bertrand SL, Joe C, Levine MI. Lumbar herniated disk disease: comparison of MRI, myelography, and post-myelographic CT scan with surgical findings. Orthopedics 1994; 17:121–127.
4. Hollis PH, Malis LI, Zappulla RA. Neurological deterioration after lumbar puncture below complete spinal subarachnoid block. J Neurosurg 1986; 64:253–256.
5. Herkowitz HN, Garfin SR, Bell GR, Bumphrey F, Rothman RH. The use of computerized tomography in evaluating non-visualized vertebral levels caudad to a complete block on a lumbar myelogram. A review of thirty-two cases. J Bone Joint Surg 1987; 69A:218–224.
6. Van Goethem JW, van den Hauwe L, Ozsarlak O, De Schepper AMA, Parizel PM. Spinal tumors. Eur J Radiol 2004; 50:159–176.
7. Amiot LP, Poulin F. Computed tomography-based navigation for hip, knee, and spine surgery. Clin Orthop 2004; 421:77–86.
8. Chen YT, Wang MS. Three-dimensional reconstruction and fusion for multi-modality spinal images. Comput Med Imaging Graph 2004; 28:21–31.
9. Obenauer S, Alamo L, Herold T, Funke M, Kopka L, Grabbe E. Imaging skeletal anatomy of injured cervical spine specimens: comparison of single-slice vs multi-slice helical CT. Eur Radiol 2002; 12:2107–2111.
10. Bradley WG, Jr., Waluch V, Yadley RA, Wycoff RR. Comparison of CT and MR in 400 patients with suspected disease of the brain and cervical spinal cord. Radiology 1984; 152:695–702.
11. Kucharczyk W, Brant-Zawadzki M, Sobel D, et al. Central nervous system tumors in children: detection by magnetic resonance imaging. Radiology 1985; 155:131–136.
12. Williams RS, Williams JP. Tumors. In: Rao KCVG, Williams JP, Lee BCP, Sherman JL, eds. MRI and CT of the Spine. Baltimore, MD: Williams and Wilkins; 1994: 347–426.
13. Masaryk TJ. Neoplastic disease of the spine. Radiol Clin North Am 1991; 29:829–845.
14. Sevick RJ, Wallace CJ. MR imaging of neoplasms of the lumbar spine. Magn Reson Imaging Clin North Am 1999; 7:539–553.
15. Li KC, Poon PY. Sensitivity and specificity of MRI in detecting malignant spinal cord compression and in distinguishing malignant from benign compression fractures of vertebrae. Magn Reson Imaging 1988; 6:547–556.
16. Nittner K. Spinal meningiomas, neurinomas and neurofibromas and hourglass tumors. In: Vinken PJ, Bruyn GW, eds. Handbook of Clinical Neurology. Ed 20. New York, NY: Elsevier North-Holland; 1976:177–322.

17. Zimmerman RA, Bilaniuk LT. Imaging of tumors of the spinal canal and cord. Radiol Clin North Am 1988; 26:965–1007.
18. Quekel LGBA, Versteege CWM. The "dural tail sign" in MRI of spinal meningiomas. J Comput Assist Tomogr 1995; 19:890–892.
19. Lowe GM. Magnetic resonance imaging of intramedullary spinal cord tumors. J Neurooncol 2000; 47:195–210.
20. Miller DJ, McCutcheon IE. Hemangioblastomas and other uncommon intramedullary tumors. J Neurooncol 2000; 47:253–270.
21. Baker KB, Moran CJ, Wippold FJ, et al. MR imaging of spinal hemangioblastoma. AJR Am J Roentgenol 2000; 174:377–382.
21a. Khanna AJ, Shindle MK, Wasserman BA, et al. Use of magnetic resonance imaging in differentiating compartmental location of spinal tumors. Am J Orthop 2005; in press.
22. Grem JL, Burgess J, Trump DL. Clinical features and natural history of intramedullary spinal cord metastasis. 1985; Cancer 56:2305–2314.
23. Riffaud L, Morandi X, Massengo S, Carsin-Nicol B, Heresbach N, Guegan Y. MRI of intramedullary spinal schwannomas: case report and review of the literature. Neuroradiology 2000; 42:275–279.
24. Chamberlain MC, Sandy AD, Press GA. Spinal cord tumors: gadolinium-DTPA-enhanced MR imaging. Neuroradiology 1991; 33:469–474.
25. Dillon WP, Norman D, Newton TH, Bolla K, Mark A. Intradural spinal cord lesions: Gd-DTPA-enhanced MR imaging. Radiology 1989; 170:229–237.
26. Fulbright R, Ross JS, Sze G: Application of contrast agents in MR imaging of the spine. J Magn Reson Imaging 1993; 3:219–232.
27. Jahre C, Sze G. Magnetic resonance imaging of spinal metastases. Top Magn Reson Imaging 1988; 1:63–70.
28. Sze G, Krol G, Zimmerman RD, Deck MDF. Intramedullary disease of the spine: diagnosis using gadolinium-DTPA-enhanced MR imaging. AJR Am J Roentgenol 1988; 151:1193–1204.
29. Parizel PM, Baleriaux D, Rodesch G, et al. Gd-DTPA-enhanced MR imaging of spinal tumors. AJR Am J Roentgenol 1989; 152:1087–1096.
30. Holder LE. Clinical radionuclide bone imaging. Radiology 1990; 176:607–614.
31. McCarthy EF. Diagnosing bone disease. In: McCarthy EF, Frassica FJ, eds. Pathology of Bone and Joint Disorders with Clinical and Radiographic Correlation. Philadelphia, PA: W. B. Saunders Company; 1998, p. 18.
32. McCarthy EF. Plasma cell dyscrasia. In: McCarthy EF, Frassica FJ, eds. Pathology of Bone and Joint Disorders with Clinical and Radiographic Correlation. Philadelphia, PA: W. B. Saunders Company; 1998, p. 188.
33. Ortiz AO, Lefkowitz D. Imaging of spinal tumors. In: Castillo M., ed. Spinal Imaging: State of the Art. Philadelphia, PA: Hanley & Belfus, Inc.; 2001: pp. 145–148.
34. Bohdiewicz PJ, Wong CY, Kondas D, Gaskill M, Dworkin HJ. High predictive value of F-18 FDG PET patterns of the spine for metastases or benign lesions with good agreement between readers. Clin Nucl Med 2003; 28:966–970.
35. Bohm P, Huber J. The surgical treatment of bony metastases of the spine and limbs. J Bone Joint Surg Br 2002; 84:521–529.
36. Pittas AG, Adler M, Fazzari M, et al. Bone metastases from thyroid carcinoma: clinical characteristic adn prognostic variables in one hundred forty-six patients. Thyroid 2000; 10:261–268.
37. Redmond J III, Friedl KE, Cornett P, et al. Clinical usefulness of an algorithm for the early diagnosis of spinal metastatic disease. J Clin Oncol 1988; 6:154–157.

11 Laboratory Studies and Diagnostic Work-Up of Bony Lesions in the Spine

KAI-UWE LEWANDROWSKI, MD, ROBERT F. MCLAIN, MD, AND HENRY J. MANKIN, MD

CONTENTS

1. THE SCOPE

Almost any time a physician treats a bony lesion or fracture pathological to the spine, the world of poor bone quality is entered. In order to improve understanding (and control) of the normal and diseased skeletal system, it is necessary to be conversant with a basic knowledge of these disorders affecting the spine. Therefore, basic laboratory tests, which can aid in the diagnostic work-up and evaluation of tumor recurrence, are reviewed in this chapter. It should be noted, though, that this chapter provides only an overview on the subject and it does not provide a complete review of all laboratory tests and prognostic factors applicable to spine tumor patients.

2. BONE AS A TISSUE

Bone is a specifically designed and uniquely ordered structure, which serves as a beautifully engineered framework for the body; it is a protector of organs, a system for movement of tissues in an orderly and structured fashion, a reservoir for the cells of the marrow and fat and type I collagen and the location of three unique cell types: the osteoblast, the osteocyte, and the osteoclast. These three types of cells are important in the development and maintenance of the bone. The cells are locally synthesized from osteoprogenitor cells, which in simple terms creates an osteoblast to make bone, an osteocyte to maintain it, and, by a less direct route, the osteoclast to destroy it. These cells are the critical components, which maintain the structure

of the bone and are very sensitive to variations in shape, weight, trauma, and a variety of disorders and diseases. Amazingly, the cells can and do very appropriately and rapidly adjust to these disorders *(1)*.

Of considerable importance is the recent recognition of an array of cytokines and glycoproteins, which for the most part affect the bone cells either to enhance production or increase the rate of destruction *(1–4)*. These include the transforming growth factor (TGF)-βs, fibroblast growth factors, the bone morphogenetic proteins, the insulin-like growth factors (IGF)-1 and -2, the interleukins (IL), especially IL-1, tumor necrosis factor, platelet-derived growth factor, parathyroid hormone (PTH), 1,25 dihydroxy vitamin D, osteoadherin, hyaluronan, osteonectin, osteopontin, and bone sialoprotein. These materials plus estrogen and androgen are thought to be responsible for the modifications in synthesis frequently encountered as well as the variation in size and structure of the bone *(1–4)*. The actual sequence by which these materials act is still not completely known, but it is thought that bone cells arise from stem cells, which under the influence of the bone morphogenetic proteins and TGF-βs, become osteoprogenitor cells. These cells become pre-osteoblasts under the action of fibroblast growth factors and platelet-derived growth factors. PTH, 1,25 dihydroxy vitamin D, the IGF-1 and -2, and the TGF-βs are responsible for conversion of the cells to active osteoblasts which synthesize bone *(4)*. Other agents (e.g., osteoadherin, hyaluronan, osteonectin, osteopontin, and bone sialoprotein) are thought to be responsible for defining the shape, texture, and turnover rates of the bone *(1–4)* and 1,25 dihydroxy vita-

From: *Current Clinical Oncology: Cancer in the Spine: Comprehensive Care.*
Edited by: R. F. McLain, K-U. Lewandrowski, M. Markman, R. M. Bukowski,
R. Macklis, and E. C. Benzel © Humana Press, Inc., Totowa, NJ

min D and PTH and parathyroid-related protein are thought to be responsible for the bone destruction *(3)*.

By a biomechanical definition, bone can be considered to be a two-phase composite. The organic phase consists of closely cross-linked, highly ordered, relatively insoluble type I collagen fibers, which in large measure define the structure and shape of the bones *(5,7)*. Impregnated within those fibers at specific sites in a quite orderly fashion *(5,7)* are extraordinarily tiny crystals of calcium hydroxyapatite having the basic formula of $Ca_{10}(PO_4)_6(OH)_2$ *(5,7,8)*. The dimensions of that crystal are extremely small, $50 \times 100 \times 200$ Å, which provides an enormous surface area *(6,9,10)*. If all the calcium and phosphate of bone were in one crystalline segment, the estimated surface area is less than two square meters. By contrast, the crystalline polyhedral structure of the tiny segments of calcium hydroxyapatite presents a reactive surface for a 60 kg person, which is estimated as greater than 100 square miles. In addition, the crystal has a hydration shell, unfilled surface spaces and is quite reactive *(8,10)*. On the basis of these observations, it should be evident that the bone mineral is in direct contact with the extracellular fluid and represents a highly reactive reservoir, both for rapid deposition of excess mineral or for almost instantaneous recovery of materials during periods of deficit or in the diseased state *(10)*.

3. CONDITIONS AFFECTING THE INTEGRITY OF BONE

Although the panoply of bone diseases must surely number in the hundreds, this chapter only consider four categories of causation of weakened bones: hyperparathyroidism; the rachitic syndromes (i.e., rickets, osteomalacia, and renal osteodystrophy); osteoporosis; and malignant diffuse skeletal disease, chiefly represented by metastatic disorders, and disorders of the hematopoietic system such as multiple myeloma. The difficulty of distinguishing them from each other on the basis of history, physical examination, and imaging is a major issue for the physician treating spinal neoplasia. The patients often have the same complaints, the identical findings and may not, on standard laboratory tests, show a great difference. One of the purposes of this chapter is to describe in more detail two of the four syndromes (hyperparathyroidism and malignancies) with consideration of appropriate diagnostic work-up of spinal lesions.

4. PRIMARY HYPERPARATHYROIDISM

Primary hyperparathyroidism is a well recognized entity and was partially identified more than a century ago by Friedrich von Recklinghausen *(11)*. He and his coworkers are responsible for the descriptive Latin appellation of osteitis fibrosa cystica (generalisata) for the entity. The histological changes are quite distinctive and, in florid disease, show fibrous replacement of the marrow, osteoclastic resorption of the bone, osteoblastic rimming on new and, often, incompletely mineralized lamellar bone trabeculae and "brown tumors," and "...areas of granulation tissue, inflammatory cells and giant cells with virtually no bone at all..." *(12)*. The disease results from an excess secretion of PTH, which mostly occurs in response to a solitary adenoma or, less commonly, a hyperplasia affecting all four glands or, in rare cases, a carcinoma of a single parathy-

roid gland *(13–18)*. Because the parathyroid gland output of PTH is believed to be almost entirely dependent on the serum and extracellular fluid values of [Ca^{++}] (it should be noted that ionized magnesium also plays a role in discharging the PTH from the glands *[32–34]*), the implication is that the diseased gland fails to recognize the signal and does not "turn off" in response to high levels of serum or extracellular fluid [Ca^{++}] and, hence, becomes a "runaway train," pouring out the PTH and not obeying or even seeing the critical message sent by the excessive calcium levels *(19–21)*.

Bone breakdown occurs partly as a result of destruction of the crystals, but more importantly as a result of osteoclastic resorption, which causes holes to occur in the bone *(22–25)*. These fill in with fibrous tissue (hence the name osteitis fibrosa) and at times become confluent to produce a large defect known as a "brown tumor" *(23,26–28)*. Because there is also a simultaneous decrease in the %TRP, a phosphate diabetes ensues and the patient becomes hyperphosphaturic *(15,16)*. The chemical findings are then an elevated serum calcium, a lowered serum phosphate, and because bone formation occurs in response to the destruction, an elevated serum alkaline phosphatase. The increase bone formation often results in a patchy increase in activity of the bone scan. It should be noted that some of the newer markers are useful in this regard and bone-specific alkaline phosphatase, osteocalcin, urinary pyridinilone, deoxypyrodinilone, and *N*-telopeptide of collagen can all be abnormal in even mild cases of hyperparathyoidism *(29)*. The serum urate elevation (reflecting tissue breakdown *[30]*), diminished %TRP, and increased urinary calcium all contribute to recognition of the presumptive diagnosis. To be certain of the diagnosis, particularly in the face of the many other causes of hypercalcemia *(15,31,32)*, an analysis of the concentration of PTH must be performed, which is not as easy a task as originally considered *(33,34)*. It has been proposed that the principal tests at present are the immunoradiometric and immunochemiluminometric assays for PTH 1-84, which have their greatest value in separating hyperparathyroidism from the hypercalcemia of malignancy. The latter involves principally PTH-related protein promoter (PTHrP), which is not ordinarily detected by these immune studies *(15,16,31,33,35,36)*.

Today, for reasons probably related to the widespread use of rapid automated laboratory screening systems, the presentation of the disorder has changed to a much blander and often much more subtle picture *(37–42)*. One rarely encounters the full-blown clinical syndrome and most often the patient is either asymptomatic or has an easy fatigability, a sense of weakness, and intellectual weariness that, according to some, has a specific psychometric pattern *(36,42,43)*. Occasionally, the patient may complain of lower back pain and on imaging the patients may be shown to have a mild to moderate osteopenia. The occurrence of renal stones formerly set at over 50% of the patients has now been reduced to less than 10% *(38)* and florid bone lesions (especially brown tumors) are rarely, if ever, seen *(28,37,39–41)*. Considering the fact that the disorder is considerably more frequent in women and increased in incidence with advanced age, the confusion with osteoporosis is common *(42)*.

The principal role of the spine surgeon in the management of patients with hyperparathyroidism is that of a "case-finder". If one has a high index of suspicion for patients with back or other bone pain coupled with a compression fracture or even just osteopenia on routine radiographs of the spine, one should obtain serum studies, which will suggest the diagnosis. The nature and extent of the disease can be easily assessed by appropriate immunoassays for PTH and other studies *(21,29, 33,42,44)*. Once the diagnosis is made the patient should be treated by people skilled in the management of metabolic bone disease and surgeons with experience in removing the parathyroid glands.

There are several genetic syndromes of which hyperparathyroidism is an essential part. These include multiple endocrine neoplasia type I (Wermer syndrome; consisting of parathyroid, pituitary, and pancreatic tumors) and type II (Sippel syndrome; consisting of thyroid carcinoma, pheochromocytomas, and hyperparathyroidism). It is unlikely that the physician will encounter these rare disorders as a primary presentation of spinal pain *(23,45)*.

5. MALIGNANCIES

In any discussion of bone lesions to the spine, one must include metastatic lesions from lung, renal, and breast primaries, as well as lesions stemming from primaries of the gastrointestinal and hematopoietic system.

5.1. PROSTATE CANCER

Early detection of prostate cancer is paramount for successful treatment of prostate cancer in the earliest, most treatable stages. The prostate-specific antigen (PSA) can be followed with a screening test that measures the amount of PSA. PSA is produced by the prostate and circulating levels in the serum increase with age. Higher than normal PSA levels are indicative of cancer in the gland *(46)*. However, high PSA levels can also be found in other conditions that are noncancerous, including prostatitis and benign prostatic hyperplasia *(46,47)*. Therefore, the use of PSA assay for prostate cancer detection is not without problems.

Other PSA derivatives have been studied to decrease false-positive results of PSA testing in men with PSA levels in the diagnostic "...gray zone..." *(46)*. The free-to-total PSA ratio (F/T PSA) has been investigated in many clinical trials *(46)*. It has been demonstrated that men with prostate cancer have a lower percentage of free PSA than men without cancer because a higher percentage of PSA is bound to various serum proteins. Optimized prostate cancer detection "...has been suggested with use of the F/T PSA; particularly in men with total PSA in the 4 to 10 ng/mL range" *(47)*. This is believed to reduce the number of unnecessary prostate biopsies. Furthermore, a decreasing F/T PSA (i.e., a negative F/T PSA slope) may itself serve as a marker for early prostate cancer detection *(47)*.

5.2. COLORECTAL CANCER

Markers for colorectal cancer (CRC) include tumor-associated antigens (TAAs) such as carcinoembryonic antigen (CEA). CEA has also been described as a marker for a variety of extraintestinal tumors such as lung, breast, ovarian, and bladder cancers *(50)*. However, CEA has poor sensitivity and specificity as a serological screening tool for early CRC detection particularly in early stage I of CRC *(48,49)*.

Another CRC tumor marker, which has been demonstrated to be useful as a screening tool for CRC, includes tumor-associated glycoprotein (TAG)-72 *(51)*. This marker is a high-molecular-weight mucin-like glycoprotein and is expressed in a variety of tumors. However, it also suffers from low sensitivity and specificity for CRC *(51)*.

Enzymes have been studied as a serum marker for CRC. These include ornithine decarboxylase (ODC), matrix metalloproteinase (MMP)-7, and urokinase-type plasminogen activator *(48)*. These enzymes are elevated in increased cellular proliferation and ODC in particular has been implicated to play an important role in the malignant transformation of skin, stomach, and colon *(52,53)*. Similarly, MMP-7, at least theoretically, is integral to the degradation and remodeling of the extracellular matrix during the process of tumor invasion and metastasis *(54–58)*. However, its role as a screening tool for CRC is currently under investigation *(51)*.

Yet another approach to development of new screening and diagnostic tools in CRC is the analysis of genomic abnormalities in cases of CRC. Chromosomal material is commonly lost in sporadic CRC *(59)*. Often these regions are located on chromosomes 5, 8, 17, and 18 *(51)*. Their loss is believed to result in deletion of tumor suppressor genes. As such, 20 to 50% of sporadic CRCs and in 30% of adenomas the 5q chromosome is lost *(58)*. This is consistent with the fact that the *adenomatous polyposis coli* (*APC*) gene is located on chromosome 5q21 *(51)*. Its loss has been implicated in CRC carcinogenesis *(51)*. However, its role as a prognostic marker in CRC is unclear. Other genetic markers are currently under investigation *(59)*.

Although screening for sporadic CRC has been limited, more formalized screening is recommended for the hereditary CRC syndromes *(51)*. Both familial adenomatous polyposis syndrome and hereditary non-polyposis CRC syndrome develop on the basis of germ line mutations *(51)*. Hence, patients develop CRC early in their lives. Genetic testing is paramount for screening first-degree relatives of affected patients *(51)*.

In sporadic CRC, genetic testing is limited. However, this may change, as shown by Ahlquist et al. *(60)*. Human mucosal cell DNA was isolated from frozen stool samples and screened for point mutations at any of 15 sites on *K-ras*, *p53*, and *APC*; *Bat-26*, a microsatellite instability marker; and highly amplifiable DNA *(51)*. These assays were highly sensitive (91% in cancer and 82% for adenomas >1 cm diameter) *(61)*.

The use of CEA as a prognostic tool in CRC has been widely studied. Preoperative CEA elevation appears to correlate with a poorer prognosis and increased tumor recurrence rate following curative CRC resection *(49)*. In fact, 5-yr survival rates are much higher (93%) if pre- and postoperative CEA levels are normal *(51)*. This compared to a 67% 5-yr survival when CEA was elevated both pre- and postoperatively *(51,60,61)*. In addition, failure of CEA to return to normal levels postoperatively following a curative resection for CRC, is a poor prognostic factor *(51)*.

Serial measurement of CEA levels may be used as a test following a curative CRC resection to detect tumor recurrence *(51)*. The nature of CEA testing makes this especially attractive. Specifically, "… it has a low cost in relation to other methods of detecting recurrence (e.g., CT [computed tomography] of the abdomen and pelvis, magnetic resonance imaging, colonoscopy)…" *(51)*. About three-fourths of patients with recurrent CRC have an elevated serum CEA level before developing symptoms *(61)*. "The use of CEA in this manner has, however, been controversial, even though early non-randomized studies suggested that surgery prompted by this method resulted in more potentially curative reoperations for recurrence," *(51)*. More recent studies have failed to show a survival advantage *(61)*.

5.3. GYNECOLOGICAL AND BREAST CANCER

Several serum tumor markers have been identified for diagnosis and follow-up for patients with gynecological malignancy or breast cancer. In epithelial ovarian cancer, CA125 has been identified as the most sensitive marker *(61)*. However, CA125 detection in the serum of patients with minimal malignant tumor has not been possible *(63)*. In addition, many nonmalignant conditions including endometriosis, menstruation, and massive ascites may elevate the CA125, and approx 50% of patients with clear cell adenocarcinoma do not show CA125 elevated above 100 U/mL *(64)*. The use of multiple tumor markers together with imaging studies is recommended to improve sensitivity and specificity in the diagnosis of ovarian cancer *(62)*.

The role of tumor markers, such as CA 15-3, tissue polypeptide-specific antigen (TPS) and CEA in diagnosis and evaluation of recurrent breast cancer is poorly understood *(65)*. Given et al. *(65)* examined the predictive value of these markers in 1448 breast cancer patients. The sensitivity, specificity, positive predictive value, and negative predictive value of CA 15-3, TPS, and CEA for visceral, bony, and regional recurrence were calculated. These studies showed that CA 15-3 was the most sensitive marker *(65)*. It was elevated in 68% of patients with visceral and in 69% of patients with bony recurrence. In comparison, TPS is 64 and 51%, and CEA is 27 and 46% for visceral and bony recurrence, respectively *(65)*. "The positive predictive value of CA 15-3 at 47% for visceral and 54% for bony recurrence was greater than that for TPS (visceral 25%, bony 21%) or CEA (visceral 18%, bony 26%). The sensitivity of CA 15-3 and TPS for regional recurrence was low at 23 and 17%, respectively" *(65)*. In addition, the authors found that the mean lead time effect in visceral recurrence for TPS and CA 15-3 were 8 and 10 mo, compared to with lead times of 7.5 and 8.25 mo for TPS and CA 15-3 in patients with bony recurrence. CA 15-3 remains the most sensitive tumor marker in breast cancer follow-up with a significantly greater positive predictive value when compared to TPS or CEA *(65)*.

Recently, tissue-based markers, such as steroid receptors and the *c-erbB-2* gene *(neu/erbB-2)* have been have been implicated in breast cancer prognosis. However, they are not predictive of all recurrences. Bull et al. *(64)* examined the prognostic value of *p53* alterations in combination with *neu/erbB-2* amplification and found that *p53* mutations occurred in 24.5% of the axillary node-negative breast carcinomas. Elevated risks of disease recurrence and overall mortality in patients with both *p53* mutation and *neu/erbB-2* amplification in their tumor com-

pared with patients with neither or only one of the alterations *(64)*. Therefore, mutations of the *p53* gene may be beneficial to identify women at higher risk of disease recurrence and death, when the tumor has *neu/erbB-2* amplification present. On the contrary, the absence of *neu/erbB-2* amplification, the presence of *p53* mutation may not provide additional independent prognostic information *(64)*.

Other potential tumor markers for breast cancer include vascular endothelial growth factor (VEGF), leptin, and prolactin *(66)*. They have been suggested to have roles in the regulation of angiogenic process. Coskun et al. *(66)* examined serum leptin, prolactin and VEGF levels in 30 metastatic, 55 non-metastatic breast cancer patients, and 25 control subjects. Whereas serum leptin and prolactin levels were found to be similar in non-metastatic, metastatic patients, and control subjects, higher serum VEGF levels (249.8 ± 154.9 pg/mL) were found in metastatic patients, when compared with the non-metastatic patients (138.7 ± 59.3 pg/mL) and control subjects (108.4 ± 47.7 pg/mL), ($p < 0.05$) *(66)*. Moreover, "…patients with visceral metastasis (337.0 ± 168.0 pg/mL) had higher serum VEGF levels, when compared with patients with bone metastasis (162.6 + 71.8 pg/mL), ($p < 0.05$)" *(66)*. These studies show that serum VEGF appears to have merit in the evaluation of the angiogenic and metastatic activity in breast cancer patients.

5.4. RENAL CELL CARCINOMA

Renal carcinoma is curable when found in the early stage. Few prognostic markers are available to identify patients at risk for the recurrence and metastasis of renal cell carcinoma. Current clinical prognostic factors, such as tumor grade, renal vein involvement, and extension to regional lymph nodes, have limited value in this respect *(67)*.

Recently, a number of adhesion molecules were investigated for their potential as prognostic markers for various neoplasms. It is believed that dysfunction of adhesion molecules, such as cadherins, play an important role in the progression tumors of epithelial origin *(68)*. Similarly, loss or abnormal expression of cadherins in tumors can promote tumor invasion and disease progression, as demonstrated for E-cadherin expression in the prostate *(69)*. The role of these adhesion molecules as a marker for renal cell carcinoma progression is less understood and is currently under investigation.

One of these adhesion molecules, cadherin-6, is expressed in kidney and renal cell carcinoma. It may have may have prognostic value in renal cell carcinoma *(68)*. Paul et al. *(69)* evaluated a total of 216 patients with renal cell carcinoma, who underwent tumor nephrectomy, by analyzing them for cadherin-6 expression by immunohistochemistry and immunoblotting. The expression pattern was correlated with known prognostic factors of renal cell carcinoma. The authors found that cadherin-6 expression in renal cell cancer correlated with known prognostic factors, such as "… pT stage ($p = 0.03$), pN stage ($p = 0.001$), histological growth pattern ($p = 0.001$), M stage ($p = 0.06$), and renal venous involvement ($p = 0.019$)," *(69)*. However, the authors did not find a correlation with tumor grading ($p = 0.74$) or tumor size ($p = 0.84$) *(69)*.

Other markers, CA 125, CD44, and epithelial membrane antigen (EMA) expression in renal cell carcinoma, have been investigated to determine their role as prognostic factors (70). CD44 is a cell adhesion molecule, and CA 125 and EMA are TAAs used in the diagnosis and monitoring of the outcome and response to treatment of various human malignancies (70). Bamias et al. (70) found positive staining for "...CA 125 in 28 patients (30.43%), CD44 in 48 patients (52.17%), and EMA in 74 patients (80.43%)...." In addition, they noted increased CA 125 expression in those with higher T stage and histological grade (70). However, EMA expression and grade were inversely related. These markers also appeared to be indicative of increased risk of recurrence (70). Furthermore, the authors' analysis showed that "...CA 125 expression predicted a significantly higher probability of death (28.6 vs 8% in patients with T1 or T2 tumors" (70). Hence, CA 125 and EMA appear to be useful prognostic markers in renal cell carcinoma.

5.5. LUNG CANCER

Traditionally, there has been a limited role of prognostic tumor markers in lung cancer patients. Recently, however, the predictive value for response to treatment and prognosis of pretreatment concentrations of tumor markers has been investigated for patients with non-small cell lung cancer (NSCLC). Trape et al. (72) determined pretreatment levels of CEA, cancer antigen 125 (CA125), and cytokeratin 19 fragment (CYFRA21-1) in 48 patients with advanced stage (IIIA–IV) NSCLC that were treated with platin-based chemotherapy. They found that the sensitivity for CYFRA21-1, CA125, and CEA was 66.7, 45.8, and 47.3%, respectively (72). Furthermore, the "...predictive factors for non-response to treatment were CA125 > 35 KU/L (OR = 5.36; $p = 0.017$) and presence of metastasis (OR = 6.92; $p = 0.007$)..." and the "....prognostic factors for survival were performance status >1 (HR = 4.22; $p = 0.0002$)..." (72). The predictive values for the presence of metastasis was (HR = 3.1; $p = 0.0028$) and CA125 > 35 KU/L (HR = 2.33; $p = 0.02$). The authors concluded that CA125 is "...a predictive factor for response to treatment and a prognostic factor for survival in patients with NSCLC treated with chemotherapy" (72).

These findings were corroborated by Ando et al. (73), who also investigated the merit of CEA, CA125, and Cyfra21-1 as a prognostic factor by analyzing their series of 584 NSCLC patients. In addition, they tested these patients for squamous cell carcinoma antigen. They found that there was, in fact, a significant correlation between the serum levels of these factors and the clinical stages. The presence of both Cyfra21-1 and CA125 appeared to correlate with a negative clinical prognosis. The authors concluded that the simultaneous expression of Cyfra21-1 and CA125 together implied the worst prognosis (73).

Another NSCLC tumor marker has been recently described. Turken et al. (74) described the c-erbB2 oncoprotein, which they found to be highly expressed in approximately one-third of NSCLC patients (74). In their series of 84 patients, they investigated *c-erbB2* expression and correlated it with disease stage, histological type, and response to treatment. They found that *c-erbB2* was overexpressed in 35% of the cases (74). In addition, adenocarcinoma patients with higher stage disease (stage IIIB–IV) were noted to express the c-erbB2 protein more often (74). However, this relationship did not remain when correlating it to response to chemotherapy (74). Nonetheless, the authors concluded that c-erbB2 overexpression may have a role as a prognostic marker for NSCLC patients, particularly for evaluation of tumor progression (74).

When evaluating patients suspected of having lung cancer, one must consider the presence of paraneoplastic syndromes, which may, in fact, be the first clinical presentation. One of the common clinical findings is that of hyponatremia because of the syndrome of inappropriate secretion of antidiuretic hormone (SIADH). The clinical symptoms of weakness, lethargy, confusion, coma, and seizures are not owing to the malignancy itself, but rather are because of the inappropriate ADH production. SIADH should be suspected if low serum sodium and low serum osmolality(<280 mOsm/kg) is coupled with a high urine osmolality (greater than serum osmolality) and high urine sodium (>20 mEq/L). Fifteen percent of patients with present with hyponatremia owing to SIADH (75). Another possible cause of hyponatremia in some small cell carcinoma patients is a tumor produced atrial natriuretic factor causing sodium loss without ADH elevation (75).

5.6. HEMATOPOETIC MALIGNANCIES
5.6.1. Non-Hodgkin's Lymphoma

Therapeutic approaches for non-Hodgkin's lymphoma are currently based on the International Prognostic Index (76). Although a number of biological prognostic factors have been investigated, serum VEGF and IL-6 have been identified as useful prognostic factors for non-Hodgkin's lymphoma. Niitsu et al. (76) found that VEGF and IL-6 levels are independent prognostic factors in patients with aggressive lymphoma. This was demonstrated by comparing serum VEGF and IL-6 levels in normal controls, which were significantly higher in patients with aggressive lymphoma or adult T-cell leukemia/lymphoma. Furthermore, the disease-free survival in patients with higher levels of VEGF or IL-6 were significantly shorter than in patients with low levels. The authors concluded that VEGF or IL-6 both were independent prognostic factors for overall survival of aggressive lymphoma (76).

5.6.2. Multiple Myeloma

As has been known for many years, there is a class of disorders known as the monoclonal gammopathies, which includes multiple disorders of varying extent and malignancy. The diseases are associated with abnormalities of the plasma cell, which either under the stimulus of some other condition (such as Gaucher disease, hypothyroidism, lupoid hepatitis, and others) will develop a clonal abnormality with the slow production of abnormal cells that produces an immunoglobulin product that migrates with these proteins on serum protein or immunoelectrophoretic studies (77–79). In addition to the monoclonal gammopathies associated with specific disorders, another rare one, Waldenstrom's macroglobulinemia, of unknown cause, may have as a feature osteopenia particularly of the spine and may result in fractures (79). But of all of these, the most frequently encountered and the most pernicious is multiple myeloma, which is believed by many to be a primary malignancy of bone and far exceeds in frequency of occurrence all other primary neoplasms including osteosarcoma (77–80).

Myeloma is a malignant disorder in which a single clone of plasma cells undergoes neoplastic conversion to "myeloma cells" characterized by unchecked growth. From a primary single or multiple separate sites spreads to involve virtually the entire bone marrow, producing a specific symptom complex and almost always leading inexorably to the patient's demise (77–80). Although myeloma is considered to be a small round cell type of tumor and, hence, may be localized to one area and present as a fairly discrete permeative lesion, it may also be generalized in its bone marrow distribution and offer imaging features resembling the osteopenic states previously described.

Clinically, patients with generalized multiple myeloma are in their mid-50s or older and generally complain of fatigue, malaise, and illness. They may be intermittently febrile and describe night sweats. The patient may complain of weight loss and poor appetite and often has poorly localized bone pain in the back, shoulders, or lower extremities (77,81). A pathological fracture of the spine or the femur may be the herald event. Examination shows the patient to appear pale, chronically ill, and in many cases complain of diffuse bone tenderness, particularly over the sternum and pelvis (81). The bone scan, although likely to be active at the site of a fracture, in 25% of the patients shows no increase even at the site of discrete lesions. A radiographic skeletal survey is recommended to search for foci of myeloma (77,82). Special imaging studies may disclose more extensive disease than can be appreciated in plain radiographs. A magnetic resonance imaging (MRI) of the spine is especially useful because it is likely to show evidence of patchy areas of altered pattern consistent with marrow element disease.

The laboratory findings in patients with myeloma can be quite extraordinary and may be very useful in arriving at a diagnosis. Most patients with diffuse disease of a sufficient degree that they present with osteopenia, will have a fairly profound normocytic, normochromic anemia often with a hematocrit less than 30. The sedimentation rate is usually more than 100 and these two tests (hematocrit and sedimentation test) are often very helpful as a screen for the disease (see Subheading 6.). Many other laboratory abnormalities may exist. Platelet deficiency, high uric acid (secondary gout), abnormal renal function, increased hydroxyproline peptides in the urine, and an abnormal serum protein electrophoresis or serum immunoelectrophoresis will provide almost certain evidence for the disease (83–85). The finding of an abnormal peak migrating with the IgA or IgG fraction is virtually diagnostic of myeloma and if the bone marrow shows more than 20% plasma cells (up to 8% is normal, between 10 and 20% is a presumptive diagnosis) there is no need to biopsy the bone lesion(s) for a diagnosis (88–88). In addition, Bence Jones proteinuria, once a valuable diagnostic test, has been recognized as occurring less than 50% of the time. A urinary protein immunoelectrophoresis may have a significantly higher yield (89).

It should be noted that myeloma is believed to stimulate osteoclastic activity possibly on the basis of lymphotoxin, IL-1, IL-6, and PTHrP activity. In addition to the anti-cancer medications there are now very favorable reports on the use of the bisphosphonates, especially calendronate and more recently risidronate (89).

6. SCREENING STUDIES

Patients presenting with nonspecific complaints of lower back pain and who demonstrate a diffuse osteopenia on standard radiographs, particularly affecting the spine and perhaps resulting in a compression fracture, present a puzzle to the physician to whom they turn for help. The problem that faces clinicians is how to screen for the presence or absence of hyperparathyroidism, metastatic lesions, or even myeloma? Some imaging studies are useful but are relatively nonspecific. The laboratory studies are of greater help, but the clinician needs to seek out tests that specifically relate to the diagnosis of the entities previously described. Differentiation is sometimes subtle and difficult but with the help of the studies outlined next the diagnosis often can be confirmed.

The neoplastic screening studies include:

1. History and physical examination.
2. Radiographs of the spine and pelvis (and hands and lateral skull if indicated).
3. Posteroanterior and right lateral radiograph of the chest.
4. Abdominal ultrasound or CT.
5. Chest CT.
6. Bone scan.
7. The basic laboratory screening series (a total of 13 tests).

    a. Complete blood count (lowered with chronic disease, marrow replacement, with chemotherapy and radiation).
    b. Erythrocyte sedimentation rate (elevated with most neoplasms, infection.
    c. Blood urea nitrogen and creatinine (elevated with renal disease).
    d. Glucose (endocrine abnormalities, paraneoplastic syndrome).
    e. Calcium (bone resorption).
    f. Phosphorus (bone resorption).
    g. Alkaline phosphatase (rest, bone resorption).
    h. SGOT (liver disease).
    i. TSH and T4 (thyroid disease).
    j. Serum immunoelectrophoresis (multiple myeloma, gammopathies).
    k. Urinanalysis (renal cell tumors, elevated cast, and blood).

If a patient with neoplastic bone diseases has enough osteopenia to be visible on routine radiographs of the spine (with or without some compression fractures) or pelvis, laboratory tests and prognostic markers may be used to distinguish the various disorders in the following manner:

6.1. HYPERPARATHYROIDISM

The calcium will be elevated, the phosphorus diminished, the alkaline phosphatase elevated, and the bone scan and radiographs of the hands and skull may show the presence of specific types of lesions (see Section 4). The second order tests for this group should include 24-h urinary calcium, PTH, uric acid, pyridinoline crosslinks of type I collagen, and plasma tartrate resistant acid phosphatase, the last two tests are designed to assess the rate of bone destruction. In addition, radiological consultation can best demonstrate an enlarged parathyroid gland by magnetic resonance and immune system imaging.

6.2. OSTEOMALACIA (OF ALL TYPES)

The calcium is likely to be low or low-normal and with the exception of renal osteodystrophy, the phosphorus is low or very low depending on the type of osteomalacia that is present. In renal osteodystrophy, the blood urea nitrogen and creatinine should reveal the nature of the process, but the phosphorus is almost invariably high and the calcium quite low. The alkaline phosphatase is usually elevated in both osteomalacia and chronic renal disease. The second order screens for this group of disorders include electrolytes, PTH, 25 hydroxy- and 1,25 dihydroxy vitamin D, serum osteocalcin, and urinary pyridinoline crosslinks. A 24-h urinary calcium is very helpful, as is on occasion analysis of the urine for sugar, amino acids, and determination of the tubular reabsorption for phosphate. A bone biopsy is often confirmatory particularly for the presence of wide osteoid seams.

6.3. OSTEOPOROSIS

This area is the most difficult because all the tests will generally be normal. The exceptions to this are the thyroid function tests (the only "curable" form of osteoporosis) and the sugar (some patients with diabetes may have a significant osteoporosis). The bone scan is almost uniformly inactive except in the presence of a fracture. Secondary screens for osteoporosis include bone specific alkaline phosphatase, serum osteocalcin, and serum type I collagen extension peptides (all of which measure synthesis), and urinary pyridinoline crosslinks and tartrate resistant acid phosphatase, which measure bone destruction. To map and trace the degree of the various disease forms, electronic measurement, such as quantitative digital radiography of the spine and hips, as well as studies of the same areas using dual photon absorptiometry should be performed. A bone biopsy is often helpful in assessing the extent of the disease.

6.4. PROSTATE CANCER

The total PSA will be elevated. The F/T PSA should be determined for optimized prostate cancer detection. The F/T PSA ratio is particularly useful in men with total PSA in the 4 to 10 ng/mL range.

6.5. COLORECTAL CANCER

Useful surveillance markers for colorectal cancer include TAAs, such as CEA, and TAG-72 (51). This marker is a high molecular weight mucin-like glycoprotein and is expressed in a variety of tumors. However, these markers suffer from low sensitivity and specificity for CRC (51). Nevertheless, serial measurement of CEA levels are recommended as a test following a curative CRC resection to detect tumor recurrence (51).

Enzymes including ODC, MMP-7, and urokinase-type plasminogen activator are indicative of cell proliferation and appear to indicate malignant transformation of CRC (52,53). Some of these tests are still investigational.

6.6. GYNECOLOGICAL AND BREAST CANCER

In epithelial ovarian cancer, CA125 has been identified as the most sensitive marker (61). The use of CA125 is recommended in conjunction with imaging studies.

In breast cancer, many markers, including CEA and CA15-3, are used and they are reported to be useful as markers for monitoring. Other TAAs include CA 19.9, CA 15.3, TAG.72, and TPS, these are also present in breast malignancies (66).

In the laboratory, tissue-based markers, such as steroid receptors and the *neu/erbB-2*, have been implicated in breast cancer prognosis. However, they are not predictive of all recurrences. The prognostic value of *p53* alterations in combination with *neu/erbB-2* amplification was recently recognized in breast cancer patients (64).

Other potential tumor markers for breast cancer include VEGF, leptin, and prolactin (66).

6.7. RENAL CELL CARCINOMA

Few prognostic markers are available to identify patients at risk for recurrence and metastasis of renal cell carcinoma. Current clinical prognostic factors (i.e., tumor grade, renal vein involvement, and extension to regional lymph nodes) have limited value in this respect (67). Adhesion molecules, such as cadherins, were investigated for their potential as prognostic markers for renal cell carcinoma. Cadherin-6 expression pattern appear to correlate with known prognostic factors of renal cell carcinoma, such as pT stage, pN stage, histological growth pattern, M stage, and renal venous involvement (69).

Other markers include CA 125, CD44, and EMA. Increased CA 125 expression was shown to correlate with higher T stage and histological grade (70).

6.8. LUNG CANCER

Traditionally, there has been a limited role of prognostic tumor markers in lung cancer patients. Recently, CEA, cancer antigen 125 (CA125), and cytokeratin 19 fragment (CYFRA21-1) have been evaluated. CA125 is considered a predictive factor for response to treatment and a prognostic factor for survival for NSCLC patient (72).

Expression of the c-erbB2 oncoprotein has also been shown and correlated with disease stage, histological type, and response to treatment, and is believed to have a role as a prognostic marker for NSCLC patients (74).

In cases of hyponatremia, SIADH owing to the inappropriate ADH production should be suspected if low serum sodium and low serum osmolality (<280 mOsm/kg) coupled with a high urine osmolality (greater than serum osmolality) and high urine sodium (>20 mEq/L) is present. SIADH is common in patients with pulmonary carcinoma. ADH or atrial natriuretic factor could be elevated (75).

6.9. MYELOMA

The complete blood count will almost always show a normocytic normochromic anemia and the erythrocyte sedimentation rate is likely to be in triple digits (>100/h). The serum immunoelectrophoresis will in approx 90% of the cases display an abnormal protein migrating with the IgG or IgA fraction. Serum calcium determinations may show an elevation. Second order confirmatory studies may include urinary immunoelectrophoresis, a skeletal survey, and a bone marrow biopsy searching for a high concentration of plasma cells (>15–20%).

7. CONCLUSIONS

The end result of a failure of calcium and phosphorus homeostatic mechanisms, whether because of neoplastic or metabolic bone disease, is quite frequently a disaster, which in many cases requires ingenuity and talent to reconstruct if it affects the spine. It is the author's hope that use of the prognostic markers detailed in this chapter may aid the spine surgeon in better determining appropriate surgical treatments for these patients by more accurately assessing tumor stage, response to treatment, and evaluation of tumor recurrence.

REFERENCES

1. Mundy, GR. Bone remodeling. In: Favus, M, ed. Primer on the Metabolic Bone Diseases and Disorders of Mineral Metabolism. 4th ed. Philadelphia, PA: Lippincott William and Wilkins; 1999:30–38.

2. Lian JB, Stein GS, Canalis E, Gehron Robey P, Boskey AL. Bone formation: osteoblast lineage cells, growth factors, matrix proteins and the mineralization process. In: Favus, M, ed. Primer on the Metabolic Bone Diseases and Disorders of Mineral Metabolism. 4th ed. Philadelphia, PA: Lippincott William and Wilkins; 1999:14–29.

3. Glimcher MJ. The nature of the mineral phase in bone. In: Avioli LV, Krane SM, eds. Metabolic Bone Diseases and Related Disorders. 3rd ed. San Diego, CA: Academic Press; 1998:23–95.

4. Khosla S, Kleerekoper M. Biochemical markers of bone turnover. In: Favus, M, ed. Primer on the Metabolic Bone Diseases and Disorders of Mineral Metabolism. 4th ed. Philadelphia, PA: Lippincott William and Wilkins; 1999:128–133.

5. Glimcher MJ. The nature of the mineral component of bone and the mechanism of calcification. In: Coe FL, Favus ME, eds. Disorders of Bone and Mineral Metabolism. New York, NY: Raven Press; 1992:265–286.

6. Broadus AE. Mineral balance and homeostasis. In: Favus, M, ed. Primer on the Metabolic Bone Diseases and Disorders of Mineral Metabolism. 4th ed. Philadelphia PA: Lippincott William and Wilkins; 1999:74–80.

7. Rodan GA. Introduction to bone biology. Bone 1992; 13:3–6.

8. Landis WJ, Glimcher MJ. Electron diffraction and electron probe micronanalysis of the mineral phase of bone tissue prepared by anhydrous techniques. J Ultrastruct Res. 1978; 63:188–223.

9. Boskey AL. Mineral-matrix interactions in bone and cartilage. Clin Orthop 1992; 281:244–274.

10. Silverberg SJ. The distribution and balance of calcium, magnesium and phosphorus. In: Favus ME, ed. Primer on Metabolic Bone Diseases and Disorders of Mineral Metabolism. Kelseyville, CA: American Society for Bone and Mineral Research; 1990:30–32.

11. von Recklinghausen FD. Die fibrose oder deformierende ostitis, die osteomalazie und die osteoplastische carcinose in ihren gegenseitigen Beziehungen. Forschr R Virchow. 1891:1–45.

12. Jaffe HL. Metabolic, Degenerative and Inflammatory Diseases of Bones and Joints. Philadelphia, PA: Lea and Febiger; 1972:301–331.

13. Bilezikian JP. Primary hyperparathyroidism. In: Favus, M, ed. Primer on the Metabolic Bone Diseases and Disorders of Mineral Metabolism. 4th ed. Philadelphia, PA: Lippincott William and Wilkins; 1999:187–191.

14. Chang CW, Tsue TT, Hermreck AS, Baxter KG, Hoover LA. Efficacy of preoperative dual-phase sestamibi scanning in hyperparathyoidism. Am Otholaryngol 2000; 21:355–359.

15. Bilezikian JP. Hypercalcemic states: their differential diagnosis and acute management. In: Coe FL, Favus ME, eds. Disorders of Bone and Mineral Metabolism. New York, NY: Raven Press; 1992:493–522.

16. Habener JF, Potts JT, Jr. Primary hyperparathyroidism. In: Avioli LV, Krane SM, eds. Metabolic Bone Disease. 2nd ed. Philadelphia, PA: WB Saunders; 1990:475–546.

17. Wynne AG, van Heerden J, Carney JA, Fitzpatrick LA. Parathyroid carcinoma: clinical and pathologic features in 43 patients. Medicine (Baltimore) 1992; 71:197–205.

18. Obara T, Fujimoto Y. Diagnosis and treatment of patients with parathyroid carcinoma; an update and review. World J Surg 1991; 15:738–744.

19. Ladenson JH. Calcium determination in primary hyperparathyroidism. J Bone Miner Res 1991; 6:S33–S41.

20. Spiegel AM. Pathophysiology of primary hyperparathyroidism. J Bone Miner Res 1991; 6:S15–S17.

21. Hellman P, Carling T, Rask L, Akerstrom G. Pathophysiology of primary hyperparathyroidism. Histo Histopathol 2000; 15:619–627.

22. Raisz, LG. Mechanisms and regulation of bone resorption by osteoclastic cells. In: Coe FL, Favus ME, eds. Disorders of Bone and Mineral Metabolism. New York, NY: Raven Press; 1992:287–311.

23. Hayes CW, Conway WF. Hyperparathyroidism. Radiol Clin North Am 1991; 29:85–96.

24. Parisien M, Silverberg SJ, Shane E, Dempster DW, Bilezikian JP. Bone disease in primary hyperparathyroidism. Endocrinol Metab Clin North Am 1990; 19:19–34.

25. Heath DA. Primary hyperparathyroidism. Clinical presentation and factors influencing clinical management. Endocrinol Metab Clin North Am 1990; 18:631–646.

26. Kappelle JW, Raymakers JA, Bosch R, Dursma SA. No short-term effects of 24,25-dihydroxycholecalciferol in healthy subjects. Bone 1989; 10:397–399.

27. Habener JF, Potts JT, Jr, Primary hyperparathyroidism. In: Avioli LV, Krane SM, eds. Metabolic Bone Disease. 2nd ed. Philadelphia, PA: WB Saunders; 1990:475–546.

28. Parisien M, Silverberg SJ, Shane E, Dempster DW, Bilezikian JP. Bone disease in primary hyperparathyroidism. Endocrinol Metab Clin North Am 1990; 19:19–34.

29. Rossini M, Gatti D, Isaia G, Sartori L, Braga V, Adami S. Effects of oral alendronate in elderly patients with osteoporosis and mild primary hyperparathyroidism. J Bone Miner Res 2001; 16:113–119.

30. Scott JT, Dixon ASTJ, Bywaters EGL. Association of hyperuricaemia and gout with hyperparathyroidism. Br Med J 1964; 1:1070–1073.

31. Lafferty, FW. Differential diagnosis of hypercalcemia. J Bone Miner Res 1991; 6:S51–S59.

32. Jorde R, Bonaa KH, Sundsfjord J. Primary hyperparathyroidism detected in a health screening. J Clin Epidemiol 2000; 53:1164–1169.

33. Nussbaum SR, Potts JT, Jr. Immunoassays for parathyroid hormone 1-84 in the diagnosis of hyperparathyroidism. J Bone Miner Res 1991; 6:S43–S50.

34. Yonemura K, Suzuki G, Fujigaki Y, Hishida A. New insights on the pathogenesis of hypercalcemia in primary hyperparathyroidism. Am J. Med Sci 2000; 320:334–336.

35. Lopez Hanninen E, Vogl TJ, Steinmuller T, Ricke J, Neuhaus P, Felix R. Preoperative contrast enhanced MRI of the parathyroid glands in hyperparathyroidism. Invest Radiol 2000; 35:426–430.

36. Potts JT, Jr. Hyperparathyroidism and other hypercalcemic disorders. Adv Intern Med 1996; 41:165–212.

37. Breslau NA, Pak CYC. Asymptomatic primary hyperparathyroidism. In: Coe FL, Favus ME, eds. Disorders of Bone and Mineral Metabolism. New York, NY: Raven Press; 1992:523–538.

38. Heath H, III, Hodgson SF, Kennedy MA. Primary hyperparathyroidism: incidence, morbidity and potential economic impact in a community. N Engl J Med 1980; 302:189–193.

39. Harrison BJ, Wheeler MH. Asymptomatic primary hyperparathyroidism. World J Surg 1991; 15:724–729.

40. Heath H, III. Clinical spectrum of primary hyperparathyroidism: evolution with changes in medical practice and technology. J Bone Miner Res 1991; 6:S63–S64.

41. Mundy GR, Cove DH, Fisken R. Primary hyperparathyroidism: changes in the pattern of clinical presentation. Lancet. 1980; 1:1317–1320.

42. Silverberg SJ. Natural history of primary hyperparathyroidism. Endocrinol Metab Clin North Am 2000; 29:451–464.

43. Neumann PJ, Torppa AJ, Blumetti AE. Neuropsychologic deficits associated with primary hpyperparathyroidism. Surgery 1984; 96:1119–1123.

44. Tanaka Y, Narue T, Funahashi H, et al. Bone metabolic analysis in patients with primary hyperparathyroidism. Biome Pahrmacother 2000;54:197–199.

45. Takami GM, Shirahama S, IkedaY, et al. Familial hyperparathyroidism. Biomed Pharmacother 2000; 54:21s–24s.

46. Stenman UH, Leinonen J, Alfthan H, Rannikko S, Tuhkanen K, Alfthan O. A complex between prostate-specific antigen and alpha 1-

antichymotrypsin is the major form of prostate-specific antigen in serum of patients with prostatic cancer: assay of the complex improves clinical sensitivity for cancer. Cancer Res 1991; 51:222–226.

47. Catalona WJ, Partin AW, Slawin KM, et al. Use of the percentage of free prostate-specific antigen to enhance differentiation of prostate cancer from benign prostatic disease: a prospective multicenter clinical trial. JAMA 1998; 279: 1542–1547.

48. Pokorny RM, Hunt L, Galandiuk S. What's new with tumor markers for colorectal cancer? Dig Surg 2000; 17:209–215.

49. Helm J, Choi J, Sutphen R, Barthel JS, Albrecht TL, Chirikos TN. Current and evolving strategies for colorectal cancer screening. Cancer Control 2003; 10:193–204.

50. Carpelan-Holmstrom M, Louhimo J, Stenman UH, Alfthan H, Haglund C. CEA, CA 19-9 and CA 72-4 improve the diagnostic accuracy in gastrointestinal cancers. Anticancer Res 2002; 22:2311–2316.

51. Crawford N, Colliver DW, Galandiuk S. Tumor markers and colorectal cancer: utility in management. J Surg Oncol 2003; 84:239–248.

52. De Young NJ, Ashman LK. Physicochemical and immunochemical properties of carcinoembryonic antigen (CEA) from different tumour sources. Aust J Exp Biol Med Sci 1978; 56:321–331.

53. Takami H, Koudaira H, Kodaira S. Relationship of ornithine decarboxylase activity and human colon tumorigenesis. Jpn J Clin Oncol 1994; 24:141–143.

54. Brown PD. Matrix metalloproteinase inhibitors: A novel class of anticancer agents. Adv Enzyme Regul 1995; 35:293–301.

55. Mori M, Barnard GF, Mimori K, Ueo H, Akiyoshi T, Sugimachi K. Overexpression of matrix metalloproteinase-7 mRNA in human colon carcinomas. Cancer 1995; 75:1516–1519.

56. Miseljic S, Galandiuk S, Myers SD, Wittliff JL. Expression of urokinase-type plasminogen activator and plasminogen activator inhibitor in colon disease. J Clin Lab Anal 1995; 9:413–417.

57. Buo L, Meling GI, Karlsrud TS, Johansen HT, Aasen AO. Antigen levels of urokinase plasminogen activator and its receptor at the tumor-host interface of colorectal adenocarcinomas are related to tumor aggressiveness. Hum Pathol 1995; 26:1133–1138.

58. McDermott U, Longley DB, Johnston PG. Molecular and biochemical markers in colorectal cancer. Ann Oncol 2002; 13:235–245.

59. Vogelstein B, Fearon ER, Hamilton SR, et al. Genetic alterations during colorectal-tumor development. N Engl J Med 1988; 319:525–532.

60. Slentz K, Senagore A, Hibbert J, Mazier WP, Talbott TM. Can preoperative and postoperative CEA predict survival after colon cancer resection? Am Surg 1994; 60:528–531.

61. McArdle C. ABC of colorectal cancer: Effectiveness of follow up. BMJ 2000; 321:1332–1335.

62. Gadducci A, Cosio S, Carpi A, Nicolini A, Genazzani AR. Serum tumor markers in the management of ovarian, endometrial and cervical cancer. Biomed Pharmacother 2004; 58:24–38.

63. Agnantis NJ, Goussia AC, Stefanou D. Tumor markers. An update approach for their prognostic significance. Part I. In Vivo 2003; 17:609–618.

64. Bull SB, Ozcelik H, Pinnaduwage D, et al. The combination of p53 mutation and neu/erbB-2 amplification is associated with poor survival in node-negative breast cancer. J Clin Oncol 2004; 22:86–96.

65. Given M, Scott M, Mc Grath JP, Given HF. The predictive of tumor markers CA 15-3, TPS and CEA in breast cancer recurrence. Breast 2000; 9:277–280.

66. Coskun U, Gunel N, Toruner FB, et al. Serum leptin, prolactin and vascular endothelial growth factor (VEGF) levels in patients with breast cancer. Neoplasma 2003; 50:41–46.

67. Maldazys JD, deKernion JB. Prognostic factors in metastatic renal carcinoma. J Urol 1986; 136:376–379.

68. Shiozaki H, Tahara H, Oka H, et al. Expression of immunoreactive E-cadherin adhesion molecules in human cancers. Am J Pathol 1991; 139:17–23.

69. Paul R, Necknig U, Busch R, Ewing CM, Hartung R, Isaacs WB. Cadherin-6: a new prognostic marker for renal cell carcinoma. J Urol 2004; 171:97–101.

70. Bamias A, Chorti M, Deliveliotis C, et al. Prognostic significance of CA 125, CD44, and epithelial membrane antigen in renal cell carcinoma. Urology 2003; 62:368–373.

71. Umbas R, Isaacs WB, Bringuier PP, et al. Decreased E-cadherin expression is associated with poor prognosis in patients with prostate cancer. Cancer Res 1994; 54:3929–3933.

72. Trape J, Buxo J, Perez de Olaguer J, Vidal C. Tumor markers as prognostic factors in treated non-small cell lung cancer. Anticancer Res 2003; 23:4277–4281.

73. Ando S, Kimura H, Iwai N, Yamamoto N, Iida T. Positive reactions for both Cyfra21-1 and CA125 indicate worst prognosis in non-small cell lung cancer. Anticancer Res 2003; 23:2869–2874.

74. Turken O, Kunter E, Cermik H, et al. Prevalence and prognostic value of c-erbB2 expression in non-small cell lung cancer (NSCLC). Neoplasma 2003; 50:257–261.

75. Carr DT, Holoye PY, Hong WK. Murray JF, Nadel JA, eds. Bronchogenic Carcinoma. Textbook of Respiratory Medicine. 2nd ed. 1994:1552–1553.

76. Niitsu N, Okamato M, Nakamine H, et al. Simultaneous elevation of the serum concentrations of vascular endothelial growth factor and interleukin-6 as independent predictors of prognosis in aggressive non-Hodgkin's lymphoma. Eur J Haematol 2002; 68:91–100.

77. Campanacci M. Plasmacytoma In Bone and Soft Tissue Tumors. New York, NY: Springer Verlag; 1990:559–574.

78. Goodman MA. Plasma cell tumors. Clin Orthop 1986; 204:86–92.

79. Waldenstrom JG. Benign monoclonal gammapathy. Acta Med Scand 1984; 216:435–447.

80. Kyle RA. Monoclonal gammapathy and multiple myeloma in the elderly. Baillieres Clin Haematol 1987; 1:533–557.

81. Jackson A, Scarffe JH. Prognostic significance of osteopenia and immunoparesis at presentation in patients with solitary myeloma of bone. Eur J Cancer 1990; 26:363–371.

82. Kyle RA. Diagnostic criteria of multiple myeloma. Hematol Oncol Clin North Am 1992; 6:347–358.

83. Dimopoulos MA, Moulopoulos A, Delasalle K, Alexanian R. Solitary plasmacytoma of bone and asymptomatic multiple myeloma. Hematol Oncol Clin North Am 1992; 6:359–369.

84. Vaickus L, Ball ED, Foon KA. Immune markers in hematologic malignancies. Crit Rev Oncol Hematol 1991; 11:267–297.

85. Kyle RA, Garton JP. Laboratory monitoring of myeloma proteins. Semin Oncol 1986; 13:310–317.

86. Martin AD, Bailey DA, McKay HA, Whiting S. Bone mineral and calcium accretion during puberty. Am J Clin Nutr 1997; 66:611–615.

87. Aitken JM, Hart DM, Anderson JB, Lindsay R, Smith DA, Speirs CF. Osteoporosis after oophorectomy for non,Ä'malignant disease in premenopausal women. Br Med J 1973; 2:325–328.

88. Genant HK, Block JE, Steiger P, Glueer CC, Ettinger B, Harris ST. Appropriate use of bone densitometry. Radiology 1989; 170:817–822.

89. Ganeval D, Lacour B, Chopin N, Grunfeld JP. Proteinuria in multiple myeloma and related diseases. Am J Nephrol 1990; 10:58–62.

12 Principles of Medical Management

Tarek Mekhail, MD, MSc, FRCSI, FRCSEd, Rony Abou-Jawde, MD, and Maurie Markman, MD

Contents

1. INTRODUCTION

In the past, patients rarely questioned the therapeutic decisions made by their physicians. Physicians, in turn, were guided by the principle of "doing onto others as you would have done onto you" and were largely limited by their clinical experiences. Today, evidence-based medicine dictates most treatment decisions, and the role of the physician in educating patients about available therapeutic options is becoming increasingly critical. The patient's autonomy has taken a more significant role in the ultimate treatment chosen.

The first, and probably the most important, decision that should be made at the initiation of cancer treatment is the identification of treatment goals. Discussing the prognosis and the goals of treatment with the patient and the family always facilitates future treatment decisions. It is very important, however, to understand the patient's values, concerns, and fears and to ensure that the goals of treatment make sense to the patient.

Traditionally, therapies with the intent to cure have been distinguished from those with palliative intent. In oncology, one almost always uses the word cure in its statistical sense based on the analysis of survival curves. Technically, cure is accomplished on the survival curve for a group of patients compared to a population of age- and sex-matched controls. However, in many cancer patients, statistical cure is unlikely and treatment is palliative in nature and directed at the prolongation of life. It is appropriate with these patients to think of cancer as a disease of chronic nature in which the duration and the quality of survival become of paramount importance. In treatments with curative intent, one might accept a higher degree of toxicity than would be acceptable for treatments of palliative intent. This might affect decisions regarding dose reduction, treatment delays, or even treatment discontinuation if quality of life is not maintained.

2. CANCER BIOLOGY

Since the 1970s, the biology and pathogenesis of cancer have begun to be elucidated. Investigators have identified many of the molecular mechanisms that lead to the development and spread of malignancies. There are two common features in the pathogenesis of all cancers: the loss of regulation of growth and the ability to locally invade tissues and metastasize. The molecular differences between normal cells and tumor cells are, thus, central to our understanding of how cancer starts and to devising optimal strategies to eliminate it. A common misconception is that cancer cells replicate faster than normal cells. Rather, the growth of malignant tumors appears to result from two factors: (1) lack of appropriate control responses to the signals that normally interrupt the cell cycle and (2) failure of cellular death programming and the response to appropriate stimuli or stresses (apoptosis). The transformation from a normal cell to a tumor cell is now considered to be dependent on mutations in gene products that are important for integrating extracellular and intracellular signals to the cell cycle and cell death machinery and on those gene products involved in directly controlling cell cycle progression. Loss of either type of function will lead to loss of regulatory cell growth signals. The discovery of oncogenes in the 1970s and their overexpression or increased activity in tumor cells led to the suggestion that the abnormality in tumor cells was the presence of too much signal that pushed the cell through the cell cycle. The discovery of tumor suppressive genes in the 1980s added to this model by suggesting that the growth abnormality of tumor cells resulted from a combination of too few cell cycle brakes, (*tumor suppressors*) and too many cell cycle accelerators (*oncogenes*).

From: *Current Clinical Oncology: Cancer in the Spine: Comprehensive Care.*
Edited by: R. F. McLain, K-U. Lewandrowski, M. Markman, R. M. Bukowski, R. Macklis, and E. C. Benzel © Humana Press, Inc., Totowa, NJ

2.1. ONCOGENES IN HUMAN CANCER

Oncogenes are generally thought of as gene products that enhance cell cycle progression. Oncogenes can result from point mutation, overexpression, or translocation. Examples of point mutation oncogenes include the RAS family of oncogenes including: *H-RAS*, *K-RAS*, and *N-RAS*. The *K-RAS* oncogene is mutated in more than 90% of pancreatic adenocarcinoma tumors and a significant number of colon cancers *(1)*. The second major mechanism of increased activity of oncogenes is over expression, which may occur through a variety of genetic mechanisms including chromosome translocation, DNA amplification, and enhanced gene transcription. Some examples include chromosome 8, 14 translocation resulting in c-*myc* oncogene in Burkitt's lymphoma, and plasmacytomas *(2)*. DNA amplification is an important example of oncogene activation in breast cancer in which the *Her-2/neu* oncogene is present in multiple copies within tumor cells of more aggressive tumors *(3)*. The third mechanism of oncogene activation is translocation and fusion. This is the mechanism involved in chronic myelogenous leukemia and the Philadelphia chromosome that results from reciprocal translocation of chromosomes 9q and 22q leading to the fusion between the *ABL* gene on chromosome 9 and the *BCR* gene on chromosome 22. The resulting protein leads to uncontrolled tyrosine kinase activity *(4)*. Another interesting translocation occurs between chromosome 15 and 17 in acute promyelocytic leukemia. As a result of the translocation, there is fusion between the PML gene on chromosome 15 and the retinoic acid receptor (RAR)-α on chromosome 17 *(4)*.

As will be described in Subheadings 4.1.–4.6., many of these oncogenes have been the targets for new therapeutic agents.

2.2. TUMOR SUPPRESSIVE GENES

In contrast to oncogenes, tumor suppressive genes normally act to slow the growth of cells. Loss of activity of such genes through mutation causes deregulation of the cell cycle thus contributing to tumor formation. The best studied of these genes are the retinoblastoma gene, p53 tumor suppressive gene, and the VHL genes *(5,6)*.

3. PRINCIPLES OF CHEMOTHERAPY

The effective use of cancer chemotherapy requires an understanding of the principles of tumor biology, cellular kinetics, pharmacology, and drug resistance. Thanks to this understanding over the last two decades, great successes have been accomplished in the treatment of some cancer types. This is exemplified in the frequently achieved cure in germ cell tumors and lymphomas.

3.1. THE CELL CYCLE

Proliferation results from a cell passing through the cell cycle, undergoing mitosis, and giving rise to two daughter cells. The cell cycle is composed of mitosis and interphase. The latter is a period between mitoses and is composed of G_1, S, and G_2 phases (Fig. 1). The S phase represents the period during which DNA is synthesized resulting in the duplication of the entire DNA content of a cell. During the S phase, the DNA content of diploid human cell goes from 2N to 4N. G_1 and G_2 are the gap phases during which a cell prepares for S phase and mitosis, respectively. During G_1 and G_2, protein and RNA syntheses occur, but the DNA content remains stable. Mitosis is the phase

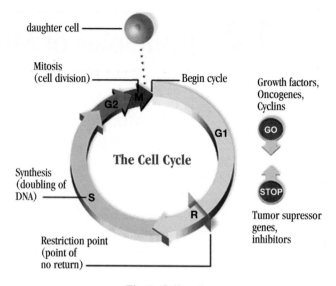

Fig. 1. Cell cycle.

in which the nuclear and cytoplasmic material of a cell are split and divided between two daughter cells. Cells that are not passing through the cell cycle are in G_0 phase. G_0 cells are metabolically active but do not proliferate. Cells may withdraw from the cell cycle in early G_1 and enter G_0 or may be stimulated to exit G_0 and enter the cell cycle at G_1. The cell cycle is a complex but ordered process that is carefully regulated during the transition from one phase of the cycle to another. Generally, one phase of the cycle cannot begin until the previous phase has been successfully completed. Such careful regulation ensures that the DNA is duplicated correctly and subsequently divided equally between two daughter cells.

The rate of growth of a tumor is a reflection of the proportion of actively dividing cells (the growth fraction), the length of the cell cycle (doubling time), and the rate of cell loss. Variations in these three factors are responsible for the variable rates of tumor growth observed among tumors of different histology, as well as among metastatic tumors, and tumors of the same histology.

Tumors characteristically exhibit a sigmoid-shaped Gompertzian growth curve in which tumor-doubling time varies with tumor size. Tumors grow most rapidly at small tumor volumes. As tumors become larger, growth slows based on a complex process depending on cell loss and tumor blood and oxygen supply. Understanding the kinetics of cell proliferation is critical to our understanding of how chemotherapeutic agents work and to the development of combination chemotherapy protocols that are most effective. Agents that are effective only during a particular phase of the cell cycle, such as the S phase of cellular DNA synthesis, are called phase specific. Agents whose effect is prolonged and independent of any specific cell cycle phase are called phase nonspecific. This distinction between specific and nonspecific agents is relative rather than absolute. Phase nonspecific agents can also be subdivided to those agents who are more effective in killing proliferating tissue as opposed to non-proliferating tissue (cycle nonspecific) vs those that show no such specificity (cycle nonspecific) *(7,8)*.

3.2. DRUG RESISTANCE

Multiple mechanisms of chemotherapeutic failure have been identified using tissue culture and many tumor models. The mechanisms are frequently interrelated because altered gene expression underlies most of the cellular and biochemical mechanisms. Cells may also exhibit reduced degree of sensitivity to drugs by virtue of their position in the cell cycle. Cells that are in the G_0 phase are generally resistant to all drugs that are active in the S phase. This phenomenon of kinetic resistance is usually temporary. However, as cells may be recruited into the actively divided compartments and if the drug concentration can be maintained long enough, all cells may eventually pass through the vulnerable phase of the cycle.

In addition, tumor cells may exhibit pharmacological resistance, in which failure to kill cells is a function of insufficient drug concentration. This may occur if the tumor cells are present in body locations where it is difficult to achieve effective drug concentrations, e.g., the central nervous system. Other factors include the altered metabolism of drugs, decreased activation or increased deactivation, or accelerated drug elimination from the cell.

3.2.1. Multiple Drug Resistance

The multiple drug resistance gene (*MDR1*) produces a transmembrane glycoprotein known as P-glycoprotein (Pgp) *(9)*. In the presence of intracellular adenosine triphosphate (ATP), these glycoproteins pump toxic chemicals from the inside of the cell to the extracellular environment. This pump affects a variety of antineoplastic agents, most prominently vinca alkaloids, anthracycline antibiotics, and dactinomycin. The hallmark of this mechanism is the simultaneous acquisition of resistance to all of these agents at the exposure to one member of the group and the lack of cross-resistance for other drugs (e.g., an anti-metabolite, alkylating agent, or bleomycin). The efflux of these agents when caused by Pgp can be inhibited by a variety of agents including calcium-channel antagonists, cyclosporin, calmodulin inhibitors, and other agents. Inhibitors of Pgp are under study in combination with chemotherapy with the aim to reverse drug resistance.

3.2.2. ATYPICAL MULTIPLE DRUG RESISTANCE

Other mechanisms of MDR include changes in drug efflux unrelated to Pgp, changes in drug uptake, and changes in drug metabolism *(10)*. Drug resistance may also occur owing to the over expression of DNA repair genes (e.g., *ERCC1*); altered gene expression; and mechanisms related to host drug interactions, such as increased drug inactivation by normal tissues, and other dose-limiting toxicities related to increased sensitivity of normal tissues to drug (toxicity).

3.3. COMBINATION CHEMOTHERAPY

Most of the successful programs of cancer chemotherapy involve the use of a combination of antineoplastic agents, often according to complex administration schedules. The major rationale for the use of such combinations is tumor cell drug resistance, resulting from biochemical or cytokinetic factors. Most of the successful programs of combination chemotherapy, however, will develop by empirical trial and error. Combination chemotherapy regimens, however, share certain features, which include:

1. Only drugs that are active against the tumor in question as a single agent are included in the combination.
2. Drugs that are generally noncross resistant.
3. Drugs that have different toxicity profiles allowing for the administration of full or nearly full doses of each of the active agents.

4. TARGETED TREATMENT IN CANCER

Although treatments for cancer have evolved significantly over the past decade, the goals of cancer drug development remained fairly constant: optimizing antitumor activity and minimizing side effects. The observation that mustard gases, used in World Wars I and II, caused lymphopenia and splenic involutions, and the findings by Osborn and Huennekens, in 1958, that aminopterin specifically inhibited dihydrofolate reductase, an enzyme essential for DNA and RNA synthesis, inspired the search for drugs that target key pathways in cell development. Advances in technology and a better understanding of the genetic factors that control normal cellular feedback mechanisms, paved the way for the development of targeted treatments with fewer side effects than traditional chemotherapy, good outcomes, and options for outpatient and oral administration.

4.1. ALL-*TRANS*-RETINOIC ACID

Acute promyelocytic leukemia (APL) accounts for approx 10% of acute myeloblastic leukemias in adults and is associated with a high mortality rate as a consequence of frequent intracranial hemorrhages *(11,12)*. In the mid-1970s, Rowley et al. *(12)* linked the occurrence of APL to a balanced and reciprocal translocation between the long arms of chromosomes 15 and 17. In 1987, the RAR-α was mapped to chromosome 17q21, *(13)* and the breakpoints on chromosome 15 clustered in the region of a promyelocytic leukemia (*PML*) gene, a growth suppressor gene *(12,14)*. RAR-α is a DNA binding transcription factor that regulates myeloid differentiation *(15)*. Therefore, the abnormal PML-RAR-α hybrid disrupts the normal function of both these genes and could explain the blast proliferation and the differentiation block at the promyelocytic stage in APL *(15)*.

All-*trans*-retinoic acid (ATRA) is present usually in the plasma at low concentrations, mostly protein bound, and derived by the intracellular oxidation of retinal (vitamin A), which is absorbed from the gastrointestinal tract *(12)*. ATRA has the ability to bind RAR-α and cause the degradation of the abnormal PML-RAR-α receptor resulting in clinical remissions *(15)*. Tallman et al. *(16)* demonstrated improved disease-free and overall survival with ATRA whether as induction or maintenance therapy, compared to chemotherapy alone in patients with newly diagnosed APL. Compared with most anticancer treatments, ATRA is generally well tolerated with few serious side effects *(12)*. These include the potential for the fatal retinoic acid syndrome, which is characterized by fever, respiratory distress, radiographic pulmonary infiltrates, pleural effusion, weight gain, and leukocytosis. The progression of retinoic acid syndrome can be controlled by early steroid administration. *(12)*.

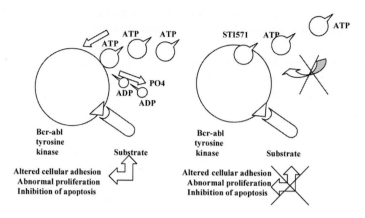

Fig. 2. Proposed mechanism of action of STI-571.

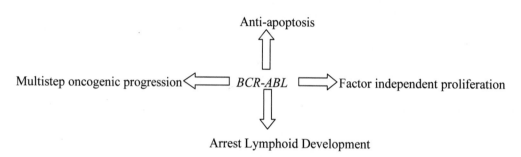

Fig. 3. Proposed function of *BCR-ABL*.

Chronic myeloid leukemia (CML) is characterized by the massive clonal expansion of myeloid cells *(17)* and occurs in three distinct phases: the chronic phase, the accelerated phase, and the blastic phase, in which leukemic cells lose the ability to differentiate. CML is characterized by the presence of the Philadelphia chromosome *(18)*, which was discovered in the 1960s and results from a reciprocal translocation between the long arms of chromosomes 9 and 22 *(17)*. Chromosome 22 carries the *BCR* gene, whereas chromosome 9 carries the *ABL* gene, and encodes for a tightly regulated tyrosine kinase, involved in signal transduction and regulation of cell growth *(19)*. The *BCR-ABL* fusion is translated into a chimeric protein called p210. In CML patients, p210 deregulates tyrosine kinase signaling downstream pathways that mediate the proliferation and transformation of CML hematopoietic progenitor cells (Fig. 2 *[12]*).

Until recently, interferon-α, either alone or in combination with cytarabine, was considered the treatment of choice for CML *(19)*. Stem cell transplantation has also become an effective treatment for a substantial proportion of CML patients, however, it is associated with significant morbidity and mortality *(19)*. Furthermore, blast crisis is highly refractory to treatment with either chemotherapy or stem cell transplantation *(18)*.

Research targeting deregulated tyrosine kinase led to the discovery of STI-571, a potent and selective inhibitor of tyrosine kinase activity. STI-571 functions by competitively inhibiting the ATP-binding site of the tyrosine kinase enzyme, leading to the inhibition of tyrosine phosphorylation of proteins involved in *BCR-ABL* signal transduction (Fig. 3 *[17]*). Therefore STI-571 causes growth arrest and apoptosis in hematopoietic cells expressing the *BCR-ABL* gene without affecting normal cells *(17)*. STI-571 has several advantages over interferon-α. It is an oral medication with faster and more frequent hematologic and cytogenetic responses *(19)*. STI-571 has also demonstrated promising results in gastrointestinal stromal tumors (GIST), which are known to be notoriously resistant to most chemotherapeutic agents. The efficacy of STI-571 in GIST may be explained by the inhibition of the activity of a mutated tyrosine kinase, the *c-kit* tyrosine kinase, which is highly expressed in GIST tumors *(20)*.

The most frequent side effects of STI-571 were nausea, edema, myalgia, and diarrhea *(17)*. Myelosuppression occurred in up to 25% of patients in one study *(17)* and was managed by temporary drug interruption or dose reduction *(17)*. The reason for myelosuppression is thought to be related either to the inhibition of the *c-kit* gene in normal cells or the compromised normal hematopoietic cells in leukemia patients *(17)*.

4.2. MONOCLONAL ANTIBODIES

Monoclonal antibodies (MAbs), "the magic bullets" for treating cancer have changed from being a fiction topic in the 1950s to real therapeutic options. In 1975, Kohler and Milstein *(21)* showed the possibility of producing MAbs capable of binding specific tumor antigens. Initially, they used hybridomas, which result from the fusion of murine splenic cells with a human myeloma cell line. Although, hybridomas were capable

Table 1
Characteristics of Desirable Monoclonal Antibodies

- Specified antigen.
- Low immunogenicity.
- Adequate half-life.
- Ability to recruit immune effector functions or conjugation to toxin or radionucleide.
- Lend themselves to commercial production.

Table 2
Characteristics of an Ideal Antigen

- Expressed only or nearly all tumor cells.
- Not present on critical host cell.
- High copy numbers on cell membranes.
- No mutation or variation.
- Required for cell survival or critical function.
- Not shed or secreted.
- Not modulated after antibody binding.

Table 3
Antibody-Induced Effects

- Direct anti-tumor effects.
  - Induces apoptosis.
  - Inhibits ligand receptor interaction.
  - Enhances the cytotoxic effect of a second agent.
  - Aids the delivery of toxic payloads.
  - Inhibits the expression of some proteins essential for neoplastic cell survival and growth.
- Induction of anti-idiotype network.
- Complement dependent cytotoxicity.
- Antibody-dependent cell-mediated cytotoxicity.

of producing large quantities of MAbs depending on the antigenic challenge, it was only after two decades of experiments that MAbs succeeded as anticancer agents. The first antibodies used in humans included murine, or rat proteins, and led to the development of human antimouse antibodies and human antirat antibodies *(22)*. Newer generation of MAbs include *chimeric* antibodies (formed of antibodies from two different species), or *humanized* antibodies (formed of human antibody containing the complementarity-determining region from a nonhuman source) *(22)*. *Primatized* antibodies are formed of a primate variable region and a human constant region *(22)*.

Antibodies maybe conjugated or unconjugated. Conjugated antibodies are generally linked to either a cytotoxic or a radioactive agent *(23)*. Conjugated antibodies must be internalized into the cells after antigen binding in order for the cytotoxic or radioactive agent to exert its effect. They are also more likely to cause allergic or hypersensitivity reactions. Unconjugated antibodies, on the other hand, remain on the cell surface and rely on the immune system to exert their effect *(23)*. The characteristics of a desirable MAb and an ideal antigen are summarized in the Tables 1 and 2.

The antibody-induced effects can be summarized in Table 3.

4.3. ANTI-CD33

In the United States, it is estimated that the annual incidence of acute myelogenous leukemia (AML) is around 2.4 per 100,000 individuals and this figure increases with age *(24)*.

In the hematopoiesis pathway, a pluripotent stem cell gives rise to a committed precursor cell, which, in turn, is responsible for the production of erythrocytes, platelets, monocytes, and granulocytes. Both, the stem cells and the precursor cells express CD34 antigen. In contrast the CD33 antigen is only present on myeloid precursors and not on the hematopoietic stem cells *(25)*. The CD33 is also present on the blast cells in at least 90% of patients with AML *(26)*, making it an attractive target for selective therapy that could potentially ablate the myeloid leukemic cells and spare the hematopoietic stem cells.

Gemtuzumab ozogamicin is an anti CD33 antibody, attached to calicheamycin, an antitumor antibiotic. Gemtuzumab ozogamicin was developed to target the CD33 antigen. When attaching to the receptor, it results in the formation of a complex that is internalized first, then releases the colicheamycin into the cell resulting in cell death *(27)*. This agent has been approved by the Food and Drug Administration (FDA) for the treatment of relapsed/refractory AML in patients ≥60 yr of age and has shown benefit in treating recurrent AML and as such may benefit many patients. However, it is not clear whether it can cure patients with AML if used as a single agent *(26)*. Several trials are ongoing using gemtuzumab ozogamicin in combination with other chemotherapeutic agents in different stages of disease. Major side effects include severe myelosuppression, with median duration for absolute neutrophil count recovery of 40.5 d and platelet recovery of 39 d in one study *(26)*.

Non-Hodgkin's lymphoma (NHL) is a relatively common form of malignancy. Approximately 80% of NHL patients have B-cell lymphoma, and of these more than 95% of cases express the CD20 differentiation antigen on their tumor cell surfaces *(22)*. CD20 is an ideal target antigen; expressed on B-cell NHL and on normal B cells but not on plasma cells, B-cell precursors, stem cells, or dendritic cells. It is not shed or internalized, and it does not undergo modification following binding to antibody *(28–30)*. The search for an anti-CD20 antigen resulted in the development of a genetically engineered MAb in 1990 *(22)*. The FDA approved Rituximab® in 1997, based on five clinical studies as a single-agent in relapsed or refractory CD20 positive B-cell low-grade or follicular NHL. Rituximab functions by mediating antibody-dependent cell-mediated cytotoxicity (ADCC); it also mediates CDC, inhibits cell growth, sensitizes chemoresistant cells to toxins and chemotherapy, and induces apoptosis in a dose-dependent manner (Fig. 4 *[22]*). Adverse events were mainly infusion related and occurred mostly with the first infusion *(22)*. The most common of these were fever, chills, nausea, fatigue, headache, angioedema, pruritus, and, infrequently, hypotension and bronchospasm *(22)*. There was no significant suppression of blood counts and no increased incidence of infections *(22)*. In patients with high tumor loads, rituximab caused rapid tumor lysis. Currently, there are encouraging results with the combination of Rituximab and standard chemotherapy with no added toxicity reported. In addition,

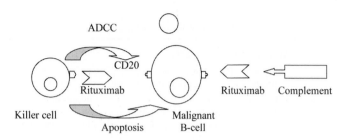

Fig. 4. Proposed mechanism of action of Rituximab®.

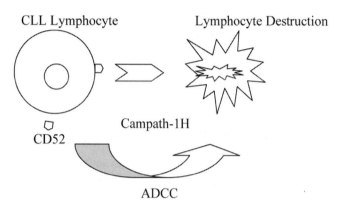

Fig. 5. Proposed mechanism of action of Campath-1H.

good responses have been reported in patients treated with anti-CD20 combined with radioactive substrates *(31)*.

4.4. RITUXIMAB ANTI-CD20 (FIG.4)

Chronic lymphocytic leukemia (CLL) is the most common form of adult leukemia in the Western world, with an estimated annual incidence of 8100 to 12,000 cases. CD52 is an antigen expressed in abundance on most normal lymphocytes both the B- and T-cell lineage as well as on malignant lymphocytes, and monocytes *(22)*, but spares hematopoietic stem cells (Fig. 5). The function of this CD52 is not yet known. Campath-1H, a humanized MAb, was approved by the FDA on May 7, 2001 for the treatment of patients with B-cell CLL who have been treated with alkylating agents and failed fludarabine therapy. It elicits cell death by ADCC after binding to the CD52 receptor on cell membranes. Campath-1H was able to elicit major tumor responses even in the presence of bulky disease, however, it is likely that this MAb will be more used in the context of minimal residual disease following regular chemotherapy or as adjuvant to high dose therapy protocols *(32)*. The most common side effects encountered are infusion related, and are markedly reduced after the first dose *(22)*. However the hematologic side effect is quite significant with prolonged lymphopenia and secondary increase risk of opportunistic infections in pretreated people *(32)*. These infections can be prevented in part by the prophylactic use of antibacterial and antifungal medications *(22)*.

Table 4
Percentage Range of EGFR Expression in Solid Tumors[a]

Tumor Type	Percentage
Bladder	90%
Cervical/uterus	90%
Head and neck	80–100%
Prostate	65%
Renal cell	50–90%
Esophageal	43–89%
Lung	40–80%
Ovarian	35–70%
Pancreatic	30–50%
Colorectal	25–77%
Breast	14–91%

[a]Source: American Cancer Society, 2000.

4.5. CAMPATH 1-H (ANTI-CD 52) (FIG. 5)

Many solid tumors express a type of receptors on their cell membranes, collectively called epidermal growth factor receptors (EGFRs). These are a family of structurally related tyrosine kinase receptors (TKRs). The TKRs integrate a multitude of external stimuli with specific internal signals and responses; the signal transduction ultimately allows the cell to respond correctly to its environment. The TKRs have an extracellular domain for binding ligands, a transmembrane domain, and an intracellular component containing the catalytic tyrosine kinase domain, which is responsible for the generation and regulation of intracellular signaling. It has been suggested and supported by experimental data, that aberrant activation of the kinase activity of these receptors plays a primary role in development and/or progression of human cancer *(33)*. The expression of EGFR in various solid tumors is outlined in Table 4.

One of the members of these EGFR is the HER2 or erbB-2 and is overexpressed in 25 to 30% of patients with breast cancer *(34)*. Patients with breast cancer that carry this overexpressed receptor were found to have a more aggressive disease, significantly shortened disease-free survival, and shortened overall survival *(34)*.

4.6. HERCEPTIN, ANTI-HER2 (FIG. 6)

Herceptin is a recombinant DNA-derived humanized MAb that was approved by the FDA on September 25, 1998 for treating metastatic breast cancer. There are two proposed mechanisms of action (Fig. 6). Herceptin either binds to the erbB2/HER2 receptor and leads to its removal from the cell surface, or causes downregulation of the receptor by internalization into the cell *(35)*. In phase 1 trials, the antibody was reported to be safe and to be confined to the tumor cells *(34)*. The efficacy of this MAb was demonstrated in HER2-positive breast cancer patients when used alone or in combination with standard therapy *(34)*. The most worrisome side effect is cardiac dysfunction, especially in patients pretreated with anthracyclines.

The EGFR is also known as erb-B1. EGFR is stimulated by several ligands, but mostly by EGF and transforming growth factor (TGF)-α *(36)*. EGFR overexpression has been implicated in the development of several solid tumors *(36)*. Activation of the EGFR by its ligands induces a signaling cascade

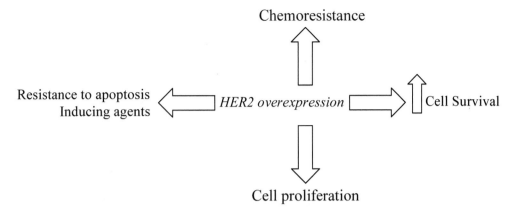

Fig. 6. Proposed *HER2* overexpression effect on tumor cells.

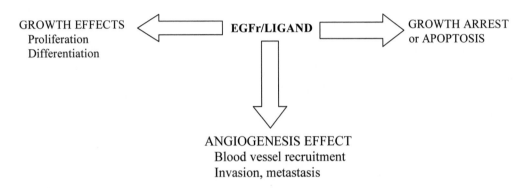

Fig. 7. Proposed function of the EGFR/ligand.

reaction carried by the inherent tyrosine kinase moiety of the receptor leading to DNA synthesis, cell proliferation, differentiation, migration, and neovascularization, all of which are important in the pathogenesis and growth of malignant tumors *(36)*. Drugs targeting this receptor or the receptor-ligand were, therefore, being explored. C225 is a chimeric MAb. It has a higher affinity to the EGFR than either TGF-α or EGF *(36)*. And as such it was used in the treatment of several solid tumors. C225 has a dual mechanism of action; it competes for the binding of the EGFR, and also removes the receptor from the cell membrane by internalization, thus disrupting the cellular process responsible for proliferation, growth, and metastasis (Fig. 7 *[36]*). Side effects with C225 are mild and much less toxic than what is seen with the traditional regimens *(36)*. Several trials are being conducted now using either C225 alone or in combination with other agents in the treatment of many of these solid tumors with favorable results so far *(36)*.

4.7. C225 (FIG. 7)

Another approach to blocking the activity of these EGFR is the use of small molecules designated to inhibit their intracellular domains, that is their tyrosine kinase activity.

By inhibiting these kinases the signal transduction mechanism can be blocked. These newer agents compete with ATP sites on the tyrosine kinase.

ZD-1839 (Iressa) is one of these newer agents. It produces numerous effects on tumor cells expressing erb-B1 (Fig. 8).

4.8. ZD-1839 (FIG. 8)

ZD-1839 has good oral bioavailability and minimal side effects. These include acneform skin eruptions, nausea, vomiting, and diarrhea. It has shown a response rate of 10% when used as monotherapy in advanced non-small cell lung cancer (NSCLC), however resulted in no advantage in terms of response rate or survival vs placebo, when used in combination with chemotherapy in first line treatment of NSCLC *(37)*.

5. SUMMARY

The understanding of tumor biology, cellular kinetics, pharmacology, and drug resistance has helped in the development of several new targeted treatments with fewer side effects, good outcomes, and options for outpatient and oral administration. Several of these targeted treatments have been approved for the treatment of different types of cancers whether as single agents or in combination with traditional chemotherapy with promising results. Ongoing research in tumor biology and signal transduction pathways may ultimately lead to the "magic bullet" and change the approach to cancer treatment.

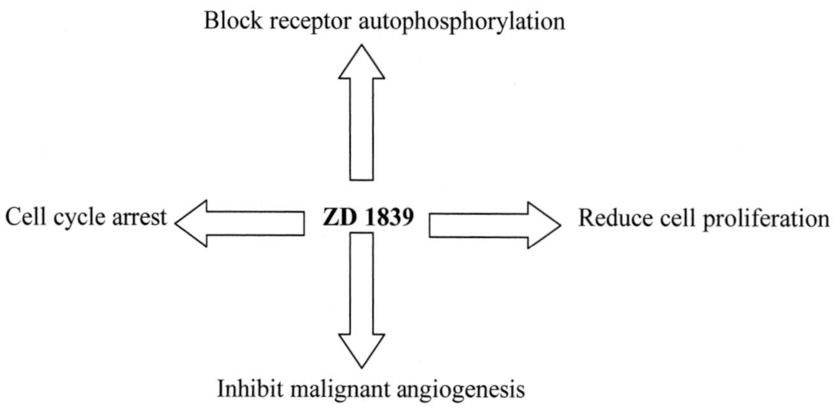

Block receptor autophosphorylation

Cell cycle arrest ⟸   **ZD 1839**   ⟹ Reduce cell proliferation

Inhibit malignant angiogenesis

Fig. 8. Proposed mechanism of action of 2D1839.

REFERENCES

1. Bos JL. Ras oncogenes in human cancer: a review. Cancer Res 1989; 49:4682–4689.

2. Rabbitts TH. Chromosomal translocations in human cancer. Nature 1994; 372:143–149.

3. Slamon DJ, Godolphin W, Jones LA, et al. Studies of the HER-2/neu proto-oncogene in human breast and ovarian cancer. Science 1989; 244:707–712.

4. Fenaux PC, Chomienne C, Degos L. Acute promyelocytic leukemia: biology and treatment. Semin Oncol 1997; 24:92–102.

5. Stanbridge, EJ. Suppression of malignancy in human cells. Nature 1976; 260:17–20.

6. Knudson AG, Jr. Mutation and cancer: statistical study of retinoblastoma. Proc Natl Acad Sci USA 1971; 68:820–823.

7. Bruce WR. The action of chemotherapeutic agents at the cellular level and the effects of these agents on hematopoietic and lymphomatous tissue. Proc Can Cancer Conf 1967; 7:53–64.

8. Valeriote F van Putten L. Proliferation-dependent cytotoxicity of anticancer agents: a review. Cancer Res 1975; 35:2619–2630.

9. Beck WT. The cell biology of multiple drug resistance. Biochem Pharmacol 1987; 36:2879–2887.

10. Moscow JA, Cowan KH. Multidrug resistance. J Natl Cancer Inst 1988; 80:14–20.

11. Stone RM, Mayer RJ. The unique aspects of acute promyelocytic leukemia. J Clin Oncol 1990; 8:1913–1921.

12. Warrell RP, Jr, de The H, Wang ZY, Degos L. Acute promyelocytic leukemia. N Engl J Med 1993; 329:177–189.

13. Mattei MG, Petkovich M, Mattei JF, Brand N, Chambon P. Mapping of the human retinoic acid receptor to the q21 band of chromosome 17. Hum Genet 1988; 80:186–188.

14. Daniel MT, Koken M, Romagne O, et al. PML protein expression in hematopoietic and acute promyelocytic leukemia cells. Blood 1993; 82:1858–1867.

15. Fenaux P, Degos L. Differentiation therapy for acute promyelocytic leukemia. N Engl J Med 1997; 337:1076–1077.

16. Tallman MS, Andersen JW, Schiffer CA, et al. All-trans-retinoic acid in acute promyelocytic leukemia. N Engl J Med 1997; 337:1021–1028.

17. Druker BJ, Talpaz M, Resta DJ, et al. Efficacy and safety of a specific inhibitor of the BCR-ABL tyrosine kinase in chronic myeloid leukemia. N Engl J Med 2001; 344:1031–1037.

18. Druker BJ, Sawyers CL, Kantarjian H, et al. Activity of a specific inhibitor of the BCR-ABL tyrosine kinase in the blast crisis of chronic myeloid leukemia and acute lymphoblastic leukemia with the Philadelphia chromosome. N Engl J Med 2001; 344:1038–1042.

19. Goldman JM, Melo JV. Targeting the BCR-ABL tyrosine kinase in chronic myeloid leukemia. N Engl J Med 2001; 344:1084–1086.

20. Joensuu H, Roberts PJ, Sarlomo-Rikala M, et al. Effect of the tyrosine kinase inhibitor STI571 in a patient with a metastatic gastrointestinal stromal tumor. N Engl J Med 2001; 344:1052–1056.

21. Kohler G, Milstein C. Continuous cultures of fused cells secreting antibody of predefined specificity. Nature 1975; 256:495–497.

22. White CA, Weaver RL, Grillo-Lopez AJ. Antibody-targeted immunotherapy for treatment of malignancy. Annu Rev Med 2001; 52:125–145.

23. Weiner LM. An overview of monoclonal antibody therapy of cancer. Semin Oncol 1999; 26:41–50.

24. Hernandez JA. Land KJ, McKenna RW. Leukemias, myeloma, and other lymphoreticular neoplasms. Cancer 1995; 75:381–394.

25. Andrews RG, Takahashi M, Segal GM, Powell JS, Bernstein ID, Singer JW. The L4F3 antigen is expressed by unipotent and multipotent colony-forming cells but not by their precursors. Blood 1986; 68:1030–1035.

26. Dinndorf PA, Andrews RG, Benjamin D, Ridgway D, Wolff L, Bernstein ID. Expression of normal myeloid-associated antigens by acute leukemia cells. Blood 1986; 67:1048–1053.

27. Naito K, Takeshita A, Shigeno K, et al. Calicheamicin-conjugated humanized anti-CD33 monoclonal antibody (gemtuzumab zogamicin, CMA-676) shows cytocidal effect on CD33-positive leukemia cell lines, but is inactive on P-glycoprotein-expressing sublines. Leukemia 2000 14:1436–1443.

28. Anderson KC, Bates MP, Slaughenhoupt BL, Pinkus GS, Schlossman SF, Nadler LM. Expression of human B cell-associated antigens on leukemias and lymphomas: a model of human B cell differentiation. Blood 1984; 63:1424–1433.

29. Press OW, Appelbaum F, Ledbetter JA, et al. Monoclonal antibody 1F5 (anti-CD20) serotherapy of human B cell lymphomas. Blood 1987; 69:584–591.

30. Einfeld DA, Brown JP, Valentine MA, Clark EA, Ledbetter JA. Molecular cloning of the human B cell CD20 receptor predicts a hydrophobic protein with multiple transmembrane domains. EMBO J 1988; 7:711–717.

31. Press OW. Radiolabeled antibody therapy of B-cell lymphomas. Semin Oncol 1999; 26:58–65.

32. Dyer MJ. The role of CAMPATH-1 antibodies in the treatment of lymphoid malignancies. Semin Oncol 1999; 26:52–57.

33. Schlessinger J. Cell signaling by receptor tyrosine kinases. Cell 2000; 103211–225.

34. Slamon DJ, Leyland-Jones B, Shak S, et al. Use of chemotherapy plus a monoclonal antibody against HER2 for metastatic breast cancer that overexpresses HER2. N Engl J Med 2001; 344:783–792.

35. Harari D, Yarden Y. Molecular mechanisms underlying ErbB2/HER2 action in breast cancer. Oncogene 2000; 19:6102–6114.

36. Waksal HW. Role of an anti-epidermal growth factor receptor in treating cancer. Cancer Metastasis Rev 1999; 18:427–436.

37. Ciardiello F, Caputo R, Bianco R, et al. Inhibition of growth factor production and angiogenesis in human cancer cells by ZD1839 (Iressa), a selective epidermal growth factor receptor tyrosine kinase inhibitor. Clin Cancer Res 2001; 7:1459–1465.

13 Multiple Myeloma and Plasmacytoma

Mohamad Hussein, MD

CONTENTS

1. INTRODUCTION

Multiple myeloma (MM) is a clonal disorder of B-cell lymphocytic lineage characterized by malignant transformation of plasma cells. It accounts for approx 10% of all the hematological malignancies and 1% of all cancers in the United States. In the year 2000, MM was diagnosed in approx 13,700 people in the United States and accounted for 20% of deaths from hematological malignancies *(1)*. The median age of onset is 68 yr. It is slightly more frequent in women and the incidence in African-Americans is twice that of Whites. Both the overall incidence and specifically the incidence in African-Americans have been rising in recent years. A recent study explored whether dietary factors contribute to the risk of MM and the twofold higher incidence among Blacks compared with Whites in the United States. Data from a food frequency questionnaire were analyzed for 346 White and 193 Black subjects with MM, and 1086 White and 903 Black controls who participated in a population-based case–control study of MM in three areas of the United States. This study concluded that the greater use of vitamin C supplements by Whites and the higher frequency of obesity among Blacks may explain part of the higher incidence of MM among Blacks compared to Whites in the United States. In addition, the increasing prevalence of obesity may have contributed to the upward trend in the incidence of MM during recent decades *(2)*.

2. ETIOLOGY

Several agents have shown an association with the development of MM though causation has not been proven. Of the possible etiological agents, ionizing radiation probably has the strongest link to the causation of MM as evidenced by the five times elevated risk of MM in atomic bomb survivors. Exposure to nickel, benzene, aromatic hydrocarbons, agricultural chemicals, and silicon are other potential risk factors. Proven contribution of each of these agents to the total number of MM cases is, however, very small.

Monoclonal gammopathy of unknown significance is considered a premalignant condition though very few of these patients actually progress to MM.

Cytogenetic studies using chromosomal banding techniques show an abnormal karyotype in only 30% of MM patients. More recent studies using a more sensitive fluorescent *in situ* hybridization show abnormalities in 80% of MM patients. Abnormalities involving chromosome 13 are the most frequent and have the worst prognosis. 13q14 was the commonest abnormality reported in one study. A single tumor suppressor gene mutation connected with malignant transformation is yet to be identified. It is possible that cumulative mutational genetic damage may finally result in malignant transformation. Families with clusters of myeloma cases are rare.

Interleukin (IL)-6 is an important cytokine in myeloma cell growth and proliferation *(3)*. Close cell-to-cell contact between myeloma cells and the bone marrow stromal cells triggers a large amount of IL-6 production, which supports the growth of these cells, as well as protects them from apoptosis induced by dexamethasone or other chemotherapeutic agents *(4)*. IL-6, however, is not an absolute requirement for the proliferation of myeloma cells and anti-IL-6 antibody has not been shown to provide much clinical benefit *(5)*. A recent study shows that vascular endothelial growth factor (VEGF), in addition to its known stimulation of bone marrow angiogenesis, also has direct effects on MM cells. The results of this study suggest that VEGF stimulates proliferation and migration of MM cells

From: *Current Clinical Oncology: Cancer in the Spine: Comprehensive Care.*
Edited by: R. F. McLain, K-U. Lewandrowski, M. Markman, R. M. Bukowski,
R. Macklis, and E. C. Benzel © Humana Press, Inc., Totowa, NJ

in both autocrine and paracrine mechanisms. Within the bone marrow, VEGF is produced by both MM cells and bone marrow stromal cells. IL-6 secreted by bone marrow stromal cells enhances the production and secretion of VEGF by MM cells; conversely, VEGF secreted by MM cells enhances IL-6 production by bone marrow stromal cells. Moreover, binding of MM cells to bone marrow stromal cells enhances both IL-6 and VEGF secretion, suggesting an autocrine VEGF loop (6). Therefore treatment strategies targeting the different cytokines involved in the growth and development of the myeloma cell is currently being investigated.

3. PATHOGENESIS OF BONE DISEASE IN MM

Osteoclasts accumulating on the surfaces adjacent to myeloma cells are responsible for the bone destruction in MM. Increased osteoclast activity is not seen in bones that are free of tumor. There is in addition of impaired osteoblast activity. Multiple potential osteoclast activating factors have been identified. These include tumor necrosis factor (TNF)-β, receptor activator of nuclear factor (NF)-κB (RANK) ligand, IL-1-β, parathyroid hormone-related protein promoter (PTHrP), hepatocyte growth factor, IL-6, TNF-α, matrix metalloproteinases (MMP1, MMP2, and MMP9), as well as insulin-like growth factors-IV. None of these factors shows consistent correlation with either bone disease or with overall disease progression. The cell–cell interaction between MM cells and the marrow stroma cell is important in the production of the osteoclast activating factor (7).

4. CLINICAL FEATURES

The presenting clinical manifestations of MM are subtle and variable. They reflect both the direct and indirect consequences of abnormal plasma cell infiltration.

Anemia is found initially in two-thirds of patients diagnosed with multiple myeloma (8). Patients with multiple myeloma and anemia can experience easy fatigability, decreased energy level, dizziness, impaired cognitive function, respiratory distress, and cardiac decompensation, all of which can diminish the patient's quality of life (9).

The cause for the anemia in multiple myeloma is likely complex and multifactorial. Its morphology is usually that of a normocytic and normochromic anemia, but megaloblastic and macrocytic anemia have been described in the literature (10–12).The cytopenias of MM are a result of multiple factors including marrow infiltration by plasma cells, renal failure, chemotherapy, anemia of chronic disease, and the inhibitory effect of cytokines such as IL-6 and IL-1. The serum erythropoietin levels are low relative to the amount of anemia. The blood smear on MM patients characteristically shows excess rouleaux formation. Bleeding manifestations are seen owing to thrombocytopenia, coagulopathy, which are more common in immunoglobulin (Ig)A myeloma and hyperviscosity syndrome.

Hypercalcemia is the presenting feature in 15 to 30% of MM cases and manifests as nausea, vomiting, constipation, thirst, polyuria, and lethargy. A low albumin level can mask true hypercalcemia, whereas abnormal calcium binding by paraproteins can cause a spurious hypercalcemia. It is prudent to measure calcium levels when in doubt. Hypercalcemia in MM patients usually is a marker of bone disease and high tumor burden. Unlike humor hypercalcemia of malignancy, parathyroid hormone-like peptide is not involved in the hypercalcemia of MM.

Hyperviscosity is more often seen in IgA myeloma owing to the tendency of these monoclonal proteins to form polymers or in IgG myeloma of subclass 3. It can manifest as renal insufficiency, neurological signs, pulmonary edema, and a bleeding disorder. Examination of retinal veins shows sluggish circulation. Measuring serum viscosity should confirm the diagnosis.

MM patients have a high risk of infections because of a poor humoral immune response with additional T-cell and natural killer (NK) cell defects, exposure to chemotherapy, and steroids. Although the encapsulated organisms such as *Streptococcus pneumoniae* and *Haemophilus influenzae* are more classically associated with MM, gram negative bacilli are, in practice, the most common isolates. Fungal infections by organisms such as *Candida* are also frequent.

MM usually involves the axial skeleton and the proximal ends of the long bones. Involvement of the distal extremities is uncommon. Almost any bone of the body can, however, be involved and almost 30% of MM patients have non-vertebral fractures. Three patterns of bone involvement have been described. The classic appearance is that of punched out osteolytic lesions. Generalized osteoporosis usually accompanies lytic lesions, but in 20% it may be the only manifestation of MM bone disease. Finally, an osteosclerotic pattern of bone disease in MM has been described in association with the polyneuropathy, organomegaly, endocrinopathy, monoclonal gammopathy, and scleroderma (POEMS) syndrome.

More than two-thirds of myeloma patients present with bone pains and, in many cases, the skeletal disease will significantly affect the quality of life. The pain is related to activity and usually does not occur at night except with movement. The pain is usually the result of pathological fractures accompanied by muscle spasms and at times because of MM cell infiltration in bones. These patients also present with radicular pain in the thoracic or lumbar regions. Rib fractures are often precipitated by coughing and can cause pleuritic pain. Skull involvement is commonly seen on radiology but it is usually clinically silent. Vertebral involvement can also present with painless compression fractures and a kyphotic deformity resulting in the loss of height. These patients will also manifest restrictive lung functions from the changes in the chest cavity.

Compression of the spinal cord may result from posterior extension of the vertebral tumor or from retropulsion of the fractured vertebral body. In 5% of patients, the cause of spinal cord compression is an extradural plasmacytoma. Warning signs of impending spinal cord compression are severe back pain, band like pain, progressive weakness and paresthesias of lower limbs, and urinary incontinence. This constitutes a medical emergency requiring or magnetic resonance imaging or computed tomography scans to determine the cause and radiotherapy or neurosurgery to decompress the spine.

Extramedullary plasmacytomas are soft tissue masses consisting of clusters of the malignant plasma cells. They are usually seen in pleura, mediastinum, or abdomen where they are also known to cause destruction of adjacent bones. Osteosclerotic myelomas usually detected when the biopsy of an osteosclerotic lesion reveals plasma cells. It is usually associated with the POEMS syndrome. The MM in these patients is characterized by low levels of plasma cells in the marrow and low levels of monoclonal proteins. Treatment is with aggressive treatment of isolated bone lesions (radiotherapy or surgery) and avoiding agents toxic to nerves in any systemic therapy.

Bone plasmacytoma is an isolated collections of clonal plasma cells with no evidence of bone disease elsewhere, absence of marrow plasmacytosis, monoclonal proteins that are either absent or disappear after treatment of the plasmacytoma, and no evidence of hypercalcemia. Local treatment with external beam radiation is the standard approach to such tumors. More than 50% of these patients will eventually develop overt MM.

5. DIAGNOSIS AND STAGING

The minimal diagnostic criteria for MM include either:

- Bone marrow plasma cells >10%.
- Solitary plasmacytoma with the typical clinical picture of MM with at least one of the following present:
  - Serum M protein (>3 gm/dL).
  - Urine M proteins (usually >1 g/dL).
  - Lytic bone lesions.

Table 1 gives the diagnostic criteria.

The median survival for MM without treatment is 7 mo. With the use of chemotherapy and good supportive care, the median survival is 36 to 48 mo and up to 7 yr in specialized centers. The standard Durie-Salmon staging system (Table 1) is based on factors that correlate with the total tumor load. Patients presenting in stage I have a low tumor load and have a median survival of 5 yr, whereas a patient in stage IIIB disease is likely to have a median survival of 15 mo. This staging system has been widely used for several years, but seems to have several shortcomings. An alternative simpler staging system (Table 2) has been proposed based on β-2-microglobulin (β2M) and albumin levels. Patients showing complex and cytogenetic abnormalities show a worse prognosis. The plasma cell labeling index is also an independent predictor of long term survival.

6. INVESTIGATIONS

Monoclonal proteins are the hallmark of MM. One percent of MM patients are unable to secrete monoclonal proteins because of a defect in the assembly or secretion mechanisms. The serum electrophoresis pattern is altered by a spike of monoclonal protein (M band) usually in the γ-globulin region and is associated with a flattening of the rest of the γ-globulin curve. (Fig. 1). Serum electrophoresis may give a fail to show a M-spike in 20%. Immunoelectrophoresis of serum and urine is much more sensitive and can quantify the monoclonal proteins. The combined use of these tests will correctly identify the paraprotein in 99% of patients. The common monoclonal proteins seen in MM are IgG (55%), IgA (25%), and light chain disease (20%). κ-light chains are secreted twice as often as λ.

The monoclonal Igs are too large to be filtered in the glomerulus and, therefore cannot be detected in the urine. The plasma

Table 1
Criteria for Multiple Myeloma Diagnosis

Major criteria

Plasmacytoma	
Marrow plasmacytosis	>30%
Monoclonal proteins	
IgG	>3.5 g/dL
IgA	>2 g/dL
Bence Jones	>1 g/24 h

Minor criteria

Marrow plasmacytosis	10–29%
Lytic bone lesions	
Monoclonal proteins present but less than	
for major criteria	
Decrease in other immunoglobulins	

Diagnosis: 2 major/1 major + 1 minor/3 minor

IgA, immunoglobulin A; IgG, immunoglobulin G.

Table 2
Durie-Slamon Staging

	Stage I	Stage II	Stage III
Hb gm/dL	>10	8.5–10	<8.5
Monoclonal proteins g/dL			
IgG	<5	5–7	>7
IgA	<3	3–5	>5
Bence Jones (24 h)	<4	4–12	>12
Calcium	Normal	>12	
Lytic lesions	–ve	–ve	+ve

β2M (mg/L)	Albumin (g/dL)	Median survival (months)
<2.5		58
2.5–5.5		38
>5.5	>3.0	25
>5.5	<3.0	16

Each stage is subclassified as A or B. Presence of abnormal blood urea nitrogen or creatinine indicates subclass B. IgA, immunoglobulin A; IgG, immunoglobulin G.

cells secrete and excessive amount of light chains, which are small enough to pass through the glomeruli and can be detected as Bence-Jones proteins in the urine. The classic methods of Bence-Jones protein detection in the urine have to be replaced by urine immune electrophoresis. Twenty-four-hour urine protein excretion is, thus, a useful surrogate marker of light chain excretion in the urine.

The patients with MM are likely to show pancytopenia with anemia occurring early and thrombocytopenia occurring in an advanced stage. Granulocytopenia is common but mild. The sedimentation rate is disproportionately high for the degree of anemia.

The patients will typically have elevated serum globulins with hypoalbuminemia and inversion of the A:G ratio. An elevated lactic acid dehydrogenase is seen in 10 to 15% of MM patients

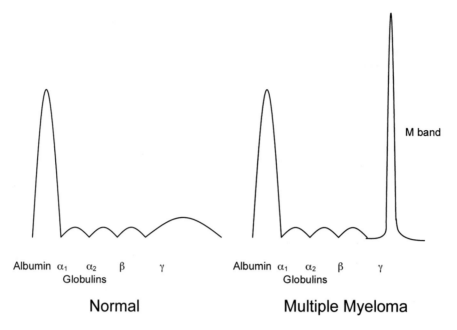

Fig. 1. Serum electrophoresis.

and correlates with a poor prognosis. Blood urea and creatinine levels reflect the presence of renal dysfunction.

The bone marrow biopsy is essential to establish the diagnosis of MM. The plasma cells characteristically will stain selectively for λ- or κ-light chains only (light chain restriction) reflecting their clonal origin. Cytogenetic studies can be performed on the biopsy specimen. A plasma cell labeling index less than or equal to 0.8% indicates a good prognosis.

At the time of diagnosis a bone survey will reveal lytic lesions in at least 70% of patients with MM, whereas 20% will show evidence of generalized bone demineralization only. Approximately 10% of the patients will have normal radiographs at presentation. An osteoblastic reaction resulting in osteoclastic myeloma is rare (1.4%). It is usually seen in the context of the POEMS syndrome as previously mentioned.

7. TREATMENT

Therapy for MM can be artificially divided in to active care and supportive care. The active care can be further divided in to an induction phase and a maintenance phase. This latter division is because of the fact that MM is an incurable disease. With this algorithm in mind, we will briefly discuss the new and upcoming aspects of each category.

7.1. ACTIVE THERAPY

7.1.1. Bone Marrow Transplant

Allogeneic bone marrow transplant for MM should be used in a research setting. More than 90% of MM patients are ineligible owing to high age, lack of human leukocyte antigen-matched sibling donor, or comorbidity. In addition, it is associated with high treatment associated morbidity and mortality (13).

The results of autologous stem cell transplants in MM are perplexing. The French myeloma group randomized 200 untreated myeloma patients to auto bone marrow transplant or conventional chemotherapy. Twenty-five precent of those randomized to the transplant arm did not receive one. The overall survival was superior in the transplant group (52 vs 12%), but was related to the β2M level suggesting that patient selection may be a bias in the results (14). A timely second high-dose therapy appears to be an important factor in the outcome of tandem transplant. When serial landmark analyses were performed at 11, 12, 13,14, 15, and 16 mo, both event-free survival and overall survival were longer among the patients who had received a second transplant within 13 mo (when nearly 85% of second transplants had been completed) compared with the others receiving their second cycle of high-dose therapy later or not at all. The proportion of high-risk patients (unfavorable cytogenetics and high β2M) was not different regardless of whether a second transplant had been performed at any of the landmarks examined. Interestingly, the difference in outcome between the group completing a second transplant and the remaining patients gradually emerged by 12 mo and was lost by 15 mo (15). This pattern supports the results of the Cox regression model that identified timelines of a second transplant as a significant variable for clinical outcome. More recently, performing a second transplant within 3 mo affects the complete remission as well as the overall outcome of therapy (16). The delay to the second transplant could be related to the cumulative toxicity of the induction and harvest regimens. Grade III/IV extramedullary toxicities was noted in one-third of the patients treated with vincristine, adriamycin, and dexamethasone (VAD) and in approximately two-thirds of those treated with high-dose Cytoxan. Further, more two-thirds of the patients treated with the first high-dose therapy utilizing Melphalan at 200 mg/m^2 experienced grade III/IV toxicity. Eliminating chemotherapy from the induction regimen, modifying the preharvest chemotherapy could potentially decrease the toxicity, and allow for a larger number of patients to receive the targeted therapy in a timely fashion. Moreover, a biological regimen that could influence the tumor biology could potentially have a major impact on the response to chemotherapy *(17)*. The Mayo and the M.D. Anderson groups investigated the role of Thalidomide with and without Dexamethasone in newly diagnosed myeloma patients. A 64 to 72% response rate with minimal toxicity was achieved *(18,19)*. Substituting this regimen for VAD should decrease toxicity, and could potentially change the tumor microenvironment and biology to allow for a better response rate. This approach is currently under investigation by our group through the South West Oncology Group.

7.1.2. Chemotherapy

Myeloma patients with signs of progression such as increasing M protein levels or evidence of anemia, hypercalcemia, renal insufficiency, lytic bone lesions, or extramedullary plasmacytomas need to be treated. There is a subgroup of patients with smoldering myeloma in stage IA who can be watched until progression.

The goal of treatment is to prolong survival and to palliate symptoms. The best measure of response in myeloma is by documenting reduction in M protein concentration in blood (objective response >25%, partial response >50%, and complete response >75%) and by documenting reduced 24-h protein excretion in the urine in association with stable or improved anemia, bone disease, and hypercalcemia. Responders to chemotherapy show a distinct survival advantage over nonresponders, but neither the speed nor response or the degree of response seemed to influence survival (20). It is now believed that achieving a disease-stabilization or a plateau phase defined as period of disease stability after chemotherapy of at least 4 to 6 mo correlates best with survival.

Conventional chemotherapy for MM consists or oral melphalan with prednisone (MP) given for 5 to 7 d every 6 wk. It usually takes three to four cycles to get to a plateau. It produces a response in 50 to 60% of patients and is fairly well tolerated. To improve the on this response rate, various combination chemotherapy therapy (CCT) regimen were developed in the 1970s and 1980s. In 1998, an overview of 6633 patients from 27 randomized trials comparing CCT with MP showed them to be equivalent in terms of survival in both low- and high-risk MM patients. There is no evidence of benefit of maintenance chemotherapy after attaining a plateau. Unnecessary chemotherapy exposes a patient to the risks of secondary leukemia and drug resistance. Several small trials have evaluated the role of interferon-α in maintenance regimen with widely conflicting results. Most of these trials were underpowered and thus an overview of the individual patient data from 24 randomized trials and 4012 patients was undertaken to resolve these conflicting results *(21)*. Median time to progression was improved with interferon, but the survival benefit was not. Any benefit of long-term interferon needs to be balanced against cost and toxicity of interferon maintenance.

The most effective treatment in patients with relapsed myeloma is a combination of VAD, which has shown a response in 50 to 60% of these patients. The response is shorter lived than in newly treated patients *(22)*.

7.1.3. Bisphosphonate Use in MM

Chemically, the bisphosphonates have a backbone of phosphorus-carbon-phosphorus, which allows it to bind to the bone mineral exposed in the resorption lacunes by the osteoclasts. The osteoclasts cell function is disrupted as they internalize the bisphosphonate present in an extremely high concentration *(23)*. The bisphosphonates have been show to induce apoptosis in the osteoclasts *(24)*. Secretion of cytokines such as IL-6, which may have a role not only in stimulating osteoclasts, but are also important for MM cell survival, is downregulated.

In a study, 62 newly diagnosed MM patients were randomly assigned to either chemotherapy with or without monthly palmidronate. Patients treated with the combination showed significant reduction of *N*-telopeptide (marker of bone resorption), IL-6, and paraprotein level in 3 mo and of β2M and skeletal events in 6 mo *(25)*. These results are confirmed after long term follow-up of stage III MM patients randomized to chemotherapy alone or combined with palmidronate. After a median follow-up of 21 mo, patients treated with palmidronate had fewer skeletal events (pathological fracture, radiation or surgery to bone, and spinal cord compression) *(26)*. Interestingly, MM patients on second-line chemotherapy at the time of trial entry lived longer in the monthly palmidronate arm of the study (14 vs 21 mo, *p* = 0.041).

Zolendronate is a new highly potent bisphosphonate. In the treatment of hypercalcemia of malignancy zolindronatic acid 4 mg was superior to palmidronate 90 mg in needing shorter infusion time, earlier response, and longer duration of response *(27)*. In Durie-Salmon stage III patients with at least one bony lesion, zolendronate was as effective as palmidronate in reducing skeletal events in 13 mo and, interestingly, was superior in reducing the bone resorption factors.

Osteoprotegerin (OPG) is an alternative to bisphosphonates in treating skeletal metastatic disease. It binds and inactivates the OPG ligand, which is an essential factor required for osteoclast differentiation. OPG has been shown to oppose the bone resorption resulting from parathyroid hormone (PTH), PTHrP, $1,25(OH)2D3$, TNF-α, and IL-1B. This compound is currently under investigation.

7.1.4. Radiation

For the majority of patients excellent pain control can be achieved with external beam radiation. The exact dose and schedule of such radiotherapy is not standardized. A single dose of 8 gy has been shown to be effective *(28)*. Usually a 30 gy dose will be given in 10 fractions.

Radiopharmaceuticals such as Stroncium[89] and Samarium[153], which is linked to the bisphosphonate ethylene diamine tetramethylene phosphonic acid are preferentially taken up at sites of new bone formation and have been studied in prostate and breast cancer patients with bone metastasis. They are not likely to be as effective in MM in which the osteoblast activity is suppressed.

7.1.5. Surgery

Patients who have long standing lytic lesions, especially the ones that are at a high risk for pathological fractures in weight bearing bones should be evaluated by an orthopedic surgeon for prophylactic fixation. Pain that increases with movement is a sign of impending fracture. The risk of fracture increases if more than 30% of the bone diameter is effected by the bone lesion. The fracture risk is a dramatic 80% if more than 50% of the bone diameter is destroyed.

Prophylactic fixation of an impending fracture is simpler and safer than surgery after a pathological fracture. This prevents unnecessary pain and morbidity for the patient and the rehabilitation is much faster. Surgery is usually followed by external beam radiation to prevent tumor regrowth.

There is no evidence that surgery predisposes these patients to tumor progression or dissemination.

Kyphoplasty is associated with early pain control, early functional recovery and restoration of vertebral body height. At the Cleveland Clinic 18 MM patients underwent 55 kyphoplasty procedures with restoration of on average 34% of height and significant improvement in SF36 scores for bodily pain, physical function, vitality, and social functioning *(24)*.

REFERENCES

1. Landis SH, Murray T, Bolden S, Wingo PA. Cancer statistics. CA Cancer J Clin 1999; 49:8–31.
2. Brown LM, Gridley G, Pottern LM, et al. Diet and nutrition as risk factors for multiple myeloma among blacks and whites in the United States. Cancer Causes Control 2001; 12:117–125.
3. Anderson KC, Lust JA. Role of cytokines in multiple myeloma. Semin Hematol 1999; 36:14–20.
4. Grigorieva I, Thomas X, Epstein J. The bone marrow stromal environment is a major factor in myeloma cell resistance to dexamethasone. Exp Hematol 1998; 26:597–603.
5. Bataille R, Barlogie B, Lu ZY, et al. Biologic effects of anti-IL-6 murine monoclonal antibody in advanced multiple myeloma. Blood 1995; 86:685–691.
6. Podar K, Tai Y, Davies FE, et al. Vascular endothelial growth factor triggers signaling cascades mediating multiple myeloma cell growth and migration. Blood 2001; 98:428–435.
7. Roodman GD. Biology of osteoclast activation in cancer. J Clin Oncol 2001; 19:3562–3571.
8. Kyle RA. Multiple myeloma: review of 869 cases. Mayo Clinic Proc 1975; 50:29–40.
9. Dammacco F, Castoldi G, Rodjer S. Efficacy of epoetin alfa in the treatment of anemia of multiple myeloma. Br J Haematol 2001; 113:172–179.
10. William JW, Beutler E, Ersler AJ, Roudles RW. Hematologia. 1st ed. 1975:968–1002.
11. Gomez AR, Harley JB. Multiple myeloma and pernicious anemia. W V Med J 1970; 66:38–41.
12. Miramon Lopez J., Ruiz Cantero A., Morales Jimenez J., Lara Fernandez A., Hita Perez J. [A new case of association of multiple myeloma and megaloblastic anemia.] An Med Interna 1999; 16:654–655.
13. Gharton G, Tura S, Svensson H, et al. Allogeneic bone marrow transplantation in multiple myeloma: an update of the EBMT registry. Boston, MA: Harvard Medical School. Sixth International Workshop on Multiple Myeloma. Syllabus, Boston, MA, 1997, June 14–18.
14. Blade J, San Miguel JF, Fontanillas M, et al. Survival of multiple myeloma patients who are potential candidates for early high-dose therapy intesification/autotransplantation and who were conventionally treated. J Clin Oncol 1996; 14:2167–2173
15. Barlogie B, Jagannath S, Desikan KR, et al. Total therapy with tandem transplants for newly diagnosed multiple myeloma. Blood 1999; 93:55–65.
16. Attal M, Harousseau JL, Facon T, et al. Single versus double transplant in myeloma: a randomized trial of the "Inter Groupe Francais Du Myélome" (IFM). Blood 1999; 94:714a.
17. Hideshima T, Chauhan D, Shima Y, et al. Thalidomide and its analogs overcome drug resistance of human multiple myeloma cells to conventional therapy Blood 2000; 96:2943–2950.
18. Rajkumar SV, Hayman S, Gertz MA, et al. Combination therapy with thalidomide plus dexamethasone for newly diagnosed myeloma. J Clin Oncol 2002; 20:4319–4323.
19. Weber D, Rankin K, Gavino M, Delasalle K, Alexanian R. Thalidomide alone or with dexamethasone for previously untreated multiple myeloma. J Clin Oncol 2003; 21:16–19.
20. Bladé J, López-Guillermo A, Bosch F, et al. Impact of response to treatment on survival in multiple myeloma: Results in a series of 243 patients. Br J Haematol 1994; 88:117–121.
21. Myeloma Trialists' Collaborative Group. Interferon as therapy for multiple myeloma: an individual patient data overview of 24 randomized trials and 4012 patients. Br J Haematol 2001; 113:1020–1034.
22. Barlogie B, Smith L, Alexanian R. Effective treatment of advanced multiple myeloma refractory to alkylating agents. N Engl J Med 1984; 310:1353–1356.
23. Rogers MJ, Watts DJ, Russell RG. Overview of bisphosphonates. Cancer 1997; 80:1652–1660.
24. Yoneda T, Michigami T, Yi B, et al. Use of bisphosphonates for the treatment of bone metastasis in experimental animal models. Cancer Treat Rev 1999; 25:293–299.
25. Terpos E, Palmermos J, Tsionos K, et al. Effect of palmidronate administration on markers of bone turnover and disease activity in multiple myeloma. Eur J Haematol 2000; 65:331–336.
26. Berenson JR, Lichtenstein A, Porter L, et al. Long-term pamidronate treatment of advanced multiple myeloma patients reduces skeletal events: Myeloma Aredia Study Group. J Clin Oncol 1998; 16:593–602.
27. Major P, Lortholary A, Hon, J et al. Zolendronic acid is superior to palmidronate in the treatment of hypercalcemia of malignancy: A pooled analysis of two randomized controlled clinical trials. J Clin Oncol 2001; 19:558–567.
28. Janjan NA. Radiation for bone metastases: conventional techniques and the role of systemic radiopharmaceuticals. Cancer 1997; 80:1628–1645.
29. Dudeney S, Hussein M, Karam MA, et al. Kyphoplasty in the treatment of vertebral compression fractures due to multiple myeloma. 8th Inernational Myeloma Workshop, Banff, Canada 2001, May 4–8: Abstract P156.

14 Lymphoma

RONALD M. SOBECKS, MD

CONTENTS

1. EPIDEMIOLOGY AND ETIOLOGY

In the year 2002 there was an estimated 60,900 new cases of lymphoma in the United States, with 53,900 cases of non-Hodgkin's lymphoma (NHL) and 7000 cases of Hodgkin's lymphoma *(1)*. Estimated deaths in 2002 for NHL and Hodgkin's lymphoma were 24,400 and 1400, respectively. The male to female ratio for both NHL and Hodgkin's lymphoma is presently 1.1:1. Although the incidence of Hodgkin's lymphoma has remained stable over the past several decades, there has been an increasing incidence of NHL in North America at a rate of approx 2 to 3% per year. NHL comprises 4% of male and female cancers in the United States, being the fifth most common malignancy among women (after breast, lung, colorectal, and uterine) and the sixth most common among men (after prostate, lung, colorectal, urinary bladder, and melanoma) *(1)*.

With the exception of Burkitt and lymphoblastic lymphoma, that are more often seen in children and young adults, the median age at presentation for NHL is older than 50 yr *(2)*. By contrast, Hodgkin's lymphoma has a bimodal age curve, with an initial age peak at 15 to 35 yr and a second smaller peak after age 50 *(3)*.

The exact etiology for both Hodgkin's lymphoma and NHL remains unknown. Epstein-Barr virus has been postulated to be involved in the pathogenesis of Hodgkin's and Burkitt's lymphoma, as well as many of the lymphomas that are related to acquired immunodeficiency syndrome (AIDS) or transplant immunosuppression *(2,3)*. Other risk factors for the development of NHL include other viruses such as human immunodeficiency virus (HIV), human T-cell leukemia virus (HTLV)-1, hepatitis C virus, human herpes virus 8, as well as congenital immunodeficiency, immunosuppression for organ transplants, and autoimmune diseases. Environmental factors such as pesticides, herbicides, organic chemicals (e.g., benzene), wood

preservatives, and prior chemotherapy or radiation therapy have been associated with the development of NHL *(4)*. In addition, chromosomal translocations and molecular rearrangements are important in the development of many lymphomas *(4)*. For instance, the t(14;18) (q32;q21) abnormality, which is found in most follicular lymphomas and some diffuse, large B-cell lymphomas results in overexpression of the BCL-2 protein, which inhibits apoptosis *(5)*.

2. CURRENT TREATMENT AND PROGNOSIS

Before formulating a treatment approach for lymphoma the disease subtype and stage must be determined. An adequate initial tissue specimen is critical to accurately classify the disease subtype. Sufficient sample should be collected for immunophenotyping, cytogenetic analysis, and molecular studies. If lymphadenopathy is present, an entire lymph node should be obtained to assess the nodal architecture by an experienced hematopathologist for further classification purposes. A needle biopsy or fine-needle aspiration alone may provide inadequate tissue that may result in diagnostic errors *(6)*. Table 1 lists the current classification of lymphomas reported by the World Health Organization *(2,3)*.

A thorough initial staging evaluation should be performed prior to instituting therapy. This should include a complete physical examination, complete blood count and differential with review of the peripheral blood smear, complete serum chemistry profile including a lactate dehydrogenase, bone marrow biopsy, and aspirate (preferably a bilateral exam), and computed tomography (CT) scans of the chest, abdomen, and pelvis. In some cases, a chest X-ray may be sufficient in place of a chest CT scan. For certain disease subtypes and presentations, further initial testing such as cytological examination of body fluids (e.g., cerebrospinal fluid, ascites, pleural fluid) as well as radionuclide and positron emission tomography scans may also be appropriate. Table 2 shows the Ann Arbor staging system for Hodgkin's lymphoma and NHL *(7,8)*.

From: *Current Clinical Oncology: Cancer in the Spine: Comprehensive Care.*
Edited by: R. F. McLain, K-U. Lewandrowski, M. Markman, R. M. Bukowski,
R. Macklis, and E. C. Benzel © Humana Press, Inc., Totowa, NJ

Table 1
World Health Organization Classification of Lymphoma

Precursor B-cell neoplasm	Precursor T-cell neoplasms
Precursor B lymphoblastic leukemia/lymphoma[a] Blastic NK cell lymphoma[a]	Precursor T lymphoblastic leukemia/lymphoma[a]

Mature B-cell neoplasms	Mature T-cell and NK-cell neoplasms
Chronic lymphocytic leukemia /small lymphocytic lymphoma[c] B-cell prolymphocytic leukemia[b] Lymphoplasmacytic lymphoma[c] Splenic marginal zone lymphoma[c] Hairy cell leukemia[c] Plasma cell myeloma Solitary plasmacytoma of bone[b] Extraosseous plasmacytoma[b] Extranodal marginal zone B-cell lymphoma of mucosa-associated lymphoid tissue (MALT-lymphoma)[c] Nodal marginal zone B-cell lymphoma[c] Follicular lymphoma (grades 1 and 2)[c] Follicular lymphoma (grade 3)[b] Anaplastic large cell lymphoma[b] Mantle cell lymphoma[b] Diffuse large B-cell lymphoma[b] Mediastinal (thymic) large B-cell lymphoma[b] Intravascular large B-cell lymphoma[b] Primary effusion lymphoma Burkitt lymphoma/leukemia[a]	T-cell prolymphocytic leukemia[b] T-cell large granular lymphocytic leukemia[c,d] Aggressive NK cell leukemia[a] Adult T-cell leukemia/lymphoma[a] Extranodal NK/T-cell lymphoma, nasal type[b] Enteropathy-type T-cell lymphoma[b] Hepatosplenic T-cell lymphoma[b] Subcutaneous panniculitis-like T-cell lymphoma Mycosis fungoides[c] Sezary syndrome[c] Primary cutaneous anaplastic large cell lymphoma[b] Peripheral T-cell lymphoma, unspecified[b] Angioimmunoblastic T-cell lymphoma[b]

Hodgkin's lymphoma	

Nodular lymphocyte predominant
Classical Hodgkin's lymphoma:
  Nodular sclerosing
  Lymphocyte-rich
	
	Mixed cellularity
	Lymphocyte depleted

[a]Very aggressive lymphoma subtype.
[b]Aggressive lymphoma subtype.
[c]Indolent lymphoma subtype.
[d]If CD56+, this is an aggressive lymphoma subtype.

After the disease subtype and stage are known, the goals of treatment for an individual patient must be determined. These goals range from cure, to improved survival and quality of life, to disease palliation and comfort measures. Treatment decisions are also influenced by whether the disease is early or advanced stage and whether the disease is indolent, aggressive, or very aggressive (see Table 1).

2.1. PROGNOSTIC SYSTEMS

An international prognostic factors project has been developed for advanced stage Hodgkin's disease (9). From an analysis of more than 5000 patients, seven independent predictors were noted for a decreased likelihood of freedom from progression. In addition, an International Prognostic Index (IPI) exists for NHL that is based on five parameters (10). After generating a score from the number of predictors or risk factors from each prognostic system outcome measures, such as freedom from progression, disease-free survival, and overall survival, can be estimated. These prognostic systems are summarized in Tables 3 and 4.

2.2. TREATMENT FOR HODGKIN'S LYMPHOMA

Early stage Hodgkin's disease includes stages I or II, no bulky disease (largest mass diameter <10 cm and mediastinal disease <1/3 of the transthoracic diameter), and no B symptoms (fever, night sweats, and >10% weight loss from baseline). For these patients, brief duration chemotherapy with adriamycin, bleomycin, vinblastine, and dacarbazine (ABVD) or vinblastine, methotrexate, and bleomycin followed by radiation therapy are highly effective treatment approaches. Disease-free survival rates achieved are 87 to 96% and overall survival rates are 97 to 100% at up to 42 mo of median follow-up duration (11–13).

For advanced stage Hodgkin's disease ABVD chemotherapy has been a standard treatment approach with 5-yr failure-free survival and overall survival rates of 61 and 73%, respectively (14). The addition of radiation therapy to chemotherapy has not improved overall survival in this group of patients (15). However, radiation therapy is often administered to bulky disease sites after chemotherapy has been com-

Table 2
Cotswold Revision of the Ann Arbor Staging Classification for Hodgkin's Lymphoma

Stage	Definition
I	Single lymph node region or lymphoid structure (e.g., spleen, thymus, Waldeyer's ring)
II	Two or more lymph node regions on the same side of the diaphragm
III	Lymph node regions or structures on both sides of the diaphragm
III$_1$	With or without splenic, hilar, celiac, or portal nodes
III$_2$	With paraaortic, iliac, or mesenteric nodes
IV	Diffuse involvement of one or more extralymphatic organs or sites

Ann Arbor Staging Classification for Non-Hodgkin's Lymphoma

Stage	Definition
I	One lymph node region
I$_E$	One extralymphatic organ or site
II	Two or more lymph node regions on the same side of the diaphragm
II$_E$	One extralymphatic organ/localized site in addition to stage II criteria
III	Lymph node regions on both sides of the diaphragm
III$_E$	One extralymphatic organ/localized site in addition to stage III criteria
III$_S$	Spleen in addition to criteria for stage III
III$_{SE}$	Spleen and one extralymphatic organ/localized site in addition to stage III criteria
IV	Diffuse or disseminated involvement of one or more extralymphatic organs ± associated lymph node involvement

A—No symptoms
B—Fever, drenching sweats, or weight loss
X—Bulky disease: .1/3 widening of the mediastinum at T5–T6; or maximum of nodal mass .10 cm.
E—Involvement of a single extranodal site, or contiguous or proximal to known nodal site of disease.

pleted. In the setting of relapsed or refractory Hodgkin's disease, autologous hematopoietic stem cell transplantation may still be curative therapy (16).

2.3. TREATMENT FOR NON-HODGKIN'S LYMPHOMA

Limited stage NHL includes Ann Arbor stages I and II, disease bulk less than 10 cm, and no B symptoms. For limited stage, indolent NHL radiation therapy alone may be curative (17). In this setting, combined modality treatment with chemotherapy and radiation therapy may also be employed (18). However, it is unknown whether radiation therapy alone or in combination with chemotherapy is better.

For advanced stage, indolent NHL the therapeutic options include watchful waiting until patients become symptomatic from their disease (19), conventional chemotherapy (e.g., cyclophosphamide, vincristine, and prednisone; single-agent chlorambucil; fludarabine or cladribine-based regimens [20–22]), interferon (with chemotherapy or as maintenance treatment after chemotherapy [23]) and monoclonal antibodies (e.g., Rituximab, Ibritumomab [24,25]). For patients with recurrent disease, autologous as well as allogeneic hematopoietic stem cell transplantation may be effective in achieving long-term, disease-free survival (26).

Radiation therapy alone for limited stage, aggressive NHL has resulted in 5-yr disease-free survival rates of 20 to 50% (27). When radiation is combined with chemotherapy cyclophosphamide, doxorubicin, vincristine and prednisone (CHOP) progression-free survival rates of 80 and 63% as well as overall survival rates of 81 and 74% have been demonstrated at 5 and 10 yr, respectively (28). Although combined radiation therapy and CHOP may improve disease-free survival and time to pro-

gression when compared with CHOP alone, there has been no difference in overall survival at 10 yr (29).

For advanced stage, aggressive NHL, the IPI (Table 4) should be used to help guide therapeutic decisions. CHOP chemotherapy may potentially cure 50 to 70% of patients with low- or low-intermediate risk disease (10). Although other more intense regimens have been used, in general these have not improved outcomes with the exception of younger patients with poor prognosis (30). For high-intermediate or high-risk disease, CHOP chemotherapy can only cure approx 25% of patients (10). These patients should therefore be considered for clinical trials. Coiffer et al. (31) performed a multicenter, French trial that randomized elderly, diffuse large B-cell NHL patients to CHOP or CHOP with Rituximab (31). The Rituximab arm had a significantly higher complete response rate (76 vs 63%, $p = 0.005$) as well as event-free and overall survivals at 2 yr median follow-up while having no increased toxicity. For younger patients with advanced stage, aggressive NHL, and higher risk IPI scores, autologous hematopoietic stem cell transplantation can be considered (32).

Patients with relapsed aggressive NHL may respond to salvage chemotherapy regimens (e.g., etoposide methyloprednisolone high-dose cytarabine cisplatin [ESHAP], ifosfamide, carboplatin, and etoposide [ICE]) (33,34). A randomized trial of such patients with chemotherapy-sensitive disease demonstrated a significant survival advantage for those receiving autologous hematopoietic stem cell transplants as compared with those receiving conventional salvage chemotherapy (35). However, for patients with primary refractory disease neither conventional chemotherapy nor autologous transplantation has

Table 3
Prognostic Scoring System for Hodgkin's Lymphoma

Gender	Age	Stage	Hemoglobin	WBC	Lymphocyte count	Albumin
Male	>45 yr	IV	<10.5 g/dL	>15 × 10⁹/L	<0.6 × 10⁹/L or <8% of the WBC count	<4 g/dL

Number of predictors	5-Yr FFP (%)
0–1	79
2–7	60
0–2	74
3–7	55
0–1	70
4–7	47

WBC, white blood cell; FFP, freedom from progression.

Table 4
The International Prognostic Index for Non-Hodgkin's Lymphoma

Age	Performance status	Stage	LDH	Number of extranodal sites
>60 yr	>2	III/IV	>normal	>1

Number of predictors	Risk category	CR(%)	5-Yr DFS (%)	5-Yr survival (%)
0–1	Low	87	70	73
2	Low-intermediate	67	50	51
3	High-intermediate	55	49	43
4–5	High	44	40	26

LDH, lactate dehydrogenase; CR, complete response; DFS, disease-free survival.

demonstrated durable responses. Such patients should therefore be considered for clinical trials.

The very aggressive lymphomas (e.g., Burkitt's and lymphoblastic) commonly involve the bone marrow and central nervous system (CNS). All treatment regimens should therefore include CNS prophylaxis with intrathecal chemotherapy. CNS radiation therapy is not routinely used in most protocols except occasionally for patients with CNS disease. Multi-agent acute lymphoblastic leukemia-like chemotherapy regimens have achieved 70 to 100% complete remission rates and 50 to 100% disease-free survival rates (36,37). Patients with disease relapse may be evaluated for hematopoietic stem cell transplantation. In contrast to treatment regimens for Burkitt/Burkitt-like NHL that may be completed in a few months, those for lymphoblastic NHL contain maintenance therapy after consolidation treatment that usually continues until patients have completed 2 yr of therapy. This often includes agents such as vincristine, methotrexate, 6-mercaptopurine, and prednisone.

3. GENERAL CHARACTERISTICS AND IMPACT OF SKELETAL INVOLVEMENT

Although the majority of lymphomas involve lymph node distributions, they may also involve extranodal sites by either direct extension to a contiguous area or by hematogenous or lymphatic spread (38). Approximately 6% of NHL patients have bone disease as a presenting sign (39). The incidence for Hodgkin's lymphoma is more rare (<1%) (40). A single site of bone disease is considered one extranodal site and therefore stage I_E, whereas diffuse involvement of one or more sites is considered stage IV disease as described in Table 2. The prognostic scoring systems consider stage IV disease and more than one extranodal site poor risk features (see Tables 3 and 4). Skeletal involvement by lymphomas may also be debilitating from pain or fractures. In addition, involvement of the bone marrow may eventually result in cytopenias that can predispose patients to life-threatening infections and hemorrhage.

4. SPINAL INVOLVEMENT

4.1. INCIDENCE

Approximately 9% of epidural spinal tumors are lymphomas *(41)*. NHL may result in spinal cord compression in approx 0.1 to 10% of patients *(42,43)*. More than half of the cases involve the thoracic spine, whereas the cervical spine is the least commonly effected *(44,45)*. Most cases of intraspinal lymphoma have systemic disease, however, approx 0.1 to 7% of these have been reported to have primary spinal epidural NHL *(43)*. Only 0.2% of such cases have been observed for Hodgkin's lymphoma *(46)*. Although lymphoma classification systems have changed with time, many of the earlier described cases of spinal epidural lymphoma (SEL) have reported that aggressive histological subtypes were usually more common than indolent subtypes. Of the 104 patients (72%) listed in Table 5, 75 had intermediate or high-grade histologies. The median age for all patients in the NHL group was 52.5 yr, whereas that the median age for those with Hodgkin's lymphoma was 54 yr. Some reports also have suggested a male predominance *(43,47)*.

4.2. SIGNIFICANCE

NHL involving the spine can be either a primary or secondary event *(48)*. Although primary SELs have been reported (Table 5), these are rare and in some cases may have developed from an undetected vertebral body or retroperitoneal lymphoma *(49)*. Many of the reports that previously described these lymphomas were made before the availability of modern neuroimaging modalities, thus, limiting an accurate assessment of the disease. However, more recent reports in which magnetic resonance imaging (MRI) was utilized have more clearly demonstrated the existence of this disease entity *(50–52)*. These patients with stage I$_E$ disease may have a favorable outcome if diagnosed and treated early in contrast to those patients who have secondary SEL *(43)*. Progressive disease, particularly if not responsive to therapy, may result in significant pain as well as neurological deficits from spinal cord and nerve root compression.

4.3. DIAGNOSTIC AND CLINICAL FEATURES

Plain films of the spine are often normal for patients with spinal NHL. However, some reports have indicated abnormalities in approx 15 to 40% of such patients *(43)*. Myelograms, CT, and CT myelography were formerly used to identify complete or partial blocks of the spinal cord in order to locate the level of the lymphoma *(45,53–55)*. However, these imaging modalities have been replaced by MRI as the initial neuroimaging method for evaluating such patients (*see* Fig. 1). Although there is no pathognomonic finding on MRI for this disease, the presence of a homogeneous isointense lesion extending over multiple vertebrae having continuity with a paraspinal soft tissue mass and with diffuse vertebral marrow signal changes is suspicious for a lymphoma *(56)*. Lyons et al. *(43)* suggested that finding a spinal epidural lesion by neuroimaging with normal plain films in patients with back pain and no history of cancer more likely represents a primary SEL than secondary disease or other malignancy.

When the mid-thoracic spine is involved, patients may have more severe neurological sequelae. This may in part be related to an increased risk of ischemia owing to the more limited vascular supply to this part of the spinal cord *(57)*. Cerebrospinal fluid analysis often demonstrates an elevated protein level, but the cytology may be normal *(44,50)*.

4.4. PRESENTATION OF SPINAL DISEASE

There have been two stages described for the presentation of SEL *(45)*. Initially, a prodromal stage often occurs in which patients may have back and radicular pain as well as paresthesias. These symptoms may exist for months before the diagnosis is established. The next stage is that of cord compression, which for some patients may occur concurrently with the prodromal symptoms. There is loss of motor function followed by sensory impairment, which is manifested by paresis, paralysis, discrete sensory levels, accentuated reflexes, and loss of sphincter control.

4.5. NATURAL HISTORY

There has been controversy as to whether primary SELs exist. Russell and Rubinstein *(58)* suggested that the epidural space contains normal lymphoid tissue. Conceivably this tissue could transform to a lymphoma. Alternatively, these lymphomas may have originated from a vertebral, paraspinal, or retroperitoneal source *(59)*. They may enter the epidural space through intervertebral foramina and extend to other vertebral bodies resulting in compression fractures, cord compression, and ischemia from interruption of the spinal cord's vascular supply *(45)*.

A thorough staging evaluation should, therefore, be performed to exclude other sites of disease. More advanced stage disease as well as more aggressive histological subtypes have had worse outcomes than that of primary SEL and more indolent subtypes, respectively *(43,59)*. Perry *(47)* and Raco *(60)* have also found that patients with lymphomas of T-cell origin have had longer survival than those with B-cell phenotypes.

4.6. RESPONSE TO MEDICAL MANAGEMENT

Patients presenting with significant neurological symptoms, such as cord compression, require urgent medical attention and therapeutic intervention before a staging evaluation can be completed. Efforts should be made to rapidly obtain a tissue diagnosis (e.g., frozen section of a biopsy specimen, bone marrow exam). The prompt institution of high-dose steroid therapy is also imperative. This provides symptomatic improvement, often in hours, by decreasing spinal cord edema. Corticosteroids also are lympholytic and therefore have had an important role in many treatment regimens for lymphoma. Doses of 60 to 100 mg iv dexamethasone followed by a taper regimen have been recommended *(53)*. In addition, the administration of analgesics such as narcotics is also appropriate for many patients.

Although earlier reports of treatment for SELs demonstrated the importance of radiation therapy, more recent evidence suggests that chemotherapy should be included as well *(42,45,61,62)* (*see* Table 5). The majority of lymphoma subtypes described have been of intermediate or high-grade histology. As such, these diseases are usually chemosensitive with high remission rates and with potential for long-term survival as described in Subheadings 2.2. and 2.3. Mora et al. *(63)* suggested that radiation therapy be avoided in growing children *(63)*. When possible, omitting radiation therapy also avoids potential myelopathies and may prevent early myelosuppression that prohibits administration of chemotherapy to treat systemic disease *(61)*.

Table 5
Primary Spinal Epidural Non-Hodgkin's Lymphoma

Reference	No. of patients	Median age (yr)	Therapy*			Histology[a]			Outcome
			S	RT	CT	Low	Intermediate	High	
67	1	51	1	1	1	—	1	—	NED at 4 yr
68	1	63	1	1	—	—	1	—	DWD at 4 mo
48	1	45	1	—	—	—	1	—	DWD at 7 mo
69	1	26	1	—	—	—	1	—	DWD at 10 mo
70	1	24	1	1	—	—	1	—	NED at 18 mo
64	10	38	10	10	—	8	2	—	7 NI MS 21 mo
42	5[b]	46	5	5	3	—	2	3	MS 27+ mo 3 patients with NED
53	3[b]	66	3	3	2	—	1	2	MS 12 mo; 3 NED
55	5	43[c]	5	5	—	2	3	—	MS 18 mo; 3 NI
66	4[b]	50	4	4	1	2	—	2	MS 12 mo; 4 DWD
54	1	59	1	1	1	—	1	—	NED at 22 mo
62	2	52[c]	2	2	2	—	2	—	2-CR[d]
65	5[b]	60	5	5	3	2	—	3	MS 6 mo; 2 DWD 1-A (11yr); 2 DWOD
47	3[b]	66	3	3	1	—	2	1	MS 3 mo; 1 DWD
71	1	59	1	1	—	—	1	—	NED at 3 yr
43	10	70	10	10	—	6	4	—	MS 42 mo; 4 relapsed 6-A (3 with relapse)
61	4[b]	36	1	1	4	1	3	—	MS 17 mo; 4 CR
72	3	59	3	3	1	1	1	1	1 NED at 4 yr[e]
41	19	53	19	16	13	3	4	12	4 A: MeS 61 mo 15 D: MeS 31 mo
60	6	9	6	6	6	—	—	6	6 A; median F/U 52 mo
63	3[b]	10	3	3	3	—	—	3	2 D at 7–8 mo; 1 CR at 12 yr
51	1	71	1	1	—	—	1	—	Relapsed at 7 mo
50	1	75	—	1	1	1	—	—	NED >8 mo
52	13[b]	62	13	13	5	3	9	1	MS 29.5 mo for IH[f] MS 103 mo for L[g]
Totals	**104**	**52.5[h]**	**100**	**96**	**47**	**29**	**41**	**34**	

*Number of patients who had received each treatment modality.

[a]Number of patients with each histological grade subgroup.

[b]Additional patients were included in the reference, but only those with likely stage I_E disease reported.

[c]Mean.

[d]One patient relapsed 32 mo after radiation therapy and then received chemotherapy with no evidence of disease for 5 yr.

[e]Patient with a high-grade lymphoma who received chemotherapy; two other patients died within 2 mo.

[f]Eight out of 10 with complete remission and one relapse.

[g]Three out of three with complete remission with two relapses.

[h]Median.

S, surgery; RT, radiation therapy; CT, chemotherapy; NED, no evidence of disease; DWD, dead with disease; NI, neurologically improved; DWOD, dead without disease; MS, median survival; A, alive, MeS, mean survival; CR, complete remission; F/U, follow-up; IH, intermediate/high-grade non-Hodgkin's lymphoma; L, low-grade non-Hodgkin's lymphoma.

Because the spinal epidural space receives its blood supply from the systemic circulation, chemotherapeutic agents may be administered without having to cross the blood–brain barrier (61). However, intrathecal chemotherapy with methotrexate and/or cytarabine has been given as well (52,54), particularly in the presence of cerebrospinal fluid lymphomatous involvement or for high-grade lymphomas.

4.7. TREATMENT OF LOCALIZED DISEASE

Localized SEL is rare and treatment approaches are described in Subheadings 2.2. and 2.3. for the different pathologic subtypes of lymphoma. The reports in Tables 5 and 6 suggest that radiation therapy doses of 3000 to 4000 cGy are

necessary for optimal response. This has been effective in reversing neurological deficits if administered promptly even after cord compression develops (43,53–55,64).

Although the role of chemotherapy is more established for secondary SELs, it has been effective for some primary cases as well (42,45,47,61,62) (see Tables 5 and 6). Until further outcome information is available, combined radiation therapy and chemotherapy have been advocated by some in order to treat the primary lesion as well as any occult systemic disease (42,47). This approach also helps avoid extensive decompressive procedures. Fifty-nine (82%) of the 72 patients in Table 5 who were treated with combined chemotherapy and radiation

A

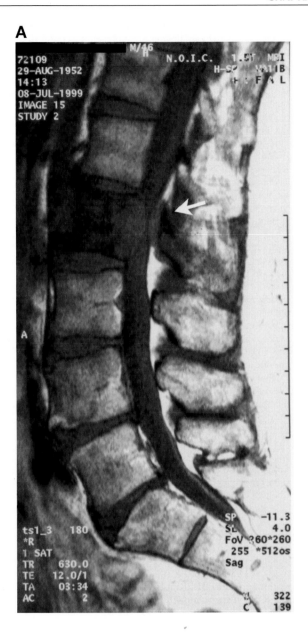

B

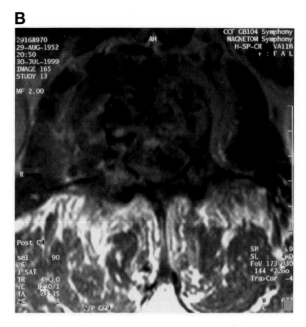

Fig. 1. Magnetic resonance imaging of the spine from a patient at the Cleveland Clinic Foundation with a primary spinal epidural large B-cell non-Hodgkin's lymphoma. (A) Sagittal T1-weighted sequences demonstrate involvement of the L2 vertebra and the ventral as well as dorsal epidural space with marked compression of the thecal sac (arrow); (B) corresponding axial T1-weighted post-contrast image again confirming epidural involvement and canal compromise by the lymphoma.

Table 6
Primary Spinal Epidural Hodgkin's Lymphoma

Reference	N	Median age	S	RT	CT	Outcome
73	1	54	1	1	—	NED at 17 mo
74	1	56	1	—	1	CR (? duration)
46	1	46	1	1	1	CR at 21 mo

S, surgery; RT, radiation therapy; CT, chemotherapy; NED, no evidence of disease; CR, complete remission.

therapy had intermediate or high-grade lymphoma histology. The median survival for the subset of patients treated with this combined modality therapy was 24.5 mo (range, 3 mo to 12 yr) and 44 (61%) of these 72 patients achieved a complete remission.

4.8. TREATMENT OF DISSEMINATED DISEASE

After a staging evaluation has documented the extent of a patient's disease appropriate systemic therapy should be instituted based on the lymphoma subtype as discussed in Subheadings 2.2. and 2.3. In this setting chemotherapy and/or immunotherapy are usually administered if patients are otherwise acceptable candidates for such treatment. The addition of radiation therapy may also be beneficial in some cases, particularly to locally control disease areas that are causing significant neurological compromise.

4.9. NEED FOR SURGICAL TREATMENT

In general, the role of surgery for lymphomas has been to provide diagnostic material. Before the availability of modern imaging techniques such as CT scans, surgery was commonly used for staging information as well (e.g., staging laparotomy). However, in the setting of truly localized stage I disease, surgical resection followed by radiation therapy may potentially be curative for some patients.

After identification of an epidural spinal mass with no other evidence of disease, decompressive laminectomy, and subtotal resection have routinely been performed (41,43,51,65). This approach is also appropriate if there is spinal cord compression and a patient is not a candidate for radiation therapy to the involved area. This includes instances in which there is a disease relapse after prior radiation therapy that prohibits additional radiation from being administered or if neurological deficits progress rapidly during radiation therapy *(53)*. Sufficient tissue should be obtained from surgery for diagnostic testing, which includes immunophenotyping, cytogenetic analysis, and molecular studies.

Perry et al. *(47)* found that of 18 undiagnosed lymphoma patients presenting with spinal cord compression none were functionally worse after laminectomy for decompression and tissue diagnosis. If surgery is necessary Margulies et al. *(53)* suggested that an anterolateral approach is preferable to one from the posterior because most lymphomas enter the epidural space anteriorly and are found anterior or anterolateral to the spinal cord.

REFERENCES

1. Jemal A, Thomas A, Murray T, Thun M. Cancer Statistics, 2002. CA Cancer J Clin 2002; 52:23–47.
2. Stein H, Delsol G, Pileri S, et al. Hodgkin lymphoma. In: Jaffe ES, Harris NL, Stein H, Vardiman JW, eds. World Health Organization Classification of Tumours. Pathology and Genetics. Tumours of Haematopoietic and Lymphoid Tissues. Lyon: IARC Press; 2001:238–253.
3. Harris NL, Müller-Hermelink HK, Catovsky D, et al. Mature B-cell neoplasms. In: Jaffe ES, Harris NL, Stein H, Vardiman JW, eds. World Health Organization Classification of Tumours. Pathology and Genetics. Tumours of Haematopoietic and Lymphoid Tissues. Lyon: IARC Press; 2001:119–235.
4. Armitage JO, Mauch PM, Harris NL, Bierman P. Non-Hodgkin's lymphomas. In: Devita VT, Hellman S, Rosenberg SA, eds. Cancer: Principles and Practice of Oncology. 6th ed. Philadelphia, PA: Lippincott Williams and Wilkins; 2001:2258–2260.
5. Cleary ML, Smith SD, Sklar J. Cloning and structural analysis of cDNAs for bcl-2 and a hybrid bcl-2 /immunoglobulin transcript resulting from the t(14;18) translocation. Cell 1986; 47:19–28.
6. Pinkus GS. Needle biopsy in malignant lymphoma. J Clin Oncol 1996; 4:2415–2416.
7. Lister TA, Crowther D, Sutcliffe SB, et al. Report of a committee convened to discuss the evaluation and staging of patients with Hodgkin's disease: Cotswolds meeting. J Clin Oncol 1989; 7:1630–1636.
8. Carbone PP, Kaplan HS, Musshoff K, Smithers DW, Tubiana M. Report of the Committee on Hodgkin's Disease Staging Classification. Cancer Res 1971; 31:1860–1861.
9. Hasenclever D, Diehl V. A prognostic score for advanced Hodgkin's disease. International Prognostic Factors Project on Advanced Hodgkin's disease. N Engl J Med 1998; 339:1506–1514.
10. The International Non-Hodgkin's Lymphoma Prognostic Factors Project. A predictive model for aggressive non-Hodgkin's lymphoma. N Engl J Med 1993; 329:987–994.
11. Santoro A, Bonfante V, Viviani S, et al. Subtotal nodal (STNI) vs. involved field (IFRT) irradiation after 4 cycles of ABVD in early stage Hodgkin's disease (HD). Proc Am Soc Clin Oncol 1996;1 5:415.
12. Klasa RJ, Connors JM, Fairey R, et al. Treatment of early stage Hodgkin's disease: Improved outcome with brief chemotherapy and radiotherapy without staging laparotomy. Annal Oncol 1996; 7:21.
13. Horning SJ, Hoppe RT, Mason J, et al. Stanford-Kaiser Permanente G1 study for clinical stage I and IIA Hodgkin's disease: subtotal lymphoid irradiation versus vinblastine, methotrexate, and bleomycin chemotherapy and regional irradiation. J Clin Oncol 1997; 15:1736–1744.
14. Canellos GP, Anderson JR, Propert KJ, et al. Chemotherapy for advanced Hodgkin's disease with MOPP, ABVD, or MOPP alternating with ABVD. N Engl J Med 1992; 327:1478–1484.
15. Loeffler M, Brosteanu O, Hasenclever D, et al. Meta-analysis of chemotherapy versus combined modality treatment trials in Hodgkin's disease. International Database on Hodgkin's Disease Overview Study Group. J Clin Oncol 1998; 16:818–829.
16. Bierman PJ, Anderson JR, Freeman MB, et al. High-dose chemotherapy followed by autologous hematopoietic rescue for Hodgkin's disease patients following first relapse after chemotherapy. Ann Oncol 1996; 7:151–156.
17. Reddy S, Saxena VS, Pellettiere EV, Hendrickson FR. Stage I and II non-Hodgkin's lymphomas; long-term results of radiation therapy. Int J Radiat Oncol Biol Phys 1989; 16:687–692.
18. Network NCC. NCCN preliminary non-Hodgkin's lymphoma practice guidelines. Oncology 1997; 11:28–46.
19. Horning SJ. Treatment approaches to the low-grade lymphomas. Blood 1994; 83:881–884.
20. Kennedy BJ, Bloomfield CD, Kiang DT, Vosika G, Peterson BA, Theologides A. Combination versus successive single agent chemotherapy in lymphocytic lymphoma. Cancer 1978; 41:23–28.
21. Saven A, Lee T, Kosty M, Piro L. Cladribine and mitoxantrone dose escalation in indolent non-Hodgkin's lymphoma. J Clin Oncol 1996; 14:2139–2144.
22. McLaughlin P, Hagemeister FB, Romaguera JE, et al. Fludarabine, mitoxantrone, and dexamethasone: an effective new regimen for indolent lymphoma. J Clin Oncol 1996; 14:1262–1268.
23. Solal-Celigny P, Lepage E, Brousse N, et al. Recombinant interferon alpha-2b combined with a regimen containing doxorubicin in patients with advanced follicular lymphoma. N Engl J Med 1993; 329:1608–1614.
24. McLaughlin P, Grillo-Lopez A, Link BK, et al. Rituximab chimeric anti-CD20 monoclonal antibody therapy for relapsed indolent lymphoma: half of patients respond to a four dose treatment program. J Clin Oncol 1998; 16:2825–2833.
25. Witzig TE, Flinn IW, Gordon LI, et al. Treatment with ibritumomab tiuxetan radioimmunotherapy in patients with rituximab-refractory follicular non-Hodgkin's lymphoma. J Clin Oncol 2002; 20:3262–3269.
26. Verdonck LF, Dekker AW, Lokhorst HM, Petersen EJ, Nieuwenhuis HK. Allogeneic versus autologous bone marrow transplantation for refractory and recurrent low-grade non-Hodgkin's lymphoma. Blood 1997; 90:4201–4205.
27. Chen MG, Prosnitz LR, Gonzalez-Serva A, Fischer DB. Results of radiotherapy in control of stage I and II non-Hodgkin's lymphoma. Cancer 1979; 43:1245–1254.
28. Shenkier TN, Voss N, Fairey R, et al. Brief chemotherapy and involved-region irradiation for limited-stage diffuse large cell lymphoma: an 18-year experience from the British Columbia Cancer Agency. J Clin Oncol 2001; 20:197–204.
29. Horning SJ, Glick JH, Kim K, et al. Final report of E1484: CHOP v CHOP + Radiotherapy (RT) for limited stage diffuse aggressive lymphoma. Blood 2001; 98:724a.
30. Fisher RI, Gaynor ER, Dahlberg S, et al. Comparison of a standard regimen (CHOP) with three intensive chemotherapy regimens for advanced non-Hodgkin's lymphoma. N Engl J Med 1993; 328:1002–1006.
31. Coiffier B, Lepage E, Briere J, et al. CHOP chemotherapy plus rituximab compared with CHOP alone in elderly patients with diffuse large B-cell lymphoma. N Engl J Med 2002; 346:235–242.
32. Haioun C, LePage E, Gisselbrecht C, et al. Benefit of autologous bone marrow transplantation over sequential chemotherapy in poor-risk aggressive non-Hodgkin's lymphoma: updated results of the prospective study LNH87-2. Group d'Etude des Lymphomes de l'Adulte. J Clin Oncol 1997; 15:1131–1137.
33. Velasquez WS, McLaughlin P, Tucker S, et al. ESHAP-an effective chemotherapy regimen in refractory and relapsing lymphoma: a 4 year follow-up study. J Clin Oncol 1994; 12:1169–1176.
34. Moskowitz CH, Bertino JR, Glassman JR, et al. Ifosfamide, carboplatin, and etoposide: a highly effective cytoreduction and peripheral-blood progenitor-cell mobilization regimen for transplant-eligible patients with non-Hodgkin's lymphoma. J Clin Oncol 1999; 17:3776–3785.
35. Philip T, Guglielmi C, Hagenbeek A, et al. Autologous bone marrow transplantation as compared with salvage chemotherapy in relapses of chemotherapy-sensitive non-Hodgkin's lymphoma. N Engl J Med 1995; 333:1540–1545.

36. Magrath IT, Adde M, Shad A, et al. Adults and children with small non-cleaved cell lymphoma have a similar excellent outcome when treated with the same chemotherapy regimen. J Clin Oncol 1996; 14:925–934.

37. Hoelzer D, Ludwig WD, Thiel E, et al. Improved outcome in adult B-cell acute lymphoblastic leukemia. Blood 1996; 87:495–508.

38. Chade HO. Metastatic tumours of the spine and spinal cord. In: Vinkers PJ, Bruyn GW, eds. Handbook of Clinical Neurology. Vol 20. Amsterdam: North Holland; 1976:415–433.

39. Spagnoli I, Gattoni F, Viganotti G. Roentgenographic aspects of non-Hodgkin's lymphomas presenting with osseous lesions. Skeletal Radiol 1982; 8:39–41.

40. Eustace S, O'Regan R, Graham D, Carney D. Primary multifocal skeletal Hodgkin's disease confined to bone. Skeletal Radiol 1995; 24:61–63.

41. Salvati M, Cervoni L, Artico M, Raco A, Ciappetta P, Delfini R. Primary spinal epidural non-Hodgkin's lymphomas: a clinical study. Surg Neurol 1996; 46:339–343.

42. Epelbaum R, Haim N, Ben-Shahar M, Ben-Arie Y, Feinsod M, Cohen Y. Non-Hodgkin's lymphoma presenting with spinal epidural involvement. Cancer 1986; 58:2120–2124.

43. Lyons MK, O'Neill BP, Kurtin PJ, Marsh WR. Diagnosis and management of primary spinal epidural non-Hodgkin's lymphoma. Mayo Clin Proc 1996; 71:453–457.

44. Haddad P, Thaell JF, Kiely JF, et al. Lymphoma of the spinal epidural space. Cancer 1976; 38:1862–1866.

45. Oviatt DL, Kirshner HS, Stein RS. Successful chemotherapeutic treatment of epidural compression in non-Hodgkin's lymphoma. Cancer 1982; 49:2446–2448.

46. Higgins SA, Peschel RE. Hodgkin's disease with spinal cord compression. A case report and a review of the literature. Cancer 1995; 75:94–98.

47. Perry JR, Deodhare SS, Bilbao JM, Murray D, Muller P. The significance of spinal cord compression as the initial manifestation of lymphoma. Neurosurgery 1993; 32:157–162.

48. Slager UT, Kaufman RL, Cohen KL, Tuddenham WJ. Primary lymphoma of the spinal cord. J Neuropathol Exp Neurol 1982; 41:437–445.

49. Iizuka H, Nakamura T, Kato M. Malignant lymphoma of the spinal epidural space: report of three cases. Neurol Med Chir 1989; 29:307–311.

50. Pels H, Vogt I, Klockgether T, Schlegel U. Primary non-Hodgkin's lymphoma of the spinal cord. Spine 2000; 25:2262–2264.

51. Barnard M, Perez-Ordonez B, Rowed DW, Ang LC. Primary spinal epidural mantle cell lymphoma: case report. Neurosurgery 2000; 47:1239–1241.

52. McDonald AC, Nicoll JA, Rampling RP. Non-Hodgkin's lymphoma presenting with spinal cord compression; a clinicopathological review of 25 cases. Eur J Cancer 2000; 36:207–213.

53. Margulies JY, Kenan S, Michowitz SD, et al. Cord compression as the presenting symptom of extradural malignant lymphoma. Arch Orthop Trauma Surg 1987; 106:291–296.

54. Toner GC, Holmes R, Sinclair RA, Tang SK, Schwarz MA. Central nervous system lymphoma: primary lumbar nerve root infiltration. Acta Haematol 1989; 81:44–47.

55. Maiuri F, Gangemi M, Giamundo A, Iaconetta G, De Chiara AR. Primary spinal epidural lymphomas. Acta Neurol (Napoli) 1988; 10:213–219.

56. Mascalchi M, Torselli P, Falaschi F, Dal Pozzo G. MRI of spinal epidural lymphoma. Neuroradiology 1995; 37:303–307.

57. Mullins GM, Flynn JP, el-Mahdi AM, McQueen JD, Owens AH Jr. Malignant lymphoma of the spinal epidural space. Ann Intern Med 1971; 74:416–423.

58. Russell DS, Rubinstein LJ. Pathology of Tumours of the Nervous System. 5th ed. Baltimore, MD: Williams and Wilkins; 1989:608–615.

59. Rao TV, Narayanaswamy KS, Shankar SK, Deshpande DH. "Primary" spinal epidural lymphomas: a clinico-pathological study. Acta Neurochir (Wien) 1982; 62:307–317.

60. Raco A, Cervoni L, Salvati M, Delfini R. Primary spinal epidural non-Hodgkin's lymphomas in childhood: a review of 6 cases. Acta Neurochir (Wien) 1997; 139:526–528.

61. Wong ET, Portlock CS, O'Brien JP, DeAngelis LM. Chemosensitive epidural spinal cord disease in non-Hodgkins lymphoma. Neurology 1996; 46:1543–1547.

62. Ron IG, Reider I, Wigler N, Chaitchik S. Primary spinal epidural non-Hodgkin's lymphoma. The contribution of nuclear magnetic resonance imaging, therapeutic approach and review of the literature. Tumori 1992; 78:397–402.

63. Mora J, Wollner N. Primary epidural non-Hodgkin lymphoma: Spinal cord compression syndrome as the initial form of presentation in childhood non-Hodgkin lymphoma. Med Pediatr Oncol 1999; 32:102–105.

64. Cappellani G, Giuffre F, Tropea R, et al. Primary spinal epidural lymphomas. Report of ten cases. J Neurosurg Sci 1986; 30:147–151.

65. Laing RJ, Jakubowski J, Kunkler IH, Hancock BW. Primary spinal presentation of non-Hodgkin's lymphoma. A reappraisal of management and prognosis. Spine 1992; 17:117–120.

66. Dimarco A, Campostrini F, Garusi GF. Non-Hodgkin's lymphomas presenting with spinal epidural involvement. Acta Oncol 1989; 28:485–488.

67. Herbst KD, Corder MP, Justice GR. Successful therapy with methotrexate of a multicentric mixed lymphoma of the central nervous system. Cancer 1976; 38:1476–1478.

68. Mitsumoto H, Breuer AC, Lederman RJ. Malignant lymphoma of the central nervous system: a case of primary spinal intramedullary involvement. Cancer 1980; 46:1258–1262.

69. Hautzer NW, Aiyesimoju A, Robitaille Y. "Primary" spinal intramedullary lymphomas: a review. Ann Neurol 1983; 14:62–66.

70. Itami J, Mori S, Arimizu N, Inoue S, Lee M, Uno K. Primary intramedullary spinal cord lymphoma: report of a case. Jpn J Clin Oncol 1986; 16:407–412.

71. Schild SE, Wharen RE Jr, Menke DM, Folger WN, Colon-Otero G. Primary lymphoma of the spinal cord. Mayo Clin Proc 1995; 70:256–260.

72. Lim CC, Chong BK. Spinal epidural non-Hodgkin's lymphoma: case reports of three patients presenting with spinal cord compression. Singapore Med J 1996; 37:497–500.

73. Citow JS, Rini B, Wollmann R, Macdonald RL. Isolated, primary extranodal Hodgkin's disease of the spine: case report. Neurosurgery 2001; 49:453–456.

74. Moridaira K, Handa H, Murakami H, et al. Primary Hodgkin's disease of the bone presenting with an extradural tumor. Acta Haematol 1994; 92:148–149.

15 Metastatic Breast Carcinoma

John Hill, MD and G. Thomas Budd, MD

Contents

1. INTRODUCTION

Carcinoma of the breast is the most frequent cancer in women in the United States and the second leading cause of cancer deaths. In the year 2005, it is estimated that more than 210,000 new cases will be diagnosed, while approx 40,000 will die from the disease. A slight decrease in mortality has been noted in recent years, attributable to improved screening practices as well as modest improvements in treatment (1).

Although widespread screening with examinations and mammography has increased the proportion of women diagnosed with breast cancer at an earlier stage, approx 5 to 10% of patients initially present with metastatic disease (2). Another substantial group of women will present with large primary tumors, nodal involvement, or other poor risk factors that put them at great risk for eventual metastatic recurrence. Although the use of adjuvant radiation, chemotherapy, and hormonal therapy has been shown to improve outcomes in this group of patients, cure remains elusive in a large percentage.

Studies have shown that more than 70% of patients with metastatic breast cancer develop bone metastases in their lifetime. Of women who experience first relapse, one in three will occur in the skeleton (3). The median survival after the first diagnosis of a metastatic bone lesion is 2 yr, although overall survival for women with metastatic breast cancer can range from months to longer than 5 yr (4). Before documented metastatic disease, lymph node involvement is the most reliable predictor of future bone recurrence (5).

Skeletal complications can be expected in approximately one-third of advanced breast cancer patients. These complications can include hypercalcemia, pathological fracture, and spinal cord compression, in addition to pain that might precede

such complications (6). When considering metastatic disease to the spine, treatment goals must include management of symptoms, prevention of complications, and treatment of complications should they arise.

Spinal cord compression owing to vertebral involvement can be a source of significant morbidity in this patient population. Any approach to management of such circumstances requires careful evaluation by physicians specialized in multiple disciplines, including radiology, medical oncology, radiation oncology, and surgery. The heterogeneity in outcomes among this group of patients requires thoughtful consideration as to the most appropriate short- and long-term management strategies.

Although all treatment in such cases is palliative in nature, many patients treated with aggressive, acute surgical management, followed by systemic therapy, can obtain long-term survival measured in years. It is imperative to determine which patients fall into this category. Although performance status is certainly an important consideration, other prognostic factors have been shown to have significance. One study found that women with metastatic disease limited to bone lived an average 6 mo longer than women who also had extra-osseus involvement. Other factors that proved to be of prognostic importance included histological grade of the tumor, estrogen receptor positivity, bone involvement at initial presentation, disease-free interval, and age. Thus, the approach to long-term management of patients with spinal cord compression, as well as other metastatic complications, must be individualized by the involved care team (7).

2. CLINICAL PRESENTATION OF SPINAL METASTASES

Detection of metastatic lesions in the spine varies widely by clinical situation. Whole body bone scans are commonly employed as part of an initial staging evaluation. Although the role of such

From: Current Clinical Oncology: Cancer in the Spine: Comprehensive Care.
Edited by: R. F. McLain, K-U. Lewandrowski, M. Markman, R. M. Bukowski,
R. Macklis, and E. C. Benzel © Humana Press, Inc., Totowa, NJ

investigations is clear in patients with symptoms of bone involvement, the role in asymptomatic patients is much less apparent. Any area of abnormality on bone scan can be more clearly defined via plain X-rays, computed tomography, or magnetic resonance imaging (MRI).

Earliest spinal involvement, without concurrent complication, may manifest as only vague, localized pain. Acute worsening of pain could indicate vertebral fracture with or without impending neurological compromise, including nerve root compression and spinal cord compression. Studies have shown that the risk for vertebral fracture in women with breast cancer is 5 to 20 times higher than that of age-matched controls, depending on stage of disease (8). If neurological structures become compromised, this can be manifested as progressive lower extremity weakness, radicular pain, altered sensation, gait disturbance, and change in bowel or bladder frequency (9). Occasionally, routine serologies may detect hypercalcemia in patients with no symptoms of bone involvement, which in this population warrants a search for osseus involvement.

In patients with pain or neurological symptoms concerning for spinal involvement, clinicians may choose to proceed by defining the extent of disease with MRI without the use of preceding bone scan. Although plain films are reliable at detecting changes in bone and pathological fractures, more sophisticated modalities, such as MRI, are sensitive in detecting extension into surrounding tissues and compromise of neurological structures. When performed, MRI should include the entire spine, as multiple levels can be involved simultaneously.

3. ROLE OF MEDICAL THERAPY

3.1. ANALGESICS

Pain is likely the first symptom that will be experienced by patients with metastatic disease to the spine. Before more definitive treatment, management of this symptom is a major priority for clinicians. Unfortunately, pain control regimens are frequently inadequate to handle the degree of pain experienced by patients. One study of patients presenting for radiation oncology evaluation revealed that nearly 80% rated pain levels as moderate or severe despite prescribed analgesics (10). On occasion, definitive radiotherapy or systemic treatment may be necessary to obtain adequate pain control. However, relief from these modalities is not immediate and may occur over several weeks.

For mild localized pain, nonopioid analgesics, such as acetaminophen or nonsteroidal anti-inflammatory drugs, may be sufficient. However, more severe pain usually requires the addition of narcotic pain medications (9). After initial titration with intravenous formulations, most patients can subsequently be converted to long-acting oral formulations with shorter acting agents used for breakthrough episodes.

Corticosteroids, such as dexamethasone, are frequently employed and are standard-of-care for patients presenting with evidence of spinal cord compression. These agents reduce the inflammation and edema associated with cord and nerve compression, thus abating further neurological compromise. Pain is diminished and neurological function may be preserved. High-dose dexamethasone, defined as 100 mg iv bolus followed by 24 mg orally four times daily for 3 d, then tapered over 10 d, has been shown to be superior to lower dose regimens in terms of pain control and in increasing the number of patients who remain ambulatory, though the latter is less consistent (11,12).

Neuropathical pain, which may be encountered when there is nerve root involvement, may be resistant to standard analgesics. Agents such as Amitriptyline, Carbamazepine, and Gabapentin have been shown to be effective in this situation (9).

3.2. BISPHOSPHONATES

Bisphosphonates, such as clodronate, pamidronate, and zoledronate, are compounds which inhibit osteoclast-mediated bone resorption (13). Many roles for this class of drugs have been clearly defined, whereas others remain in question. Pamidronate, given as a 90-mg dose intravenously over 2 to 4 h, is routinely used in the acute treatment of hypercalcemia, along with aggressive hydration with normal saline (9). Also, studies have shown that similar dosing of pamidronate, repeated every 4 wk, significantly reduces skeletal morbidity in breast cancer patients with documented osteolytic lesions. Reductions were noted in pathological fractures, hypercalcemia, and need to radiate bone for pain relief (14).

In patients with pain syndromes secondary to bone lesions, pamidronate has been shown to have modest benefit in pain control when given in combination with systemic chemotherapy or hormonal therapy. However, treatment with bisphosphonates should not displace routine analgesia, radiotherapy, or surgical intervention if indicated in the acute management of cancer pain (15).

Attention has been given towards using bisphosphonates in the adjuvant setting for patients with no evidence of metastatic bone lesions. One such study using clodronate in patients with primary breast cancer found a significant decrease in appearance of both visceral and osseus metastases (13). However, a subsequent study of node-positive patients found no such improvement (3). The reason for this disparity is possibly related to the inclusion criteria of each study, with the first study requiring evidence of tumor cells in the bone marrow. It is possible that such patients, who are at high risk for developing symptomatic bone metastases, will benefit from adjuvant bisphosphonates, whereas those without marrow involvement may not. Another explanation for the disparity in these studies could be the small size of the study populations.

3.3. CHEMOTHERAPY

Subsequent to acute management of complications from spinal metastases, definitive systemic treatment with chemotherapy, hormonal manipulation, or biological agents has been shown to improve survival, although the vast majority of women with metastatic involvement will die from their disease (16). Multiple chemotherapeutic agents have been shown to be active in metastatic breast cancer, including cyclophosphamide (C), anthracyclines (Adriamycin [A]; Epirubicin [E]), methotrexate (M), and 5-flurouracil (F). Traditional treatment regimens have included combinations of these agents, such as CMF, FAC, FEC, and AC (17).

Recent meta-analysis of randomized clinical trials in metastatic breast cancer arrived at several conclusions. It found that combination chemotherapy yielded significantly higher response rates and improved overall survival compared to monotherapy. However, this survival advantage has not been proven in most randomized studies. Also, chemotherapy delivered at higher doses was associated with higher response rate and, perhaps, improved survival compared to less intensive dosing. However, these findings have been hard to reproduce and must be balanced by the fact that polychemotherapy and dose-intensive regimens are associated with a higher degree of toxicity. Finally, although anthracycline-containing regimens showed superiority in response rate, they did not seem to significantly improve survival over regimens not including an anthracycline (17).

Newer classes of agents have introduced that also have significant activity in this disease. These include the taxanes, paclitaxel, and docetaxel; a third-generation vinca alkaloid, vinorelbine; an orally active pro-drug of 5-fluorouracil, capecitabine; and gemcitabine among others (16,18,19). Until very recently, these drugs were typically employed as second-line agents or in the setting of anthracycline resistance. However, some of these agents, especially the taxanes, are now being used more frequently as first-line treatment for metastatic disease (16).

The apparent improved response rates and survival with higher doses of chemotherapy have led investigators to examine the role of chemotherapy at doses that are, in fact, myeloablative, followed by autologous or allogeneic stem cell support. Though preliminary data showed promise, this has not been proven to be an effective approach in this population and remains investigational (16).

3.4. BIOLOGICAL AGENTS

The discovery that up to 25% of human breast cancers overexpress HER2 has led to intense research into using this as a target for treatment. The HER2 gene product is a transmembrane receptor possessing partial homology with the epidermal growth factor receptor. It possesses an intrinsic tyrosine kinase activity that may play a direct role not only in the pathogenesis of tumors, but also in the apparent clinical aggressiveness of tumors that overexpress HER2. Recombinant humanized monoclonal antibodies directed against this receptor were initially shown to have activity as single agents with metastatic breast cancer in which HER2 was overexpressed (20).

Subsequent studies have looked to improve on this response rate by adding one such monoclonal antibody, trastuzumab, to chemotherapy in women with metastatic breast cancer overexpressing HER2. It has now been demonstrated in randomized trials that the combination of antibody plus chemotherapy is associated with longer time to disease progression, higher rate of response, longer duration of response, and longer survival as first-line therapy in this patient population. This effect was noted in regimens that contained anthracycline and those that employed single-agent paclitaxel. Of note, however, was the increase in cardiac dysfunction noted most prominently in women treated with the anthracycline, cyclophosphamide, and trastuzumab combination (21).

3.5. HORMONAL THERAPY

Hormonal therapy is the initial treatment of choice in women with estrogen-receptor-positive tumors if they are asymptom-

atic and have limited disease. Specific medical treatments have supplanted ablative procedures such as oopherectomy. These include progestins, gonadotropin-releasing-hormone analogs, antiestrogens, and aromatase inhibitors. Of women with metastatic breast cancer, 20–35% respond to first-line hormonal therapy. Of those who initially respond and subsequently progress, many will respond to a second-, third-, or fourth-line hormonal agent (16).

Tamoxifen, which acts by blocking the binding of estrogen to its receptor, has been recognized as the standard first-line treatment for advanced breast cancer in postmenopausal women. Aromatase inhibitors, which block a critical step in the production of estrogens, have been historically employed as second-line agents after failure of tamoxifen. However, recent studies have shown that one such agent, anastrazole, is at least as effective as tamoxifen for first-line treatment, and associated with fewer side effects (22). Letrozole, another agent in the aromatase inhibitor family, has been shown to be superior to tamoxifen in a randomized trial (23). Therefore, these agents are considered a suitable first-line therapy.

Studies have also investigated the relative efficacy of aromatase inhibitors vs progestins. Anastrazole, letrozole, and exemestane were each compared to megestrol acetate in randomized trials and found to be superior in efficacy (24–26).

4. ROLE OF SURGICAL INTERVENTION

As previously stated, the heterogeneity of this patient population must prompt the clinician to individualize any intervention based on each particular patient's treatment goals. Patients who respond to initial systemic therapy have a good chance of survival at 3 yr, with up to one-fifth surviving at 5 yr. By contrast, patients with extensive, unresponsive disease who have limited life expectancy may not be appropriate for aggressive surgical intervention. This stresses the importance of a multidisciplinary approach to individual patients. Unfortunately, some retrospective reviews have found that orthopedic surgeons were consulted less than 50% of the time when it was appropriate to do so (9).

Some patients who might benefit from early orthopedic evaluation include those with pain exacerbated by movement and relieved by rest, possibly indicating spinal instability. Vertebral bodies that show 50% destruction with associated pain are at high risk for fracture and also warrant surgical evaluation. Patients with moderate deformity and collapse of vertebral bodies also fall into this category. Of course, patients with documented spinal cord or nerve root compression must be seriously considered for decompression followed by spinal stabilization. Again, factors such as site and number of levels effected, whether the compression is partial or complex, fixability, duration, performance status, and predicted survival must be taken into account prior to proceeding with any surgical intervention (9).

Drainage of the breasts via the azygous system contributes to the propensity for metastases to the thoracic and lumbar regions. Anterior decompression and reconstruction are the most commonly employed surgical interventions in these situations. The rate of neurological improvement with this approach has been noted to be near 78%, compared to only 23% with laminectomy alone. Posterior procedures may also be necessary if anterior stabilization is not sufficient or feasible. This is particularly true when instrumentation is required at the cervicothoracic or lumbosacral junctions (27).

Other small series have evaluated the outcomes of surgical interventions for patients with metastatic disease to the spine. One study looked at 55 patients with thoracic and lumbar instability owing to spinal metastases treated with surgical stabilization. Forty-nine patients obtained complete pain relief. Of the 28 patients who showed clinical evidence of cord compression or cauda equina syndrome, 20 had major recovery of neurological function. Although this group of patients carried a wide range of diagnoses, breast was the leading primary site of malignancy, occurring in 31 of the studied patients (28).

5. ROLE OF RADIOTHERAPY

Depending on the clinical scenario, radiation therapy may be appropriate as single modality palliation, in concert with systemic treatment, or as a postoperative adjunct in patients with breast cancer metastatic to the spine. In terms of relieving local pain from bone metastases, radiotherapy typically yields some response in 70 to 80% of patients (9). If surgical intervention is deemed unwarranted or inappropriate, radiotherapy may be useful in the prevention or delay of compression fracture, as well as in palliation of patients with cord compression. In patients with spinal cord compression, cauda equina syndrome, or other nerve compression syndrome, radiation treatment and steroid therapy should be initiated within 12 to 24 h if the patient is not a surgical candidate. Primary treatment goals with radiotherapy include pain relief, maintaining function, and prevention of further neurological compromise (10).

Several investigators have considered the utility of radiation therapy in this clinical setting. One prospective study analyzed 130 consecutive patients with cord compression secondary to metastatic disease. Twelve patients were initially approached surgically because of spinal instability. Of 105 evaluable cases that were treated with radiation alone, 80% showed improvement in back pain, and nearly 50% of those with motor dysfunction showed some improvement in symptoms. More than 30% of those without motor disability showed no deterioration over the 15-mo median follow-up period. Of the 105 patients, 44 were noted to have breast as the primary source of disease. These patients tended to be more likely to respond to radiation therapy and showed longer survival times, owing to the relative radiosensitivity and chemosensitivity of the disease (29).

Postoperative radiotherapy is generally recommended after fixation of pathological fractures, stabilization of impending fractures, or spinal decompression and stabilization. Treatment with external beam radiotherapy should begin 2 to 4 wk after surgery, depending on the speed of wound healing. Radiation after surgical procedures for previously unirradiated long bones and acetabular lesions has been shown to decrease the need for repeat surgeries and improve functional status (10). It is possible that this may hold true for spinal lesions as well.

6. SUMMARY

Although progress has been made in prevention and treatment of breast cancer, the vast majority of patients with metastatic disease will eventually die from the illness. The main goals of treatment remain palliation of symptoms and prolongation of survival. Chemotherapy, hormonal manipulation, radiation, and surgical intervention all play important roles in achieving these goals (16). Cooperation among medical oncologists, radiation oncologists, and surgeons is vital in determining the appropriate use of these tools.

REFERENCES

1. Jemal A, Thomas A, Murray T, Ward E, et al. Cancer statistics, 2002. CA Cancer J Clin 2002; 55:10–30.
2. Dignam J. Differences in breast cancer prognosis among African-American and caucasian women. CA Cancer J Clin 2000; 50:50–64.
3. Saarto T, Blomqvist C, Virrkunen P, Elomaa I. Adjuvant clodronate treatment does not reduce the frequency of skeletal metastases in node-positive breast cancer patients: 5-year results of a randomized controlled trial. J Clin Oncol 2001; 19:10–17.
4. Brown H, Healey J. Metastatic Cancer to the Bone. In: DeVita V, Hellman S, Rosenberg S, eds. Cancer Principles & Practice of Oncology. 6th ed. Philadelphia, PA: Lippincott Williams and Wilkins; 2001:2713–2729.
5. Colleoni M, O'Neill A, Goldhirsch A, et al. Identifying breast cancer patients at high risk for bone metastases. J Clin Oncol 2000; 18:3925–3935.
6. Domchek SM, Younger J, Finkelstein DM, Seiden MV. Predictors of skeletal complications in patients with metastatic breast carcinoma. Cancer 2000; 89:363–368.
7. Coleman RE, Smith P, Rubens RD. Clinical course and prognostic factors following bone recurrence from breast cancer. Br J Cancer 1998; 77:336–340.
8. Kanis JA, McCloskey EV, Powles T, Paterson AH, Ashley S, Spector T. A high incidence of vertebral fracture in women with breast cancer. Br J Cancer 1999; 79:1179–1181.
9. The Breast Specialty Group of the British Association of Surgical Oncology. The management of metastatic bone disease in the United Kingdom. Eur J Surg Oncol 1999; 25:3–23.
10. Frassica DA, Thurman S, Welsh J. Radiation therapy. Orthop Clin North Am 2000; 31:557–566.
11. Sorensen S, Helweg-Larsen S, Mouridsen H, Hansen HH. Effect of high-dose dexamethasone in carcinomatous metastatic spinal cord compression treated with radiotherapy: a randomised trial. Eur J Cancer 1994; 30A:22–27.
12. Heimdal K, Hirschberg H, Slettebo H, Watne K, Nome O. High incidence of serious side effects of high-dose dexamethasone treatment in patients with epidural spinal cord compression. J Neurooncol 1992; 12:141–144.
13. Diel IJ, Solomayer E, Costa S, et al. Reduction in new metastases in breast cancer with adjuvant clodronate treatment. N Engl J Med 1998; 339:357–363.
14. Theriault RL, Lipton A, Hortobagyi G, et al. Pamidronate reduces skeletal morbidity in women with advanced breast cancer and lytic bone lesions: a randomized, placebo-controlled trial. J Clin Oncol 1999; 17:846–854.
15. Hillner BE, Ingle JN, Berenson JR, et al. American Society of Clinical Oncology guidelines on the role of bisphosphonates in breast cancer. J Clin Oncol 2000; 18:1378–1391.
16. Hortobagyi, GN. Treatment of breast cancer. N Engl J Med 1998; 339:974–984.
17. Fossati R, Confalonieri C, Torri V, et al: Cytotoxic and hormonal treatment for metastatic breast cancer: a systemic review of published randomized trials involving 31,510 women. J Clin Oncol 1998; 16:3439–3460.

18. Chevallier B, Fumoleau P, Kerbrat P, et al. Docetaxel is a major cytotoxic drug for the treatment of advanced breast cancer: a phase II trial of the clinical screening cooperative group of the European Organization for Research and Treatment of Cancer. J Clin Oncol 1995; 13:314–322.

19. Blum JL, Jones SE, Buzdar AU, et al. Multicenter phase II study of capecitabine in paclitaxel-refractory metastatic breast cancer. J Clin Oncol 1999 17:485–493.

20. Baselga J, Tripathy D, Mendelsohn J, et al. Phase II study of weekly intra venous recombinant humanized anti-p185^{HER2} monoclonal antibody in patients with HER2/*neu*-overexpressing metastatic breast cancer. J Clin Oncol 1996; 14:737–744.

21. Slamon DJ, Leyland-Jones B, Shak S, et al. Use of chemotherapy plus a monoclonal antibody against HER2 for metastatic breast cancer that overexpresses HER2. N Engl J Med 2001; 344:783–792.

22. Bonneterre J, Thurlimann B, Robertson JF, et al. Anastrozole versus tamoxifen as first-line therapy for advanced breast cancer in 668 postmenopausal women: results of the tamoxifen or arimidex randomized group efficacy and tolerability study. J Clin Oncol 2000; 18:3748–3457.

23. Mouridsen H, Gershanovich M, Sun Y, et al. Superior efficacy of letrozole versus tamoxifen as first-line therapy for postmenopausal women with advanced breast cancer: results of a phase III study of the International Letrozole Breast Cancer Group. J Clin Oncol 2001; 19:2596–2606.

24. Buzdar AU, Jonat W, Howell A, et al. Anastrozole vs megestrol acetate in the treatment of postmenopausal women with advanced breast carcinoma: results of a survival update based on the combined analysis of data from two mature phase III trials: Arimidex Study Group. Cancer 1998; 83:1142–1152.

25. Dombernowsky P, Smith I, Falkson G, et al. Letrozole, a new oral aromatase inhibitor for advanced breast cancer: double-blind randomized trail showing a dose effect and improved efficacy and tolerability compared with megestrol acetate. J Clin Oncol 1998; 16:453–461.

26. Kaufmann M, Bajetta E, Dirix LY, et al. Exemstane is superior to megestrol acetate after tamoxifen failure in postmenopausal women with advanced breast cancer: results of a phase III randomized double-blind trial. J Clin Oncol 2000; 18:1399–1411.

27. Wetzel FT, Phillips FM. Management of metastatic disease of the spine. Orthop Clin North Am 2000; 31:611–621.

28. Galasko CSB. Spinal instability secondary to metastatic cancer. J Bone Joint Surg (Br) 1991; 73B:104–108.

29. Maranzano E, Latini P, Checcaglini F, et al. Radiation therapy in metastatic spinal cord compression: a prospective analysis of 105 consecutive patients. Cancer 1991; 67:1311–1317.

16 Genitourinary Oncology

Prostate, Renal, and Bladder Cancer

ROBERT DREICER, MD, FACP

CONTENTS

1. INTRODUCTION

Among the major genitourinary neoplasms, prostate and renal cell carcinomas rank high among all epithelial neoplasms in the relative incidence of both bone metastases and spinal cord compression (1,2). Although advanced urothelial cancers (primarily bladder cancer) represent a relatively small number of patients, this neoplasm too has a relatively high predilection to spread to bone (3). Although the fundamental management issues of skeletal metastases are similar within these neoplasms, the systemic therapies utilized to treat these diseases are very different; hormonal therapy for prostate cancer, immunotherapy for renal cell cancer, and systemic chemotherapy for advanced urothelial cancers. The relative effectiveness of these diverse therapies impact on some important aspects of the management of metastatic disease to the spine in patients with these neoplasms.

2. PROSTATE CANCER

2.1. EPIDEMIOLOGY AND ETIOLOGY

In 2005, it is estimated that there will be approx 232,000 new diagnoses of prostate cancer in the United States representing 33% of all cancer cases affecting men and more than 30,000 deaths related to this disease (4).

The etiology of prostate cancer is complex and multifactorial, involving a spectrum of genetic and environmental factors. Several prostate cancer susceptibility and aggressiveness loci have been reported, however, the current available data suggests that no major gene accounts for a large proportion of susceptibility to the disease (5). Although recognized only recently, prostate cancer like many other common epithelial neoplasms has a recognized familial component (6). Men with a father or brother affected with prostate cancer have a life-time

relative risk (RR) of 2 of developing the disease. The RR increases to 3 if either brother or father are younger than 60 at diagnosis and to a RR of 4 if both are affected at an early age (7).

Androgens such as testosterone are known to be strong tumor promoters, activating via the androgen receptor to stimulate cell division and enhance the effect of endogenous and exogenous carcinogens. Prostate cancer risk is more than 50% higher in African-American men than in Caucasian Americans, and two- to threefold lower in native Chinese and Japanese men. In part, these differences may be explained by ethnic differences in circulating levels of free testosterone or genes associated with androgen synthesis (8).

2.2. THERAPY OPTIONS FOR ADVANCED PROSTATE CANCER

In the era prior to prostate-specific antigen (PSA), the majority of patients presenting with advanced disease had evidence of bone metastases with symptoms of pain, progressive fatigue, and anorexia. One of the more remarkable consequences of the widespread clinical application of PSA testing in the management of prostate cancer has been a significant stage migration with a dramatic decline in the numbers of patients presenting with clinically advanced disease (9). With the presumption that earlier diagnosis and therapy may result in an increased likelihood of cure, a substantial number of patients are undergoing curative intent therapy (i.e., radical prostatectomy, radiotherapy). Approximately one-third of prostate cancer patients with clinically localized disease treated with radical prostatectomy develop evidence of biochemical failure during long-term follow-up (10). Thus, the downstream impact of our current prostate cancer screening and therapeutic strategies has created a new subset of prostate cancer patients, those with evidence of disease recurrence, biochemically (PSA) defined, potentially representing thousands of patients per year in the United States alone (11). Some of these patients are being treated with hormonal therapy before the demonstration of clinical metastatic disease resulting in another subset of patients,

From: Current Clinical Oncology: Cancer in the Spine: Comprehensive Care.
Edited by: R. F. McLain, K-U. Lewandrowski, M. Markman, R. M. Bukowski,
R. Macklis, and E. C. Benzel © Humana Press, Inc., Totowa, NJ

those with PSA-only evidence of disease who are androgen-independent. Ultimately most patients with evidence of biochemical failure will likely develop disease progression and hormonal therapy has been the primary therapeutic modality for 60 yr (12,13).

Androgen ablation options for patients with advanced prostate cancer include orchiectomy, luteinizing hormone-releasing hormone analogs (LHRH), combined androgen ablation, antiandrogen monotherapy, and intermittent hormonal therapy (14). Although a complete review of these approaches is beyond the scope of this chapter, there are some points relevant to the management of patients with metastatic disease to the spine. Although bilateral orchiectomy and medical castration with LHRH analogs has been demonstrated to be therapeutically equivalent, LHRH analogs have become the defacto standard of care for men with metastatic prostate cancer and are typically administered via either subcutaneous or intramuscular 3 or 4 mo depot injections (15). These agents may cause an initial surge in testosterone (testosterone flare) in 5 to 10% of men that can be mitigated by concomitant administration of antiandrogens. Castrate levels of testosterone are typically obtained between d 14 and 21. Given the time to development of castrate levels of testosterone, patients presenting with impending or frank spinal cord compression should be managed with bilateral orchiectomy given evidence that serum testosterone reaches castrate levels in a mean of 3 h (16).

Although androgen deprivation therapy for metastatic prostate cancer is a highly effective therapy with response rates in the 70 to 90% range, it is not a curative intervention, with median duration of response in the 12–18 mo range. Once the disease process becomes refractory to hormonal therapy (with clinical progression, i.e., bone and soft tissue metastases) median survival is in the 6 to 9 mo range. Any current discussion of survival of patients with prostate cancer needs to be within the context of the dramatic stage migration that has occurred over the past 10 to 15 yr as previously discussed. Patients with evidence of biochemical, i.e., PSA failures following definitive therapy, may have prolonged survival periods, with a recent experience reporting a median survival from PSA failure to death from prostate cancer being a median of 13 yr (12).

2.3. SPINAL INVOLVEMENT

Bone is the primary site of metastatic disease in prostate cancer as evidenced by an incidence of 85 to 100% in patients who die of the disease (17). The most common site of bone metastases in prostate cancer is the spine, followed by the femur, pelvis, ribs, sternum, skull, and humerus (18). Although bone metastases from prostate cancer are typically osteoblastic, histological and biochemical studies clearly indicate an increase of both bone formation and bone resorption (19).

Given the high rate of bone metastases in prostate cancer with a predilection for the spine as a primary location, elucidating the underlying mechanism of this somewhat unusual phenomenon has long been of interest to clinicians and investigators. More than 60 yr ago Baston suggested that prostate carcinoma cells reach the lumbar vertebrae via the vertebral venous plexus (Batson's plexus). This hypothesis was based both on the observation of an unusually high prevalence of lower spine metastases from autopsy series and cadaver experiments showing that contrast liquid could flow from the prostatic veins to higher segments of the spine in the setting of increased intra-abdominal pressure (20). Although a few subsequent reports supported Batson's hypothesis, other investigators concluded that a systemic route of spread for metastases was more likely (21). More recent work has focused on tumor specific features that may enhance either metastatic potential or site specific microenvironmental factors that may provide a selective advantage for tumor invasiveness and growth (21).

2.4. SPINAL METASTASES, CORD COMPRESSION, CLINICAL ISSUES

2.4.1. Clinical Presentation, Radiographic Evaluation

Patients with spinal metastases from prostate cancer most frequently present with complaints of pain. Given that the most men with prostate cancer present in their 60s and 70s, comorbid conditions, such as osteoarthritis, are prevalent complicating the initial clinical evaluation of patients. The most problematic presentation of spinal metastases is in association with spinal cord compression, which develops most commonly as a result of metastases that involve the vertebral body and with extension into the spinal canal. Spinal cord compression has been reported to occur in approx 10% of prostate cancer patients at some time during the disease course (22,23). Prostate cancer patients with spinal cord compression typically present with pain, weakness, autonomic dysfunction, and sensory loss (24). Pain is unequivocally the most common presenting symptom with retrospective prostate cancer series reporting this finding in 75 to 100% of patients with spinal cord compression. However, in one prospective study, 41% of patients were pain free at the time a spinal cord compression was documented (23).

The radiographic evaluation of patients with advanced prostate cancer and back pain is guided in part by the patient's disease status and the history and physical exam. Newly diagnosed patients with advanced prostate cancer (with screening and stage migration, a relatively uncommon presentation today) typically will undergo radionucleotide bone imaging to assess the extent of bone involvement. Although sensitive, bone scans have a low specificity. False-positive scans can occur because of trauma, degenerative disease, or Paget's disease. In patients with newly diagnosed, clinically organ-confined disease however, the likelihood of a positive bone scan due to metastases has been demonstrated to be 0.6 and 2.6% for those with serum PSA concentrations between 10.1 and 15 ng/mL and 15.1 and 20 ng/mL, respectively (25). On the basis of these studies, many urologists will not obtain a baseline bone scan in patients with newly diagnosed, early-stage, asymptomatic prostate cancer who have serum PSA concentrations of less than 15 to 20 ng/mL. Therefore, when some of these patients develop disease progression and present with new back pain a previous bone scan will frequently not be available.

When a patient with prostate cancer presents in the office with new or worsening, chronic back pain, the initial radiographic evaluation should consist of plain radiographs of the spine (Fig. 1). These films can typically be obtained the same day and may provide information regarding concomitant degenerative disease, the presence of obvious blastic or lytic metastases

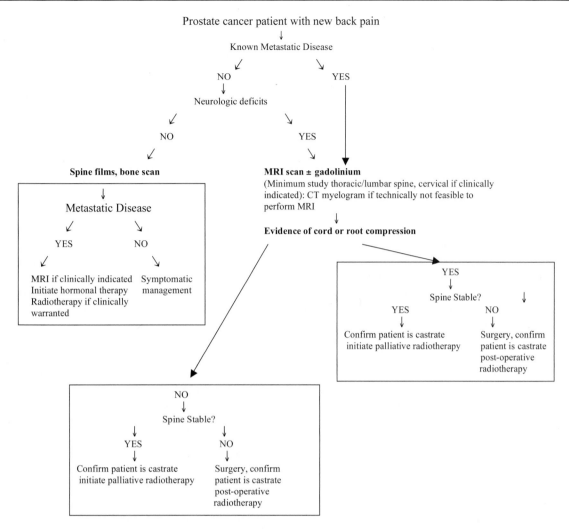

Fig. 1. Treatment algorithm for prostate cancer patients with back pain.

and/or evidence of bony destruction. Although plain radiographs are more than 90% sensitive and 85% specific for demonstration of abnormalities in patients with symptomatic spinal metastases, false-positive rates may be as high as 20% and autopsy series indicate that as many as 25% of spinal lesions are invisible on radiography (26,27). Subsequent bone scan imaging will allow a more thorough evaluation for the presence of metastatic disease.

If the patient presents with moderate-severe pain, neurological deficits on exam, a history of loss of bowel or bladder function, plain films demonstrating bony destruction, or if the clinicians index of suspicion suggests the potential for a spinal cord compression, then an magnetic resonance imaging (MRI) is required on a urgent basis. The MRI scan is the gold standard for the evaluation of the spine. Generic recommendations for patients with any neoplasm with suspected spinal cord compression typically include complete spine MRI, especially when there is high risk for skip lesions. In some centers, the cervical spine is not imaged routinely in this setting (in the absence of clinical or plain film findings) because it adds significantly to acquisition time. Some have advocated obtaining scout whole-spine sagittal MRI images to avoid missing noncontiguous sites

(21). In prostate cancer patients with suspected spinal cord compression (without cervical spine symptoms, clinical findings, or plain film evidence of bony destruction) MRI of the thoracic and lumbar-sacral spine with and without gadolinium should be the minimum study obtained. Given the high frequency of involvement of both the lumbar and thoracic spine, failure to image both areas may compromise radiotherapy if untreated lesions become symptomatic and are detected at a later time.

2.4.2. Therapy of Spine Metastases, Spinal Cord Compression

The initial therapeutic maneuver in the hormone naïve patient who presents with new bone or soft tissue metastases is to initiate androgen ablation therapy to induce castrate levels of testosterone. Androgen ablation options for patients with advanced prostate cancer include, LHRH or bilateral orchiectomy. Although orchiectomy remains the gold standard, patients are increasingly opting for medical therapy with LHRH analogs in part because of the psychological implications of surgical castration. Although therapeutically equivalent to LHRH analogs, orchiectomy remains the treatment of choice for patients presenting with spinal cord compression or diffuse, painful bone metastases as it leads to the rapid achievement of castrate levels of testosterone (hours) compared to the 14 to 21 d required for LHRH analogs *(16)*. Patients who opt for medical castration despite the issues previously noted, must be started concomitantly on an antiandrogen or other agents to block the potential testosterone flare seen in approx 10% of patients who initiate therapy with an LHRH analog *(14)*.

For the majority of patients who are androgen-independent, management of spine metastases in the absence of spinal cord compression involves consideration of the patient's current disease status, clinical condition, and prior therapy. Patients with bone metastases from prostate cancer may experience periods of pain followed by near or total resolution without specific intervention. Initial evaluation will typically include plain radiographs and a bone scan. Although nonsteroidal anti-inflammatory agents may be helpful initially, most patients will require opioids analgesics with an appropriate prophylactic bowel regimen while the evaluation is underway.

External beam radiotherapy has been the mainstay of the management of painful bone metastases for decades. Radiotherapy has a proven role in palliation of pain from bone metastases with numerous randomised trials obtaining response rates in the 70 to 90% range *(28)*. Although the efficacy of radiotherapy is not in doubt, the optimal dose and fractionation schema remains controversial. Advocates of a single large radiotherapy fraction (8–10 gy) point to the potential for rapid response and convenience, critics note an increased toxicity profile and that a decrease in total dose may compromise the duration of response. Prolonged schedules (40 gy in 20 fractions/50 gy in 25 fractions) result in less acute toxicity and may provide longer control but are problematic for many patients. Typical treatment schedules in North America consist of 20 gy in 5 or 30 gy in 10 fractions *(28)*.

Patients with multiple bony sites of metastatic disease or those with progression in areas previously treated with external-beam therapy may benefit from systemic therapies including chemotherapy or bone-seeking radioisotopes.

Historically, chemotherapy for advanced prostate cancer was widely held to be toxic and without any clinically meaningful benefit *(29)*. In 1996, Canadian investigators reported the results of a phase III study in which patients with symptomatic advanced prostate cancer were randomized to receive either prednisone alone or mitoxantrone and prednisone. This trial was unique in that the primary end-point of this study was a palliative response defined by decrease in pain and analgesic requirements. A palliative response was observed in 29% of patients treated with mitoxantrone and prednisone vs 12% in those treated with prednisone alone. Although patients treated in the chemotherapy-containing arm demonstrated a significantly longer period of palliation (43 vs 18 wk), no survival difference was demonstrated *(30)*. Subsequently, the results of Canadian study were confirmed by a second multicenter phase III trial leading to an Food and Drug Administration (FDA) indication for advanced prostate cancer for mitoxantrone *(31)*. Mitoxantrone is typically administered with a short iv infusion once every 3 wk as an outpatient with 10 mg of prednisone in divided doses administered daily. Palliation of bone pain and other disease-related symptoms (fatigue, cachexia, and so on)

may be seen relatively promptly. Patients without a clinical response after one to two cycles of therapy are not likely to obtain symptomatic improvement.

Although mitoxantrone-based therapies have the ability to palliate a subset of patients, the response rates are modest with a low objective response rate and no evidence of survival. Given the low response objective response rates with mitoxantrone, other antineoplastics with alternative mechanisms of actions were explored. Phase II trials with taxane-based therapies with targeted microtubular function demonstrated intriguing levels of activity leading to two landmark randomized phase III studies that compared these regimens to mitoxantrone plus prednisone. TAX327 compared docetaxel plus prednisone to mitoxantrone plus prednisone. The study included both a tri-weekly (75 mg/m^2 every 21 d) and a weekly (30 mg/m^2 weekly for 5 wk, repeated every 6 wk) docetaxel arm. A survival advantage was reported for triweekly docetaxel plus prednisone (but not weekly docetaxel plus prenisone) over mitoxantrone plus prednisone. Median survival was 18.9 mo for triweekly docetaxel plus prednisone and 16.4 mo for mitoxantrone and prednisone, a 24% reduction in the hazard of death ($p = 0.009$). Pain response was also more common with triweekly docetaxel (35%) than with mitoxantrone (22%, $p = 0.01$) *(32)*. SWOG 9916 compared triweekly docetaxel plus estramustine (docetaxel 60 mg/m^2 escalated to 70 mg/m^2 on d 2 and estramustine 280 mg three times daily on d 1–5 administered on a 21-d cycle) to mitoxantrone and prednisone and also demonstrated a survival advantage for the docetaxel-containing arm (median 18 mo vs 16 mo, 20% reduction in the hazard of death, $p = 0.01$). In both studies, grade 3 or 4 toxicity was somewhat more common with docetaxel than with mitoxantrone. These two studies are the first to show a survival benefit with chemotherapy in AIPC and establish docetaxel administered every 21 d as a standard drug in AIPC *(33)*.

Radiopharmaceuticals represent another systemic therapy option for patients with multiple painful bony metastatic sites. Strontium-89, the first radiopharmaceutical approved for use in the United States is a pure β-emitting radioactive analog of calcium that selectively irradiates metastatic sites in bone while generally sparing normal bone tissue. Other radiopharmaceuticals either approved or in clinical trials include samarium 153 ethylenediaminetetramethylene phosphonate, rhenium 186 hydroxyethylidene diphosphonate, and tin 117m (4+) diethylene triaminepentacetic acid. Studies suggest that 60 to 80% of patients with prostate cancer derive a palliative benefit from systemic administration of bone-seeking β-emitting radiopharmaceuticals *(34)*.

Recently, the concept of "bone-targeted" therapy has emerged, involving a combination of chemo-hormonal therapy with bone-specific agents, such as Strontium-89, with one early clinical trial suggesting a potential impact on survival of this approach in advanced prostate patients *(35)*.

3. RENAL CELL CARCINOMA CANCER

3.1. EPIDEMIOLOGY AND ETIOLOGY

Malignant tumors of the renal pelvis and kidney (the vast majority being renal cell carcinoma) represent approx 2% of

Table 1
Randomized Trials of Biological Response Modifier-Based Therapies in Metastatic Renal Cell Carcinoma

Therapy	Reference	No. of patients	Overall response rate (%)	Survival benefit
IFN-α	63	167	16	Yes ($p = 0.011$)
Medroxyprogesterone		168	2	
IFN-α + vinblastine	64	79	16	Yes ($p = 0.0049$)
Vinblastine			2	
IFN-γ	65	98	4.4	No ($p = 0.54$)
Placebo		99	6.6	
IL-2 + IFN-α	46	70	1	No ($p = 0.1$)
IL-2 + IFN-α + 5 Fluorouracil		61	5	
IL-2	66	138	6.5	No ($p = 0.55$)
IFN-α		147	7.5	
IL-2 + IFN-α		140	18.6	

IL, interleukin-2; IFN, interferon.

new cancer diagnoses in the United States with an estimated 22,500 new cases and 8000 cancer deaths (4). The highest incidence is in individuals in the seventh decade with a median age at diagnosis of 66 yr and there is an approx 60:40 male predominance. There has been a significant increase in the incidence of renal cell carcinoma over the past 40 yr with evidence of a stage migration with increasing numbers of patients with localized tumors (36). This phenomenon may be partially explained by the discovery of increasing numbers of asymptomatic tumors as a consequence of the ubiquitous application of non-invasive abdominal imaging including computed tomography, ultrasound, and MRI (37).

Like breast cancer, colon cancer, and retinoblastoma, renal cancer occurs in both a sporadic (nonhereditary) and a hereditary form with at least four forms of hereditary renal cell carcinoma currently recognized. In 1993, the von Hippel-Lindau (VHL) gene was first identified and has been found to be mutated in a high percentage of tumors and cell lines from patients with sporadic (nonhereditary) clear cell renal carcinoma (38,39).

3.2. THERAPY OPTIONS FOR ADVANCED RENAL CANCER

Although progress against many of the major epithelial neoplasms has been achieved over the last decade, the outlook for patients with metastatic renal cell carcinoma remains very poor with a 5-yr survival rate of less than 10% (40).

In contrast to the utility of chemotherapy in many epithelial cancers, to date the results have been dismal in renal cell carcinoma with the majority of studies reporting response rates in the 5 to 10% range (41). Resistance to these agents has been ascribed to high levels of expression of P-glycoprotein (the multi-drug resistance [MDR] gene product-1), however studies performed with MDR inhibiting agents have not demonstrated improvements in response rates with antineoplastics agents such as vinblastine (42).

Renal cell carcinoma has long been seen as a model for the investigation of biological response modifier therapy because of the long-recognized biological "eccentricities" of this disease manifested by well documented cases of spontaneous regression of metastatic disease and the occasional patient with metastatis who does well for long time periods without any specific therapeutic intervention.

Two cytokines, interferon (IFN)-α and interleukin (IL)-2 produce tumor regressions in 10 to 15% of patients with metastatic disease (43). In a review of IFN-α in 1042 patients, the overall response rate was 12% (44). Responses are typically confined to patients with good performance status and lung-predominant metastatic disease, other factors, such as prior nephrectomy and longer disease-free progression interval, are also predictive of response. Randomized trials (Table 1) comparing IFN vs medroxyprogresterone or vinblastine suggests a modest survival advantage for patients treated with IFN-α (43).

High-dose IL-2 was approved by the FDA for use in advanced kidney cancer based on results of studies conducted by the IL-2 working group demonstrating a 7% complete and 8% partial response rate in 255 patients. Median survival was 16.3 mo for all patients with 10 to 20% alive at 5 to 10 yr following therapy (42). High-dose IL-2 is associated with significant toxicities and requires an experienced group of physicians and nurses providing supportive care for optimal results. Lower dose regimens of IL-2 have been evaluated with response rates reported in the 15 to 20% range (42). The von Hippel-Kindau gene inactivation and subsequent vascular endothelial growth factor (VEGF) overproduction has been increasingly identified as an important target in clear cell carcinoma of the kidney (45). Three agents that affect various aspects of VEGF activity have been demonstrated to have intriguing levels of anti-tumor activity in renal cancer, these include bevacizumab (avastin), SU-11248 (Sutent) and Bay 43-9006 (sorafenib). Phase III trials of these agents of ongoing and may lead to a new treatment paradigm of this difficult epithelial cancer (45).

The role of nephrectomy in patients with metastatic disease has, until recently, been limited to very small numbers of patients with intractable pain or bleeding, however, recent evidence from two randomized trials suggests that patients with optimal performance status who are planning to receive biological response modifier therapy may have improved outcomes after undergoing resection of the primary renal neoplasm (46,47).

3.3. RENAL CARCINOMA: SPINAL INVOLVEMENT, CORD COMPRESSION, CLINICAL MANAGEMENT

Osseous metastases occur in 25 to 50% of patients with metastatic renal cell, ranking fourth in spinal metastatic incidence behind, lung, breast, and prostate cancer (48,49). In patients with bone metastases the spine is the most common location (49%) followed by ribs (39%), ileum (30%), and femur (27%) (50). The incidence of spinal cord compression in patients with renal cell carcinoma is not well defined with one large retrospective series identifying only 3 such patients among more than 161 patients with renal cell carcinoma cancer diagnosed over a 9-yr period (51).

Initial evaluation of patients with suspected osseous metastatases should include a bone scan and directed plain radiographs. Patients presenting with signs and symptoms worrisome for epidural cord compression should be evaluated with contrast MRI studies of the spine.

Although historically considered a relatively radio-resistant neoplasm (52), there is both experimental and clinical evidence of the effectiveness of external beam radiotherapy in the management of painful bone metastatic sites (53). In patients with a known diagnosis of metastatic renal cell carcinoma with a stable spine who present with spinal cord compression, radiotherapy represents an effective therapeutic intervention.

In patients with epidural compression in previously irradiated areas or those with unstable spinal lesions or painful metastatic sites unresponsive to radiotherapy, there is evidence to support the role of surgical therapy. Jackson et al. (54) reported on 79 patients with metastatic renal cell carcinoma to the spine managed with a variety of anterior, posterior, or combined approaches. Preoperative embolization and radiotherapy was utilized in approx 50% of the patients, all but three underwent internal fixation. Significant pain reduction was reported in 89% of patients with neurological improvement in 65% of 66 patients (54).

4. BLADDER CANCER

4.1. EPIDEMIOLOGY AND ETIOLOGY

In 2005, it is estimated that there will be approx 47,000 new diagnoses of bladder cancer with approx 9000 deaths because of the disease (4). Bladder cancer is the fourth most common cancer in men and the seventh most common in women. The incidence of bladder cancer increases with age with a peak incidence in the seventh decade of life. The reason for this increasing prevalence among older patients is not known, however, various factors including greater potential duration of exposure to carcinogens and diminished ability to repair DNA damage has been proposed (55). Cigarette smoking is the most important risk factor, although work in the dye, rubber, or leather industries is also strongly associated with bladder cancer (56). Women in the United States have incidence and mortality rates from bladder cancer that are approximately one-quarter to one-third those of men (57).

Bladder cancer in North America and Western Europe presents predominantly as transitional cell carcinoma and can be thought of as two interrelated disease processes. The majority of patients (approx 75%) present with superficial disease (not invading musclaris propria) and are managed for recurrent dis-

Table 2
Randomized Trials of Chemotherapy in Metastatic Urothelial Cancer

Therapy	Reference	No. of patients	Overall response rate (%)	Survival benefit
Cisplatin	67	126	39	
MVAC		120	12	Yes ($p = 0.0002$)
CISCA	68	48	46	
MVAC		54	65	Yes ($p = 0.000315$)
Gemcitabine + cisplatin	69	203	49	No ($p = 0.75$)
MVAC		202	46	

MVAC, methotrexate, vinblastine, doxorubicin, cisplatin; CISCA, cyclophosphamide, doxorubicin, cisplatin.

ease on an ongoing basis with cystoscopic examination, resection, and, in selected patients with intravesical, administration of chemotherapy or biological response modifiers. Although 20 to 25% of patients with superficial bladder cancer will progress into muscle invasion, the majority (up to 90%) of patients presenting with muscle-invasive disease have this finding at their initial presentation without a previous history of superficial bladder cancer (58).

4.2. THERAPY OPTIONS FOR ADVANCED BLADDER CANCER

Metastatic transitional cell carcinoma of the bladder is an aggressive neoplasm characterized by rapid growth and dissemination with a median survival typically less than 1 yr. Despite the availability of a myriad of antineoplastics with moderate-significant anti-tumor activity yielding overall response rates in the 40 to 80% range, randomized trials continue to demonstrate median survival rates in the 13 to 14 mo range, with very limited long-term survival (59).

Advanced transitional cell carcinoma is a moderately chemosensitive neoplasm. Although the methotrexate, vinblastine, doxorubicin, cisplatin (MVAC) regimen has been the standard of care for more than a decade, the limitations of this regimen was recently highlighted by the update of the Intergroup trial which compared cisplatin and MVAC in patients with advanced urothelial cancer. With a minimum follow-up of 6 yr, only 3.7% of patients treated on the MVAC arm were alive and disease-free, emphasizing the need to seek alternative therapeutic options (60). The optimal choice of chemotherapy for previously untreated patients with metastatic disease remains controversial. Cisplatin-based regimens such as MVAC produce response rates in the 40 to 70% range with some patients, albeit a very limited number, achieving long-term survival (Table 2). The toxicity profile associated with this regimen is well known and includes relatively high rates of mucositis and myelosuppression and the use of this and other cisplatin-based regimens are limited to patients with relatively normal renal function. In the last 5 to 10 yr, newer agents have been brought into clinical practice including paclitaxel and gemcitabine. These drugs have significant single-agent activity in previously untreated patients with response rates of 42% and 20 to 30%, respectively (2,3). Chemotherapy combinations widely utilized to treat advanced disease include MVAC, gemcitabine plus cisplatin, and carboplatin plus paclitaxel. In selected patients with primarily soft-tissue metastatic disease achieving significant clinical response, adjunctive surgical resection may improve patient outcome (61).

4.3. SPINAL INVOLVEMENT, CORD COMPRESSION, CLINICAL MANAGEMENT

Bone is second only to lymph nodes as the most common metastatic site for transitional cell carcinoma of the urothelium with one large series reporting up to 35% of patients developing osseous metastatic disease (3). In the series reported by Sengelov et al. (3), the spine was the most common location for bone metastases (40%) followed by the pelvis (26%), femurs (10%), and ribs (10%). The incidence of spinal cord compression in patients with urothelial carcinoma is poorly characterized with one large retrospective series identifying only 1 patient among more than 772 patients with urothelial neoplasms cancer diagnosed over a 9-yr period (51).

Initial evaluation of patients with suspected osseous metastatases is typical of that of other solid tumors and should include a bone scan and directed plain radiographs. Patients presenting with signs and symptoms worrisome for epidural cord compression should be evaluated with contrast MRI studies of the spine.

Patients with spinal bone metastases without evidence of a spinal cord compression are typically managed with involved field radiotherapy. Chemotherapy may be palliative in patients with multiple sites of metastatic disease, however, bone metastases is a poor prognostic factor in terms of chemotherapy response rates and survival (62).

Patients with evidence of spinal cord compression with a stable spine no prior radiotherapy to the area involved should be managed with radiotherapy. Patients with prior radiotherapy or those whose disease progresses while receiving radiotherapy require surgical management.

REFERENCES

1. Sioutos PJ, Arbit E, Meshulam CF, Galicich JH. Spinal metastases from solid tumors. Analysis of factors affecting survival. Cancer 1995; 76:1453–1459.
2. Ratanatharathorn V, Powers WE. Epidural spinal cord compression from metastatic tumor: diagnosis and guidelines for management. Cancer Treat Rev 1991; 18:55–71.
3. Sengelov L, Kamby C, von der maase H. Pattern of metastases in relation to characteristics of primary tumor and treatment in patients with disseminated urothelial carcinoma. J Urol 1996; 155:111–114.
4. Jemal A, Murray T, Ward E, et al. Cancer Statistics 2005. CA Cancer J Clin 2005; 55:10–30.
5. Nwosu V, Carpten J, Trent JM, Sheridan R. Heterogeneity of genetic alterations in prostate cancer: evidence of the complex nature of the disease. Hum Mol Genet 2001; 10:2313–2318.
6. Carter BS, Beaty TH, Steinberg GD, Childs B, Walsh PC. Mendelian inheritance of familial prostate cancer. Proc Natl Acad Sci USA 1992; 89:3367–3371.
7. Bratt O. Hereditary prostate cancer. BJU Int 2000; 85:588–598.
8. Ross RK, Pike MC, Coetzee GA, et al. Androgen metabolism and prostate cancer: establishing a model of genetic susceptibility. Cancer Res 1998; 58:4497–4504.
9. Smith DS, Catalona WJ, Herschman JD. Longitudinal screening for prostate cancer with prostate specific antigen. JAMA 1996; 276:1309–1315.
10. Pound CR, Partin AW, Epstein JI, Walsh PC. Prostate-specific antigen after anatomic radical retropubic prostatectomy: patterns of recurrence and cancer control. Urol Clin North Amer 1997; 24:395–406.
11. Laufer M, Pound CR, Carducci MA, Eisenberger MA. Management of patients with rising prostate-specific antigen after radical prostatectomy. Urology 2000; 55:309–315.
12. Pound CR, Partin AW, Eisenberger MA, Chan DW, Pearson JD, Walsh PC. Natural history of progression after PSA elevation following radical prostatectomy. JAMA 1999; 281:1591–1597.
13. Lytton B. Prostate cancer: a brief history and the discovery of hormonal ablation treatment. J Urol 2001; 165:1859–1862.
14. Dreicer R. The evolving role of hormone therapy in advanced prostate cancer. Cleve Clin J Med 2000; 67:720–722.
15. Peeling WB. Phase III studies to compare Goserelin (Zoladex) with Orchiectomy and with Diethylstilbestrol in treatment of prostatic carcinoma. Urology 1989; 33:45–52.
16. Maatman TJ, Gupta MK, Montie JE. Effectiveness of castration versus intravenous estrogen therapy in producing rapid endocrine control of metastatic cancer of the prostate. J Urol 1985; 133:620–621.
17. Whitmore WF. Natural history and staging of prostate cancer. Urol Clin North Am 1984; 11:209–220.
18. Galasko CSB. The anatomy and pathways of skeletal metastases. In: Weiss L, Gilbert HA, eds. Bone Metastasis. Boston, MA: Hall Medical Publishers; 1981:49–63.
19. Garnero P. Markers of bone turnover in prostate cancer. Cancer Treat Rev 2001; 27:187–192.
20. Batson OV. The function of the vertebral veins and their role in the spread of metastases. Ann Surg 1940; 112:138–149.
21. Chen TC. Prostate cancer and spinal cord compression. Oncology 2001; 15:841–855.
22. Kuban DA, el-Mahdi AM, Sigfred SV, Schellhammer PF, Babb TJ. Characerictics of spinal cord compression in carcinoma of the prostate. Urology 1986; 28:364–369.
23. Bayley A, Milosevic M, Blend R, et al. A prospective study of factors predicting clinically occult spinal cord compression in patients with metastatic prostate carcinoma. Cancer 2001; 92:303–310.
24. Osborn JL, Getzenberg RH, Trump DL. Spinal cord compression in prostate cancer. J Neurooncol 1995; 23:135–147.
25. Oesterling JE, Martin SK, Bergstralh EJ Lowe FC. The use of prostate-specific antigen in staging patients with newly diagnosed prostate cancer. JAMA 1993; 269:57–60.
26. Wong DA, Fornasier VL, MacNab I. Spinal metastases: the obvious, the occult and the imposters. Spine 1990; 15:1–4.
27. Posner JB. Neurologic complications of cancer. In: Davis FA, ed. Contemporary Neurology Series. Philadelphia, PA: FA Davis; 1995:122.
28. Catton CN, Gospodarowicz MK. Palliative radiotherapy in prostate cancer. Sem Urol Oncol 1997; 15:65–72.
29. Tannock IF. Is there evidence that chemotherapy is of benefit to patients with carcinoma of the prostate? J Clin Oncol 1985; 3:1013–1021.
30. Tannock IF, Osaba D, Stackler MR, et al. Chemotherapy with mitoxantrone plus prednisone or prednisone alone for symptomatic hormone-resistant prostate cancer: a Canadian randomized trial with palliative end points. J Clin Oncol 1996; 14:1756–1764.
31. Kantoff PW, Halabi S, Conaway M, et al. Hydrocortisone with or without mitoxantrone in men with hormone-refractory prostate cancer: results of the cancer and leukemia group B 9182 study. J Clin Oncol 1999; 17:2506–2513.
32. Tannock I, de Wit R, Berry W, et al. Docetaxel plus prednisone or mitoxantrone plus prednisone for advanced prostate cancer. N Engl J Med 2004; 351:1502–1512.
33. Petrylak D, Tangen C, Hussain M, et al. Docetaxel and estramustine compared with mitoxantrone and prednisone for advanced refractory prostate cancer. N Engl J Med 2004; 351:1513–1520.
34. McEwan AJB. Unsealed source therapy of painful bone metastases: an update. Semin Nucl Med 1997; 27:165–182.
35. Tu SM, Millikan RE, Mengistu B, et al. Bone-targeted therapy for advanced androgen-independent carcinoma of the prostate: a randomised phase II trial. Lancet 2001; 357:336–341.

36. Chow WH, Devesa SS, Warren JL, Fraumeni JF Jr. Rising incidence of renal cell cancer in the United States. JAMA 1999; 281:1628–1631.

37. Pantuck AJ, Zisman A, Belldegrun AS. The changing natural history of renal cell carcinoma. J Urol 2001; 166:1611–1623.

38. Latif F, Tory K, Gnarra J, et al. Identification of the von Hippel-Lindau disease tumor suppressor gene. Science 1993; 260:1317–1320.

39. Shuin T, Kondo K, Torigoe S, et al. Frequent somatic mutations and loss of heterozygosity of the von Hippel-Lindau tumor suppressor gene in primary human renal cell carcinomas. Cancer Res 1994; 54:2852–2855.

40. Motzer RJ, Bander NH, Nanus DM. Renal-cell carcinoma. N Engl J Med 1996; 335:865–875.

41. Motzer RJ, Russo P. Systemic therapy for renal cell carcinoma. J Urol 2000; 163:408–417.

42. Figlan RA. Renal cell carcinoma: management of advanced disease. J Urol 1999; 161:381–387.

43. Bukowski RM. Cytokine therapy for metastatic renal cell carcinoma. Semin Urol Oncol 2001; 19:148–154.

44. Wirth MP. Immunotherapy for metastatic renal cell carcinoma. Urol Clin North Am 1993; 20:283–295.

45. Rini BI, Small EJ. Biology and clinical development of vascular endothelial growth factor-targeted in renal cell carcinoma. J Clin Oncol 2005; 23:1028–1043.

46. Flanigan RC, Salmon SE, Blumenstein BA, et al. Nephrectomy followed by interferon alfa-2b compared with interferon alfa-2b alone for metastatic renal-cell cancer. N Engl J Med 2001; 345:1655–1659.

47. Mickisch GHJ, Garin A, van Poppel H, et al. Radical nephrectomy plus interferon-alfa-based immunotherapy compared with interferon alfa alone in metastatic renal-cell cancer: a randomised trial. Lancet 2001; 358:966–970.

48. Saitoh H, Hida M. Metastatic processes and a ptoetnital indication of treatment for metastatic lesions of renal adenocarcinoma. J Urol 1982; 128:916–918.

49. Skinner DG, Colvin RB. Diagnosis and management of renal cell carcinoma: a clinical and pathological study. Cancer 1971; 28:1165–1177.

50. Swanson DA, Orovan WL, Johnson DE, Giacco G. Osseous metastases secondary to renal cell carcinoma. Urology 1981; 18:556–561.

51. Liskow A, Chang CH, Desanctis P, Benson M, Fetell M, Housepian E. Epidural cord compression in association with genitourinary neoplasms. Cancer 1986; 58:949–954.

52. Seitz W, Karcher KH, Binder W. Radiotherapy of metastatic renal cell carcinoma. Sem Surg Oncol 1988; 4:100–102.

53. DiBiase SJ, Valicenti RK, Schultz D, Xie Y, Gomella LG, Corn BW. Palliative irradiation for focally sumptomatic metastatic renal cell carcinoma: support for dose escalation based on a biological model. J Urol 1997; 158:746–749.

54. Jackson RJ, Gokaslan ZL, Loh SC. Metastatic renal cell carcinoma of the spine: surgical treatment and results. J Neurosurg 2001; 94:18–24.

55. Baumgart J, Zhukovskaya NV, Anisimov VN. Carcinogenesis and aging. VIII. Effect of host age on tumour growth, metastatic potential, and chemotherapeutic sensitivity to 1.4-benzoquinone-guanylhydrazonethiosemicarbazone (ambazone) and 5-fluorouracil in mice and rats. Exp Pathol 1988; 33:239–248.

56. Silverman DT, Levin LI, Hoover RN, et al. Occupational risks of bladder cancer in the United States: I. White men. J Natl Cancer Inst 1989; 81:1472–1480.

57. Ross RK, Jones PA, MC Y. Bladder cancer epidemiology and pathogenesis. Sem Oncol 1996; 23:536–545.

58. Kryger JV, Messing E. Bladder cancer screening. Sem Oncol 1996; 23:585–597.

59. Vaughn DJ, Malkowicz SB. Recent advances in bladder cancer chemotherapy. Cancer Invest 2001; 19:77–85.

60. Saxman SB, Propert KJ, Einhorn LH, et al. Long-term follow-up of a phase III intergroup study of cisplatin alone or in combination with methotrexate, vinblastine, and doxorubicin in patients with metastatic urothelial carcinoma: a cooperative group study. J Clin Oncol 1997; 15:2564–2569.

61. Dreicer R. Locally advanced and metastatic bladder cancer. Curr Treat Options Oncol 2001; 2:431–436.

62. Bajorin DF, Dodd PM, Mazumdar M, et al. Long-term survival in metastatic transitional cell carcinoma and prognostic factors predicting outcome of therapy. J Clin Oncol 1999; 17:3173–3181.

63. Medical Research Council Renal Cancer Collaborators.: Interferon-a and survival in metastatic renal carcinoma: early results of a randomised controlled trial. Lancet 1999; 353:14–17.

64. Pyrhonen S, Salminen E, Ruutu M, et al. Prospective randomized trial of interferon alfa-2a plus vinblastine versus vinblastine alone in patients with advanced renal cell cancer. J Clin Oncol 1999; 17:2859–2867.

65. Gleave ME, Elhilali M, Fradet Y, et al. Interferon gamma-1b compared with placebo in metastatic renal-cell carcinoma. N Engl J Med 1998; 338:1265–1271.

66. Negrier S, Escudier B, Lasset C, et al. Recombinant human interleukin-2, recombinant human interferon alfa-2a, or both in metastatic renal-cell carcinoma. N Engl J Med 1998; 338:1272–1278.

67. Loehrer PJ, Einhorn LH, Elson PJ, et al. A randomized comparison of cisplatin alone or in combination with methotrexate, vinblastine, and doxorubicin in patients with metastatic urothelial carcinoma: A cooperative group study. J Clin Oncol 1992; 10:1066–1073.

68. Logothetis CJ, Dexeus FH, Finn L, et al. A prospective randomized trial comparing MVAC and CISCA chemotherapy for patients with metastatic urothelial tumors. J Clin Oncol 1990; 8:1050–1055.

69. von der Maase H, Hansen SW, Roberts JT, et al. Gemcitabine and cisplatin versus methotrexate, vinblastine, doxorubicin, and cisplatin in advanced or metastatic bladder cancer: results of a large, randomized, multinational, multicenter, phase III study. J Clin Oncol 2000; 18:3068–3077.

17 Spinal Metastases From Gastrointestinal Malignancies

MELLAR P. DAVIS, MD, FCCP

CONTENTS

1. INTRODUCTION

Among 965,000 new patients with cancer occurring yearly in the United States, bone metastases will eventually develop in 30 to 70% (1). The most common site of metastases is the spine occurring in 50 to 70% of those with bone metastases (1). In adults, malignant bone tumors arise most frequently from extraosseous epithelial primaries, whereas children usually have primaries from within bone (2). Primaries most commonly associated with bone metastases are breast, prostate, lung, kidney, and thyroid carcinoma (1,3). Pain occurs in some, but not all, bone metastases as 33 to 50% of patients with skeletal metastases do not have pain (4). The experience of pain is not particular to gender or primary tumor-related, nor is it predictable based on radiological appearance. The primary site of malignancy remains unidentified in 10% of patients with skeletal and spinal metastases. In most series of bone and spinal metastases, gastrointestinal primaries make up a similar percentage of those with unknown primaries (3). The distribution of metastases within the spine follows the same pattern regardless of the primary site with few exceptions (3). Spinal cord compression is the most feared complication of spinal metastases and the distribution of metastases within the spine does not correlate with the same risk of cord compression. The thoracic spine is most vulnerable.

Spinal metastases from gastrointestinal cancers have not been systematically reviewed. The available literature is piecemeal among retrospective reviews and case series of bone metastases and epidural spinal cord compression (ESCC) associated with solid tumors. As a result, a review of the subject will be limited by bias associated with reporting small series of patients, case reports, and retrospective reviews. With the available literature, the characteristic features pertaining to incidence, prevalence, clinical and radiographic findings, as well as prognosis will be reviewed. Treatment is not uniquely developed for gastrointestinal spinal metastases but falls into the category of radio-resistant- and chemotherapy-resistant tumors. Radio-resistance and chemotherapy resistance has important prognostic and perhaps therapeutic implications. Several important points will be made in this regard.

2. PATHOPHYSIOLOGY

2.1. GENETICS

Multiple genetics and epigenetic alterations in oncogenes, tumor supressor genes, cell cycle regulators, cell adhesion molecules, growth factor receptors, and mismatch repair genes are involved in the genesis of gastrointestinal cancers. None are unique to a particular cancer and none predict or are associated with the development of bone metastases (5). Genetic instability is associated with the initial step in gastric and colorectal cancers but rarely found with esophageal cancers (5). Increased telomerase activity is found in most gastrointestinal cancers, as is the activation of *P53* gene and anomalous expression CD_{44}. Amplification of cyclin D_1 is commonly found with gastric

From: *Current Clinical Oncology: Cancer in the Spine: Comprehensive Care*.
Edited by: R. F. McLain, K-U. Lewandrowski, M. Markman, R. M. Bukowski,
R. Macklis, and E. C. Benzel © Humana Press, Inc., Totowa, NJ

cancer and cyclin E in gastric and colorectal cancer *(5)*. Reduced expression of cyclin-dependent kinase inhibitors p16[MTSI] and P27[KIPI] is often found. Amplification of the oncogene *C-met* and *K-sam* preferentially occurs in poorly differentiated gastric cancers where amplification of *C-erbB$_2$* and loss of heterogenity of the *P73* genes are particularly found in well differentiated gastric cancers *(5)*. Knowing the molecular "fingerprint" of a particular primary gastrointestinal cancer provides an improved histopathological identification of metastases and, hopefully, will provide information about behavior and allow for selective targeted therapy in the future.

2.2. MICROSCOPIC PATHOLOGY

Micrometastasis of tumor cells to the bone marrow occur in 25 to 75% of patients with common malignancies *(6)*. Not all micrometastases grow to become clinically significant lesions. The formation of metastases depends in part on the synergistic relation between cancer cells, osteoclasts, and tumor-associated macrophages. Malignant cells secrete factors that stimulate osteoclastic cells both directly and indirectly *(7)*. Cancer cells release parathyroid hormone-related protein promoter, transforming growth factor-β, interleukin (IL)-1, IL-6, and IL-11, epidural growth factor, as well as tumor necrosis factor-β and -α, which stimulates osteoclasts leading to bone lysis *(6,7)*. Bone metastases will depend on elaboration of these mediators. Osteoblasts have receptors for several cellular growth factors and also control bone resorption by influencing osteoclasts *(7)*. Release of bone-derived growth factors and cytokines from resorbing bone attracts cancer cells and stimulates their growth and division *(7)*.

2.3. ANATOMY

Metastatic bone disease produces a greater visualized skeletal damage than suspected for tumor burden at that site *(7)*. The vertebrae is the most frequent site of bony metastases. Autopsy series indicate that 70% of patients with skeletal metastases have vertebral deposits *(8)*. This is owing, in part, to the well-vascularlized hematopoietic bone marrow found in vertebral bodies. The spread of tumor cells occurs directly and most frequently as a result of hematogenous spread rather than by retrograde flow through the venous plexus of Batson draining the epidural space. Five to ten percent of venous blood, derived from abdominal viscera from both the portal and caval systems, drains into the valveless paravertebral venous plexus that functions as a portosystemic shunt *(8)*. Increases in intraabdominal pressure associated with cough, sneeze, vomiting, or Valsalva maneuver spreads gastrointestinal tumor cells in a retrograde fashion to the epidural space because of the valveless nature of Batson's venous plexus *(2)*. Contrary to this theory of tumor spread through Batson's plexus, is the theory that such drainage pattern should result in predominately extraosseous epidural metastases, which is an unusual clinical finding *(9,10)*. Most epidural metastases are a result of direct tumor extension from the vertebral body into epidural space, which would not be expected if Batson's plexus is the original tributary of tumor spread to the spine. The preponderance of metastatic thoracic spinal disease associated with spinal cord compression when compared to cervical spine and lumbar spinal metastases in many series is related to: (1) a greater number of vertebral bodies in the thoracic spine; (2) the narrowness of the thoracic spinal canal compared to cervical spine and lumbar spine; and (3) presence of a physiological kyphosis *(3)*. Fifty-nine percent of spinal metastases are found in the thoracic spine and most involve multiple vertebra *(2,3)*. Not all series have demonstrated that thoracic metastases occur with greater frequency than other areas of the spine *(8,11)*, but most have note that the thoracic spine is the most frequent location for symptomatic spinal cord compression. Sites of metastases are not solely determined by blood flow when expressed as a percentage of cardiac output and calculated as perfusion per kilogram of tissue matched for distribution of metastases. Distinctly more common are skeletal metastases than predicted for the relatively low overall perfusion rate of bone compared to percentage of cardiac output directed to other organs *(12)*. The peripherally directed nutrient arteries of bone divide into capillaries at the endosteal margin of bone and form an open sinusoidal system, which has an intermittently discontinuous basement membrane that allows hematopoietic cells to enter circulation but also provides a landing zone for metastatic tumor cells *(12)*. Metastatic deposits usually originate in the posterior vertebral body, which is the best-vascularized portion of the vertebra *(11)*. Bone lesions, initially found at the time of cord compression, arise from within posterior vertebral body in 45%, in the posterior arch in 41%, in the entire vertebra in 14%, the extradural space in only 5%, and intradural in 1 to 2% *(13)*. Extension of tumor through the posterior vertebral cortex results in anterior compression of the thecal sac (ESCC) *(2)*. Spinal cord compression results from: (1) pathological vertebral fracture with dislocation in 50%; (2) pressure because of an enlarging extradural deposit in 39%; (3) spinal angulation following vertebral collapse in 11%; and by (4) intradural extramedullary metastases; or (5) intramedullary metastases *(8,14)*; or (6) by tumor extension through the spinal foramen *(9)*. Spinal cord compression at two or more sites will occur in 17% sometime during the course of disease *(3,15)*. The distribution of gastrointestinal malignancies follows the usual distribution found with other solid tumors except for rectal cancer, which produces a preponderance of lumbar vertebral metastases *(2,10,15)*. Most patients will have more than one level of spinal involvement at diagnosis and, in general, as with asymptomatic metastases, the primary tumor does not correlate with the site of the symptomatic vertebral involvement *(8,9,16)*. Most series have combined cauda equina lesions and spinal cord lesions because outlook is the same and, therefore, they are not separated in this chapter.

2.4. NEUROPATHOLOGY

The early histology of cord compression usually consists of posterior and lateral wedge-shaped areas of demyelination with the base toward the cord surface *(17)*. Gray matter is initially spared. With time, lesions appear multifocal and eventually become transverse. Epidural tumors usually extend to the anterior cord from the posterior aspect of the affected vertebral body, and compress the dural membrane, which abuts the cord affecting the interior cord *(3,17)*. Rarely is the pathology because of direct compression of the anterior spinal artery. More often, an epidural tumor compresses small radicals within the spinal cord

Table 1
Vertebral Metastases or Epidural Cord Compression Caused by Gastrointestinal

Reference	GI primaries	Total no.
62	9	235
63	4	43
41	6	104
64	9	141
21	12	345
19	23	101
60	6	83
42	8	100
68	9	92
Totals	98	1589

from anterior spinal artery, which when occluded precipitates neurological deficits *(17)*. Alternatively, venous occlusion may lead to vascular congestion, hemorrhage, and edema within spinal cord substance *(9)*.

3. PREVALENCE OF GASTROINTESTINAL CANCERS

3.1. CAUSES OF VERTEBRAL METASTASES AND SPINAL CORD COMPRESSION (TABLE 1)

In most series, gastrointestinal primaries make up a small percentage of solid tumors that metastasize to the spine *(2)*. Gastrointestinal cancers are the cause of spinal cord compression in 6.6% of all patients ranging from 0 to 23% *(18,19)*. The variable percentage of patients with spinal metastases owing to gastrointestinal malignancies in each series is influenced by referral, ethnic prevalence of gastrointestinal malignancies, and a clinical- or autopsy-based series. For example, in a clinical series from St. Mark's Hospital between 1943 and 1986, only 48 of 4000 patients with colon cancer were found to have bone metastases *(15)*. In an autopsy series of 528 patients extended over 10 yr, skeletal metastases were found in 11.7% of patients dying with colon cancer and 19.4% of patients dying with rectal cancer *(20)*. Most gastrointestinal cancers that spread to bone and/or vertebra remain occult and usually do not produce spinal cord compression. In a series of 600 patients treated for spinal cord compression or spinal root compression, overall, 4.8% of patients had gastrointestinal primaries (7% of men, 2% of women) *(13)*. In the Sorensen series of patients, 4% of patients with metastatic cord compression or cauda equina syndrome had gastrointestinal cancers *(21)*.

In 10 reports gathered from the literature of patients with vertebral metastases or epidural cord compression, 5.8% of the primaries were of gastrointestinal origin. This is consistent with the series reported by Grant *(9)*.

4. PREVALENCE OF BONE AND SPINAL METASTASIS

4.1. GASTRIC CANCER

A retrospective review of 234 bone scans preformed on patients with gastric cancers from a total of 17,176 gastric cancer patients, metastatic lesions were found in 106 patients (45% of those having bone scans, <1% of the entire series). Spinal

metastases were found in 66% of patients with bone scan evidence of metastases *(22)*. From the same group, 162 of 328 patients with gastric cancer who had bone scans for clinical reasons had evidence of metastases. There is no information about the total number of gastric cancer patients seen during the period of the study or the reasons for the bone scans *(23)*. In another series, postmortem radiographic appearances of bone metastases occurred in 70 gastric cancer patients within a series of 537 solid tumor patients with bone metastasis *(24)*. In an autopsy series reported by Johnston *(12)*, 40 of 653 patients (6%) with skeletal metastases had gastric cancer. In an autopsy series of patients who died with solid tumors, 65 had gastric cancers and of these patients 13 were found to have spinal metastases (20%) *(25)*. From an autopsy series of 1000 patients, 13 of 119 patients with gastric cancer had bone metastases, and 6 of 85 patients with lumbar spine metastases had gastric cancer *(24)*. In a series of patients treated for spinal metastases without surgery, 8 of 101 patients with spinal cord compression had gastric cancer *(19)*. In another series of 52 patients with metastatic spinal disease, one had gastric cancer *(26)*. Scintographic detection of spinal metastases occurred in 48 of 158 patients (30%) reported by Tatsui *(27)*. In summary, 6 to 30% of gastric cancer patients dying of their disease will be found to have spinal metastases, 2 to 8% of patients will have symptomatic spinal cord compression *(26)*.

4.2. COLON CANCER (TABLE 2)

In an autopsy series involving 118 patients dying of colon cancer, 11 were found to have bone metastases *(24)*. From a subgroup of 20 patients surgically treated reported by Kleinmann *(28)*, from a total group of 77 patients with spinal metastases, 1 had colon cancer *(28)*. In a series from Memorial Sloan-Kettering Cancer Center *(29)*, 53 of 765 patients with disseminated metastatic colon cancer had skeletal metastases and most were located in the spine. In this series, only 14 (1.8%) had bone only metastases as most had additional non-osseous metastases *(29)*. In a retrospective series of patients with thoracic spinal metastases requiring surgery over a 14-yr period of time, 9 of 109 patients had colon cancer *(30)*. In another series, 2 of 99 patients with extradural extension of spinal metastases had colon cancer primaries *(31)*. Colon cancer was responsible for 4 of 101 spinal metastases treated non-surgically as reported by Katagirl *(19)*. In a retrospective series involving patients with spinal metastases from a general hospital, 2 of 131 patients had colon cancer *(10)*. Lumbar spine involvement was found in 1 of 59 patients from an autopsy series reported by Fonrnasier *(24)*. Finally, bony metastases in colorectal cancer occurs in 33 to 61% of patients when radionuclide scanning was used *(32)*. This is much higher than the commonly accepted frequencies of 5% from other radiographic or autopsy series.

In summary, although autopsy findings of colon cancer bone metastases are common, clinical evidence of cord compression from spinal metastases occurs as a result of colon in 3.4% of all patients with extradural spinal cord compression from solid tumors.

4.3. RECTAL CANCER (TABLE 3)

Rectal cancer was responsible for spinal cord compression in 1 of a series of 52 patients reported by Smith *(26)*. From a

Table 2
Spinal Metastasis From Colon Cancer

Reference	No. with colon cancer	Total
28	1	77
30	2	109
31	2	99
19	4	101
10	2	131
24	1	59
Totals	18	517

Table 3
Rectal Cancer and Spinal Metastases and/or Spinal Cord Compression

Reference	No. with rectal cancer	Total
26	1	52
10	3	131
28	3	20
Totals	7	203

Table 4
Spinal Metastases From Pancreatic Cancer

Reference	No. with pancreatic cancer	Total
24	11	500
10	1	131
26	1	52
Totals	13	683

Table 5
Hepatocellular Carcinoma-Associated Bone and Spine Metastases

Reference	No. with hepatocellular carcinoma	Total
19	9	101
66	1	131
67	3	103
68	1	84
69	7	231
Totals	21	650

series reported by investigators from Memorial Sloan Kettering (29), 8.9% of patients with rectal cancer had osseous metastases, the majority of which were vertebral. Bone metastases were confirmed in 48 patients treated for rectal cancer and occurred predominately in the lumbar spine and pelvis (29). Four thousand patients were treated for rectal cancer during this period of time (15). A case series reported from a London hospital between 1968 and 1978 that includes patients with spinal metastases and neurological deficits, 3 of 131 had rectal cancer (10). Kleinmann (28) reported a group of 20 patients requiring surgery owing to ESCC and acute neurological deficits, 3 patients had rectal cancer (28). In an autopsy series from Malmo (20), 26 of 134 patients dying with rectal cancer had skeletal metastases. The percentage of patients with vertebral metastases from the group is not known, although most patients would be assumed to have spinal metastases judging from other series. Of 131 patients presenting with spinal metastases with or without cord compression, six had colorectal cancer (33). Colon and rectal primaries were not separately reported (33).

The diverse prevalence of rectal cancer associated vertebral metastases is owing to patient selection (i.e., surgical, clinical, or autopsy series). Approximately 5% of all symptomatic vertebral metastases associated with solid tumors are because of rectal cancer.

4.4. BILE DUCT CANCER (TABLE 4)

Out of 500 patients in an autopsy series of patients with lumbar spine metastases, 11 had pancreatic primaries (24). Two of the 11 patients had additional bone metastases besides their lumbar spine metastases. Another autopsy series demonstrated bone metastases in 4 of 32 patients dying from pancreatic cancer. In a series reported by Young (34), six patients with pancreatic cancer underwent postmortem examination two had gross evidence of spinal metastases in which one had radiographic evidence of spinal involvement ante-mortem. In a sec-

ond study involving a comparison between clinical and radiographic findings with postmortem evidence of disease, one of six patients had clinical evidence of spinal metastases, an additional one of six had postmortem radiographic evidence of vertebral metastases, two of six had postmortem histological findings of spinal metastases. There was a poor correlation between gross findings and radiographic (pre-magnetic resonance imaging [MRI]) evidence of metastases. In a series of patients presenting with spinal metastases, only 1 of 131 patients had pancreatic cancer (10). In a series of 52 surgically treated patients, 1 had pancreatic metastases to the spine (25). Johnston (12) reported that pancreatic cancer was known to have spread to the skeleton in 5 of 40 patients (12%). Overall, approx 6% of patients with pancreatic cancer will have skeletal metastases (12).

Gall bladder cancer rarely metastases to the spine. Out of 100 patients in a series of vertebral metastases, two had gallbladder primaries (19). In an autopsy series of 734 patients, 21 had gallbladder cancers and no skeletal or spinal metastases were found (25). Katagirl (19) found two of 101 patients with spinal metastases had gallbladder primaries.

Approximately 1.9% of patients with spinal metastases and ESCC have pancreatic primaries. However, 6% of patients with pancreatic cancers will have bone metastases. The frequency will again depend on the type of series.

4.5. HEPATOCELLULAR CARCINOMA (TABLE 5)

Vertebral metastases from hepatocellular carcinoma have been reported anecdotally. Autopsy series have a prevalence of bone metastases ranging between 3 and 12% (35). Several series reviewed by Byrne demonstrated a prevalence of 3 per 103 patients, 1 of 84 patients, and 7 of 231 patients with solid tumor spinal metastases had hepatocellular primaries (35). Stark (10) found one patient with hepatocellular carcinoma among 131 patients presenting to a community hospital with spinal metastases. In a series of patients treated nonsurgically, 9 patients had hepatocellular carcinoma from a total of 101 patients with spinal cord compression (19). This series originated from Japan where hepatocellular carcinoma is relatively common.

The prevalence of hepatocellular carcinoma as a cause of metastases to the bone or spine is 3.3%, however, several large series of patients with spine metastases found no patients with hepatocellular carcinoma (35). Therefore, the prevalence is probably less than 3%.

4.6. SUMMARY

The prevalence of gastrointestinal cancer as a cause of vertebral metastases is less than 10%. Gastric cancer and colorectal cancer are more common primaries to spread to the vertebrae. The prevalence is subject to bias based on the case series (whether clinical or autopsy series). Cultural factors will also play a role because of the prevalence of disease among the various ethnic groups. Autopsy findings do not correlate well with series reported on the basis of clinical or radiographic findings. The prevalence of vertebral metastases will be higher in autopsy series. The distribution of metastases along the spine does not predict the location of the primary with the exception of rectal cancer, which more frequently involves lumbar spine.

5. PROGNOSIS IN SPINAL METASTASES: GASTROINTESTINAL CANCER

Most patients with gastrointestinal cancers have visceral metastases at presentation so that even if all else is favorable (absence of pathological fracture, solitary skeletal metastases) survival is likely to be 25% or less at 1 yr. In a second series, Bauer (37) found that survival closely related to tumor burden. No patients who had visceral or brain metastases were alive at 1 yr (37).

Klekamp (38) also found that patients who had spinal and extraosseous metastases had a poor prognosis. Survival in this series did not appear to correlate with preoperative neurological function. Most patients with gastrointestinal cancers would have a poor outlook because most have a high tumor burden and visceral metastases.

Sioutos (30) published the survival of a small number of patients with colon and spinal metastases (30). A mean survival was 15.8 mo and the median survival was 7 mo (range 2–39 mo). The factors influencing survival of all solid tumors patients in this series were preoperative neurological deficits, extent of disease, the number of vertebral bodies involved, tumor location (posterior or anterior in the vertebral body), primary cancer site, and age of patient. By this scoring system, most gastrointestinal cancers will have two to three adverse factors because most will have multiple metastases outside of the primary site in addition to vertebral metastases (i.e., tumor beyond primary site and vertebral body) and most patients will be older. Anteriorly located metastases in the vertebral body are associated with poor surgical outcomes (31). The anterior approach to surgery may alter this prognostic factor.

Tatusi (27) evaluated the interval from diagnosis to onset of spinal metastases and survival in large series of patients with spinal tumors (27). Gastric cancer patients had a mean interval from diagnosis to onset of spinal metastases of 6.9 mo. Nearly two-thirds of these patients had multiple metastases at relapse. The survival at 6 mo was only 15% and none survived 1 yr (27). Because the outlook was so poor for these patients, the author recommended radiation alone. Patients who have both multiple bone metastases from gastric cancer and either disseminated intravascular coagulation and/or microangiopathic hemolytic anemia have a median survival time of only 2 mo (39). Such a dismal outlook would suggest a conservative approach to management.

Bone metastases from rectal cancer is associated with a median survival of 4 mo (range 1–26 mo) with only 1 of 48 patients alive beyond 6 mo as reported by Talbot (15). The bone metastases were symptomatic with widespread metastases as seen in 75% of patients. Bone metastases were generally diffuse and occurred more frequently in patients with an initial advanced stage primary (15).

Tabbara (40), in a 30-yr retrospective review, found the median survival of colorectal cancer patients with spinal cord compression 7 and 5 wk for patients with esophageal cancer and spinal metastases (40). Patients with hepatocellular carcinoma and spinal metastases have a survival of less than 25% at 6 mo and less than 10% at 1 yr (19). The prognosis for patients with spinal metastases from primaries poorly responsive to radiation and chemotherapy was unfavorable in this series (19).

The mean postoperative survival of patients with gastrointestinal cancer and spinal epidural metastases as reported by Dunn (41) was 151 d compared to 388 d for prostate cancer, 203 d for breast cancer, 249 d for renal cancer, and 520 d from myeloma (41). Survival was not related to surgical outcome or neurological improvement.

In summary, the outlook for patients with gastrointestinal cancer and vertebral metastases with or without spinal cord compression is poor. Except for perhaps colon cancer as reported by Sioutos (30) and rectal cancer by Tokuhashi survival is less than 6 mo and particularly for primaries arising from the upper gastrointestinal tract. Surgery and radiation do not influence the prognosis. The poor outlook is because of widespread extraosseous metastases, involvement of multiple vertebral bodies, and the chemotherapy and radiation resistant nature of most gastrointestinal cancers.

6. TREATMENT

The purpose of treatment for spinal metastases is palliative particularly in the case of metastases arising from the gastrointestinal tract. The primary goals of therapy are restoration and maintenance of neurological function, relief of pain, local tumor control, and spinal stabilization (3). Guidelines for managing spinal metastases have not been established owing to lack of systematic and carefully controlled studies, great variability of patient characteristics, tumor burden and origin, and therapeutic limitations because of potential cord injury (3).

Therapeutic options include radiation, vertebreplasty, posterior instrumentation with laminectomy, and corpectomy (vertebrectomy) via anterior or posterior lateral approach (3,30). The outlook for patients with spinal metastases from gastrointestinal primaries is poor and only slightly better than spinal metastases from lung cancer, therefore surgical corpectomy is rarely an option. Most patients have high tumor burdens with additional bone metastases and visceral metastases.

Gastrointestinal cancers are chemotherapy-resistant and only a minority respond to systemic multi-agent therapy and those that do, do so only temporarily. Additionally, gastrointestinal cancers are relatively radio-resistant. It is unknown whether surgery adds to the palliative benefit of radiation in the setting of a short expectant survival. Differences of opinion have been expressed *(30,42)*. Patients with poorly responsive tumors with spinal metastases but without neurological impairment and no evidence of vertebral collapse may do just as well with radiation alone *(19)*. Patients with poorly responsive tumors and neurological deficits do poorly with radiation alone *(19)*. Surgical treatment should be instituted if (1) life expectancy is greater than 6 mo, (2) spinal lesions are relatively solitary and localized by MRI and stabilization is possible, (3) tumor burden is low (i.e., few to no visceral metastases), (4) patient is not a Frankel type A (complete paralysis), and (5) general condition and comorbidities are compatible with aggressive surgery and general anesthesia *(19)*. Other indications for surgery with or without postoperative radiation are:

1. Diagnosis is in doubt.
2. Spinal instability or cord compression by bony deformity or fragments caused by vertebral collapse.
3. Tumor fails to respond to radiation and an there is expected survival long enough to enjoy the fruits of surgery.
4. Relapse in a previously radiated vertebral site and a good expected survival (i.e., >3–6 mo).
5. High cervical cord compression, which can be life threatening.
6. Radio-resistant tumor with a rapid onset of signs and symptoms of cord compression and anatomically complete block (with a reasonable expectation of survival) *(3)*.

6.1. CHEMOTHERAPY

Chemotherapy has been beneficial in treating ESCC associated with Hodgkin's disease, non-Hodgkin's lymphoma, seminoma, and Ewing's sarcoma *(9)*. Benefits are directly related to the chemotherapy and radiation sensitivity of the underlying primary. Unfortunately most, if not all, gastrointestinal cancers respond poorly to chemotherapy *(43)*. Most responses observed are partial and temporary. Cisplatin chemotherapy has been used for esophageal and gastric cancers (combined with of 5-fluorouracil [5FU]), gemcitabine or 5FU with pancreatic cancer and 5FU, capcitabine, CPT-11, or oxaliplatin for colon cancer. Indications for their use include palliation after treatment of ESCC, for patients with a good performance status and adequate renal and hepatic function. Chemotherapy for gastrointestinal cancers should not be the primary treatment of ESCC. Chemotherapy should be considered only in a desperate situation, when both surgery and radiation have been exhausted as treatment of ESCC and after a clear discussion about the goals of care. Chemotherapy should not be added to aggressive radiation in the treatment of ESCC.

The detrimental effects of chemotherapy to wound healing particularly in patients who have had surgery, radiation, and are on corticosteroids, should be considered. Surgical wounds, which when opened, will fail to heal or heal slowly in patients on chemotherapy, leading to a significant risk for infection, particularly during periods of myelosuppression.

7. MANAGEMENT OF ADVANCED GASTROINTESTINAL CANCERS

7.1. ESOPHAGEAL CANCER

The disease stage is highly predictive of survival: 80% of patients with pathological stage I disease survive 5 yr, whereas patients with stage II or III disease have a 5-yr survival rate of 34 and 15%, respectively. Adenocarcinoma has become more prevalent for unknown reasons. However, this does not significantly altered treatment. Primary treatment consists of surgery or chemoradiation (usually 5FU and cisplatin) with or without surgery. Palliation of local symptoms can be achieved by radiation, chemoradiation, or by placement of an esophageal stent, brachytherapy, or photodynamic therapy, or a combination of these treatments. Patients who have advanced disease may benefit temporarily from a course of 5FU- and cisplatin-based chemotherapy for the purpose of palliating symptoms. Recently, paclitaxel as either a single agent or in combination with cisplatin has produced objective responses in patients with advanced esophageal cancer *(44)*. Patients with advanced disease need to be strong enough and have adequate liver and kidney function in order to receive chemotherapy. The goal of therapy in advanced disease is palliation and should take into account quality of life.

7.2. GASTRIC CANCER

Regardless of the extent of the surgical procedure used to treat gastric cancer, the effectiveness of surgery to cure gastric cancer, particularly node positive cancer, is poor. The overall 5-yr survival of node positive gastric cancer is at best 30% and in most series much lower. A variety of chemotherapy combinations have been used to palliate advanced disease:

- FAM (5FU, doxorubicin, mitomycin-c).
- FAXTx (5FU, doxorubicin, methotrexate).
- ELF (etoposide, leucovorin, 5FU).
- EAP (etoposide, doxirubicin, cisplatin).
- PLEF (cisplatin, leucovorin, etoposide, 5FU).

Short-term survival may be significantly prolonged, however, overall survival is not *(45)*. Adjuvant use of chemotherapy improves the results of surgery. A recent randomized trial using adjuvant 5FU, leucovorin, and radiation postoperatively in a group of patients at risk for relapse (85% of whom were node positive) found that the adjuvant therapy increased the mean time to relapse from 19 to 30 mo and the median survival from 27 to 42 mo *(46)*. Postoperative adjuvant chemoradiation should be discussed with patients who are at high risk for relapse.

7.3. PANCREATIC CANCER

Pancreatic cancer is usually locally advanced or metastatic at the time of diagnosis and rarely amenable to surgical resection. Palliative biliary and gastric surgical bypass procedures are frequently preformed or alternatively endoscopic biliary stenting. Because a large percentage of patients develop distant metastatic disease (usually liver or peritoneum), improved local tumor control using 5FU-based chemotherapy plus radiation will translate, at best, into a small improvement in survival. More effective systemic agents are needed. Gemcitabine produces a response in 10 to 15% of patients and more frequently produces a subjective symptomatic benefit in the absence of tumor response. Gemcitabine is superior to 5FU in this regard (47). Combination therapy with 5FU and gemcitabine does not improve survival more than single agent gemcitabine (48). Patients with advanced pancreatic cancer with adequate hepatic function and good performance score could be considered for either palliative gemcitabine or investigational chemotherapy.

7.4. HEPATOCELLULAR CARCINOMA

Hepatic resection or liver transplants are the only potential curative therapies for hepatocellular carcinoma. However, 80% are inoperable at diagnosis. Nonsurgical management include radiofrequency thermoablation or ethanol injection, which both produce tumor necrosis in greater than 80% of patients and may influence short-term survival. Embolization or chemoembolization using the hepatic artery may palliate pain and also produce short-term tumor control. Internal radiation using intra-arterial iodine-131-lableled lipidol has also favorably influenced survival (49). Systemic chemotherapy has been disappointing because of both tumor resistance or poor patient tolerance. Chemotherapy alone rarely reduces tumor burden or palliates symptoms and does not prolong survival (50).

7.5. COLORECTAL CANCER

Adjuvant 5FU and leucovorin are standard therapy for pathological stage III colon cancer and 5FU and radiation for T3 or node positive rectal cancer (51,52). Pre-operative radiation and 5FU may allow resection for locally advanced rectal cancer and also palliate locally recurrent cancer. Isolated metastatic recurrences to liver or lung should be resected if possible (53). A significant proportion of patients (30%) will be 5-yr survivors. Anastomotic recurrences should also be resected and patient closely watched for second colorectal primaries with repeated colonoscopies.

Four drugs have activity in advanced colorectal cancer: 5FU, capcitabine, CPT-11, and oxaliplatin (54–56). Weekly 5FU and leucovorin as a single day infusion appear to be more tolerable than bolus 5FU with leucovorin given on five consecutive days each month. Both CPT-11 and oxaliplatin have demonstrated anti-tumor activity as second line single agents (55,56). Responses are higher when combining either of these two agents with 5FU, but the degree of toxicity is also higher. Present treatment involves a combination of 5FU with either CPT-11 or oxaliplatin as initial therapy in patients with metastatic disease. A greater survival or palliative benefit occurs, more so than using each agent sequentially. The purpose of chemotherapy in advanced colon cancer is palliative and significant drug toxicity is a detriment to the quality of life in patients who have incurable illness.

8. SYMPTOM MANAGEMENT

Pain is a significant problem for patients with spinal metastases and the guidelines for pain management should follow the World Health Organization stepladder guidelines. Opioids should be utilized with either corticosteroids or nonsteroidal anti-inflammatory drugs for moderate or severe pain. Yoshioka (57) in a retrospective review, reported the use of morphine in 28 patients with bone pain from spinal metastases and 28 patients with malignant tumor induced sciatica. The mean daily oral dose of

morphine used for bone pain was 103 mg, median 85 mg. Patients with sciatica received a mean daily dose was 539 mg and median 164 mg. The patients with rectal cancer and sciatica required significantly higher doses of morphine per day (mean 1007 mg, median 192 mg) than other cancer patients with sciatica.

8.1. RADIATION AND SURGERY

Murai (58) reported the radiation pain response in 68 patients. Relief of pain occurred in 78%. Seventy-five percent of patients with gastric cancer and 100% of patients with hepatocellular cancer experienced relief. Other studies have shown that 80% of patients with back pain from spinal cord compression respond to radiation (19). In the series reported by Katagirl (19), 67% of patients found pain relief. The rapidity of pain relief differs between the group with radio-responsive and less responsive primaries.

Surgery will also relieve pain in 70 to 90% of patients (3,42,59). Radiation and surgery did not palliate pain as well for thoracic spine metastases as they did for cervical and lumbar spine in the series reported by Kleinman (28). It was thought that this was owing to the limited cross-sectional area of the thoracic spine and the poor blood supply to the thoracic spine limiting radiation response (28).

Pain relief may be prognostic. Half of the patients without pain relief survived less than 3 mo in a series reported by Katagirl (19). Radiation is also unlikely to relieve pain in patients with major vertebral fractures and bony deformity causing ESCC or with spinal angulation (10). Surgery is preferred in these situations.

8.2. CO-ANALGESICS

Corticosteroids play an important role in the early management of ESCC. Pain reduction occurs in 64% with the use of corticosteroids usually within the first day of treatment (2). Pain reduction is more rapid when high doses of dexamethasone (100 mg/d) are started simultaneously with high-dose fractionated radiation (60). However high doses vs standard doses of dexamethasone at the onset of radiation does not ultimately produce any significant difference in long-term pain relief or neurological improvement (61). Several dosing regimens have been previously published: dexamethasone 100 mg followed by 24 mg four times daily for 3 d then taper; and dexamethasone 10 to 16 mg bolus then 4 mg four times daily for 3 to 7 d. The chances of morbidity is small if steroids can be tapered over several weeks (2,3). Short-term morbidity includes hyperglycemia, psychosis, confusion, and infection. Wound healing may be delayed if corticosteroids cannot be tapered.

Patients who have a major neurological deficit associated with paralysis should be considered for prophylactic heparin in order to avoid the significant risk of venous thrombosis if no contraindication exist (9). Intermittent compression stockings should be used otherwise.

8.3. BISPHOSPHONATES

Bisphosphonates bind to expose bone mineral around osteoclasts. Once released from bone mineral they are internalized by osteoclasts, disrupting bone resorption and inducing osteoclast apoptosis. Bisphosphonates may also have a direct anti-tumor effect on cancer cells (7). Bisphosphonates are the treatment of choice for malignancy-related hypercalcemia. The skeletal morbidity is reduced for patients with multiple myeloma and breast cancer. Pain relief occurs independent of the nature of the underlying tumor or radiographic appearance (7). The relief of metastatic bone pain correlates with the reduced rate of bone absorption. There is little data on the use of bisphosphonates in patients with bone metastases from gastrointestinal cancers. Clinical trials need to be done to quantify benefits. Usual doses of pamidronate are 60 to 90 mg parenteral every 3 to 4 wk and zolendronate 4 mg every 4 wk.

8.4. RADIOPHARMACEUTICALS

Radiopharmaceuticals are now available to palliate metastatic bone pain. Strontium-89 is a β-emitter, which reduces pain associated with prostate cancer and breast cancer. Strontium is taken up at sites of new bone formation and hence is most effective for osteosclerotic metastases. The half-life of strontium-89 precludes dosing more frequently than at 3-mo intervals. Samarium-153 is a γ- and β-particle-emitting radioisotope, which allows imaging and therapy simultaneously (7). As with strontium, samarium is taken up at sites of new bone formation. Samarium can be given as an outpatient and will significantly reduce bone pain and analgesic consumption. The half-life of samarium is shorter and, thus, can be given at more frequent intervals if necessary. Drawbacks to radiopharmaceutics include myelosuppression, cost, delayed onset to analgesia, and handling. Repeated dosing can be done depending on response, half-life of the radiopharmaceutical, and blood counts and bone marrow reserve.

8.5. END-OF-LIFE CARE

Patients with spinal metastases from gastrointestinal malignancies have a poor outlook and a short life expectancy. It is imperative that the managing physicians clearly outline the goals of care and avoid nebulus medical terms. A compassionate and honest discussion of outlook, the goals of care, and advice about advanced care planning are essential for patients informed choice and future planning. This should be done in a quiet atmosphere, with ample time for questions. Goal orienting both the patient and family will provide a sense of hope. If the goal is not a cure, then it is relief of pain and improvement in neurological deficits. The patient needs to live as well as she or he is able to until death occurs. "There is nothing more we can do" should never be said.

9. CONCLUSION

Gastrointestinal cancers are responsible for less than 10% of all spinal metastases. Spinal metastases occur in the face of advancing intra-abdominal disease and high tumor burden and, thus, portend a poor outlook. Only patients with spinal metastases from lung cancer have a worse outlook. The main treatment is radiation despite the relative radio-resistant nature of most gastrointestinal cancers. This is because of prognosis and lack of evidence that surgery followed by radiation improves neurological function or pain compared to radiation alone. However, there are selected indications for surgery. Surgical procedures can be appropriately chosen based on modern imaging. Chemotherapy has a very limited role in the treatment of symptomatic spinal metastases. Palliation of symptoms and advanced care planning need to be combined with directed antitumor therapy.

ACKNOWLEDGMENT

The author would like to thank Robert Pelley, MD for his reviewing this manuscript.

REFERENCES

1. Toma S, Venturino A, Sogno G, et al. Metastatic bone tumors. Clin Orthop Relat Res   295:246–251.
2. Boogerd W, van de Sande J. Treatment of complications. Cancer Treat Rev 1993; 19:129–150.
3. Ratanatharathorn V, Powers WE. Epidural spinal cord compression from metastatic tumor: diagnosis and guidelines for management. Cancer Treat Rev 1991; 18:55–71.
4. Galasko CSB. Diagnosis of skeletal metastases and assessment of response to treatment. Clin Orthop and Relat Res 1995; 312:64–75.
5. Yasui W, Yokozaki H, Shimamoto F, Tahara H, Tahara E. Molecular-pathological diagnosis of gastrointestinal tissues and its contribution to cancer histopathology. Pathol Int 1999; 49:763–774.
6. Orr FW, Lee J, Duivenvoorden WCM, Singh G. Pathophysiologic interactions in skeletal metastasis. Cancer 2000; 88:2912–2918.
7. Coleman RE. Metastatic bone disease: clinical features, pathophysiology and treatment strategies. Cancer Treat Rev 2001; 27:165–176.
8. Nottebaert M, Exner GU, von Hochstetter AR, Schreiber A. Metastatic bone disease from occult carcinoma: a profile. Int Orthop 1989; 13:119–123.
9. Grant R, Papadopoulos SM, Greenberg HS. Metastatic epidural spinal cord compression. Neurol Clin 1991; 9:825–841.
10. Stark RJ, Henson RA, Evans SJW. Spinal metastases: a retrospective survey from a general hospital. Brain 1992; 105:189–213.
11. Algra PR, Heimans JJ, Valk J, Nauta JJ, Lachniet M, Van Kooten B. Do metastases in vertebrae begin in the body or the pedicles. AJR Am J Roentgenol 1992; 158:1275–1279.
12. Johnston AD. Pathology of metastatic tumors in bone. In: Urist MR, ed. Clinical Orthopaedics and Related Research. Philadelphia, PA: JB Lippincott; 1970:8–32.
13. Constans JP, De Divitiis E, Donzelli R, Spaziante R, Meder JF, Haye C. Spinal metastases with neurological manifestations. J Neurosurg 1983; 59:111–118.
14. Perrin RG. Symptomatic spinal metastases. Am Fam Physician1989; 39:165–172.
15. Talbot RW, Irvine B, Jass JR, Dowd GS, Northover JM. Bone metastases in carcinoma of the rectum: a clinical and pathological review. Eur J of Surg Oncol 1989; 15:449–452.
16. van der Sande JJ, Kroger R, Boogerd W. Multiple spinal epidural metastases; an unexpectedly frequent finding. J Neurol Neurosurg Psychiatry 1990; 53:1001–1003.
17. Shibasaki K, Harper CG, Bedbrook GM, Kakulas BA. Vertebral metastases and spinal cord compression. Paraplegia 1983; 21:47–61.
18. Ruff RL, Lanska DJ. Epidural metastases in prospectively evaluated veterans with cancer and back pain. Cancer 1989; 63:2234–2241.
19. Katagiri H, Takahashi M, Inagaki J, et al: Clinical results of nonsurgical treatment for spinal metastases. Int J Radiat Oncol Biol Phys 1998; 42:1127–1132.
20. Berge T, Ekelund G, Mellner C, Pihl B, Wenckert A. Carcinoma of the colon and rectum in a defined population. Acta Chir Scand Suppl 1973; 438:1–86.
21. Sorensen PS, Borgesen SE, Rasmusson B, et al. Metastatic epidural spinal cord compression. Cancer 1990, 65:1502–1508.
22. Choi CW, Lee DS, Chung JK, et al: Evaluation of bone metastases by Tc-99m MDP imaging in patients with stomach cancer. Clin Nucl Med 1993; 20:310–314.
23. Kim SE, Kim DY, Lee DS, Chung JK, Lee MC, Koh CS. Absent or faint renal uptake on bone scan. Clin Nucl Med 1991; 8:545–549.
24. Fornasier VL, Horne JG. Metastases to the vertebral column. Cancer 1975; 36:590–594.
25. Ortiz Gomez JA. The incidence of vertebral body metastases. Int Orthopaedics 1995; 19:309–311.
26. Smith R. An evaluation of surgical treatment for spinal cord compression due to metastatic carcinoma. J Neurol Neurosurg Psychiatry 1965 ; 28:152–158.

27. Tatsui H, Onomura T, Morishita S. Survival rates of patients with metastatic spinal cancer after scintigraphic detection of abnormal radioactive accumulation. Spine 1996; 21:2143–2148.

28. Kleinman WB, Kiernan HA, Michelsen WJ. Metastatic cancer of the spinal column. Clin Orthop Relat Res 1978; 136:166–172.

29. Besbeas S, Stearns MW. Osseous metastases from carcinomas of the colon and rectum. Dis Colon Rectum 1978; 21:266–268.

30. Sioutos P, Arbit E, Meshulam CF, Galicich JH. Spinal metastases from solid tumors. Cancer 1995 ; 76:1453–1459.

31. Brice J, McKissock W. Surgical treatment of malignant extradural spinal tumours. Br Med J 1965; 1:1339–1342.

32. Vider M, Maruyama Y, Narvaez R. Significance of the vertebral venous (Batson's) plexus in metastatic spread in colorectal carcinoma. Cancer 1977; 40:67–71.

33. Bernat JL, Greenberg ER, Barrett J. Suspected epidural compression of the spinal cord and cauda equina by metastatic carcinoma. Cancer 1983; 51:1953–1957.

34. Young JM, Funk FJ. Incidence of tumor metastasis. J Bone Joint Surg 1953; 34:55–64.

35. Byrne MJ, Scheinberg MA, Mavligit G, Dawkins RL. Heptocellullar carcinoma: presentation with vertebral metastases and radicular compression. Cancer 1972; 30:202–205.

36. Bauer HC, Wedin R: Survival after surgery for spinal and extremity metastases. Prognostication in 241 patients. Acta Orthop Scand 1995; 66:143–146.

37. Bauer HCF. Posterior decompression and stabilization for spinal metastases: analysis of sixty-seven consecutive patients. J Bone Joint Surg Am 1997; 79A:514–522.

38. Klekamp J, Samii H. Surgical results for spinal metastases. Acta Neurochir 1998; 140:957–967.

39. Etoh T, Baba H, Taketomi A, et al. Diffuse bone metastasis with hematologic disorders from gastric cancer: clinicopathological features and prognosis. Oncol Rep 1999; 6:601–605.

40. Tabbara IA, Sibley DS, Quesenberry PJ. Spinal cord compression due to metastatic neoplasm. Southern Med J 1990; 83:519–523.

41. Dunn RC, Kelly WA, Wohns RNW, et al: Spinal epidural neoplasia: a 15 year review of the results of surgical therapy. J Neurosurg 1980, 52:47-51.

42. Livingston KE, Perrin RG. The neurosurgical management of spinal metastases causing cord and cauda equina compression. J Neurosurg 1978; 49:839–843.

43. Bhardwaj S, Holland JF. Chemotherapy of metastatic cancer in bone. Clin Orthop Relat Res 1982; 169:28–37.

44. Weiner L. Paclitaxel in the treatment of esophageal cancer. Semin Oncol 1999; 20:106–108.

45. Wils J. The treatment of advanced gastric cancer. Semin Oncol 1996; 23:397–406.

46. MacDonald J, Smalley S, Benedetti J, et al. Postoperative combined radiation in chemotherapy improves disease-free survival (DFS) and overall survival (OS) in resected adenocarcinoma of the stomach and GE junction. Results of the intergroup study INT-0116 (SWOG 9008). Proceedings of ASCO 2000, 1911A.

47. Burris H, Moore M, Andersen J, et al. Improvement in survival in clinical benefit with gemcitabine as first-line therapy for patients with advanced pancreatic cancer: a randomized trial. J Clin Oncol 1997; 15:2403–2413.

48. Berlin J, Katalano J, Thomas J. A phase III study of gemcitabine in combination with 5FU versus gemcitabine alone in patients with advanced pancreatic cancer (E2297): an Eastern Cooperative Oncology Group (ECOG) trial. Proceedings of ASCO 2001, 19:127A.

49. Bergsland E, Venook A. Hepatocellular carcinoma. Curr Opin Oncol 2000; 12:357–361.

50. Leung TWT, Johnson PJ. Systemic therapy for hepatocellular carcinoma. Semin Oncol 2001; 28:514–520.

51. Moore HCF, Haller DG. Adjuvant therapy of colon cancer. Semin Oncol 1999; 26:545–555.

52. Minsky BD. Adjuvant therapy of rectal cancer. Semin Oncol 1999; 26:540–544.

53. Fong Y, Salo Y. Surgical therapy of hepatic colorectal metastasis. Semin Oncol 1999; 26:514–523.

54. Becouarn Y, Rougier P. Clinical efficacy of oxaliplatin monotherapy: phase II trials in advanced colorectal cancer. Semin Oncol 1998; 2523–2531.

55. Bleiberg H, da Gramont A. Oxaliplatin plus 5-fluorouracil: clinical experience in patients with advanced colorectal cancer. Semin Oncol 1998; 25:32–39.

56. Rougier P, Bugat R. CPT-11 in the treatment of colorectal cancer: clinical efficacy and safety profile. Semin Oncol 1996; 23:34–41.

57. Yoshioka H, Tsuneto S, Kashiwagi T. Pain control with morphine for vertebral metastases and sciatica in advanced cancer patients. J Palliat Care 1994; 10:10–14.

58. Murai N, Koga K, Nagamachi S, et al. Radiotherapy in bone metastases — with special reference to its effect on relieving pain. Gan No Rinsho 1989; 35:1149–1152.

59. Harrington KD. Orthopaedic surgical management of skeletal complications of malignancy. Cancer 1997; 80:1614–1627.

60. Greenberg HS, Kim JH, Posner JB. Epidural spinal cord compression from metastatic tumor: results with a new treatment protocol. Ann Neurol 1980; 8:361–366.

61. Vecht CJ, Haaxma-Reiche H, van Putten WL, de Visser M, Vries EP, Twijnstra A. Initial bolus of conventional versus high dose dexamethasone in metastatic spinal cord compression. Neurology 1989; 39:1255–1257.

62. Gilbert RW, Kim JH, Posner JB. Epidural spinal cord compression from metastatic tumor: diagnosis and treatment. Ann Neurol 1978; 3:40–51.

63. Portenoy RK, Galer BS, Salamon O, Freilich M, Finkel JE, Milstein D. Identification of epidural neoplasm. Radiography and bone scintigraphy in the symptomatic and asymptomatic spine. Cancer 1989; 64:2207–2213.

64. Rodichok LD, Ruckdeschel JC, Harper GR, Cooper G, Prevosti L, Fernando L. Early detection and treatment of spinal epidural metastases: the role of myelography. Ann Neurol 1986; 20:696–702.

65. Nottebaert M, Exner GU, von Hochstetter AR, Schreiber A. Metastatic bone disease from occult carcinoma: a profile. Int Orthop 1989; 13:119–123.

66. Stern WE. Localization and diagnosis of spinal cord tumors. Clin Neurosurg 1978; 25:480–494.

67. Kennady JC, Stern WE. Metastatic neoplasms of the vertebral column producing compression of the spinal cord. Am J Surg 1962; 104:155–168.

68. Wright RL. Malignant tumors in the spinal extradural space: results of surgical treatment. Ann Surg 1963; 157:227–231.

69. Arseni CN, Simionesacu MD, Horwath L. Tumors of the spine. A follow-up study of 350 patients with neurosurgical considerations. Acto Psychiatr Scand 1959; 34:398–410.

18 Lung Cancer

Jigar Shah, MD and Tarek Mekhail, MD, MSc, FRCSI, FRCSEd

Contents

1. INTRODUCTION

In the United States, 172,570 new cases of lung cancer will be diagnosed in the year 2005 and 163,510 of these patients will die of the disease *(1)*. Lung cancer is currently the leading cause of cancer death in men and has now surpassed breast cancer in women *(2–7)*. The median age at diagnosis is approx 60 yr. The highest incidence of lung cancer is noticed among Hawaiians and African-Americans in United States, and in Scotland and Wales, worldwide *(8)*.

Although the frequency of lung cancer in both men and women increased for many decades, the age-adjusted lung cancer mortality rates have decreased by 3.6% between 1990 and 1995 *(9)*. The frequency of lung cancer in men decreased by 1.4% annually through 1996, the frequency in women declined by 1.3% per year from 1994 to 1995 *(5)*. However, owing to the increased longevity and increased population size, the absolute number of lung cancer deaths and new cases of lung cancer have increased annually over the last 50 yr. The overall survival rate for lung cancer at 5 yr is estimated to be 14% *(1)*.

This chapter focuses on the etiology, risk factors, pathology, clinical presentation, staging, and treatment of lung cancer. Special emphasis is placed on bone metastasis.

2. ETIOLOGY AND RISK FACTORS

2.1. TOBACCO

Cigarette smoking is responsible for approx 87% of all cases of lung cancer *(8)*. Estimate of relative risk for developing lung cancer in a smoker is 10- to 30-fold higher in comparison with the lifetime nonsmoker. Compared to nonsmokers, lung cancer related risks of dying are 22 times higher for male smokers and 12 times higher for female smokers *(10)*. The risk of lung cancer increases with the number of years of smoking and the number of cigarettes smoked per day *(5)*.

The increased lung cancer risk for current smokers is directly proportional to the estimated milligrams of tar consumed per day. Stellman and Garfinkel *(11)*, in the more recent American Cancer Society Fifty State Study, indicated that doubling the cigarette tar yield resulted in a 40% increase in the relative risk of dying of lung cancer, independent of the number of cigarettes smoked or depth of inhalation. According to Federal Trade Commission estimates, the tar content of the current average cigarette sales in the United States is 12–13 mg of tar per cigarette compared with nearly 40 mg in the early 1950s *(7)*. After adjusting the difference in the amount of cigarettes smoked, lifelong smokers of filter cigarette experienced 20 to 40% lower risk of lung cancer then lifelong nonfilter smokers *(12–13)*.

Overall there has been a decline in the incidence of cigarette smoking over the years. The risk of lung cancer in ex-smoker remains higher than that in nonsmoker for at least 25 yr *(10)*. Nonsmokers living in a household with a smoker have a 30% increased incidence of lung cancer compared to nonsmokers who do not reside in such an environment *(10,14)*.

2.2. OCCUPATIONAL AND ENVIRONMENTAL EXPOSURE

Arsenic, asbestos, beryllium, Bis (chloromethyl) ether, chromium, nickel, vinyl chloride, coal combustion products, polycyclic aromatic compounds, and radiation are known occupational

From: *Current Clinical Oncology: Cancer in the Spine: Comprehensive Care.*
Edited by: R. F. McLain, K-U. Lewandrowski, M. Markman, R. M. Bukowski, R. Macklis, and E. C. Benzel © Humana Press, Inc., Totowa, NJ

carcinogens *(15)*. Asbestos exposure is the culprit behind approx 3 to 4% of lung cancers *(16)*. In 1955, Doll et al. *(17)* published the first study documenting an increased risk for lung cancer in individuals exposed to asbestos. The risk of lung cancer in people exposed to air-borne fibers increases with the amount of exposure and is even synergistic in exposed smokers *(18)*. The risk for lung cancer by non-occupational asbestos exposure is not well established but has succeeded in garnering significant public attention.

Originally termed "miner's phthisis" in the 19th century, uranium exposure in miners is particularly associated with small-cell lung cancer (SCLC) *(10)*. Saccomanno et al. *(19)* discovered a remarkably high incidence of SCLC in Colorado miners with high levels of exposure to uranium. The well-established increased risk for lung cancer seen in uranium miners leads to the suggestion that indoor radon exposure may cause lung cancer *(20,21)*.

Several nonmalignant lung diseases including chronic obstructive pulmonary diseases, idiopathic pulmonary fibrosis, pneumoconiosis, and tuberculosis have been associated with an increased risk of lung cancer *(22)*.

Although there is no conclusive data, some dietary substances, such as vitamin C and E and selenium, have been implicated in lung cancer prevention. β-carotene, however, was associated with an increased lung cancer incidence in two large randomized trials, most likely because of its negative interaction with cigarette smoke *(23)*.

2.3. GENETIC FACTORS

Carriers of α_1-antitrypsin deficiency allele may be at greater risk for lung cancer *(24)*. Genetic factors have also been implicated in lung cancer. The gene families implicated in lung carcinogenesis include dominant oncogenes and tumor suppressor genes *(25,26)*. Amplification of the c-*myc* oncogene has been associated with SCLC *(27)*. The *ras* family of oncogenes are among the most common activated oncogenes found in human malignancies. The mutations in *K-ras* gene have been noted in 24 to 50% of adenocarcinomas arising in heavy smokers *(28)*. The *erbB2* gene is also found to be activated in non-small-cell lung cancer (NSCLC). In one study, adenocarcinomas showed high levels of *erbB2* mRNA, whereas SCLC cells did not express *erbB2* *(29)*. In another study, investigators noted that *erbB2* expression in adenocarcinoma is independently correlated with diminished survival *(30)*.

The high frequency of chromosomal deletions in both SCLC and NSCLC implies that loss of specific gene function may be a critical step in the development of lung cancer. Two tumor suppressor genes implicated in lung cancer are the *p53* and *Rb* *(10)*. *p53* gene mutation is found in more than than 50% of lung cancers *(28)*. These mutations occur in both NSCLC and SCLC cell lines. Mutations in *p53* positively correlate with lifetime cigarette consumption *(31)*. Radon exposure is also associated with *p53* mutation that differs from those seen in tobacco-associated lung malignancies *(32)*.

3. PATHOLOGY

The currently used primary lung cancer histological classification was initially developed by the World Health Organization and later modified in 1981 *(33)*.

3.1. NON-SMALL-CELL CARCINOMA

This category includes adenocarcinoma, squamous cell carcinoma (SCC), bronchoalveolar carcinoma (BAC), large-cell carcinoma (LCC), and pulmonary carcinoids. Adenocarcinoma is the most common type of NSCLC, comprising approx 30 to 40% of cases *(34)*. It is most likely to occur in nonsmokers or former smokers and in women *(5)*. They tend to grow towards the lung with a high propensity to metastasize to both regional lymph nodes as well as distant sites *(35)*. Because of their location, quite frequently these tumors produce no symptoms. Besides T1N0 tumors, it appears that stage-by-stage adenocarcinoma has a somewhat worse prognosis than does SCC. Immunohistochemistry and electron microscopy have been increasingly used by pathologists to identify adenocarcinoma as these cells stain positive for carcinoembryonic antigen and mucin *(36)*.

SCC comprises of approx 30% of all lung cancers in the United States *(37)*. In North America, SCC has not seen the marked increase observed with adenocarcinoma. Two-thirds of SCC present as central lung tumors, whereas one-third present as peripheral tumors. It is the most likely of all lung tumors to cavitate and remain localized *(38)*. They tend to grow slowly and it is estimated that up to 3 to 4 yr are required from the development of *in situ* carcinoma to a clinically apparent tumor *(35)*. Histologically, most well-differentiated tumors demonstrate keratin pearls, whereas the more poorly differentiated SCC have positive keratin staining *(38)*.

BAC, a subtype of adenocarcinoma, has increased in incidence over the last decade. BAC arise from type 2 pneumocytes. It can present as multiple scattered nodules, a pneumonic infiltrate, or as a single nodule. BAC growth is in lepidic fashion along the alveolar septa without invasive growth indicating that these patients may be cured by surgical resection *(39)*.

LCC accounts for 10 to 15% of all lung carcinomas with the tendency to occur as a peripheral lesion with a shorter doubling time *(35,37,38)*. They have a high propensity to metastasize to regional lymph nodes and distant sites. Many tumors previously diagnosed as undifferentiated large-cell carcinoma can now be classified as poorly differentiated adenocarcinoma or squamous cell carcinoma with immuno-histochemical staining, electron microscopy, and monoclonal antibodies. This is probably the reason for decreasing incidence of LCC.

Bronchial carcinoids represent 2% of cases of carcinoid tumors *(40)*. These tumors have not been linked to smoking history. Pulmonary carcinoids are classified as typical carcinoid (also called bronchial carcinoid and Kulchitsky cell carcinoma-I and atypical carcinoid (also called well-differentiated neuroendocrine carcinoma and Kulchitsky cell carcinoma -II). Typical carcinoids are quite indolent in nature. They rarely metastasize and carry a good prognosis. The most important variables affecting the prognosis of typical carcinoids are increasing age, tumor diameter larger than 3 cm, T-stage, and N-stage. Poor prognostic pathological features for all pulmonary carcinoids include increased mitotic count, nuclear pleomorphism, undifferentiated growth pattern, lymphatic, and vascular invasion *(41)*. Patients with carcinoids are at increased risk of developing a synchronous adenocarcinoma and the development of a second malignancy is associated with a worse prognosis *(42)*.

Pulmonary carcinoids have direct access to the systemic circulation, thus, they may produce symptoms associated with carcinoid syndrome without hepatic metastases *(43,44)*. Symptoms of carcinoid syndrome include flushing, diarrhea, wheezing, pain, pellagra, and carcinoid heart disease. The flushes with bronchial carcinoids are frequently prolonged for days, reddish in color, associated with salivation, lacrimation, diaphoresis, facial swelling, palpitations, deep furrowing of the forehead, diarrhea, and hypotension *(45,46)*. After repeated flushing of this type patients may develop a constant red or cyanotic discoloration.

3.2. SMALL-CELL CARCINOMA

In 1926, Barnard *(47)* initially recognized SCLC as a separate entity. SCLC represented approx 15% of the total annual cases of lung cancers in the United States in 2001 *(48)*. SCLC tumors most commonly present as submucosal endobronchial lesions with hilar enlargement. Two-thirds of the patients have detectable distant metastasis at the time of diagnosis. The diagnosis is confirmed by histological analysis of bronchoscopic biopsy specimen or by cytologic analysis of percutaneous transbronchial fine-needle aspirations.

Although SCLC diagnosis rests primarily on morphologic assessment, immunocytochemistry, and electron microscopy are of occasional value in difficult cases. Virtually all SCLCs are immunoreactive for keratin and epithelial membrane antigen *(49)*. Neuroendocrine differentiation markers like chromogranin, neuron-specific enolase, Leu-7, and synaptophysin can be detected in approx 75% of SCLC either singly or in combination *(49)*. Neuroendocrine differentiation markers by themselves may not be diagnostic of SCLC because 10 to 20% of NSCLC also exhibit neuroendocrine differentiation. Electron microscopic features of SCLC include closely apposed cells, high nuclear to cytoplasmic ratio, finely clumped chromatin uniformly dispersed within the nucleus, and only occasional uniformly small dense core granules located in the cytoplasm *(50)*.

4. CLINICAL PRESENTATION

There are no signs or symptoms that are specifically diagnostic of lung cancer. Cough is present in 45 to 75% of all patients with lung cancer *(51)*. In patients with chronic cough, a change in character and quantity of cough should be sought from history. Approximately 25 to 35% of lung cancer patients may have associated hemoptysis. Dyspnea may occur in one-third to one-half of lung cancer patients *(51)*. Chest pain, often secondary to rib invasion, may occur in approx 25 to 50% of all patients. Unilateral wheezing, when present, is most often owing to an underlying bronchogenic carcinoma producing fixed obstruction of a major airway. Inspiratory stridor may result when obstruction occurs by a tumor located in the upper trachea. Weight loss is a frequent presenting complaint in patients with lung cancer.

When a lung tumor directly extends to pleura or when a mediastinal node or a lymphatic vessel is involved, dyspnea secondary to pleural effusion may occur. Pericardial effusion may occur if tumor extends to the pericardium and epicardium. Left-sided lung tumors may involve the left recurrent laryngeal nerve causing hoarseness *(51)*. Headaches, dyspnea, facial and upper extremity swelling, plethora, dilated neck veins, and a prominent venous pattern on upper chest can be the result of superior vena cava (SVC) syndrome. SVC syndrome results from a compression or invasion of the SVC by mediastinal lymph node metastases or by tumor itself. SCLC is noted to be the most commonly associated histologic type with SVC syndrome.

Pancoast tumor, described by Pancoast in 1924, is a superior sulcus tumor of the lung and often involves the brachial plexus. Pancoast syndrome is characterized by Horner's syndrome, rib destruction, atrophy of hand muscles, shoulder pain, and pain in the distribution of C8, T1, and T2 nerve roots on the side of the lung lesion *(52,53)*. Because of the peripheral location of the tumor, pulmonary symptoms such as cough, hemoptysis, and dyspnea are uncommon until late in the disease. Superior sulcus tumors may produce a phrenic or recurrent laryngeal neuropathy, or SVC syndrome in 5 to 10% of cases *(54–55)*.

5. PARANEOPLASTIC SYNDROMES

5.1. NON-SMALL-CELL LUNG CANCER

Non-metastatic systemic symptoms may result from lung tumors. Clinically significant syndromes occur in approx 20% of BAC patients. Mechanism by which these syndromes are produced is not clearly understood. Nonbacterial thrombotic endocarditis (NBTE or marantic endocarditis) and migratory thrombophlebitis are the two most notable cardiovascular paraneoplastic manifestations of BAC. The incidence of NBTE in adenocarcinoma and BAC is approx 7% and it commonly involves mitral valve *(56,57)*. Migratory thrombophlebitis can be associated with arterial thrombosis *(10)*. Lung cancer has been implicated in altered coagulation resulting in thrombotic and hemorrhagic diatheses. A hypercoagulable state is noted in 10 to 15% of lung cancer cases *(10)* and it is often associated with thrombocytosis and hyperfibrinogenemia.

Tumors of squamous cell histology may produce parathyroid hormone-related peptide (PTHrP), quite frequently resulting in hypercalcemia. Hypercalcemia may, however, be related to bony metastasis. Digital clubbing and hypertrophic pulmonary osteoarthropathy are most commonly associated with adenocarcinoma and least frequently with SCLC. LCC may cause gynecomastia and milky nipple discharge secondary to the production of human chorionic gonadotropin or related peptides *(10)*.

5.2. SMALL-CELL LUNG CANCER

SCLC tumors produce biologically active amines by decarboxylating amino acids and may also promote synthesis of antidiuretic hormone and adrenocorticotrophic hormone (ACTH). Overproduction of such hormones results in a syndrome of inappropriate antidiuretic hormone (SIADH) and hypercortisolism respectively. SIADH occurs in approx 10%, whereas hypercortisolism occurs in approx 1% of SCLC patients *(8)*. Hyponatremia is the hallmark of SIADH and the rate of decline in sodium levels is typically prolonged in SCLC. The clinical manifestations of hyponatremia, such as mental status changes, seizures, or lethargy, may often be absent in SCLC despite significantly low sodium levels. Similarly ectopic ACTH syndrome in SCLC rarely results in the typical Cushingoid features *(10)*.

SCLC is the most common type of lung cancer associated with paraneoplastic autoimmune neurological syndromes. The severity of the neurological symptoms is unrelated to tumor bulk. Eaton-Lambert syndrome is commonly associated with SCLC. It is characterized by proximal limb muscle weakness and fatigue. Clinically this syndrome is distinguished from myasthenia gravis by little or no involvement of the bulbar or extra-ocular muscles. The antibody mediated impairment of presynaptic neuronal calcium channel activity, which impairs the nerve stimulus induced release of acetylcholine, has been the implicated defect in neuromuscular transmission in this syndrome (10).

The most characteristic peripheral neuropathy associated with SCLC is subacute sensory neuropathy. Progressive impairment of all sensory modalities with areflexia and marked sensory ataxia followed by stabilization over a period of weeks are characteristics of SCLC associated subacute sensory neuropathy. It may precede the diagnosis of SCLC by several months (58). Limbic encephalopathy, necrotizing myelopathy, and intestinal dysmotility syndrome are among other SCLC-associated neurological syndromes (59–61). Limbic encephalopathy, associated with inflammatory infiltrate in the hippocampal and medial temporal lobe regions, is characterized by memory loss and behavior changes that often antedate the diagnosis of cancer. Relatively acute, rapidly ascending paraplegia that progresses to rapid deterioration and death is characteristic of necrotizing myelopathy. In SCLC patients with peripheral neuropathy and these rare neurological paraneoplastic syndromes, type 1 antineuronal nuclear antibody (ANNA-1), also known as anti-Hu, is a valuable serologic marker (62). Several investigators have reported cases of paraneoplastic intestinal dysmotility syndrome associated with SCLC in patients with serum antibodies to myenteric and submucosal neural plexuses of the jejunum and stomach (61,63).

6. STAGING

6.1. NON-SMALL-CELL LUNG CANCER

The extent of disease, location of the primary tumor, and associated clinical complications determine the staging of lung cancer. It is important to include assessment of extra pulmonary intrathoracic and extrathoracic metastasis for staging. Staging can be classified as clinical and/or pathological. Clinical staging is defined on the basis of the assessment of the extent of the anatomic extent of disease prior to institution of definitive therapy. Such assessment may include a medical history, physical examination, various imaging procedures, and the results of selected studies such as bronchoscopy, esophagoscopy, mediastinoscopy, thoracentesis, and thoracoscopy. Information from exploratory thoracotomy is not included in clinical staging and such patients found unresectable should be pathologically staged.

The International System for Staging Lung Cancer (64) was adopted by the American Joint Committee on Cancer and the International Union Against Cancer in 1997 (65,66) and has had wide spread application since its adoption. Tables 1 and 2 illustrate the definitions and the stage grouping of the tumor-node-metastases subsets (65,67). Invasion of phrenic nerve secondary to direct extension of lung tumor is classified as T3.

Lung tumors located in the periphery directly invading the chest wall and ribs are also classified as T3. T4 includes pleural tumor foci that are separate from direct pleural invasion by the primary tumor. A separate lesion outside the parietal pleura, in the diaphragm, or in the chest wall is designated as M1. Vocal cord paralysis (resulting from involvement of the recurrent laryngeal nerve), superior vena caval obstruction, or compression of the trachea or esophagus secondary to direct extension of the primary tumor or to lymph node involvement should be classified as T4-stage IIIB. For "Pancoast" tumors, if there is evidence of invasion of the vertebral body or extension into the neural foramina, the tumor should be classified as T4. Discontinuous tumor foci, that is only histologically detectable, would be reflected in the pathological staging and would not affect the clinical staging.

6.2. SMALL-CELL LUNG CANCER

Rather than tumor-node-metastases staging, SCLC is divided into limited and extensive disease. A tumor that can be encompassed within a single, tolerable radiation port defines limited disease, whereas all other tumors are characterized as extensive. Given higher propensity for SCLC for early metastasis, all patients should undergo detailed history and physical examination, a basic laboratory evaluation, chest computed tomography (CT), bone scanning, and brain imaging. Although controversial, bone marrow biopsy may play a role in overall staging work up of selected SCLC.

7. DIAGNOSIS

A complete medical history and physical examination are essential parts of the diagnostic process in the evaluation of lung cancer. In smokers, it is important to note any change in the amount or consistency of the sputum. Patient should always be questioned about exposure to environmental toxins and irritants, such as asbestos and smoking. Shortness of breath, wheezing, chest pain, blood in the sputum, or frequent respiratory infections, bone pain, fatigue, and unintentional weight loss can also increase the index of suspicion. Chest radiograph is often one of the first tests used to evaluate patient suspected of having lung cancer. Comparison with previous radiograph is often helpful in such cases. It is important to note that patients with persistent symptoms of cough and dyspnea with normal chest radiograph may be hiding a central lesion that is not obvious on chest radiograph. In such cases a CT scan of the chest including the liver and the adrenal glands is of great utility to further define the primary tumor and to identify lymphatic or parenchymal metastases. Apical tumors (Pancoast's tumors) may also be difficult to detect on a chest radiograph, but are usually readily detectable on a CT scan. An enlarged adrenal gland should be biopsied because it may be the sole site of metastatic disease in up to 10% of patients with NSCLC (38).

For a centrally located lesion, sputum cytologies for three consecutive days can provide cytologic diagnosis. Bronchoscopy can establish the cytological and/or histological diagnosis in 80 to 85% of patients with a centrally located lesion (38). The false-negative rates of bronchoscopic diagnosis of a peripherally located lesions range from 20 to 50% (38). A CT-guided needle biopsy can diagnose up to 90% of such peripheral lesions. Mediastinoscopy may be needed in those patients whose CT

Table 1
TNM (Tumor, Regional Lymph Nodes, Metastasis) Definition (65,71)

Primary tumor (T)

TX	Primary tumor cannot be assessed. Tumor cannot be visualized by imaging or bronchoscopy but can be proven by the presence of malignant cells in sputum or bronchial washings.
T0	No signs of primary tumor.
Tis	Carcinoma *in situ*.
T1	Tumor is ≥3 cm in greatest dimension. Tumor is surrounded by lung or visceral pleura. No bronchoscopic evidence of invasion more proximal than the lobar bronchus (not the main bronchus). The uncommon superficial tumor of any size with its invasive component limited to the bronchial wall with extension proximal to the main bronchus can also fall under T1.
T2	Tumor with any of the following features: >3 cm in greatest dimension, main bronchus involvement, ≥2 cm distal to carina, visceral pleural invasion, associated with atelectasis or obstructive pneumonitis that extends to the hilar region without involvement of the entire lung.
T3	Any size tumor with direct invasion of any of the following: Diaphragm, mediastinal pleura, parietal pericardium, chest wall (including superior sulcus tumors); or tumor in the main bronchus <2 cm from carina, but without involvement of the carina; or associated atelectasis or obstructive pneumonitis of the entire lung.
T4	Any size tumor with invasion of any of the following: Heart, great vessels, trachea, esophagus, vertebral body, carina, mediastinum; or separate tumor nodules in the same lobe; or tumor with a malignant pleural effusion. When multiple cytopathologic examinations of effusion are negative for tumor and when clinical judgement indicate that the effusion is not related to tumor, the effusion should be excluded as a staging element and the patient should be staged as T1, T2, or T3.

Regional nodes (N)

NX	Regional nodes cannot be assessed.
N0	No evidence of regional nodal metastasis.
N1	Ipsilateral peribronchial and/or ipsilateral hilar nodal and intrapulmonary nodal (including involvement by direct extension of the primary tumor) metastasis.
N2	Ipsilateral mediastinal and/or subcarinal nodal metastasis.
N3	Contralateral mediastinal, contralateral hilar, ipsilateral or contralateral scalene, or supraclavicular lymph nodal metastasis.

Distant metastasis (M)

MX	Distant metastasis cannot be assessed.
M0	No evidence of distant metastasis.
M1	Presence of distant metastasis. This includes separate tumor nodule(s) in a different lobe (ipsilateral or contralateral).

scans are not conclusive regarding mediastinal lymph node involvement and is essential in patients who are considered candidates for surgery. The subaortic and aortopulmonary window regions are inaccessible by standard cervical mediastinoscopy. Thoracentesis should be performed in individuals who have pleural effusions. Video-assisted thoracoscopic surgery is the next option in patients in whom thoracentesis does not show malignant cells. Tumor markers have no role in the staging of NSCLC at the current time.

Once the diagnosis is confirmed, it is important to assess any presence of distal metastasis. Patients with clinical stage I and II NSCLC who have normal blood chemistry and blood counts have a low chance of brain and bone metastasis, thus,

brain and bone imaging may be omitted in the absence of symptoms. Brain and bone scans, however, should be obtained as part of evaluation and staging of SCLC.

Over the past several years, positron emission tomographic (PET) scanning with 2-fluoro-2-deoxy-D-glucose has emerged as an important noninvasive test for mediastinal assessment (68). The combination of PET and CT appears to have even better sensitivity and specificity than the use of either method alone. In patients with suspected or proven NSCLC considered resectable by standard staging procedures, PET can prevent non-therapeutic thoracotomy in a significant number of cases. PET use for mediastinal staging should not be relied on as a sole staging modality, and positive findings should be confirmed by

Table 2
Lung Cancer Staging With Respective Treatment and Prognosis (1)

Stage	Tumor (T)	Node (N)	Metastasis (M)	Primary treatment	Outcome
Non-small-cell lung cancer					
Local					
IA	T1	N0	M0	Surgery and adjuvant chemotherapy	5-yr survival: >60–70%
IB	T2	N0	M0		
IIA	T1	N1	M0	Chemotherapy with or without radiotherapy	5-yr survival: >40–50%
Locally advanced					
IIB	T2	N1	M0	Chemotherapy with or without radiotherapy	5-yr survival: >40–50%
	T3	N0	M0		
IIIA	T1	N2	M0	Resectable IIIA: Neoadjuvant chemotherapy followed by surgery Nonresectable IIIA/IIIB: Concurrent chemotherapy and radiotherapy	Resectable IIIA: 5-yr survival: 15–30% Nonresectable IIIA/IIIB: 5 yr survival: 10–20%
	T2	N2	M0		
	T3	N1	M0		
	T3	N2	M0		
IIIB	Any T	N3	M0		
Advanced					
IIIB	T4	Any N	M0	Chemotherapy with 2 agents for 3–4 cycles Surgery for solitary brain metastasis	Median survival: 8–10 mo 1-yr survival: 30–35% 5-yr survival: 10–20%
IV	Any T	Any N	M1		
Small-cell lung cancer					
Limited disease	Tumor confined to ipsilateral hemithorax; can be encompassed by a single radiation port			Chemotherapy with concurrent radiotherapy	5-yr survival: 15–25%
Extensive disease	All other diseases, including metastatic disease			Chemotherapy	5-yr survival: <5%

mediastinoscopy. Metastatic disease, especially a single site, identified by PET requires further confirmatory evaluation *(69)*. The gold standard for mediastinal evaluation is still lymph node biopsy either by means of bronchoscopy or, if needed, mediastinoscopy.

8. BONE METASTASES

Approximately 25% of the four million people who die in the United States each year, die from cancer and approx 70% of these have either breast, lung, or prostate cancer *(70)*. In the United States, more than 350,000 people die annually from bone metastasis and if patients in the European Union and Japan are included, the previous number would be two to three times higher. The incidence of bone metastasis also depends on the longevity of a patient with a particular malignancy. There is higher prevalence of bone metastasis in patients with breast and prostate cancer who live longer with their respective malignancies as compared to those patients with lung malignancies. There are different patterns of bone metastasis in patients with cancer, ranging from osteolytic, as in breast cancer and myeloma, to mostly osteoblastic, as in prostate cancer. Although lung cancer can metastasize to many parts of body, this section would concentrate primarily on bone metastasis.

Bone metastasis is frequently associated with severe intractable bone pain. The mechanism of pain is not completely understood, however, evidence suggests osteolysis as a possible etiology *(71)*. This is supported by the observation that bone-resorption inhibitors like osteoprotegrin (OPG) or bisphosphonates may be used to alleviate bone pain *(72)*. Bone metastasis may result in pathological fractures, which often occur in weight-bearing bones. Leukoerythroblastic anemia, bone deformity, hypercalcemia, and nerve-compression syndromes are some of the other consequences of bone metastasis *(73)*. The initial steps in the development of bone metastasis include primary tumor invading their surrounding normal tissue followed by travel to distant sites. During this process, the cancer cells that survive enter the wide-channeled sinusoids of the bone-marrow cavity and become a potential site for bone metastasis. These cells must have the capacity to migrate across the sinusoidal wall, invade the marrow, generate their own blood supply, and travel to the endosteal bone surface where they stimulate osteoclast or osteoblast activity.

Traditionally it has been thought that bone metastases are either osteolytic or osteoblastic, but morphological analysis has revealed that in most patients bone metastases have both osteolytic and osteoblastic elements. In osteolytic lesions, the main mediator is PTHrP, whereas in osteoblastic lesions, endothelin-1 and platelet-derived growth factor are the known mediators *(73)*. Osteoclast stimulation by known mediators lead to osteolysis and not the direct effects of cancer cells on bone *(74)*. Even when lesions appear grossly to be osteolytic, there is usually also a local bone formation response reflected by an increase in levels of serum alkaline phosphatase and increased uptake of bone-scanning agents at the site of lesion.

It has been shown that human osteolytic breast cancer cells express PTHrP in vivo, which is the main mediator of osteoclast activation. When tumor cells are present at the metastatic bone site, PTHrP expression is greater than when tumor cells are present in soft-tissue (75). This implies that PTHrP is a specific mediator of osteolysis in metastatic breast cancer, and is likely to be the mediator in most other osteolytic malignancies (76,77). The role of PTHrP in mediating osteolysis is complex. One hypothesis is that tumor cells expressing high levels of PTHrP are selected for their ability to metastasize to bone alternatively, the bone microenvironment may increase PTHrP expression from malignant cells that have spread there (73). Henderson et al. (78) demonstrated that PTHrP expression by primary tumors is associated with a more favorable outcome, whereas other preclinical and clinical data have associated PTHrP production with increased bone metastatic potential. However, despite the complexity regarding the role of PTHrP in inducing osteolysis, osteolysis induced by human breast cancer metastasis has been shown to be blocked by neutralizing antibodies against PTHrP (79). In vivo, compounds that specifically decrease PTHrP expression have been shown to inhibit osteolysis caused by human cancer cells (73).

Hypercalcemia secondary to extensive bone destruction as commonly seen in patients with lung, breast, renal, ovarian, and pancreatic malignancies along with myeloma, is mostly owing to the production of PTHrP by the tumor (80), after which PTHrP acts on PTH receptors leading to increased bone resorption and increased renal tubular calcium reabsorption (81). Neutralizing antibodies to PTHrP have also been shown in preclinical studies to be effective treatment of such hypercalcemia. PTHrP stimulates osteoclasts also by stimulating production of the cytokine receptor activator of nuclear factor-κB ligand (RANKL), which, in turn, binds and activates RANK as expressed by osteoclasts. OPG and bisphosphonates can prevent bone destruction as they block the association of RANKL, as well as other ligands, with RANK. Mostly all other mediators of osteoclastic bone resorption also signal through RANKL. However, experimental results obtained from blocking RANKL activity do not reveal the importance of the tumor-specific production of RANKL. There is an ongoing debate about the exact role of RANKL in the osteolytic bone activity that is associated with human solid tumors and myeloma. Gene mutations encoding mutant estrogen receptors, interleukin-8, and the receptor for PTH have also been associated with bone metastasis (73).

Multiple factors have been identified that stimulate bone formation associated with metastatic tumors. Endothelin-1 is the ubiquitous growth factor that is implicated in stimulating bone formation and osteoblast proliferation in bone organ cultures. Studies have shown that in patients with osteoblastic metastasis endothelin-1 is increased in circulation (82,73). This is further strengthened by the evidence that endothelin-A-receptor antagonists have been shown in vivo to inhibit osteoblast proliferation and bone metastasis (73). Transforming growth factor-β2 has also been shown to stimulate the proliferation of osteoblasts in vitro, and bone formation in vivo, implicating it as a candidate mediator of osteoblastic metastasis (73). An

amino-terminal fragment of serine protease urokinase (uPA) has been shown to have mitogenic activity for osteoblasts. An overexpression of uPA by rat prostate cancer cells has been shown to induce bone metastasis in vivo (73). Izbicka et al. (83) have demonstrated that osteoblasts can be activated by human tumor cell line producing extended form of basic fibroblast growth factor (FGF)-2, subsequently causing bone formation in vivo. There is also some evidence that platelet-derived growth factor-BB has a role as mediator of the osteoblastic response in some tumor types (74).

Currently available as well as under investigation therapeutic options for bone metastasis include bisphosphonates, OPG, RANK-Fc, PTHrP antibodies, vitamin D analogs, and endothelin-A-receptor antibodies (Table 3) (73). So far there has been little research done eliciting factors that might be responsible for osteolysis in tumors other than breast and prostate cancers and myeloma. Although the answer is still nonconclusive, it seems likely that bisphosphonates may be effective in treating bone metastasis from other malignancies as cellular mechanisms responsible for osteolysis are fundamentally identical.

9. TREATMENT

9.1. NON-SMALL-CELL LUNG CARCINOMA

It has been generally agreed by all investigators that resection of the lobe containing the tumor is the standard treatment for clinically staged IA, IB, IIA, and IIB NSCLC. A similar consensus exists for patients with stage IV NSCLC emphasizing nonoperative treatment except for a rare case of patient with a solitary brain metastasis. Multi-modality therapy is recommended for stage IIIA and IIIB disease, but its exact nature and sequence still remain controversial. In resectable cases, lobectomy is the procedure of choice given higher incidence of recurrence with lower 5-yr survival with wedge or segmental resection. Five-year survival rates for respective pathological stage are illustrated in Table 2.

Table 3
Novel Approaches to Treating Bone Metastases

Treatment	Mechanism
Bisphosphonates	Block bone resorption. May block tumor-cell mitosis and stimulate tumor-cell apoptosis. May alleviate the bone pain.
Osteoprotegerin	Prevents RANKL from binding its receptor thus preventing osteoclast stimulation.
RANK-Fc	Prevents RANKL from binding its receptor and osteoclast stimulation.
PTHrP antibodies	Neutralize PTHrP.
Vitamin D analogs	Decrease PTHrP production.
Endothelin-A receptor antagonists	Blocks endothelin-1 activity thus inhibiting ostoblast proliferation and bone metastasis.

RANK-Fc, receptor activator of nuclear factor-κB-fragment crystal 2a; RANKL, receptor activator of nuclear factor-κB ligand; PTHrP, parathyroid hormone-related peptide.

Table 4
Active Chemotherapy Agents for Lung Cancer

Drug	Type of agent
Platinum agents	
Cisplatin	Atypical alkylator
Carboplatin	Atypical alkylator
Nonplatinum agents	
Etoposide	Topoisomerase II inhibitor
Topotecan	Topoisomerase I inhibitor
Irinotecan	Topoisomerase I inhibitor
Gemcitabine	Antimetabolite
Paclitaxel	Microtubule inhibitor
Docetaxel	Microtubule inhibitor
Vinorelbine	Microtubule inhibitor
Vincristine	Microtubule inhibitor
Doxorubicin	Anthracycline antibiotic
Cyclophosphamide	Alkylating agent
Ifosfamide	Alkylating agent

9.1.1. Adjuvant Radiotherapy

Adjuvant radiotherapy has been considered with the theory of eliminating small deposits of malignant cells adjacent to or draining from the primary tumor site. The results of adjuvant radiotherapy have been quite variable (84–86). In 1998, a large meta-analysis suggested that adjuvant radiotherapy was detrimental, with a 21% increase in the relative risk of death (87). However, modern radiotherapy and staging techniques were not included in this dated meta-analysis data. In 1986, the Lung Cancer Study Group demonstrated that, in N2 disease, adjuvant radiotherapy prevented local recurrence but did not improve overall survival (OS) (84). The rationale for the use of adjuvant radiation in otherwise healthy patients with N2 disease is based on this study. Unless the surgical margins are positive and repeated resection is not feasible, adjuvant radiotherapy has no role outside of a clinical trial for any other type of patients.

9.1.2. Adjuvant Chemotherapy

Even with adequate surgical resection, the prognosis for early NSCLC patients is sub-optimal, probably owing to undetectable microscopic metastasis at diagnosis. Chemotherapy with cytotoxic agents in theory may improve survival by eliminating micro-metastases. The most active chemotherapy agents (Table 4) against NSCLC are platinum agents, thus, becoming the rationale for most modern trials using platinum-based regimens. Most trials have failed to show a statistically significant benefit of adjuvant chemotherapy in NSCLC (88–91). A few trials did show a 10 to 15% survival advantage many years after diagnosis in patients with stage III or incompletely resected tumors (92,93). In 1995, a large meta-analysis evaluated data from adjuvant chemotherapy trials from 1965 to 1991 (94). It demonstrated that adjuvant therapy with alkylating agents (cyclophosphamide and nitrosourea) was detrimental, whereas treatment with cisplatin-based therapy resulted in a 13% reduction in the risk of death, but statistical significance was not reached with $p = 0.08$. Similarly, the Eastern Cooperative Oncology Group failed to show a benefit of adjuvant therapy with cisplatin, etoposide, and radiotherapy (88). Recently published results of the International Adjuvant Lung Cancer Trial (IALT), a randomized study of 1867 NSCLC patients compar-

ing cisplatin-based adjuvant chemotherapy to no adjuvant therapy, showed an absolute benefit of 5% for disease-free survival (DFS) at 5 yr ($p < 0.003$) and of 4% for OS ($p < 0.03$) (95). Adjuvant platinum-based chemotherapy should be considered in selected patients with stage I, II, or IIIA NSCLC based on the IALT and aforementioned meta-analysis results.

9.1.3. Locally Advanced Unresectable (Stage IIIB) NSCLC

Radiation treatment dose of 60 Gy used to be the mainstay of treatment for unresectable NSCLC. The long-term survival remains poor (96). In 1990, a landmark study assessing the role of combined modality treatment for stage III NSCLC patients demonstrated increased 3-yr survival rates (23 vs 11%) and long-term survival in the favor of treatment with chemotherapy and radiotherapy compared to radiotherapy alone (97,98). Pritchard and Anthony (99) in a meta-analysis showed a significant decrease in the relative risk of death at 1- and 3-yr with combined therapy for unresectable disease. Similarly, a second meta-analysis showed a 24% risk reduction of death at 1 yr and a 30% reduction at 2 yr with combined cisplatin-based chemotherapy and radiotherapy (100). In 1999, Furuse et al. (101) first showed that concurrent chemotherapy and radiotherapy improved survival when compared to sequential therapy in stage III unresectable NSCLC. These results were later confirmed by Radiation Therapy Oncology Group 9410 trial as reported in 2003 (102).

9.1.4. Locally Advanced Resectable NSCLC

Neoadjuvant chemoradiotherapy followed by complete resection is the preferred approach to Pancoast's tumor. These tumors have the tendency to invade surrounding thoracic inlet structures. Pancoast's tumors are associated with a high incidence of local recurrence as tumor free margins cannot be obtained. Among these patients receiving adjuvant radiotherapy alone, historical 2-yr survival rates have been approx 20% (103). The 2-yr survival rate with combined neoadjuvant chemotherapy and radiotherapy followed by surgical resection is in the range of 50 to 70% (104,105). Aggressive multimodality therapy have shown significant survival advantage even in patients with vertebral invasion by the tumor (106).

The success of neoadjuvant combined modality therapy in patients with unresectable (N2) tumors has resulted in its use in patients with resectable N2 tumors. In 1989, a small study, assessing the role of neoadjuvant cisplatin-based chemotherapy followed by surgery and radiotherapy in patients with resectable stage III disease, reported median survival of 32 mo and the 1-yr survival rate of 75%, both of which were higher than previously reported rates (107). In 1994, a randomized trial of 60 patients with Stage IIIA NSCLC comparing neoadjuvant six cycles of cisplatin based therapy to surgery alone, reported median survival of 64 mo in neoadjuvant arm vs 11 mo in surgery only arm with the 3-yr survival rates of 56 and 15%, respectively (108). In 1994, another randomized study of 60 patients with resectable NSCLC compared surgery alone to neoadjuvant cisplatin-based chemotherapy followed by surgery and radiotherapy (109). Long-term follow up in both of these studies supported superiority of combined modality treatment approach (110,111). On the other hand, Depierre and colleagues (112) in a study of 355 patients with early NSCLC who were randomized to receive either neoadjuvant chemotherapy followed by surgery or surgery alone, found a nonsignificant ($p = 0.15$) trend towards a survival advantage for combined therapy group. Subgroup analysis failed to show any benefit of combined therapy in patients with N2 disease. The risk of distant recurrence was noted to be lower in the chemotherapy group, whereas no significant difference was noted in the risk of locoregional relapse.

To further investigate the role of surgery in stage IIIA NSCLC, Albain et al. (113) reported a phase III study comparing definitive concurrent chemotherapy and radiotherapy (CT/RT) to induction CT/RT followed by surgery. The initial results suggested superior DFS for the group receiving induction CT/RT followed by surgery ($p = 0.02$). Although there was a trend towards improved OS favoring the surgery group, the difference had not yet reached statistical significance at 3-yr follow up (113). Taking everything together, it is likely that multimodality protocols are the best treatment option for patient with locally advanced but resectable NSCLC.

9.1.5. Advanced Disease

Chemotherapy is the backbone of treatment for metastatic NSCLC. Response rates, however, are low with poor survival. Compared with supportive care, moderate gains of 2 to 4 mo increase in survival have been reported with chemotherapy. An increase of 10 to 20% in 1-yr survival rates have been reported with the use of chemotherapy to treat patients with advanced disease (94,100). Studies have suggested benefits in terms of time to disease progression and the quality of life (114–116). These benefits were noted in NSCLC patients with good functional status.

Single agent platinum therapy remained the mainstay therapy for advanced NSCLC until 1990. With the development of taxanes, gemcitabine, and vinorelbine, several randomized trials evaluated newer agents in combination with cisplatin as compared to cisplatin alone (117–121). These trials demonstrated higher response rates and acceptable toxicity with combination chemotherapy (117–121). In 2000, the first trial showing better response rate with modern combination of paclitaxel and cisplatin compared to older regimen of etoposide and cisplatin was reported (122). In 2002, Schiller et al. (123) compared four commonly used two-drug regimens for advanced NSCLC. The four platinum-based chemotherapy regimens showed similar efficacy (123). A summary of major trials in NSCLC has been illustrated in Table 5. Several trials have evaluated three-drug regimens and none of these showed superiority to platinum-based doublets. Increased toxicity was registered with three-drug regimens and, thus, such regimens should not be used (124,125). Several trials have demonstrated that the elderly have similar rates of tolerance and benefit from chemotherapy as much as younger patients (126,127). Currently, patients with advanced NSCLC, without contraindications, should receive a two-drug chemotherapy regimen (128).

The optimal duration of therapy in patients with advanced NSCLC was evaluated by randomized trials that compared three cycles of cisplatin-based therapy with six cycles (129,130). These trials found only increased toxicity with prolonged chemotherapy administration, thus, leading to a conclusion that patients with advanced NSCLC should initially be limited to only three to four cycles of two-drug chemotherapy (129,130). Ultimately all patients will progress. The results of several randomized studies suggest that docetaxel may offer some survival benefit in a second line setting when compared to supportive care and other agents (131,132).

Surgery has a beneficial role in NSCLC patients with a solitary metastasis. For patients undergoing resection of a solitary brain metastasis followed by whole brain radiotherapy, the 5-yr survival rate can reach 10 to 20% (133,134). Although the data is less conclusive, resection of solitary adrenal metastasis may increase long-term survival (135,136).

Novel treatment paradigm calls for development of targeted therapies for NSCLC. The Genotypic International Lung Trial is first of a kind trial in which patient genotypes would determine their respective treatment plan. This trial plans on enrolling over 400 patients with stage IV NSCLC. Patients with only β-*tubulin* mutations will receive gemcitabine and cisplatin; those with *ERCC1* overexpression alone will receive gemcitabine and docetaxel; those with both aberrations will receive gemcitabine and CPT-11; and those with no alterations will receive docetaxel and cisplatin as the control arm. The shift toward more specific, biochemically targeted cancer therapies is the current trend in the design of clinical trials and drug developments.

10. TARGETED THERAPY

The overall cure rate of lung cancer is dismal, primarily because of a delayed stage at diagnosis and inability of conventional chemotherapy to cure systemic disease. Targeted therapy with novel agents, such as epidermal growth factor receptor inhibitors including cetuximab and ABX-EGF, or tyosine kinase inhibitors including gefitinib and erlotinib, have been a very active area of basic and translational research in the past few years. Phase II monotherapy trials employed gefitinib in second- and third-line setting in patients with recurrent NSCLC showing response rate ranging from 11 to 18%. Based on these results, gefitinib was approved by US Food and Drug Administration for treatment of refractory metastatic NSCLC that progressed after platinum-based and docetaxel chemotherapy (137). Phase III trials comparing combination of gefitinib and chemotherapy in chemo-naïve patients with advanced NSCLC showed no survival advantage over chemotherapy alone (138). The role of these agents in early stage lung cancer is currently under investigation. Development of new targeted agents for the treatment of lung cancer has been challenging. Better understanding of the disease, careful patient selection, and proper clinical trial design are needed before we can sort out a myriad of potential targets in our search for a few that may have an impact on this deadly disease (138).

10.1. SMALL-CELL LUNG CANCER
10.1.1. Limited Disease

Although the majority of patients with SCLC present with advanced stage disease, approximately one-third of SCLC patients present with disease that is limited to the thorax. During the 1970s, the relative sensitivity of SCLC to chemotherapy became apparent. Chemotherapy is now the mainstay for treatment of SCLC. Several studies have showed superior-

Table 5
Selected Trials in Non-Small-Cell Lung Cancer

Regimens	Results
Adjuvant chemotherapy and radiotherapy	
cAC vs immunotherapy (92).	Increased survival with adjuvant chemotherapy.
EC plus RT vs RT alone (88).	No advantage of chemotherapy.
Cisplatin based adjuvant therapy vs observation (95).	4% absolute increase in OS with adjuvant chemotherapy at 5 yr.
RT vs no therapy (85).	No survival advantage; decreased local recurrence rate only among N2 patients.
Role of chemotherapy plus radiotherapy in inoperable cancer	
CV plus RT vs RT alone (97,98).	Chemoradiotherapy group: 7 yr MS = 13.7 mo (p = 0.012); 7 yr OS = 13%.
	Radiotherapy group: 7 yr MS = 9.6 mo; 7 yr OS = 6%.
Concurrent CVM plus RT vs sequential CVM plus RT (101).	Concurrent group: MS = 16.5 mo (p = 0.03998); 5 yr OS = 15.8%.
	Sequential group: MS = 13.3 mo; 5 yr OS = 8.9%.
Concurrent CV plus RT vs sequential CV and RT (102).	Increased survival with concurrent radiotherapy.
	Concurrent group: OS = 25%; Sequential group: OS = 4% (p = 0.046).
Stage IIIA: neoadjuvant chemotherapy	
Neoadjuvant cEC followed by surgery vs surgery alone (108,110).	Neoadjuvant cheomtherapy group: 3 yr OS = 56%; MS = 64 mo.
	Surgery alone: 3 yr OS = 15%; MS = 11mo.
Neoadjuvant MIC and RT vs surgery and RT (109,111).	Increased MS neoadjuvant chemotherapy group (22 vs 10 mo).
Neoadjuvant concurrent EC plus RT f/u by surgery vs concurrent EC plus RT (112).	Surgery group: DFS = 14 mo; 3 yr OS = 38%.
	Concurrent EC plus RT alone: DFS = 11.7 mo; 3 yr OS = 33%.
Stages I, II, IIIA: neoadjuvant chemotherapy	
Neoadjuvant MIC and radiotherapy vs surgery and radiotherapy (113).	Small survival advantage for N0 or N1 disease at 1 and 4 yr. No benefit for N2 disease.
Advanced diseases: chemotherapy	
CT vs CG and CD and carboplatin plus T (123).	Equivocal results for all regimens.

c, cyclophosphamide; A, doxorubicin; C, cisplatin; E, etoposide; V, vinblastine; M, mitomycin; I, ifosfamide; G, gemcitabine; T, paclitaxel; D, docetaxel; yr, year; N, node; mo, month; OS, overall survival; MS, median survival; RT, radiotherapy; f/u, followed by; DFS, disease-free survival.

Table 6
Randomized Trials of Small-Cell Lung Cancer

Trials	Results
Extensive disease	
EC vs cAV vs EC alternating with cAV (141).	Alternating regimens failed to show any advantage. Patients in EC group more likely to have a response to therapy.
EC vs cAV vs. EC alternating with cAV (142).	No difference in survival among groups. Alternating regimens failed to show any advantage.
EC vs. Irinotecan plus C (148).	EC group: MS = 12.8 mo; 2 yr OS = 19.5%.
	Irinotecan plus C group: MS = 9.4 mo; 2 yr OS = 5.2%.
Limited disease	
Concurrent EC plus RT vs Sequential EC plus RT (145).	Improved 2- and 5-yr OS rates with concurrent therapy.
Chemotherapy with once daily RT vs chemotherapy with twice daily RT (146).	5 yr OS rate with twice daily RT: 26%.
	5 yr OS rate with once daily RT: 16%.

E, etoposide; C, cisplatin; A, doxorubicin; V, Vincristine; c, cyclophosphamide; MS, median survival; yr, year, mo, month; OS, overall survival; RT, radiotherapy.

ity of combination chemotherapy compared to single agent therapy (139,140). The combination of etoposide and cisplatin (EC) is currently the most commonly used regimen because it compared favorably with an older regimen of cyclophosphamide, doxorubicin, and vincristine (141,142).

For limited diseases, a reasonable current standard is to deliver thoracic radiation concurrent with combination chemotherapy. A 15% risk reduction of death with combination chemo-therapy and radiotherapy when compared to chemotherapy alone in patients with limited stage SCLC has been suggested by two meta-analyses (143,144). Concurrent chemotherapy and radiotherapy resulted in superior 5-yr survival compared to sequential therapy (145). Turrisi et al. (146) reported results of a randomized trial showing improved 5-yr survival with minimal additional toxicity with hyper-fractionated radiotherapy with the same total dose of 45 Gy.

SCLC is associated with high risk of development of brain metastasis. Prophylactic cranial irradiation (PCI) remains controversial as most trials have shown a reduction in central nervous system (CNS) relapse rates but a little effect on survival (8). The current recommendations with regards to PCI in patients with limited stage SCLC indicated that PCI should be used only when patients have achieved a complete or near-complete remission of disease outside of the CNS.

10.1.2. Extensive Disease

Approximately two-thirds of SCLC patients have extensive disease at diagnosis and without treatment, the median survival in this group of patients is 6 to 8 wk. Treatment with combination chemotherapy increases median survival duration to approx 8 to 10 mo. The most commonly used regimen is EC (Table 6). One study had suggested that carboplatin is equivalent to cisplatin in extensive stage NSCLC (147). A recently reported randomized trial compared EC to irinotecan and cisplatin (IC) regimen in patients with extensive disease (148). The IC group had increased median survival and 2-yr survival rate with less severe hematologic toxicity but a high incidence of diarrhea (148). Addition of paclitaxel to EC regimen for extensive SCLC patients failed to show significant survival advantage while increasing toxicity (149,150). Topotecan has

been shown to have beneficial activity as second line therapy in patients with SCLC (151).

Radiation therapy remains the most appropriate modality for the treatment of SVC syndrome, spinal cord compression, brain metastasis, and localized bone pain. However, patients with more extensive disease without local exigencies should be considered for palliative chemotherapy as it may relieve local symptoms as well as possibly prolong survival.

11. MANAGEMENT OF BONE METASTASIS

Standard management of bone metastasis includes radiotherapy and bisphosphonates for pain control or prevention of pathological fractures and observation for asymptomatic patients. In addition, orthopedic surgical procedures are used to prevent or correct pathological fractures in weight-bearing areas. Osteoclast function inhibitors, including bisphosphonates and gallium nitrate, have been shown in clinical trials to decrease bone-related complications. Recently, bisphosphonates have become an integral part of the management of bone metastasis (152–156).

Improved biological understanding of osteoclastogenesis has facilitated identification of OPG or bisphosphonate as a critical modulator of osteoclast activity (72,157). In 2003, Tchekmedyian et al. (152) reported results of a phase III trial assessing long-term safety and efficacy of zoledronic acid in reducing skeletal complications in patients with bone metastasis from solid tumors other than breast or prostate cancer. Fewer zoledronic acid treated patients developed skeletal-related event (SRE) compared with placebo treated patients (152). The majority (57%) of the study population had lung cancer and it demonstrated 31% risk reduction of developing a skeletal event with zoledronic acid compared to placebo. This was the first trial to demonstrate long-term safety and efficacy of bisphosphonate therapy in patients with bone metastasis from lung cancer. In 2003, Yano et al. (156) reported beneficial effects of combination therapy with bisphophonate and chemotherapy for SCLC patients with multiple organ metastasis including bone metastasis.

Radiotherapy and bisphosphonates can provide pain relief, however, neither has been shown to prolong survival *(155)*. New treatments are needed for known bone metastasis and for patients who are at high risk for developing such metastasis. Enzyme pro-drug gene therapy treatment strategies currently are being investigated for their potential benefit in designing novel therapies for bone cancer.

REFERENCES

1. Jemal A, Murray T, Ward E, et al. Cancer Statistics, 2005. CA Cancer J Clin 2005; 55:10–30.
2. Travis WD, Lubin J, Ries L, Devesa S. United States lung cancer incidence trends. Cancer 1996; 77:2464–2470.
3. Parkin DM, Pisani P, Perlay J. Estimates of the worldwide incidence of eighteen major cancers in 1985. Int J Cancer 1993; 54:594–606.
4. Parkin DM, Pisani P, Perlay J. Estimates of the worldwide mortality from eighteen major cancers in 1985: implications for prevention and projections of future burden. Int J Cancer 1993;55:891–903.
5. Cersosimo RJ. Lung cancer: a review. Am J Health Syst Pharm 2002; 59:611–642.
6. Jemal A, Thomas A, Murray T, Thun M. Cancer Statistics, 2002. CA Cancer J Clin 2002; 52:23–47.
7. Schottenfeld D. Etiology and epidemiology of lung cancer. In: Pass HI, Mitchell JB, Johnson DH, et al,. eds. Lung Cancer: Principles and Practice. 2nd ed. Philadelphia, PA: Lippincott Williams and Wilkins 2000:367–388.
8. Glisson BS, McKenna RJ, Movsas B. Small-cell lung cancer. In: Pazdur R, Coia LR, Hoskins WJ, et al. eds. Cancer Management: A Multidisciplinary Approach, 7th ed. New York, NY: The Oncology Group; 2003;107.
9. Cole P, Rodu B. Declining cancer mortality in the United States. Cancer 1996; 78:2045–2048.
10. Vaporciyan AA, Kies MS, Stevens CW, et al. Cancer of the lung. In: Kufe DW, Pollock RE, Weichselbaum RR, et al., eds. Cancer Medicine, 6th ed. Spain, BC Decker Inc 2003; 1385.
11. Stellman SD, Garfinkel L. Smoking habits and tar levels in a new American Cancer Society prospective study of 1.2 million men and women. J Natl Cancer Inst 1986; 76:1057–1063.
12. Lubin JH, Blot WJ, Berrino F, et al. Patterns of lung cancer risk according to type of cigarette smoked. Int J Cancer 1984; 33:569–576.
13. Wilcox H, Schoenberg J, Mason T, Bill JS, Stemhagen A. Smoking and lung cancer: risk as a function of cigarette tar content. Prev Med 1988; 17:263–272.
14. US Environmental Protection Agency. Respiratory health effects of passive smoking: Lung Cancer and other disorders. 1992.
15. Coultas DB, Samet JM. Occupational lung cancer. Clin Chest Med 1992; 13:341–354.
16. Omenn GS, Merchant J, Boatmann E, et al. Contribution of environmental fibers to respiratory cancer. Environ Health Prespect 1986; 70:51–56.
17. Doll R. Mortality from lung cancer in asbestos workers. Bri J Intern Med 1955;12:81–86.
18. Kjuus H, Skjaerven R, Langard S. A case-referent study of lung cancer, occupational exposure, and smoking II: role of asbestos exposure. Scand J Work Environ Health 1986; 12:203–209.
19. Saccomanno G, Archer VE, Saunders RP, Auerbach O, Klein MG. Early indices of cancer risk among uranium miners with reference to modifying factors. Ann NY Acad Sci 1976; 271:377–383.
20. Gilliland FD, Hunt WC, Pardilla M, Key CR. Uranium mining and lung cancer among Navajo men in New Mexico and Arizona: 1969-1993. J Occup Environ Med 2000; 42:278–283.
21. Lubin JH, Boice JD, Edling C, et al. Lung cancer in radon-exposed miners and estimation of risk from indoor exposure. J Natl Cancer Inst 1995; 87:817–827.
22. Schottenfeld D. Epidemiology of lung cancer. In: Pass HI, Mitchell HB, Johnson DH, et al., eds. Lung Cancer: Principles and Practice, Philadelphia, PA: Lippincott-Raven; 1996:305–321.
23. Goodman GE. Prevention of lung cancer. Crit Rev Oncol Hematol 2000; 33:187–197.
24. Yang P, Wentzlaff KA, Katzmann JA, et al. Alpha₁ antitrypsin deficiency allele carriers among lung cancer patients. Cancer Epidemiol Biomarkers Prev 1998; 8:461–465.
25. Bishop JM. Molecular themes in oncogenesis. Cell 1991; 64:235–248.
26. Weinberg RA. Tumor suppressor genes. Science 1991; 254: 1138–1146.
27. Little CD, Nau MM, Carney DN, Gazdar AF, Minna JD.. Amplification and expression of the c-myc oncogene in human lung cancer cell lines. Nature 1983; 306:194–196.
28. Hecht SS. Tobacco smoke carcinogens and lung cancer. J Natl Cancer Inst 1999; 91:1194–1210.
29. Schneider PM, Hung MC, Chiocca SM, et al. Differential expression of the c-erbB-2 gene in human small cell and non-small-cell lung cancer. Cancer Res 1989 ;49:4968–4971.
30. Weiner DB, Nordberg J, Robinson R, et al. Expression of the neu gene-encoded protein (P185neu) in human non-small-cell carcinomas of the lung. Cancer Res 1990; 50:421–425.
31. Suzuki H, Takahashi T, Kuroishi T, et al. p53 mutations of non-small-cell lung cancer in Japan : association between mutations and smoking. Cancer Res 1992; 52:734–736.
32. Vahakangas KH, Samet JM, Metcalf RA, et al. Mutations of p53 and ras genes in radon-associated lung cancer from uranium miners. Lancet 1992; 339:576–580.
33. The World Health Organization histological typing of lung tumors. Second edition. Am J Clin Pathol 1982; 77:123–136.
34. Travis WD. Pathology of lung cancer. Clin Chest Med 2002; 23: 65–81.
35. Geddes DM. The natural history of lung cancer: a review based on rates of tumor growth. Br J Dis Chest 1979; 73:1–17.
36. Hammar SP, Bolan JW, Bockus D, Remington F, Friedman S. Ultrastructural and immunohistochemical features of common lung tumors: an overview. Ultrastruct Pathol 1985; 9:283–318.
37. Travis WD, Travis LB, Devesa SS. Lung cancer. [Published erratum appears in Cancer 1995; 75:2979]. Cancer 1995; 75:191–202.
38. Ginsberg RJ, Vokes EE, Rosenzweig K. Non-small cell lung cancer. In DeVita VT, Hellman S, Rosenberg SA, eds. Cancer: Principles and Practice of Oncology, 6th ed. Philadelphia, PA: Lippincott Williams and Williams; 2001:925–983.
39. Noguchi M, Morikawa A, Kawasaki M, et al. Small adenocarcinoma of the lung: histologic characteristics and prognosis. Cancer 1995; 75:2844–2852.
40. Hasleton PS, Gomm S, Blair V, Thatcher N. Pulmonary carcinoid tumours: a clinicopathological study of 35 cases. Br J Cancer 1986;54: 963–967.
41. Jensen RT, Norton JA. Carcinoid tumours and the carcinoid syndrome. In: De Vita VT Jr, Hellman S, Rosenberg SA, eds. Cancer: Principles and Practice of Oncology, 5th ed. Philadelphia, PA: Lippincott-Raven; 1997:1704–1723.
42. Greenberg RS, Baumgarten DA, Clark WS, Isacson P, McKeen K. Prognostic factors for gastrointestinal and bronchopulmonary carcinoid tumors. Cancer 1987; 60:2476–2483.
43. Soga J, Yakuwa Y, Osaka M. Carcinoid syndrome: a statistical evaluation of 748 reported cases. J Exp Clin Cancer Res 1999; 18:133–141.
44. Ricci C, Patrassi N, Massa R, Mineo C, Benedetti-Valentini FJ. Carcinoid syndrome in bronchial adenoma. Am J Surg 1973; 126:671–677.
45. Feldman JM. Carcinoid tumors and the carcinoid syndrome. Curr Probl Surg 1989; 26:835–885.
46. Grahame-Smith DG. The carcinoid syndrome. Am J Cardiol 1968; 21:376–387.
47. Johnson BE. Management of small cell lung cancer. Clin Chest Med 2002; 23:225–239.
48. Greenlee RT, Hill-Harmon MB, Murray T, et al. Cancer statistics: 2001. CA Cancer J Clin 2001; 51:15–36.
49. Guinee DG Jr, Fishback NF, Koss MN, Abbondanzo SL, Travis WD. The spectrum of immunohistochemical staining of small-cell lung carcinoma in specimens from transbronchial and open-lung biopsies. Am J Clin Pathol 1994; 102:406–.414
50. Murren J, Glatstein E, Pass HI. Small cell lung cancer. In: De Vita VT Jr, Hellman S, Rosenberg SA, eds. Cancer: Principles and Prac-

tice of Oncology, 6th ed. Philadelphia, PA: Lippincott Williams and Wilkins; 2001:983–1018.

51. Kraut M, Wozniak A. Clinical presentation. In: Pass HI, Mitchell JB, Johnson DH, et al. eds. Lung Cancer: Principles and Practice, 2nd ed. Philadelphia, PA: Lippincott Williams and Wilkins; 2000:521–534.

52. Pancoast HK. Importance of careful roentgen-ray investigations of apical chest tumors. JAMA 1924; 83:1407–1411.

53. Pancoast HK. Superior sulcus pulmonary tumor: Tumor characterized by pain, Honrner's syndrome, destruction of bone, and atrophy of hand muscles. JAMA 1932; 99:1391–1396.

54. Arcasoy SM, Jett RJ. Superior pulmonary sulcus tumors and Pancoast's syndrome. N Engl J Med 1997; 337:1370–1376.

55. Komaki R. Preoperative radiation therapy for superior sulcus lesions. Chest Surg Clin North Am 1991; 1:13–35.

56. MacDonald RA, Robbins SL. The significance of nonbacterial thrombotic endocarditis: an autopsy and clinical study of 78 cases. Ann Intern Med 1957; 46:255–273.

57. Anderson HA, Prakash UBS. Diagnosis of symptomatic lung cancer. Semin Respir Med 1982; 3:165–169.

58. Graus F, Elkon KB, Cordon-Cardo C, et al. Sensory neuropathy and small cell lung cancer. Am J Med 1986; 80:45–52.

59. Brennan LV, Craddock PR. Limbic encephalopathy as a nonmetastatic complication of oat cell lung cancer: its reversal after treatment of the primary lung lesion. Am J Med 1983; 75:518–520.

60. Ojeda VJ. Necrotizing myelopathy associated with malignancy: a clinicopathologic study of two cases and literature review. Cancer 1984; 53:1115–1123.

61. Schuffler MD, Baird HW, Fleming CR, et al. Intestinal pseudo-obstruction as the presenting manifestation of small-cell carcinoma of the lung: a Paraneoplastic neuropathy of the gastrointestinal tract. Ann Intern Med 1983; 98:129–134.

62. Kimmel DW, O'Neil BP, Lennon VA. Subacute sensory neuropathy associated with small cell lung carcinoma: diagnosis aided by authimmune serology. Mayo Clin Proc 1988; 63:29–.

63. Sodhi N, Camilleri M, Camoriano JK, Low PA, Fealey RD, Perry MC. Autonomic function and motility in intestinal pseudo obstruction caused by paraneoplastic syndrome. Dig Dis Sci 1989; 34:1937–1942.

64. Mountain CF. Revisions in the international system for staging lung cancer. Chest 1997; 111:1710–1717.

65. American Joint Committee on Cancer (AJCC): Lung. In: Fleming ID, Cooper JS, Hensen DE, et al. eds. Cancer Staging Manual. 5th ed. Philadelphia, PA: Lippincott-Raven; 1997:127.

66. International Union Against Cancer (UICC): Lung and Pleural Tumors. In: Hermanek P, Hutter RVP, Sobin L, eds. TNM Atlas. 4th ed. New York, NY: Wiley-Liss; 1997.

67. Mountain CF. Staging classification of lung cancer: a critical evaluation. Clin Chest Med 2002; 23:103–121.

68. Fischer BMB, Mortensen J, Hojgaard L. Positron emission tomography in the diagnosis and staging of lung cancer: a systematic, quantitative review. Lancet Oncol 2001; 2:659–666.

69. Reed CE, Harpole DH, Posther KE, et al. Results of the American College of Surgeons Oncology Group Z0050 trial: the utility of positron emission tomography in staging potentially operable non-small cell lung cancer. J Thorac Cardiovasc Surg 2003; 126:1943–1951.

70. Wingo PA, Tong T, Bolden S. Cancer statistics. Cancer J Clin 1995; 45:8–30.

71. Mantyh PW, Clohisy DR, Koltzenburg M, Hunt SP. Molecular mechanisms of cancer pain. Nat Rev Cancer 2000; 2:201–209.

72. Honore P, Luger NM, Sabino MA, et al. Osteoprotegerin blocks bone cancer-induced skeletal destruction, skeletal pain, and pain-related neurochemical reorganization of the spinal cord. Nat Med 2000; 6:521–528.

73. Mundy GR. Metastasis to bone: causes, consequences, and theraputic opportunities. Nat Rev Cancer 2002; 2:584–593.

74. Boyde A, Maconnachie E, Reid SA, Delling G, Mundy GR. Scanning electron microscopy in bone pathology: review of methods, potential and applications. Scan Electron Microsc 1986; 4:1537–1554.

75. Powell GJ, Southby J, Danks JA, et al. Localization of parathyroid homrone related protein in breast cancer metastases: increased incidence in bone compared with other sites. Cancer Res 1991; 51:3059–3061.

76. Bryden AA, Hoyland JA, Freemont AJ, et al. Parathyroid hormone related peptide and receptor expression in paired primary prostate cancer and bone metastases. Br J Cancer 2002; 86:322–403.

77. Miki T, Yano S, Hanibuchi M, Sone S. Bone metastasis model with multiorgan dissemination of human small-cell lung cancer (SBC-5) cells in natural killer cell-depleted SCID mice. Oncol Res 2001; 12:209–217.

78. Henderson M, Danks J, Moseley J, et al. Parathyroid hormone-related protein production by breast cancers, improved survival, and reduced bone metastases. J Natl Cancer Inst 2001; 93:234–237.

79. Guise TA, Yin JJ, Taylor SD, et al. Evidence for a causal role of parathyroid hormone-related protein in the pathogenesis of human breast-cancer-mediated osteolysis. J Clin Invest 1996; 98:1544–1549.

80. Moseley JM, Kubota M, Diefenbach-Jagger H, et al. Parathyroid hormone-related protein purified from a human lung cancer cell line. Proc Natl Acad Sci USA 1987; 84:5048–5052.

81. Yates AJ, Gutierrez GE, Smolens P, et al. Effects of a synthetic peptide of a parathyroid hormone-related protein on calcium homeostasis, renal tubular calcium reabsorption and bone metabolism. J Clin Invest 1988; 81:932–938.

82. Nelson JB, Hedican SP, George DJ, et al. Identification of endothelin-1 in the pathophysiology of metastatic adenocarcinoma of prostate. Nat Med 1995; 1:944–949.

83. Izbicka E, Dunstan C, Esparza J, Jacobs C, Sabatini M, Mundy GR. Human amniotic tumor which induces new bone formation in vivo produces a growth regulatory activity in vitro for osteoblasts identified as an extended from of basic fibroblast growth factor (bFGF). Cancer Res 1996; 56:633–636.

84. The Lung Cancer Study Group. Effects of postoperative mediastinal radiation on completely resected stage II and stage III epidermoid cancer of the lung. N Engl J Med 1986; 315:1377–1381.

85. Lafitte JJ, Ribet ME, Prevost BM, Gosselin BH, Copin MC, Brichet AH. Postresection irradiation for T2N0M0 non-small cell carcinoma: a prospective, randomized study. Ann Thorac Surg 1996; 62:830–834.

86. Stephens RJ, Girling DJ, Bleehen NM, Moghissi K, Yosef HM, Machin D. The role of post-operative radiotherapy in non-small-cell lung cancer: a multicenter randomized trial in patients with pathologically staged T1-2, N1-2, M0 disease. Br J Cancer 1996; 74:632–639.

87. PORT Meta-analysis Trialists Group. Postoperative radiotherapy in non-small-cell lung cancer: sytematic review and meta-analysis of individual patient data from nine randomized controlled trials. Lancet 1998; 352:257–263.

88. Keller SM, Adak S, Wagner H, et al. A randomized trial of postoperative adjuvant therapy in patients with completely resected stage II or IIIA non-small-cell lung cancer. N Engl J Med 2000; 343:1217–1222.

89. Ohta M, Tsuchiya R, Shimoyama M, et al. Adjuvant chemotherapy for completely resected stage III non-small-cell lung cancer: results of a randomized prospective study. J Thorac Cardiovasc Surg 1993; 106:703–708.

90. Dautzenberg B, Chastang C, Arriagada R, et al. Adjuvant radiotherapy versus combined sequential chemotherapy followed by radiotherapy in the treatment of resected nonsmall cell lung carcinoma: a randomized trial of 267 patients. Cancer 1995; 76:779–786.

91. The Study Group of Adjuvant Chemotherapy for Lung Cancer. A randomized trial of postoperative adjuvant chemotherapy in non-small cell lung cancer (the second cooperative study). Eur J Surg Oncol 1995; 21:69–77.

92. Holmes EC, Gail M. Surgical adjuvant therapy for stage II and stage III adenocarcinoma and large-cell undifferentiated carcinoma. J Clin Oncol 1986; 4:710–715.

93. Xu G, Rong T, Lin P. Adjuvant chemotherapy following radical surgery for non-small-cell lung cancer: a randomized study on 70 patients. Chin Med J (Eng) 2000; 113:617–620.

94. Non-small Cell Lung Cancer Collaborative Group. Chemotherapy in non-small cell lung cancer: a meta-analysis using updated data on individual patients from 52 randomized clinical trials. BMJ 1995; 311:899–909.

95. The International Adjuvant Lung Cancer Trial Collaborative Group. Cisplatin-based adjuvant chemotherapy in patients with completely resected non-small-cell lung cancer. N Engl J Med 2004; 350:351–360.

96. Perez CA, Pajak TF, Rubin P, et al. Long-term observations of the patterns of failure in patients with unresectable non-oat cell carcinoma of the lung treated with definitive radiotherapy: report by the Radiation Therapy Oncology Group. Cancer 1987; 59:1874–1881.

97. Dillman RO, Seagren SL, Propert KJ, et al. A randomized trial of induction chemotherapy plus high-dose radiation versus radiation alone in stage III non-small-cell lung cancer. N Engl J Med 1990; 323:940–945.

98. Dillman RO, Herndon J, Seagren SL, Eaton WL Jr, Green MR. Improved survival in stage III non-small-cell lung cancer: seven-year follow-up of Cancer and Leukemia Group B (CALGB) 8433 trial. J Natl Cancer Inst 1996; 88:1210–1215.

99. Pritchard RS, Anthony SP. Chemotherapy plus radiotherapy compared with radiotherapy alone in the treatment of locally advanced, unresectable, non-small-cell lung cancer: a meta-analysis. Ann Intern Med 1996; 125:723–729. (Erratum, Ann Intern Med 1997; 126:670.)–

100. Marino P, Preatoni A, Cantoni A. Randomized trials of radiotherapy alone versus combined chemotherapy and radiotherapy in stage IIIa and IIIb non small cell lung cancer: a meta-analysis. Cancer 1995; 76:593–601.

101. Furuse K, Fukuoka M, Kawahara M, et al. Phase III study of concurrent versus sequential thoracic radiotherapy in combination with mitomycin, vindesine, and cisplatin in unresectable stage III non-small-cell lung cancer. J Clin Oncol 1999; 17:2692–2699.

102. Curran WJ, Scott CB, Langer CJ, et al. Long-term benefit is observed in a phase III comparison of sequential vs. concurrent chemo-radiation for patients with unresected stage III NSCLC: RTOG 9410. Proc Am Soc Clin Oncol 2003; 22:621.

103. Attar S, Krasna MJ, Sonett JR, et al. Superior sulcus (Pancoast) tumor: experience with 105 patients. Ann Thorac Surg 1998; 66:193–198.

104. Rusch VW, Giroux DJ, Kraut MJ, et al. Induction chemoradiation and surgical resection for non-small cell lung carcinomas of the superior sulcus: initial results of Southwest Oncology Group Trial 9416 (Intergroup Trial 0160). J Thorac Cardiovasc Surg 2001; 121:472–483.

105. Barnes JB, Johnson SB, Dahiya RS, Temes RT, Herman TS, Thomas CR Jr. Concomitant weekly cisplatin and thoracic radiotherapy for Pancoast tumors of the lung: pilot experience of the San Antonio Cancer Institute. Am J Clin Oncol 2002; 25:90–92.

106. Gandhi S, Walsh GL, Komaki R, et al. A multidisciplinary surgical approach to superior sulcus tumors with vertebral invasion. Ann Thorac Surg 1999; 68:1778–1784.

107. Skarin A, Jochelson M, Sheldon T, et al. Neoadjuvant chemotherapy in marginally resectable stage III M0 non-small cell lung cancer: long-term follow-up in 41 patients. J Surg Oncol 1989; 40:266–274.

108. Roth JA, Fossella F, Komaki R, et al. A randomized trial comparing perioperative chemotherapy and surgery with surgery alone in resectable stage IIIA non-small-cell lung cancer. J Natl Cancer Inst 1994; 86:673–680.

109. Rosell R, Gomez-Codina J, Camps C, et al. A randomized trial comparing peroperative chemotherapy plus surgery with surgery alone in patients with non-small-cell lung cancer. N Engl J Med 1994; 330:153–158.

110. Roth JA, Atkinson EN, Fossella F, et al. Long-term follow-up of patients enrolled in a randomized trial comparing perioperative chemotherapy and surgery with surgery alone in resectable stage IIIA non-small-cell lung cancer. Lung Cancer 1998; 21:1–6.

111. Rosell R, Gomez-Codina J, Camps C, et al. Preresectional chemotherapy in stage IIIA non-small-cell lung cancer: a 7-year assessment of a randomized controlled trial. Lung Cancer 1999; 26:7–14.

112. Dipierre A, Milleron B, Moro-Sibilot d, et al. Preoperative chemotherapy followed by surgery compared with primary surgery in resectable stage I (except T1N0), II, and IIIa non-small-cell lung cancer. J Clin Oncol 2002; 20:247–253.

113. Albain KS, Scott CB, Rusch VR, et al. Phase III comparison of concurrent chemotherapy plus radiotherapy (CT/RT) and CT/RT followed by surgical resection for stage IIIA (pN2) non-small cell lung cancer (NSCLC): initial results from intergroup trial 0139 (RTOG 93-09). Proc Am Soc Clin Oncol 2003;22:621a.

114. Helsing M, Bergman B, Thaning L, Hero U. Quality of life and survival in patients with advanced non-small cell lung cancer receiving supportive care plus chemotherapy with carboplatin and etoposide or supportive care only: a multicenter randomized phase III trial. Eur J Cancer 1998; 34:1036–1044.

115. Ellis PA, Smith IE, Hardy JR, et al. Symptom relief with MVP (mitomycin C, vinblastine, and cisplatin) chemotherapy in advanced non-small-cell lung cancer. Br J Cancer 1995; 71:366–370.

116. Cullen MH, Billingham LJ, Woodroffe CM, et al. Mitomycin, ifosfamide, and cisplatin in unresectable non-small-cell lung cancer: effects on survival and quality of life. J Clin Oncol 1999; 17:3188–3194.

117. Sandler AB, Nemunaitis J, Denham C, et al. Phase III trial of gemcitabine plus cisplatin versus cisplatin alone in patients with locally advanced or metastatic non-small-cell lung cancer. J Clin Oncol 2000; 18:122–130.

118. Gatzemeier U, von Pawel J, Gottfried M, et al. Phase III comparative study of high dose cisplatin versus a combination of paclitaxel and cisplatin in patients with advanced non-small-cell lung cancer. J Clin Oncol 2000; 18:3390–3399.

119. Wozniak AJ, Crowley JJ, Balcerzak SP, et al. Randomized trial comparing cisplatin with cisplatin plus vinorelbine in the treatment of advanced non-small-cell lung cancer: a Southwest Oncology Group Study. J Clin Oncol 1998; 16:2459–2465.

120. Lilenbaum RC, Herndon J, List M, et al. Sing-agent (SA) versus combination chemotherapy (CC) in advanced non-small cell lung cancer (NSCLC): a CALGB randomized trial of efficacy, quality of life (QOL) and cost-effectiveness. Prog Proc Am Soc Clin Oncol 2002; 21:1a.

121. Georgoulias V, Ardavanis A, Agelidou M, et al. Preliminary analysis of a multicenter phase III trial comparing docetaxel (D) versus docetaxel/cisplatin (DC) in patients with inoperable advanced and metastatic non-small cell lung cancer (NSCLC). Prog Proc Am Soc Clin Oncol 2002; 21:291a.

122. Bonomi P, Kim K, Fairclough D, et al. Comparison of survival and quality of life in advanced non-small-cell lung cancer patients treated with two dose levels of paclitaxel combined with cisplatin versus etoposide with cisplatin: results of an Eastern Cooperative Oncology Group trial. J Clin Oncol 2000; 18:623–631.

123. Schiller JH, Harrington D, Belani CP, et al. Comparison of four chemotherapy regimens for advanced non-small-cell lung cancer. N Engl J Med 2002; 346:92–98.

124. Kelly K, Mikhaeel-Kamel N, Pan Z, Murphy J, Prindiville S, Bunn PA Jr. A phase I/II trial of paclitaxel, carboplatin, and gemcitabine in untreated patients with advanced non-small cell lung cancer. Clin Cancer Res 2000; 6:3474–3479.

125. Frasci G, Panza N, Comella P, et al. Cisplatin, gemcitabine, and paclitaxel in locally advanced or metastatic non-small-cell lung cancer: a phase I-II study. J Clin Oncol 1999; 17:2316–2325.

126. The Elderly Lung Cancer Vinorelbine Italian Study Group. Effects of vinorelbine on quality of life and survival of elderly patients with advanced non-small-cell lung cancer. J Natl Cancer Inst 1999; 91:66–72.

127. Gridelli C, Perrone F, Gallo C, et al. Chemotherapy for elderly patients with advanced non-small-cell lung cancer: the Multicenter Italian Lung Cancer in the Elderly Study (MILES) phase III randomized trial. J Natl Cancer Inst 2003; 95:362–372.

128. Ettinger DS. Is there a preferred combination chemotherapy regimen for metastatic non-small cell lung cancer? Oncologist 2002; 7:226–233.

129. Smith IE, O'Brien ME, Talbot DC, et al. Duration of chemotherapy in advanced non small-cell lung cancer: a randomized trial of three versus six courses of mitomycin, vinblastine, and cisplatin. J Clin Oncol 2001; 19:1336–.

130. Socinski MA, Schell MJ, Peterman A, et al. Phase III trial comparing a defined duration of therapy versus continuous therapy followed by second-line therapy in advanced-stage IIIB/IV non-small-cell lung cancer. J Clin Oncol 2002; 20:1335–1343.

131. Shepherd FA, Dancey J, Ramlau R, et al. Prospective randomized trial of docetaxel versus best supportive care in patients with non-small-cell lung cancer previously treated with platinum-based chemotherapy. J Clin Oncol 2000; 18:2095–2103.

132. Fossella FV, DeVore R, Kerr RN, et al. Randomized phase III trial of docetaxel versus vinorelbine or ifosfamide in patients with advanced non-small-cell lung cancer previously treated with platinum-containing chemotherapy regimens. J Clin Oncol 2000;18:2354–2362.

133. Magilligan DJ Jr, Duvernoy C, Malik G, Lewis JW Jr, Knighton R, Ausman JI. Surgical approach to lung cancer with solitary cerebral metastasis: twenty-five years' experience. Ann Thorac Surg 1986; 42:360–364.

134. Patchell RA, Tibbs PA, Walsh JW, et al. A randomized trial of surgery in the treatment of single metastases to the brain. N Engl J Med 1990; 322:494–500.

135. Raviv G, Klein E, Yellin A, Schneebaum S, Ben-Ari G Surgical treatment of solitary adrenal metastases from lung carcinoma. J Surg Oncol 1990; 43:123–124.

136. Reyes L, Parvez Z, Nemoto T, Regal AM, Takita H. Adrenalectomy for adrenal metastasis from lung carcinoma. J Surg Oncol 1990; 44:32–34.

137. Johnson DH. Gefitinib (Iressa) trials in non-small cell lung cancer. Lung Cancer 2003; 41:S23–S28.

138. Kukunoor R, Shah J, Mekhail T. Targeted therapy for lung cancer. Current Oncol Rep 2003; 5:326–333.

139. Aisner J, Alberto P, Bitran J, et al. Role of chemotherapy in small cell lung cancer: a consensus report of the International Association for the Study of Lung Cancer workshop. Cancer Treat Rep 1983; 67:37–43.

140. Seifter EJ, Ihde DC. Therapy of small cell lung cancer: a perspective on two decades of clinical research. Semin Oncol 1988; 15:278–299.

141. Fukuoka M, Furuse K, Saijo N, et al. Randomized trial of cyclophosphamide, doxorubicin, and vincristine versus cisplatin and etoposide versus alternation of these regimens in small-cell lung cancer. J Natl Cancer Inst 1991; 83:855–861.

142. Roth BJ, Johnson DH, Einhorn LH, et al. Randomized study of cyclophosphamide, doxorubicin, and vincristine versus etoposide and cisplatin versus alternation of these two regimens in extensive small-cell lung cancer: a phase III trial of the Southeastern Cancer Study Group. J Clin Oncol 1992; 10:282–291.

143. Pignon JP, Arriagada R, Ihde DC, et al. A meta-analysis of thoracic radiotherapy for small-cell lung cancer. N Engl J Med 1992; 327:1618–1624.

144. Arriagada R, Pignon JP, Ihde DC, et al. Effect of thoracic radiotherapy on mortality in limited small cell lung cancer: a meta-analysis of 13 randomized trials among 2,140 patients. Anticancer Res 1994; 14:333–335.

145. Takada M, Fukuoka M, Kawahara M, et al. Phase III study of concurrent versus sequential thoracic radiotherapy in combination with cisplatin and etoposide for limited-stage small-cell lung cancer: results of the Japan Clinical Oncology Group Study 9104. J Clin Oncol 2002; 20:3054–3060.

146. Turrisi AT 3rd, Kim K, Blum R, et al. Twice-daily compared with once-daily thoracic radiotherapy in limited small-cell lung cancer treated concurrently with cisplatin and etoposide. N Engl J Med 1999; 340:265–271.

147. Kosmidis PA, Samantas E, Fountzilas G, Pavlidis N, Apostolopoulou F, Skarlos D.. Cisplatin/etoposide versus carboplatin/etoposide chemotherapy and irradiation in small cell lung cancer: a randomized phase III study: Hellenic Cooperative Oncology Group for Lung Cancer Trials. Semin Oncol 1994; 21:23–30.

148. Noda K, Nishiwaki Y, Kawahara M, et al. Irinotecan plus cisplatin compared with etoposide plus cisplatin for extensive small-cell lung cancer. N Engl J Med 2002; 346:85–91.

149. Niell HB, Herndon JE, Miller AA, et al. Randomized Phase III intergroup trial (CALGB 9732) of etoposide (VP-16) and cisplatin (DDP) with or without paclitaxel (TAX) and G-CSF in patients with extensive stage small cell lung cancer (ED-SCLC). Prog Proc Am Soc Clin Oncol 2002; 21:293a.

150. Mavroudis D, Papadakis E, Veslemes M, et al. A multicenter randomized clinical trial comparing paclitaxel-cisplatin-etoposide versus cisplatin-etoposide as first-line treatmetnt in patients with small-cell lung cancer. Ann Oncol 2001; 12:463–470.

151. Ardizzoni A, Hansen H, Dombernowsky P, et al. Topotecan, a new active drug in the second-line treatment of small-cell lung cancer: a phase II study in patients with refractory and sensitive disease. J Clin Oncol 1997; 15:2090–2096.

152. Tchekmedyian S, Rosen LS, Gordon D, et al. Long-term efficacy and safety of zoledronic acid in reducing skeletal complications in patients with bone metastases from solid tumors. Proc Am Soc Clin Oncol 2003;22:630a.

153. Lipton A. Bone metastases in breast cancer. Curr Treat Options Oncol 2003; 4:151–158.

154. Eaton CL, Coleman RE. Pathophysiology of bone metastases from prostate cancer and the role of bisphosphonates in treatment. Cancer Treat Rev 2003; 29:189–198.

155. Hillner BE, Ingle JN, Berenson JR, et al. American Society of Clinical Oncology guideline on the role of bisphosphonates in breast cancer. J Clin Oncol 2000; 18:1378–1391.

156. Yano S, Zhang H, Hanibuchi M, et al. Combined therapy with a new bisphosphonate, minodronate (YM529), and chemotherapy for multiple organ metastases of small cell lung cancer cells in severe combined immunodeficient mice. Clinc Cancer Res 2003; 9:5380–5285.

157. Hortobagyi GN. Novel approaches to the management of bone metastases. Semin Oncol 2003; 30:161–166.

19 Medical Management of Thyroid Cancer

AJAY SOOD, MD AND S. SETHU REDDY, MD

CONTENTS

1. INTRODUCTION

Thyroid cancer, the most common endocrine malignancy, accounts for 1.1% of all the newly diagnosed malignancies in the United States (1). It occurs three times more commonly in women. Its annual incidence has increased over the last few decades, possibly in part owing to improved diagnosis and cancer registration (2). However, the mortality rates owing to thyroid cancer have decreased by 20% between the years 1973 and 1996, because of early diagnosis, and better surveillance and treatment.

The various types of thyroid cancers are listed in Table 1 (3). Differentiated thyroid cancers (DTCs), which include papillary and follicular thyroid cancers, comprise 90% of all thyroid cancers (4). They originate from the follicular cells of the thyroid. They are also responsible for 70% of the mortality owing to thyroid cancers. Because papillary and follicular thyroid cancers are the main types, and are treated in a similar fashion, most of the subsequent discussion will be centered on these, while highlighting the difference between the two.

1.1. METASTATIC BONE DISEASE

Thyroid cancer can spread to lymph nodes or metastasize to distant sites such as lungs, bones, liver, and brain. Only 1 to 3% of the patients have distant metastasis at the time of initial diagnosis (5). Seven to twenty-three percent of the patients develop distant metastasis during their lifetime. Bone metastasis occurs in 4 to 13% of the cases (5–7). Half of these patients have bone metastasis at the initial presentation. One-third to half of those with bone involvement have multiple bone metasta-

Table 1
Types of Thyroid Cancer[a]

Primary tumor
  Differentiated[b]
    Papillary
    Follicular
  Poorly differentiated (insular)
  Anaplastic
  Hurthle cell
  Medullary
  Miscellaneous epithelial tumor
    Squamous cell, adenosquamous, mucin producing, mucoepidermoid, hyalinizing trabecular, teratoma, clomunar cell
  Non-epithelial tumor
    Lymphoma
    Sarcoma
Secondary (metastatic) tumor
  Melanoma, renal cell carcinoma, breast cancer, lung cancer

[a]Adapted from ref. 3.
[b]There are different variants of papillary and follicular cancer.

sis, and one-third have other site involvement (5,7,8). Bone involvement can be a risk factor for occurrence of cerebral metastasis (9). Vertebrae are the most commonly affected site for bone metastasis, occurring in nearly 50% of the patients, followed by pelvis, ribs, femur, skull, humerus, clavicle, and scapula (5).

Two-thirds to three-fourths of all bone metastasis are symptomatic. Symptoms usually include pain and/or swelling, but may also include fractures (in 5% of the patients) and cord compression (3.5%). The "visible" bone metastasis are invari-

From: Current Clinical Oncology: Cancer in the Spine: Comprehensive Care.
Edited by: R. F. McLain, K-U. Lewandrowski, M. Markman, R. M. Bukowski,
R. Macklis, and E. C. Benzel © Humana Press, Inc., Totowa, NJ

ably osteolytic lesions *(7)*, although osteosclerotic lesions have also been reported *(10)*. Of patients with bone metastasis, 28–60% present with symptoms related to bone metastasis *(5,7,8)*.

All symptomatic lesions are visible on radiographic studies *(5,8)*. The remaining bone metastases may be picked up by other imaging techniques like radioactive ^{131}I whole body scan, ^{99}Tc bone scan and sestamibi scan. The majority of patients with bone metastasis (86–93%) have follicular thyroid cancer, with the rest being papillary thyroid cancer *(7,8)*. However, Tickoo et al. *(11)* reported that among patients of thyroid cancer with bone involvement seen at a tertiary referral center, 28% were papillary, 22% follicular, 20% insular, 13% anaplastic, 11% Hurthle cell, and 6% were medullary cancer. Two-thirds of these patients had similarly differentiated and one-third had better differentiated metastatic tumor as compared to the primary tumor. The patients with bone metastasis also tend to be older at the time of diagnosis, 87% being older than 45 yr of age *(5)*. Metastatic thyroid tumors may rarely synthesize thyroid hormone *(12)*.

1.2. SPINE

As previously mentioned, the spine is a frequent site of bone metastasis for thyroid cancer. About 12% of consecutive patients with spinal metastasis were reported to be from thyroid cancer *(13)*. However, in an autopsy review of 140 cases of vertebral metastasis reported in 1975, only 1 case of thyroid cancer was reported *(14)*. The spinal metastasis can be asymptomatic; or can cause spinal cord compression *(15,16)*, which can present as Brown-Sequard syndrome *(17)* or distal cord compression *(18)*. DTC can also metastasize to the epidural space without vertebral involvement *(19)*, or cause isolated enlargement of intervertebral foramen *(20)*, or present as intramedullary spinal cord metastasis *(21)*. Spinal metastasis can also present as paravertebral mass *(22)* or can extend extraspinally *(23)*.

2. CLINICAL EVALUATION

The diagnosis of thyroid cancer is usually confirmed by fine-needle aspiration of the thyroid *(24)*. Other evaluations include clinical assessment of the extent of lesion by palpation of the thyroid, carotids, sternocleidomastoids, and lymph nodes, and by ultrasound. Indirect laryngoscopy is performed to evaluate vocal cords and, thereby, recurrent laryngeal nerve involvement. If lymph nodes are present, needle aspiration of the lymph nodes may be carried out.

Staging of the thyroid cancer is important for risk-stratification and prognostication. Staging is based on the tumor-node-metastases (TNM) system (Table 2) *(25,26)*. Age is an important part of staging as it is a significant factor in the determination of prognosis, prognosis being better in patients younger than 45 yr of age.

3. PROGNOSTIC FEATURES

The outcome of thyroid cancers can be assessed in terms of long-term survival and recurrence rate of the cancer with treatment. Mortality is higher in patients who are over 40 yr of age at the time of diagnosis. Recurrence rates are high when age of diagnosis is less than 20 yr or more than 60 yr *(26,27)*. Although men develop thyroid cancer less frequently, they have twice the mortality as compared to women. In fact the decline in mortal-

Table 2
TNM Classification and Staging of Thyroid Cancer

Tumor[a]	Tx	Primary tumor cannot be assessed
	T0	No evidence of primary tumor
	T1	≤1 cm and limited to thyroid
	T2	>1 cm ≤4 cm and limited to thyroid
	T3	>4 cm and limited to thyroid
	T4	Any size extending beyond thyroid capsule
Nodes[b]	Nx	Regional nodes cannot be assessed
	N0	No metastasis to regional nodes
	N1	Metastasis to regional nodes present
Metastasis	Mx	Presence of metastasis cannot be assessed
	M0	No distant metastasis
	M1	Distant metastasis present
Staging		
	Stage I	<45 yr age, any T, any N, M0
		≥45 yr age, T1N0M0
	Stage II	>45 yrs age, any T, any N, M1
		≥45 yrs age, T2N0M0
	Stage III	≥45 yrs age, T3N0M0 or any T,N1M0
	Stage IV	≥45 yrs age, any T, any N, M1

[a]Tumor size is greatest diameter of single nodule or largest nodule.
[b]Regional lymph nodes are bilateral cervical and upper mediastinal nodes.

ity over the last couple of decades has been seen only in women *(2)*. Other poor prognostic factors include: a family history of thyroid cancer, tumors less than 4 cm in diameter, bilateral disease, extrathyroidal extension, vascular invasion, regional lymph node involvement, presence of nuclear atypia, tumor necrosis, and distal metastasis *(26)*. Tumors that do not or poorly concentrate radioiodine have poorer prognosis. Follicular thyroid cancers seem to have more distant metastasis as well as higher mortality as compared to papillary thyroid cancers *(28)*. Hurthle cell, tall cell, columnar cell, diffuse sclerosis, and insular variants do poorly, as opposed to encapsulated papillary, papillary microcarcinoma, and cystic papillary variants, which have moderate to low risk. Other types such as undifferentiated, anaplastic, and medullary carcinomas have worse outcomes.

3.1. PROGNOSTIC VARIABLES AMONG PATIENTS WITH METASTASIS

Among the patients of thyroid cancer with distant metastasis, patients with bone metastasis have worse prognosis *(29)*. Long-term, patients with lung metastasis do better than patients with bone involvement *(30)*. Patients who had metastatic tissue with radioactive iodine uptake had better survival as compared to those with metastatic tissue that did not take up iodine *(5,29)*. Among the subgroup of patients with metastatic disease, older patients and follicular tumors had poorer prognosis.

Among the patients with bone metastasis, detection of metastasis as a revealing symptom of thyroid carcinoma, absence of nonosseous metastases, radioiodine uptake, and Hurthle cell subtype seemed to be associated with improved prognosis *(5,6)*. There seems to be no difference in survival in patients with single bone lesion compared to those with multiple bone lesions *(5)*.

4. MODALITIES OF TREATMENT

Because thyroid cancer is an uncommon disorder and has a prolonged course, there are no prospective randomized controlled trials to evaluate various modalities of treatment. Most of the information and guidelines are based on retrospective analysis of survival and recurrence data.

Various strategies for treatment of thyroid cancer include: surgery, radioblation, external radiation, thyroxine suppression, and chemotherapy. Most of the time these modalities are used together in a patient. National Comprehensive Cancer Network guidelines on the treatment of thyroid cancer is the most recent consensus statement of the experts in the field *(31)*.

4.1. SURGERY

All patients of thyroid cancer should have thyroidectomy. If the diagnosis of thyroid cancer is known before surgery, total thyroidectomy or near-total thyroidectomy is the procedure of choice *(26,27)*. If the diagnosis of thyroid cancer was made post-lobectomy of thyroid for thyroid nodule, then completion total thyroidectomy is required for patients with likelihood of recurrence, including patients with tumor size greater than 4 cm, tumor with metastases, multifocal tumor, vascular invasion, recurrent cancer, and tumor with involvement of resected margins *(28,32)*. Lobectomy alone may be sufficient for tumor size less than 1 cm. Experts disagree regarding completion thyroidectomy for patients with tumor size between 1 and 4 cm, although this procedure offers long-term advantage in the management of the patient. Total thyroidectomy may decrease the recurrence of tumor and increase survival; would lead to easier radioablation of the remaining thyroid tissue and thus unmask any metastasis. Leaving less than 2 g of thyroid tissue during surgery makes postoperative radioablation of the thyroid easier *(33)*.

Patients with lymph node involvement should undergo bilateral central compartment dissection or lateral modified radical neck dissection in addition to total thyroidectomy *(26)*. Complications of permanent hypoparathyroidism and residual recurrent laryngeal nerve injury occur in 2.6 and 3% of patients undergoing total thyroidectomy *(34)*, but tend to be lower with experienced surgeons.

4.2. RADIOIODINE TREATMENT

Radioactive iodine (^{131}I) is used for ablation of normal residual thyroid tissue after surgery, and to localize and ablate cancer tissue.

4.2.1. Thyroid Remnant Ablation

Some normal thyroid tissue invariably remains after total thyroidectomy *(25)*. Radioiodine is used to ablate this tissue. This helps in enhancing uptake in metastatic thyroid tissue *(35)*, as thyroid cancer and metastatic tissue is about 10 times less avid in uptake of iodine as compared to normal thyroid tissue *(36)*. Destruction of the remaining thyroid tissue also allows the patient to be followed up by serial serum thyroglobulin measurements, because thyroid tissue (benign or malignant) is the only source of thyroglobulin. In addition, it also destroys the potential site of development of new tumor. Radioablation of thyroid remnant is shown to improve survival *(37)*. Many clinicians use 30 mCi of ^{131}I for ablation, a dose that was convenient to use in the pre-1997 era, when use of larger ^{131}I doses

in ambulatory patients was not allowed. Some centers prefer to use larger doses, usually 50 to 150 mCi, as the use of 30 mCi may fail to ablate all of the residual thyroid tissue in nearly half the patients, as compared to failure in one-fourth of the patients with larger doses *(38)*. The thyroid remnant ablation is usually carried out 4 to 8 wk after surgery. The patient may require a second ablation, if more than 0.5% uptake at 48 h is seen on a diagnostic whole body scan done 6 to 12 mo later *(26)*. While using bigger doses of ^{131}I, one has to be careful about occurrence of radiation thyroiditis, especially in patients with larger thyroid remnant tissue.

4.2.2. Whole Body Scan

Whole body scans using ^{131}I are performed to look for thyroid cancer metastasis. The rationale for this is that once competing normal thyroid tissue is removed by surgery and ablation, uptake in cancer tissue would be visualized. The whole body scan can be performed in two ways: *diagnostic scan* and *post-therapy scan*.

4.2.2.1. Diagnostic Scan

The *diagnostic scan* is performed at the time when the patient is hypothyroid after stopping thyroxine, which is usually being taken to suppress tumor growth *(26)*. Usually 2mCi of ^{131}I, is administered. Larger doses may be more sensitive in picking up metastatic tissue, especially pulmonary metastases, but they may cause "thyroid stunning" effect and may decrease the effectiveness of subsequent radioiodine for ablation of metastatic cancer tissue *(39)*. Using ^{123}I may improve the image, but is expensive.

The uptake of ^{131}I by cancer tissue is thyroid-stimulating hormone (TSH)-driven, and the results are not good if the serum TSH is less than 30 mU/mL. Therefore oral thyroxine is discontinued for 4 to 6 wk before scan, to let endogenous serum TSH rise. However, by the time serum TSH is sufficiently elevated, the patient is hypothyroid and usually uncomfortable. The duration of hypothyroidism in patients who have to undergo total body scan can be reduced by switching the patient from thyroxine to oral triiodothyronine (T3), which then needs to be stopped for only 3 wk, because of its shorter half life. Theoretically, prolonged elevation of TSH can also stimulate tumor growth. To obviate these problems of the traditional protocol related to symptomatic hypothyroidism and prolonged duration of elevated TSH, commercially available recombinant human TSH (rTSH) injections can be used for diagnostic scanning *(40)*. Recombinant TSH is administered as a 0.9-mg intramuscular injection on two consecutive days, without discontinuing thyroxine. This is followed by the administration of 4 mCi of ^{131}I on the third day, and whole body scan and serum thyroglobulin measurement on the fifth day. Higher doses of ^{131}I is required for diagnostic scan in patients in whom rTSH is used as they have a higher renal clearance of iodine as compared to hypothyroid patients after thyroxine withdrawal. To be reliable, the scanning has to be long enough to collect sufficient counts. Using this protocol, the sensitivity of whole body scan was not found to be very different from the traditional way of performing a whole body scan *(41)*. rTSH can also be useful in patients with thyroid cancer who have insufficient endogenous TSH production because of secondary hypothyroidism caused by pituitary or hypothalamic disease *(42)*. rTSH injections are well tolerated, with one-tenth of the patients complaining of transient headache and nausea.

[131]I whole body scans can sometimes be falsely positive (43). Iodine can be secreted into many body secretions such as the nasopharynx, sweat, saliva, urine, and tears, which can contaminate skin, hair, and clothes, especially saliva drooled over chest, sweat into braided hair and urine on skin. Iodine can also be concentrated in areas of inflammation and by certain other malignancies. Vertebral hemangiomas may concentrate ^{131}I and mimic metastasis to the spine (44). Eosophageal retention of swallowed ^{131}I can give an artificial picture of uptake of ^{131}I in the vertebral column (45). However, this can be eliminated with repeat imaging after ingestion of food and water.

4.2.2.2. Post-Therapy Scan

The *post-therapy scan* is carried out 7 to 10 d after the ^{131}I radioablation for thyroid metastatic disease. Because larger doses of ^{131}I are administered during radioablation, this scan is more likely to pick up metastatic foci not shown by other studies such as diagnostic whole body scan, ultrasound, computed tomography (CT), magnetic resonance imaging (MRI), or other scans such as whole body ^{99}Tc scan or positron emission tomography (PET) scan (46,47). Post-therapy scan, by showing the presence or absence of metastasis, may change the risk classification of the patient. However, it is not clear if this changes the subsequent treatment, as these patients are already known to have metastasis, are being treated with ^{131}I, and are likely to be followed up by diagnostic whole body scan. This is one of the few situations in medicine that the treatment may occasionally precede the diagnosis.

4.2.2.3. Other Scans

Other scans such as [201]thallium, ^{18}F-FDG PET, [99]Tcm-tetrofosmin, and [99]Tcm-sestamibi whole body scans have been investigated for their role in the management of thyroid cancer patients (48–51). Thallium, PET, and tetrofosmin scans seem to be equally sensitive in detecting metastatic disease (48,49), although they may be more effective than ^{131}I scan in picking up lymph node spread (49). Setamibi scan may be less effective in delineating thyroid remnant or lung metastasis and may also be more sensitive for lymph node metastasis (51). Combining these scans with ^{131}I whole body scan may increase the sensitivity (48,49). These scans may be useful in patients who have had partial thyroidectomy and have residual thyroid tissue which may decrease the sensitivity of the ^{131}I whole body scan, and also in patients who have elevated serum thyroglobulin but negative ^{131}I scan (49). The use of these scans has yet to be validated in larger studies.

4.2.3. Radioiodine Treatment for Residual Disease

The unique ability of thyroid cancer tissue to concentrate iodine allows high levels of radioactivity to be delivered specifically to malignant tissue, which results in its destruction. However, only half to two-thirds of metastases concentrate iodine. The inability to concentrate iodine is seen more in elderly patients and in Hurthle cell tumors (26). Pulmonary metastases with negative diagnostic ^{131}I scan but elevated thyroglobulin can also be treated effectively (46). The use of radioiodine therapy improves survival and decreases recurrences (27).

Radioiodine is administered after thyroxine is withdrawn and the patient is hypothyroid. The method of calculating the dose of ^{131}I varies in different centers. The most common method is to administer fixed doses depending on the type of metastasis: lymph node (100–175 mCi), cancer growing through the capsule (150–200 mCi), and distant metastases including pulmonary metastases (200 mCi) (26). Alternatively and more elegantly, the dose can be calculated depending on the radiation that needs to be delivered to the malignant tissue while keeping in mind the safe limits for the blood and the whole body (52). Starting a low iodine diet of 50 µg/d 2 wk before therapy can increase the intake of radioiodine and therefore its therapeutic effect (53). The simultaneous administration of lithium retains iodine in the malignant tissue longer and prolongs the effect of radioiodine (54).

The acute complications of radioiodine therapy include mild radiation sickness causing headache, nausea, vomiting; radiation induced soft tissue reactions such as edema, hemorrhage and pain; radiation thyroiditis causing neck pain and thyrotoxicosis; radiation sialadenitis, glossodynia, dysguesia; and mild bone marrow suppression (26). Late complications include mild impairment of ovarian function (but no loss of fertility), decreased spermatogenesis, a slight increase in the risk for bladder cancer, colorectal cancer, and leukemia; and pulmonary fibrosis in patients with diffuse lung metastases.

4.3. EXTERNAL RADIATION

External radiotherapy has a limited role in the management of differentiated thyroid cancer (55). It may be beneficial in patients who have postsurgically developed macroscopic residual disease and in a subgroup of patients who have papillary tumor with microscopic residual disease after surgery, where it may be used with or without radioiodine ablation (56). It may also be used for palliation if thyroidectomy is not possible for some reason as well as for the treatment of skeletal, brain, hepatic, pulmonary, or subcutaneous metastases, especially if they do not concentrate radioiodine. External radiation may help in the local control of disease. Follicular tumors are less radio-sensitive than papillary cancer. It is also used in patients with anaplastic thyroid cancer, medullary carcinoma, and lymphoma of the thyroid.

4.4. CHEMOTHERAPY

This has a limited role and is used in the treatment of differentiated thyroid cancers that are recurrent, inoperable, metastatic, and do not concentrate [131]I (57). Chemotherapy is mainly palliative and there is no change in survival with its use. Doxorubicin, bleomycin, and cisplatin are the main chemotherapeutic agents used. Patients who respond to one agent are more likely to respond to another agent in case of relapse. Combined use of chemotherapy and external radiation may be helpful for palliation in locally advanced cancer. It may have some beneficial effect in patients with anaplastic carcinoma, medullary carcinoma, and lymphoma of thyroid.

4.5. THYROXINE SUPPRESSIVE THERAPY

Because thyroid cancer seems to be dependent on TSH for growth, all patients of thyroid cancer receive doses of thyroxine to suppress TSH below normal level (58). The extent to which serum TSH should be suppressed is controversial, most centers prefer to lower serum TSH to just below the normal range. There is an apprehension that the suppression of serum TSH to below normal levels for many years may cause osteoporosis (59), although not all studies have supported this contention (60,61). Nevertheless it is prudent to ensure adequate calcium and vitamin D intake. Similarly low serum TSH is associated with higher cardiovascular mortality (62). However, this has not yet been documented in the patients on thyroxine suppressive therapy. Recent studies by Cooper et al. (63) suggest that high-risk patients, such as those with bone metastasis have the most to gain from aggressive thyroid hormone suppressive therapy.

5. FOLLOW-UP OF THE PATIENTS

Usually the patient with thyroid cancer would undergo a total thyroidectomy, followed by ablation of the remnant thyroid tissue. Post-therapy whole body scan after radioiodine given for thyroid remnant ablation and measurement of serum thyroglobulin level is carried out. Then the patient is started on suppressive doses of thyroxine. Six to 18 mo later, a diagnostic whole body scan and serum thyroglobulin levels are repeated after withdrawing thyroxine or post rTSH administration. If there is any evidence of residual or metastatic disease then this may require treatment with radioiodine ablation or surgery. This process of screening for disease is repeated yearly, until two consecutive scans are negative and serum thyroglobulin level is suppressed. Subsequently, the patient is followed by yearly clinical examination and serum thyroglobulin. Some centers would repeat whole body diagnostic scan after 3 to 5 yr. During the clinical examination, special emphasis is placed on neck, lymph node, and chest examination. Some clinicians prefer a yearly chest X-ray. If any metastasis is suspected appropriate imaging such as radiograph, CT, or MRI may be carried out. The protocol for follow up may vary among the centers.

Serum thyroglobulin after thyroxine withdrawal or rTSH stimulation is a good indicator of residual disease. It is used in conjunction with results of whole body scan (64,65), although recent publications suggest that basal and rTSH stimulated thyroglobulin may be used alone without whole body scan to follow up selected patients with low risk thyroid cancer (66,67). Serum anti-thyroglobulin antibodies can interfere with serum thyroglobulin assay and are therefore always estimated simultaneously (65). Most patients who are disease free would have undetectable serum thyroglobulin. The levels of acceptable thyroglobulin levels during suppressive therapy have changed over the last decade. Most would now target the thyroglobulin to be less than 2 ng/mL while on suppressive therapy. A 72-hr post-rTSH thyroglobulin greater than 5 ng/mL would be a consideration for a withdrawal scan and ^{131}I therapy.

6. MANAGEMENT OF BONE METASTASES

The presence of bone metastases is a poor prognostic factor, and these are difficult to treat (8). Only 55% of whole body scan positive X-ray-negative bone metastses and none of the X-ray-positive metastases show complete response to ^{131}I therapy (7). Only 17% of bone metastases that take up iodine and 7% of all bone metastases can be cured by radioactive iodine. Complete surgical removal of bone metastses provide the best chance of cure and improved survival (6,7). If the metastases does not take up radioiodine and is not completely resectable, external radiation therapy can be used for palliative purpose (55). In such a situation, it has been suggested that the radiation dose already received by the spine from previously administered radioactive iodine may have to be taken into account (69). Embolization of bone metastases (70) and vertebral metastases (71) have been successfully carried out leading to relief of neurological symptoms in the latter patients. Patients with spinal metastases and neurological symptoms can also benefit from reconstructive and stablization surgery (14,72).

7. LONG-TERM OUTCOME

In general patients treated for thyroid cancer have good long-term survival. Ten-year survival for papillary and follicular cancer is 93 and 85%, respectively (4). For patients having bone metastases with differentiated carcinoma the survival from the time of diagnosis of thyroid cancer is poorer with 5- and 10-yr survival rates being 41 and 15% in one study (6) and 53 and 35% in another (5). If survival is measured from the time of the diagnosis of bone metastases then the 5- and 10-yr figures are 25 and 13% (Fig. 1) (5).

8. OTHER TYPES OF THYROID CANCERS

Thyroid cancers other than differentiated thyroid cancer occur only in 10% of the patients. Medullary carcinoma of thyroid, the malignancy of C-cell of the thyroid is treated with total thyroidectomy, external radiation, and chemotherapy (73). It usually does not take up radioiodine, however, radioiodine ablation has been successfully used in some patients as adjacent follicular cells trap iodine.

The most important aspect of medullary thyroid carcinoma is to carry out genetic analysis for *ret* protooncogene mutation, and if positive to screen the family members for the presence of the mutation and medullary carcinoma and plan for prophylactic thyroidectomy (74). Patients can be followed up by the measurement of plasma calcitonin, which is secreted by medullary carcinoma. The patients should also be screened for hyperparathyroidism and pheochromocytoma, which can occur as a part of multiple endocrine neoplasia. The overall 10-yr survival for medullary carcinoma is about 63%.

Anaplastic carcinoma has usually spread beyond the thyroid when diagnosed and the median survival is 6 mo. Surgery is carried out if possible, and both external radiation and chemotherapy give limited palliative benefit (75).

9. FUTURE TREATMENT STRATEGIES

Immunotherapy using radioisotopes coupled to monoclonal antibodies against medullary carcinoma cells (76), gene therapy to induce interleukin secretion in tumor cells or express enzyme to make tumor cell sensitive to antiviral therapy gangciclovir (77), and modulating or inducing the expression of sodium iodide symporter gene (78) to increase radioiodine uptake are some of the areas being investigated to further improve the outcome, especially in thyroid cancer other than the differentiated thyroid cancer.

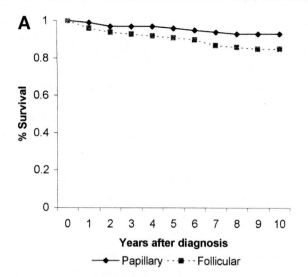

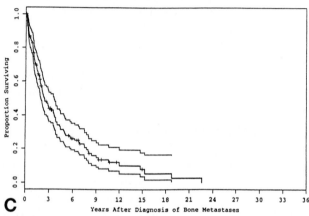

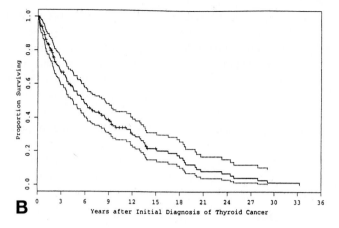

Fig. 1. Survival in **(A)** all patients of differentiated papillary and follicular thyroid cancer (adapted from ref. *4*). **(B)** Patients of thyroid cancer with bone metastasis (i) survival from the time of initial diagnosis of thyroid cancer (ii) survival from the time of diagnosis of bone metastasis. (Reproduced with permission from ref. *5*.)

REFERENCES

1. Parker SL, Tong T, Bolden S, Wingo PA. Cancer statistics, 1996, CA 1996; 46:5–27.
2. Ries LAG, Eisner MP, Kosary CL, et al. SEER cancer statistics review, 1973-1997. Bethesda, MD: National Cancer Institute; 2000.
3. Oertel J, Oertel Y. Classification of thyroid malignancies. In: Wartofsky, L, ed. Thyroid Cancer: A Comprehensive Guide to Clinical Management. Totowa, NJ: Humana Press; 2000:117–119.
4. Hundahl SA, Fleming ID, Freanger A, Merck HR. A national cancer data base report on 53,856 cases of thyroid carcinoma treated in the U.S., 1985-1995. Cancer 1998; 83:2638–2648.
5. Pittas AG, Adler M, Fazzari M, et al. Bone metastases from thyroid carcinoma: clinical characteristics and prognostic variables in one hundred forty-six patients. Thyroid 2000; 10:261–268.
6. Bernier MO, Leenhardt L, Hoang C., et al. Survival and therapeutic modalities in patients with bone metastases of differentiated thyroid carcinomas. J Clin Endocrinol Metab 2001; 86:1568–1573.
7. Marcocci D, Pacini F, Elisei R, et al. Clinical and biologic behavior of bone metastases from differentiated thyroid carcinoma. Surgery 1989; 106:960–966.
8. Proye CAG, Dromen DHR, Carnaille BM, et al. Is it still worthwhile to treat bone metastases from differentiated thyroid carcinoma with radioactive iodine? World J Surg 1922; 16:640–646.
9. Salvarti M, Frati A, Rocchi G, et al. Single brain metastasis from thyroid cancer: report of twelve cases and review of literature. J Neurooncol 2001; 51:33–40.
10. Mohan V, Bhushan B, Sahai SB, Arora MM. Osteosclerotric metastasis from thyroid carcinoma. Australs Radiol 1987; 31:204–207.
11. Tickoo SK, Pittas AG, Adler M et al. Bone metastases from thyroid carcinoma: a histopathologic study with clinical correlates. Arch Pathol Lab Med 2000; 124:1440–1447.
12. Lawrence E, Lord ST, Leon Y, et al. Tall cell paprillary thyroid carcinoma metastatic to femur: evidence for thyroid hormone synthesis within the femur. Am.J. Med. Sci 2001; 322:103–108.
13. Chen LH, Chen WJ, Niu CC, Shih CH. Anterior reconstructive spinal surgery with Zielke Instrumentation for metastatic malignancies of the spine. Arch Orthop Trauma Surg 2000; 120:27–31.
14. Fornasier VL, Horne JG. Metastases to the vertebral column. Cancer 1975; 36:590–594.
15. Ganly I, Crowther, J. Insular carcinoma of thyroid precenting as cervical cord compression. J Laryngol Otol 2000; 114:808–810.
16. Shortliffe EH, Crapo LM. Thyroid carcinoma with spinal cord compression. JAMA 1982; 247:1565–1566.
17. Masmiquel L, Simo R, Galofre P, Mesa J. Differentiated thyroid carcinoma as a cause of cervical spinal injury. J. Cancer Res Clin Oncol 1995; 121:189–191.
18. Goldstein SI, Kaufman D, Abati AD. Metastatic thyroid carcinoma presenting as distal spinal cord compression. Ann Otol Rhinol Laryngol 1988; 97:393–396.
19. Koranda P, Ryznar V, Dockal M, Chrolok J, Houdek M. Papillary adenocarcinoma of the thyroid gland metastasizing in to the epidural space of the upper thoracic spine, without vertebral Involvement–case report. Acta Univ Palacki Olomuc Fac Med 1993; 135:31–32.
20. Roberts L Jr, Drayer BP, Apple JS, Martinez S. An unusual presentation of thyroid papillary Carcinoma: enlargement of a cervical intervertebral foramen. Comput Radiol 1986; 10:45–49.
21. Hashizume Y, Hirano A. Intramedullary spinal cord metastasis. Pathologic findings in five autopsy cases. Acta Neuropathol (Ber) 1983; 61:214–218.
22. Zeidman A, Sender BZ, Badear J, Fradim Z. Follicular carcinoma of the thyroid presenting as back pain and paravertebral mass. Israel Med Assoc J Imaj 2000; 2:720–721.
23. Kashab M, Boker DK. Indication for surgery of spinal metastases within the cervical region. Neurosurg Rev 1988; 11:95–97.
24. Oertel YC. Fine-needle aspiration and the diagnosis of thyroid cancer. Endocrinol Metab Clin North Am 1996; 25:69–91.
25. Loh KC, Greenspan FS, Gee L, Miller TR, Yeo PPB. Pathological tumor–node–metastasis (pTNM) staging for papillary and follicular thyroid carcinomas: a retrospective analysis of 700 patients. J Clinical Endocrinol Metab 1997; 82:3553–3562.
26. Mazzaferri EL, Kloos RT. Current approaches to primary therapy for papillary and follicular thyroid cancer. J Chin Endocrinol Metab 2001; 86:1447–1463.
27. Samaan NA, Schultz PN, Hickey RC, et al. The results of various modalities of treatment of well differentiated thyroid carcinoma: a

retrospective review of 1599 patients. Clin Endocrinol Metab 1992; 75:714–720.

28. Mazzaferri EL, Jhiang SM. Long-term impact of initial surgical and medical therapy on papillary and follicular thyroid cancer. Am J Med 1994; 97:418–428.

29. Casara D, Rubello D, Saladin, G, Gallo V, Masarott G, Busnardo B. Distant metastases in differentiated thyroid cancer: long-term results of radioiodine treatment and statistical analysis of prognostic factors in 214 patients. Tumori 1991: 77:432–436.

30. Brown AP, Greening WP, McCready VR, Shaw HJ, Harmer CL. Radioiodine treatment of metastatic thyroid carcinoma: the Royal Marsden Hospital experience. Br J Radiol 1984; 57:323–327.

31. Mazzaferri EL. NCCN thyroid carcinoma practice guidelines. National Comprehensive Cancer Network Proceedings 1999, Oncology 1999; 13: 391–442.

32. Baudin E, Travagli JP, Ropers J, et al. Microcarcinoma of the thyroid gland–The Gustave -Roussy Institute Experience. Cancer 1998; 83:553–559.

33. Maxon HR, Englaro EE, Thomas SR, et al. Radioiodine–131 therapy for well-differentiated thyroid cancer–a quantitative radiation dosimetric approach: outcome and validation in 85 patients. J Nucl Med 1992; 33:1132–1136.

34. Udelsman R, Lakatos E, Ladenson P. Optimal surgery for papillary thyroid carcinoma. World J Surg 1996; 20:88–93.

35. Wartofsky L, Sherman SI, Gopal J, Schlumberger M, Hay ID. The use of radioactive iodine in patients with papillary and follicular thyroid cancer. J Clin Endocrinal Metab 1998; 83:4195–4199.

36. Hunt WB, Crispell KR, McKee J. Functioning metastatic carcinoma of the thyroid producing clinical hyperthyroidism. Am J Med 1960; 28:995–1001.

37. Mazzaferri EL. Thyroid remnant 131I ablation for papillary and follicular thyroid carcinoma. Thyroid 1997; 7:265–271.

38. Doi SA, Woodhouse NJ. Ablation of the thyroid remant and 131I dose in differentiated thyroid cancer. Clin Endocrinal (Orf) 2000; 52 765–773.

39. Muratet JP, Dave, A, Minier JF, Larra F. Influence of scanning doses of iodine–131 on subsequent first ablative treatment outcome in patients operated on for differentiated thyroid carcinoma. J Nucl Med 1998; 39:1546–1550.

40. Haugen BR, Pacini F, Reiners C, et al. A comparision of recombinant human thyrotropin and thyroid hormone withdrawal for the detection of thyroid remnant or cancer. J Clin Endocrinol Metab 1999; 84:3877–3885.

41. McDougall IR, Weigel RJ. Recombinant human thyrotropin in the management of thyroid cancer. Curr Opinion Oncol 2001; 13:39–43.

42. Luster M, Reinhardt W, Korber C, et al. The use of recombinant human TSH in a patient with metastatic follicular carcinoma and insufficient endogenous TSH production. J Endocrinol Invest 2000; 23:473–475.

43. Maxon HR III, Smith HS. Radioiodine–131 in the diagnosis and treatment of metastatic well differentiated thyroid cancer. Endo Metab Clinc N. Amer 1990; 19:685–718.

44. Laguna R, Silva F, Vazquez-Selles J, Orduna E, Flores C. Vertebral hemangioma mimicking a metastatic bone lesion in well-differentiated thyroid carcinoma. Clin Nucl Med 2000; 25:611–613.

45. Barzel US, Chun KJ. Artifact of I-131 whole body scan with thoracic vertebral uptake in a patient with papillary thyroid carcinoma. Clin Nucl Med 1997; 22:855.

46. Schlumberger M, Mancusi F, Baudin E, Pacini F. 131-I therapy for elevated thyroglobulin levels. Thyroid 1997; 7:27-–276.

47. Fatourechi V, Hay ID, Mullan BP, et al. Are posttherapy radioiodine scans informative and do they influence subsequent therapy of patients with differentiated thyroid cancer? Thyroid 2000; 10:573–577.

48. Shiga T, Tsukamoto E, Nakuda K, et al. Comparison of (18) F-FDG, (131) I-Na, and (201) Tl in diagnosis of recurrent or metastatic thyroid carcinoma. J. Nucl Med 2001; 42:414–419.

49. Nishiyama Y, Yamamoto Y, Ono Y, et al. Comparison of 99 Tcm-tetrofosmin with 201 Tl and 131I in the detection of differentiated thyroid cancer metastases. Nucl Med Commum 2000: 21:917–923.

50. Rubello D, Mazzarotto R, Casara D. The role of technetium–99 m methoxyisobutylisonitrile scintigraphy in the planning of therapy and follow-up of patients with differentiated thyroid carcinoma after surgery. Eur J Nucl Med 2000; 27:431–440.

51. Ng DC, Sundoam FX, Sin AE. 99m Tc-sestamibi and 131I whole-body scintigraphy and initial serum thyroglobulin in the management of differentiated thyroid carcinoma. J. Nucl Med 2000; 41:631–635.

52. Bushnell DL, Boles MA, Kaufman GE, Wades MA, Barnes WE. Complications, sequela and dosimetry of iodine-131 therapy for thyroid carcinoma. J. Nucl Med 1992; 33:2214–2221.

53. Lakshmanan M, Schaffer A, Robbins J, Reynolds J, Norton J. A simplified low iodine diet in I-131 scanning and therapy of thyroid cancer. Clin Nucl Med 1988; 13:866–868.

54. Koogn SS, Reynolds JC. Movius EG, et al. Lithium as a potential adjuvant to the 131I therapy of metastatic, well differentiated thyroid carcinoma. J Clin Endocrinol Metab 1999; 84:912–916.

55. Brierley JD, Tsang RW. External radiation therapy in the treatment of thyroid malignancy. Endocrinol Metab Clin N Am 1996; 25:141–157.

56. Tsang RW, Brierley JD, Simpson WJ, Panzarella T, Gospodarowicz MK, Sutcliffe SB. The effects of surgery, radioiodine, and ezternal radiation therapy on the clinical outcome of patients with differentiated thyroid carcinoma. Cancer 1998; 82:375–388.

57. Lessin LS, Min M. Chemotherapy of differentiated (papillary or follicular) thyroid carcinoma. In: Wartofsky L, ed. Thyroid Cancer. A Comprehensive Guide to Clinical Management. Totowa, NJ: Humana Press; 2000:221–223.

58. Pujol P, Daure JP, Nsakala N, Baldet L, Bringer J, Jaffiol C. Degree of thyrotropin suppression as a prognostic determinant in differentiated thyroid cancer. J Clin Endocrinal Metal 1996; 81:4318–4323.

59. Sijanovic S, Karner I. Bone loss in preminopausal women on long-term suppressive therapy with thyroid hormone. Medscape Womens Health 2001; 6:3.

60. Rosen HN, Moses AC, Garber J, et al. Randomized trial of pamidronate in patients with thyroid cancer: bone density is not reduced by suppressive does of thyroxine, but is increased by cyclic intravenous pamidronate. J Clin Endocrinol Metab 1998: 83:2324–2330.

61. Frusciante V, Carnevale V, Scillitani A, et al. Global skeletal uptake of technicium-99m methylene disphosphonate in female patients receiving suppressive doses of L-thyroxine and differentiated thyroid cancer. Eur J Nucl Med 1998; 25:139–143.

62. Parle JV, Maisonneuve P, Sheppard MC, Boyle P, Franklyn JA. Prediction of all-cause and cardiovascular mortality in elderly people from one low serum thyrotropin result: a 10-year cohort study. Lancet 2001; 358:861–865.

63. Cooper DS, Specker B, Ho M, et al. Thyrotropin suppression and disease progression in patients with differentiated thyroid cancer: results from the National Thyroid Cancer Treatment Cooperative Registry. Thyroid 1998; 8:737–744.

64. Carilleux AF, Baudin E, Travagli JP, Richard M, Schlumberger M. Is diagnostic iodine-131 scanning useful after total thyroid ablation for differentiated thyroid cancer? J Clin Endocrinol Metab 2000; 85:175–178.

65. Grunwald F, Menzel C, Fimmes R, Zamoro PO, Briersack HJ. Prognostic value of thyroglobulin after thyroidectomy before ablative radioiodine therapy in thyroid cancer. J Nucl Med 1996; 37:1962–1964.

66. Wartofsky L. Using baseline and recombinant human TSH-stimulated Tg measurements to manage thyroid cancer with diagnostic 131I scanning. J Clin Endocrinol Metab 2002; 87:1486–1489.

67. Robbins RJ, Chon JT, Fleischer M, Larson SM, Tuttle RM. Is the serum thyroglobulin response to recombinant human thyrotropin sufficient by itself, to monitor for residula thyroid carcinoma? J Clin Endocrinol Metab 2002; 87:3242–3247.

68. Spencer CA, Takeuchi M, Kazarosyan M, et al. Serum thyroglobulin antoantibodies: Prevalence, influence on serum thyroglobulin measurements, and prognostic significance in patients with differentiated thyroid carcinoma. J Clin Erndocrinol metal 1998; 83:1121–1127.

69. Stabin MG. Radiation dose to the upper spine from therapeutic administrations of iodine–131-sodium iodide. J Nucl Med 1993; 34:695–696.

70. VanTol KM, Hew JM, Jager PL, Verney A, Dullaart RP, Links TP. Embolization in combination with radioiodine therapy for bone metastases from differentiated thyroid carcinoma. Clin Endocrinal (Oxf) 2000; 52:653–659.

71. Smit JW, Vielvoye GJ, Goslings BM. Embolization for vertebral metastases of follicular thyroid carconoma. J Clin Endocrinol Metab 2000; 85:989–994.

72. Shirakusa T, Motonaga R, Yoshimine K, et al. Anterior rib strut grafting for the treatment of malignant lesions in the thoracic spine. Arch Orthop Trauma Surg 1989; 108:268–272.

73. Gimm O, Sutter T, Dralle H. Diagnosis and therapy of sporadic and familial medullary thyroid carcinoma. J Cancer Res Clin Oncol 2001: 127:156–165.

74. Lips CF, Hoppener JW, Thijssen JH. Medullary thyroid carcinoma: role of genetic testing and calcitonin measurement. Ann Clin Biochem 2001; 38:168–179.

75. Ain KB. Anaplastic thyroid carcinoma: behavior biology, and therapeutic approaches. Thyroid 1998; 8:715–726.

76. Behr TM, Wulst E, Radetzky S, et al. Improved treatment of medullary thyroid cancer in a nude mouse model by combined radioimmunotheraapy: doxorubicin potentiates the therapeutic efficacy of radiolabelled antibodies in a radioresistant tumor type. Cancer Res 1997; 57:5309A–5319A.

77. DeGroot LJ, Zhang R. Gene therapy for thyroid cancer; where do we stand? J Clin Endocrinol Metab 2001; 86:2923–2928.

78. Spitzweg C, Harrington KJ, Pinke LA. Vile RG, Morris JC. The sodium iodide symporter and its potential role in cancer therapy. J Clin Endocrinol Metab 2001; 86:3327–3335.

20 Carcinoma of the Unknown Primary

Thomas E. Hutson, do, PharmD and Ronald M. Bukowski, md

Contents

INTRODUCTION
EPIDEMIOLOGY AND EVALUATION
CURRENT TREATMENT AND PROGNOSIS
GENERAL CHARACTERISTICS AND IMPACT OF SKELETAL INVOLVEMENT
SPINAL INVOLVEMENT
REFERENCES

1. INTRODUCTION

The presence of metastatic cancer without evidence of its source is a common clinical entity representing between 3 and 15% of all cancer diagnoses. Patients with cancer of unknown primary (CUP) are heterogenous, having a wide variety of clinical presentations and pathological findings, resulting in diagnostic and treatment dilemmas for both the patient and clinician. Despite having a widely varying prognosis, with optimal treatment, some patients have the potential for long-term survival, whereas others are unlikely to respond to any type of treatment.

2. EPIDEMIOLOGY AND EVALUATION

Before 1970 *(1)*, little was published about CUP. Since then, several published series have resulted in the recognition of CUP as a distinct and frequently occurring oncological process *(2– 12)*. From these studies, the incidence of CUP appears to vary depending on practice location. In a community oncology practice, the incidence is approx 3% *(5)* increasing to greater than 15% in cancer referral centers *(4,8)*. This variance in the incidence of CUP is partly explained by the lack of a uniform definition *(8)* and by the inaccurate reporting to tumor registries of primary sites on a "best guess" basis, without proof of a tumor's origin *(13)*. The median age of patients with CUP is between 50 and 60 yr. Men and women are affected equally, with men predominating in some series *(13)*. About 10% of patients have a history of another antecedent cancer *(4,13,14)*. Of patients with CUP, 97% present with symptoms related to their metastasis, whereas the remainder are detected incidentally *(1,13)*. Symptoms are commonly multiple and present for 1 to 4 mo before the diagnosis of metastatic carcinoma and reflect the particular areas of involvement. In addition, constitutional symptoms, such as anorexia, weight loss, weakness, and fatigue, are common.

The most common sites of metastatic involvement include lymph nodes in approx 30% of cases, lungs in 20%, abdomen (i.e., liver, stomach, peritoneum) in 20%, bone in 15%, and brain in 5% *(8,9,15–17)*. The exact frequencies vary from series to series owing to referral bias of the reporting institutions and distribution of histological types. For example, in series that report all histological types of CUP, the most common initial site of metastatic involvement is lymph nodes in 30% and abdomen in 15% of cases. However, in a report by Le Chavalier et al. *(8)*, the most common sites of initial metastatic presentation were lymph nodes (37 %), lung (18%), and bone (12%).

The goals of the diagnostic evaluation of a patient with CUP are: (1) to document that cancer is present (i.e., by biopsy of a liver mass, biopsy, or removal of a lymph node); (2) to find any primary sites that may have important therapeutic implications (i.e., cancers in which treatment can either prolong survival or, in rare cases, be curative); and (3) to confirm any abnormalities that need to be treated to prevent immediate harm to the patient such as a fungating, bleeding, or partially obstructing cancer of the colon or stomach *(18)*. The initial evaluation of a patient with suspected CUP should be limited and is shown in Table 1. In general, if a limited evaluation does not reveal the primary cancer site, neither will an extensive workup.

Critical to the initial evaluation of patients with CUP is an optimal pathological evaluation, which can allow for the identification of the primary site, unsuspected cancer types (i.e., lymphoma), and identification of patient subsets with specific treatment implications. The initial light microscopic examination can separate patients into four histologic types that may serve as a guide to further evaluation: (1) adenocarcinoma (60%), (2) poorly differentiated adenocarcinoma or carcinoma (30%), (3) poorly differentiated malignant neoplasm (5%), and (4) squamous cell carcinoma (5%) *(6,7,19)*. In patients with adenocarcinoma, additional pathological evaluation is unlikely to identify the primary site definitively *(6,7)*. An exception is adenocarcinoma of the prostate, which can be identified by

From: *Current Clinical Oncology: Cancer in the Spine: Comprehensive Care.*
Edited by: R. F. McLain, K-U. Lewandrowski, M. Markman, R. M. Bukowski,
R. Macklis, and E. C. Benzel © Humana Press, Inc., Totowa, NJ

Table 1
Evaluation of Patients Presenting With Cancer of Unknown Primary Site

Detailed history
Complete physical examination
Complete blood count
Tumor markers:
    PSA
    CEA
    α-FP
    β-HCG
    CA-125
Liver function tests
Serum chemistry panel
Urinalysis
Stool test for occult blood
Review of pathology specimens
Chest X-ray

Additional tests as indicated: immunohistochemical stains, electron microscopy, and hormone receptors

PSA, prostate-specific antigen; CEA, carcinoembryonic antigen; α-FP, α-fetoprotein; β-HCG, β-human chorionic gonadotropin.

Table 2
Poor Prognostic Factors Influencing Outcome and Survival in Cancer of Unknown Primary Site

General characteristics	Histologic subtypes
Age >60	Well-differentiated
Male sex	adenocarcinoma
Multiple metastatic sites	Moderately differentiated
Poor performance status	adenocarcinoma
Supraclavicular lymphadenopathy	

fails to identify the primary tumor in up to 30% of patients. Autopsy studies have shown, however, that for patients whose primary sites were not documented in life, the most likely primary site is the pancreas if the metastasis occurred below the diaphragm, or the lung if the metastasis occurred above the diaphragm *(18)*.

3. CURRENT TREATMENT AND PROGNOSIS

The prognosis for most patients with CUP is dismal with a median survival of 1 to 4 mo, and only 20% and less than 10% are alive at 1 and 5 yr, respectively *(12,13)*. However, some patients with certain histological subtypes may have prolonged survival and, rarely, be cured with therapy. Nearly all long-term survivors are found in two groups: (1) patients who presented with peripheral lymphadenopathy as the sole manifestation of cancer and (2) patients with poorly differentiated or neuroendocrine carcinomas, women with peritoneal carcinomatosis, and men with poorly differentiated carcinoma in a midline lymphoadenopathic distribution *(13)*. The latter group represents histological subtypes that historically are extremely sensitive to chemotherapy. In all series, discovery of the primary site has not altered the prognosis and survival.

Several series have identified prognostic factors associated with poor outcome and survival (Table 2). Unfavorable prognostic groups include those with multiple metastatic sites, age older than 60, male sex, supraclavicular lymphadenopathy, and a histology of well-differentiated or moderately differentiated adenocarcinoma *(11,23)*. Performance status also affects survival. In one series, patients with a good performance status (ECOG performance status of 0/1) had a median survival of 6 to 10 mo vs 2 mo for those patients with a poor performance status *(24)*.

Certain histological subtypes and clinical presentations may have dramatic responses to treatment and long term survival. The recognized clinicopathological subsets and treatment considerations are outlined in Table 3. The reader is also referred to the corresponding sections of this handbook for further information. Histological subtypes in which treatment may impact on the natural history of CUP and prolong survival include: *adenocarcinoma*: women with isolated axillary lymphadenopathy or peritoneal carcinomatosis, men with bone metastasis, and patients with a single metastatic site; *squamous cell carcinoma*: patients with cervical or inguinal lymphadenopathy; and, *poorly differentiated carcinoma*: young men with extragonadal germ-cell cancer syndrome and patients with poorly differentiated carcinoma.

positive tissue staining for prostate-specific antigen (PSA). All patients with poorly differentiated carcinoma or poorly differentiated malignant neoplasm require additional specialized pathological evaluation, which in some cases, may include electron microscopy, immunohistochemistry, and cytogenetic analysis. These additional tests are useful in detecting undifferentiated cancers, such as melanoma, sarcoma, germ-cell tumors, and lymphoma.

Besides chest X-ray, further radiographic studies and/or endoscopic evaluation have failed to improve the diagnostic yield and several thousand dollars can be spent in a futile search for the primary site *(20)*. In one series of 31 patients with CUP, computed tomography found the primary site in 58% of patients, but was unhelpful or wrong in 23% *(21)*. Whereas, in a small series, positron emission tomography scanning detected primary sites in 7 of 29 patients (24%), however, survival was not altered by discovery of the primary tumor *(22)*.

The pattern of metastasis may help narrow the possible primary sites. For instance, in patients with bone metastasis as the initial manifestation of CUP, likely primary tumors include breast, lung, Hodgkin's disease, multiple myeloma (lytic lesions), and prostate (blastic lesions). However, the primary site can not always be predicted based on typical patterns of metastatic spread. Bony metastasis develop in 30 to 50% of cases when lung carcinoma presents with an evident primary site, but in only 5% of cases that present as CUP. Similarly, cancers of the pancreas and liver usually involve the bone in only 5 to 10% of cases, but when they present as CUP, they may involve the skeleton in up to 30% of cases.

The primary site of origin is determined in less than 15% of patients presenting with CUP, no matter what diagnostic efforts are undertaken. When identified, the most common sites of primary tumor are pancreas (25%), lung (23%), lower bowel (8%), hepatobiliary (8%), kidney/urinary tract (7%), upper bowel (6%), and ovary (5%) *(13)*. Even after death, autopsy

Table 3
Recommended Treatment for Patients With Recognized Clinicopathological Subsets

Histological type	Clinical subset	Treat as
Adenocarcinoma	Women with isolated axillary lymphadenopathy	Stage II breast cancer
	Women with peritoneal carcinomatosis	Stage III ovarian cancer
	Men with blastic bone metastasis and increased serum PSA	Stage IV prostate cancer
	Single metastatic site	Local excision/radiation
Squamous cell carcinoma	Cervical adenopathy	Head and neck cancer
	Inguinal adenopathy	Node dissection/radiation
Poorly differentiated carcinoma	Young men with mediastinal or retroperitoneal mass	Extragonadal germ cell tumor
	Neuroendocrine features by IHC	Small cell cancer
	All others with good PS	Small cell cancer

PSA, prostate-specific antigen; IHC, immunohistochemical statining; PS, performance status.

Table 4
Common Chemotherapy Regimens for the Empiric Treatment of Cancer of Unknown Primary

Regimen	Dose	
PCE	Paclitaxel	200 mg/m^2 iv over 1 hr on d 1
	Carboplatin	AUC of 6, iv on d 1
	Etoposide	50 mg alternating with 100 mg PO on d 1–10
		Repeat cycle every 21 d
EP	Etoposide	100 mg/m^2 iv on d 1–5
	Cisplatin	100 mg/m^2 iv on d 1
		Repeat cycle every 21 d
PEB	Cisplatin	20 mg/m^2 iv on d 1–5
	Etoposide	100 mg/m^2 iv on d 1–5
	Bleomycin	30 units iv on d 1, 8, and 15
		Repeat cycle every 21 d

Systemic therapy for patients not included in the subgroups aforementioned is difficult. Unfortunately, this group includes the majority of patients presenting with CUP. Table 4 includes the most commonly used chemotherapy regimens. Multiple trials incorporating predominantly Platinum-based chemotherapy regimens have resulted in only 20 to 35% response rates which are usually of short duration (24–29). The median survival from these trials averages between 5 and 8 mo. The advent of new chemotherapy agents, primarily the taxanes (docetaxel and paclitaxel), gemcitabine, and topoisomerase I inhibitors (topotecan and irinotecan) have resulted in renewed interest in empiric therapy for patients with CUP. Most experience with these regimens suggest higher response rates and longer median survivals than with older regimens. In addition, the toxicity of taxane/carboplatin regimens is reduced when compared to previous cisplatin-based regimens (30–33). Long-term follow-up of patients treated with paclitaxel/carboplatin/etoposide shows actual 2- and 3-yr survivals of 20 and 14%, respectively. At present, there remains no standard therapy for patients with CUP. Empiric chemotherapy regimens should incorporate newer agents with reduced toxicity and possibly greater anti-tumor activity.

In summary, patients with CUP who fit into a treatable subgroup warrant consideration for aggressive systemic therapy.

Results from numerous studies support this approach, and some patients may achieve long-term survival and cure. The role of empiric systemic chemotherapy for all other patients should be based on the patients' wishes and performance status, after a formal discussion of the limitations with currently available therapy and the associated toxicities with their use.

4. GENERAL CHARACTERISTICS AND IMPACT OF SKELETAL INVOLVEMENT

The skeleton is a common metastatic site for several cancers. Cancer of the breast and prostate are the most common sources of metastasis when the primary site is known (34). However, between 10 and 23% of patients presenting with CUP have skeletal metastasis as the first lesions to be detected (1–11). The primary location is often not identified despite extensive investigation, and rarely does its discovery influence the natural history or improve survival.

There are few studies of CUP that have separated patients with skeletal metastasis from those patients with metastasis in nonskeletal sites (35–41). Metastasis usually occur in the axial or proximal appendicular skeleton, in patients who are older than 40 yr old, whereas primary bone tumors usually occur in the appendicular skeleton in patients younger than age 40. In one study of 46 patients with skeletal metastasis of unknown origin (41), 11 metastatic carcinomas were located in the femur, 9 in the pelvis, 8 in the spine, 5 in the scapula, 3 each in the humerus, ribs, and skulls, 2 in the tibia, and 1 each in the radius and sternum. The most common histological type was adenocarcinoma.

The standard workup for patients with skeletal manifestations should parallel that for all patients presenting with CUP. On evaluation, the majority of patients (approx 75%) will be found to have multiple visceral metastatic sites. Some authors have advocated the addition of computer tomographic scans of the chest, abdomen, and pelvis in the initial workup of CUP as a means to increase the ability of detecting the primary site of origin (38,41). The most common identified primary sites from these series were lung, kidney, pancreas, prostate, breast, and thyroid. However, the cost effectiveness of this approach has been questioned.

The natural history of patients with skeletal metastasis of unknown primary parallels that of all patients with CUP. The median overall survival is 1 to 4 mo. Treatment should focus on palliation of symptoms and treatment of areas requiring immediate attention (i.e., spinal cord compression, pathological fractures). The primary palliative treatment modalities used in patients with skeletal metastasis include localized external beam radiotherapy, corticosteroids (for spinal cord compression), and, in selected cases of isolated skeletal metastasis, surgical resection. In patients with skeletal metastasis of unknown primary, in whom serum PSA is elevated, or in whom immunohistochemical studies of tumor specimens are positive for PSA should be treated with androgen deprivation therapy (Chapter 16). Likewise, women with tumor specimens expressing estrogen/progesterone receptors (Chapter 15), and patients with specimens suggesting lymphoma (Chapter 14) may derive benefit from hormonal therapy and chemotherapy, respectively. The use of bisphosphonates may provide additional palliation and reduce the incidence of pathological fracture. It is evident from both preclinical and most clinical trials that bisphosphonates (i.e., clodronate, pamidronate, and zolendronate) cause a decrease in tumor burden in bone metastatic sites. These agents have been evaluated in several phase III clinical trials in patients with metastatic breast and prostate cancers and their use should be considered in all patients with skeletal metastasis.

5. SPINAL INVOLVEMENT

The spine is a very common site of bony metastasis, with up to 75% of vertebral metastasis originating from the following primary tumors: breast, prostate, renal, and thyroid (42). In a review of 130 patients presenting to a general hospital with neurological symptoms deriving from spinal metastasis, the primary site of tumor was the lung in 33%, breast in 28%, other sites in 25%, and CUP in 14% (40). However, in actual clinical practice, it has been suggested that CUP accounts for only 3 to 4% of spine metastasis (1,35,38,43).

Spinal or radicular pain followed by neurological symptoms are the initial complaint in the majority of patients presenting with metastasis to the spine, whether a primary site is identified or not (40). In a review of patients presenting with spinal metastasis, the spine produced the first evidence of malignant disease in nearly 50% of the cases. Leg weakness and sphincter disturbance is the most common reason for referral.

After tissue diagnosis of cancer is obtained either surgically or by needle aspiration, a diligent search for a primary site should be performed. Common age and gender related cancers should be evaluated (i.e., mammography for women and digital rectal examination with serum PSA level for men). The evaluation of patients suspected to have a CUP is outlined in Table 1. If a limited evaluation does not reveal the primary cancer site, neither will an extensive workup.

In a series of patients who presented with spinal metastasis, the best predictor of outcome was the site of the primary tumor. Only 17% of patients with lung cancer, in this series, responded well to treatment and only 2% were alive 1 yr after treatment; 51% of patients with breast cancer responded well and 36% were alive at 1 yr (40). Excluding those patients with limited spinal involvement, the prognosis for patients presenting with spinal metastasis from unknown primary sites is poor. The median survival is similar to patients presenting with CUP in visceral sites.

Treatment for spinal metastasis from an unknown primary site should be palliative and include surgical decompression or radiotherapy in an attempt to alleviate pain, stabilize pathological fractures, or as treatment for spinal cord compression. A prognostic scoring system for vertebral metastasis has been developed by Tokuhashi et al. (44) in an attempt to identify those patients in which surgical excision of spinal metastasis be performed. However, a recent review suggests that patients with spinal metastasis of unknown primary sites fair poorly with curative intent surgical resection (40).

The use of systemic therapy may alleviate pain or even prolong life in selected cases. In patients suspected of having metastatic prostate cancer, the role of androgen deprivation therapy may prolong survival, whereas the use of chemotherapy (i.e., mitoxantrone and prednisone) may alleviate pain (Chapter 16). In women with suspected metastatic breast cancer, the use of anti-estrogen therapy may be equally efficacious with an improvement in long term survival (Chapter 15). The role of bisphosphonates in the treatment of metastatic cancer to bone continues to evolve, however, their use may alleviate pain and decrease pathological fractures in some patients with spinal metastasis.

REFERENCES

1. Holmes FF, Fouts TL. Metastatic cancer of unknown primary site. Cancer 1970; 26:816–820.
2. Nystrom JS, Weiner JM, Wolf RM, et al. Identifying the primary site in metastatic cancer of unknown origin. JAMA 1979; 241:381–383.
3. Osteen RT, Kopf G, Wilson RE. In pursuit of the unknown primary. Am J Surg 1978; 135:494–498.
4. Altman E, Cadman E. An analysis of 1539 patients with cancer of unknown primary site. Cancer 1986; 57:120–124.
5. Briasoulis E, Pavlidis N. Cancer of unknown primary origin. Oncologist 1997; 2:142–152.
6. Greco FA, Hainsworth JD. Tumors of unknown origin. CA Cancer J Clin 1992; 42:96–115.
7. Greco FA, Hainsworth JD. Cancer of unknown primary site. In: DeVita VT Jr, Hellman S, Rosenberg SA, eds. Cancer: Principles and Practice of Oncology. 6th ed. Philadelphia, PA: Lippincott; 2000:2537–2560.
8. Le Chavalier T, Cvitkovic E, Caille P, et al. Early metastatic cancer of unknown primary origin at presentation: a clinical study of 302 consecutive autopsied patients. Arch Intern Med 1988; 148:2035–2039.
9. Jordan WE 3rd, Schildt RA. Adenocarcinoma of unknown primary site. The Brooke Army Medical Center experience. Cancer 1985; 55:857–860.
10. Maiche AG. Cancer of unknown primary: a retrospective study based on 109 patients. Am J Clin Oncol 1993; 16:26–29.
11. Didolkar MS, Fanous N, Elias EG, Moore RH. Metastatic carcinomas from occult primary tumors: a study of 254 patients. Ann Surg 1977; 186:625–630.
12. Abbruzzese JL, Abbruzzese MC, Lenzi R, et al. Unknown primary carcinoma: natural history and prognostic factors in 657 consecutive patients. J Clin Oncol 1994; 12:1272–1280.
13. Casciato DA. Metastasis of unknown origin. In: Haskell CM, Berek JS, eds. Cancer Treatment, 5th ed. Philadelphia, PA: WB Saunders; 2001:1556-1578.
14. Gaber AO, Rice P, Eaton C, et al. Metastatic malignant disease of unknown origin. Am J Surg 1983; 145:493–497.
15. Lyman GH, Priesler HD. Carcinoma of unknown primary: natural history and response to therapy. J Med 1978; 9:445–459.
16. Schildt RA, Kennedy PS, Chen TT, et al. Management of patients with metastatic adenocarcinoma of unknown origin. A Southwest Oncology Group study. Cancer Treat Rep 1983; 67:77–79.

17. Krementz ET, Cerise EJ, Foster DS, Morgan LR. Metastasis of undetermined source. Curr Probl Cancer 1979; 4:4–37.

18. Markman M. The dilemma of evaluating and treating cancer of unknown primary site. Cleve Clin J Med 1997; 64:73–75.

19. Hainsworth JD, Greco FA. Treatment of patients with cancer of an unknown primary site. N Engl J Med 1993; 329:257–263.

20. Schapira DV, Jarrett AR. The need to consider survival, outcome, and expense when evaluating and treating patients with unknown primary carcinoma. Arch Intern Med 1995; 155:2050–2054.

21. Gorich J, Beyer-Enke SA, Muller M, et al. The value of computed tomography in the search for an unknown primary tumor. Rofo Fortschr Geb Rontgenstr Nuklearmed 1988; 149:277–279.

22. Kole AC, Nieweg OE, Pruim J, et al. Detection of unknown occult primary tumors using positron emission tomography. Cancer 1998; 82:1160–1166.

23. Lenzi R, Hess KR, Abbruzzese MC, et al. Poorly differentiated carcinoma and poorly differentiated adenocarcinoma of unknown origin: favorable subsets of patients with unknown primary carcinoma? J Clin Oncol 1997; 12:2056–2066.

24. Woods RL, Fox RM, Tattersall MH, Levi JA, Brodie GN. Metastatic adenocarcinomas of unknown primary site: a randomized study of two combination chemotherapy regimens. N Engl J Med 1980; 303:87–89.

25. Goldberg RM, Smith FP, Ueno W, et al. Fluorouracil, Adriamycin and mitomycin in the treatment of adenocarcinoma of unknown primary. J Clin Oncol 1986; 4:395–399.

26. Eagan RT, Thernean TM, Rubin J, et al. Lack of value for cisplatin added to mitomycin-doxorubicin combination chemotherapy for carcinoma of unknown primary site. Am J Clin Oncol 1987; 10:82–85.

27. Fiorre JJ, Kelsen DP, Gralla RJ, et al. Adenocarcinoma of unknown primary origin: treatment with vindesine and doxorubicin. Cancer Treat Rep 1985; 69:591–594.

28. Anderson H, Thatcher N, Rankin E, et al. VAD (vincristine, Adriamycin and cyclophosphamide) chemotherapy for metastatic carcinoma from an unknown primary site. Eur J Cancer Clin Oncol 1983; 19:49–52.

29. Hainsworth JD, Johnson DH, Greco FA. Cisplatin-based combination chemotherapy in the treatment of poorly differentiated carcinoma and poorly differentiated adenocarcinoma of unknown primary site: results of a 12-year experience. J Clin Oncol 1992; 10:912–922.

30. Hainsworth JD, Erland JB, Kalman LA. Carcinoma of unknown primary site: Treatment with one hour paclitaxel, carboplatin and extended schedule etoposide. J Clin Oncol 1997; 15:2385–2394.

31. Briasoulis E, Kaloforous H, Bafalovkos D, et al. Carboplatin plus paclitaxel in unknown primary carcinomaL A phase II study of the Hellenic Cooperative Oncology Group. J Clin Oncol 2000; 17:3101–3107.

32. Greco FA, Erland JB, Morrissey LH, et al. Carcinoma of unknown primary site: Phase II trials with docetaxel plus cisplatin or carboplatin. Ann Oncol 2000; 11:211–215.

33. Greco FA, Erland JB, Patton JF, et al. Carcinoma of unknown primary site: Long-term follow-up after taxane-based chemotherapy (abstract). Proc Am Soc Clin Oncol 2000; 19 597a.

34. Mirra JM. Metastases. In: Mirra, J. M., ed. Bone Tumors: Clinical, Radiologic, and Pathologic Correlations. Philadelphia, PA: Lea and Febiger: 1989:1499.

35. Enkaoua E, Doursounian L, Chatellier G, et al. Vertebral metastasis: a critical appreciation of the preoperative tokuhashi score in a series of 71 cases. Spine 1997; 22:2293–2298.

36. Neilan BA. Metastatic spinal cord compression. AFP 1983; 27: 191–194.

37. Baron MG, Gandara I de la, Espinosa E, et al. Bone metastasis as the first manifestation of a tumour. Int Orthop 1991; 15:373–376.

38. Rougraff BT, Kneisl JS, Simon M. Skeletal metastasis of unknown origin: a prospective study of a diagnostic strategy. J Bone and Joint Surg 1993; 75:1276–1281.

39. Saengnipanthkul S, Jirarattanaphochai K, Rojviroj S, et al. Metastatic adenocarcinoma of the spine. Spine 1992; 17:427–430.

40. Stark RJ, Henson RA, Evans SJW. Spinal metastasis: a retrospective survey from a general hospital. Brain 1982; 105:189–213.

41. Simon MA, Bartucci EJ. The search for the primary tumor in patients with skeletal metastases of unknown origin. Cancer 1986; 58: 1088–1095.

42. Harrington KD. The use of methylmetacrylate for vertebral body replacement and anterior stabilization of pathologic fracture dislocation of the spine due to metastatic malignant disease. J Bone Joint Surg 1981; 63:36–47.

43. Steckel RJ, Kagan AR. Diagnostic persistence in working up metastatic cancer with an unknown primary site. Radiology 1980; 134:367–369.

44. Tokuhashi Y, Matsuzaki H, Toriyama S, et al. Scoring system for the preoperative evaluation of metastatic spine tumor prognosis. Spine 1990; 15:1110–1113.

21 Primary Tumors of the Spine

Rex C. Haydon, MD, PhD and Frank M. Phillips, MD

Contents

1. INTRODUCTION

Primary neoplasms of the spine encompass a broad spectrum of tumors, ranging in their tissue of origin, local behavior, and potential for metastasis. The diagnosis and treatment of these disorders is accordingly varied. As a category, non-myeloproliferative primary tumors of the spine are rare, accounting for approx 5% of all bone tumors, when one excludes hemangiomas *(1,2)*. In frequency, therefore, they are much less common than metastatic and/or myeloproliferative neoplasms involving the spine, as well as non-neoplastic processes such as infection, metabolic disorders, and other pathologies. The diagnosis of primary tumors of the spine, therefore, must occur with careful consideration of other more common entities. In this chapter, we discuss the common benign and malignant tumors that afflict the spinal column, and describe the appropriate algorithm for evaluating and treating these conditions.

2. DIAGNOSIS AND EVALUATION OF PRIMARY TUMORS OF THE SPINE

2.1. CLINICAL HISTORY AND PRESENTING SYMPTOMS

The most common presenting symptom among patients with primary tumors of the spine is pain, occurring in approx 84% of patients at initial visit *(1)*. The length of symptoms depends largely on the behavior of the individual tumor, and may be helpful in diagnosis. Typically, tumors with a more rapid onset of pain reflect more aggressive tumors. In contradistinction to other spinal causes of back and neck pain, pain caused by neoplasm is not positional, and can be especially pronounced at night. Benign, or more slow-growing tumors, may be characterized by gradually increasing pain spanning several months to years. Sudden increases in pain suggest pathological fractures through abnormal bone. In eliciting a history of pain, specific attention should be paid to its location, relationship to position, quality, and severity. Furthermore, response to nonsteroidal anti-inflammatory agents may suggest osteoid osteoma.

Another common presenting symptom is neurological compromise, occurring when either nerve roots or the spinal cord itself is compressed by the expanding tumor or retropulsed bone as a result of pathological fracture. Depending on the precise location and size of the tumor, neurological symptoms can range from subtle motor-sensory deficits to paraplegia. In subtle cases, patients are often unaware of neurological dysfunction, underscoring the need for a complete and thorough physical exam at initial presentation. Neurological changes can be identified at diagnosis in approx 55% of patients with malignant tumors and 35% of patients with benign tumors *(1)*, although this is rarely the complaint that they present with on initial evaluation. The neurological findings are dependent on the location of the tumor as well. In sacral tumors, for example, autonomic dysfunction, such as the loss of bowel and bladder control, is more common. The presence of neurological compromise should prompt the physician to perform a rapid evaluation of the underlying tumor, so that treatment can be initiated and further progression halted.

Other presenting symptoms are considerably less common, however, may be important in planning treatment. Scoliotic deformities, for example, may occur in up to 70% of patients with osteoid osteoma and osteoblastoma *(3–5)*. Changes in the alignment of the spine are thought to occur in response to pain-induced paravertebral spasm. Given that most idiopathic scoliotic curves are painless, the presence of pain with deformity is highly suggestive of tumors. Recognition of spinal deformities early in patients with spine tumors is important given that they can progress quickly, requiring corrective surgery. Other important causes of kyphoscoliotic deformities include pathological fractures or instability caused by compromise of weight-bearing

From: *Current Clinical Oncology: Cancer in the Spine: Comprehensive Care.*
Edited by: R. F. McLain, K-U. Lewandrowski, M. Markman, R. M. Bukowski,
R. Macklis, and E. C. Benzel © Humana Press, Inc., Totowa, NJ

Table 1
Locational Preference of Primary Tumors

	Anterior elements	Eccentric	Posterior elements
Child	Eosinophilic granuloma	Osteochondroma	Aneurysmal bone cyst
	Osteosarcoma	Chondroblastoma	Osteoid osteoma
	Ewing's sarcoma	Osteoblastoma	Chondroblastoma
Adult	Multiple myeloma	Chondrosarcoma	Aneurysmal bone cyst
	Metastatic disease	Chondrosarcoma	
	Giant cell tumor		
	Chordoma		
	Fibrous dysplasia		

columns within the spine. Finally, localized masses are relatively uncommon in primary tumors of the spine, but may be present in benign lesions that develop over a long period of time.

A complete history should not be limited to the spine, given that cancer is often a systemic disease, with clinical manifestations outside the environs of the spinal column. A careful history should, therefore, also include constitutional symptoms such as weight loss, fevers/chills, and lethargy, as well as a complete past medical history, including any previous history of malignancy in the patient or his/her family. Several lesions such as osteochondromas, eosinophilic granuloma, and neurofibromas can be multifocal. A thorough review of systems may help to identify other manifestations of such disorders and assist with diagnosis.

2.2. PHYSICAL EXAMINATION

Similar to any patient who presents with back/neck pain and/or neurological symptoms, a complete neurological examination is essential. Palpation along the spine may help to identify the specific vertebral level causing symptoms, and may therefore, help to guide radiographic assessment. Similarly, evidence of spinal deformity should be assessed.

One must keep in mind that some primary tumors of the spine may be multifocal, or may be part of syndromes that encompass a number of physical findings outside of the spine. Typically, multifocal lesions are uncommon in primary spine tumors, and suggest conditions with widespread disease such as metastatic cancer, multiple myeloma, and myeloproliferative disorders. Still, cases have been described of multi-focal giant cell tumor of bone (6,7), and in the case of malignant bone tumors, such as chondrosarcoma and osteosarcoma, skip lesions, and/or distant metastases, may occur (6,8–11). Tumor-like entities such as eosinophilic granuloma (i.e., Hand-Schüller-Christian and Letterer-Siwe), fibrous dysplasia (i.e., McCune-Albright and Campanacci syndrome), and neurofibromatosis can result in lesions at multiple sites. Evaluation of the skin, in the case of McCune-Albright syndrome, may reveal the characteristic café-au-lait spots (irregular coast of Maine border) seen in this disorder. Similarly, neurofibromatosis can cause neurological symptoms and often demonstrate café-au-lait spots (smooth coast of California border).

2.3. RADIOLOGICAL IMAGING

In any patient with symptoms of back and neck pain and/or neurological changes, radiographic evaluation generally begins with plain films. Important properties of the lesion such as its location, bony and soft tissue extent, zone of transition, and internal characteristics can be discerned from plain films alone, and may be sufficient for diagnosis in certain cases. In evaluating the lesion, it is important to note whether it involves the anterior or posterior elements, given that many benign and malignant lesions have a special predilection for one or the other, as noted in Table 1. For tumors involving the spine, certain classic radiographic signs have been described such as the "winking owl," in which the pedicle has been eroded by an expanding tumor, or vertebra plana, where there is vertebral body collapse. Although these are considered to be classic radiographic signs for spinal lesions, most tumors are far more subtle, and can be missed on plain films. Given the limitations in visualizing soft tissue anatomy, as well as the difficulty in visualizing areas such as the upper thoracic spine, additional imaging studies are usually necessary.

The most common adjunctive study to plain radiographs in the evaluation of spine tumors is magnetic resonance imaging (MRI). MRI provides not only unparalleled soft tissue detail, but also essential information on the compression and/or compromise of neural elements. MRI can reveal important tissue characteristics of the tumor, such as its density, vascular perfusion, and necrosis, as well as the its effects on surrounding structures. In the case of primary bone tumors, MRI is the most precise study to identify the extent of marrow involvement, as well as soft tissue extent. For all of these reasons, it is an excellent modality to use for presurgical planning, not only to identify regions for biopsy, but also to delineate the margins of the tumor in anticipation of wide resection.

One limitation of MRI is its inability to provide excellent imaging of cortical bone. Computed tomography (CT) scans, either alone or in combination with myelography, provide superior imaging of cortical integrity, and may be critical to determine the extent and precise location of spine tumors. Given that primary tumor involvement of the spine may lead to spinal instability requiring surgical treatment, CT scans are also helpful for assessing the extent of bony involvement and destruction by tumor.

An additional study to evaluate patients with subtle lesions on plain film and MRI, or to stage patients with malignant tumors, is bone scintigraphy using technetium diphosphonate 99 mTc. By targeting osteoblasts that take up technetium-99, this study identifies regions undergoing rapid bone turnover. Therefore, primary bone tumors or lesions that result in local remodeling will usually demonstrate significant signal on bone scans. Although extremely sensitive, it is generally nonspecific, and rarely of diagnostic help for the purposes of primary tumors of the spine. It is primarily used to identify additional areas of skeletal involvement in multifocal diseases, although in selected tumors such as multiple myeloma and eosinophilic granuloma, bone scans are often unable to detect the osseous lesion.

Myelography used to be an important imaging study before the advent of CT scans and MRI, however, its use today is primarily limited to evaluating patients with neurological compromise. In combination with CT scans, it provides detailed information on the compression of either nerve roots or the spinal cord, and may therefore, be a helpful adjunctive study for preoperative planning.

Additional studies may be of value in individual cases. For example, nuclear studies such as tagged white blood cell scans can be helpful to distinguish infection from neoplastic processes. Similarly, angiography may be helpful for certain tumors if they are highly vascular and preoperative embolization would be of help. Additional radiological studies such as positron emission tomography scans are currently being investigated in the evaluation of tumors. Although they are not in widespread use, positron emission tomography scans may provide invaluable information regarding the metabolic activity of a given tumor, including the degree and extent of necrosis within the lesion. In sum, a variety of radiographic modalities can be used in the evaluation of spine tumors. The selection of appropriate studies is ultimately dependent on the individual needs for each case.

2.4. LABORATORY STUDIES

For the purposes of diagnosis, several laboratory studies can be an important addition to radiographic and other diagnostic modalities. Although they rarely identify primary bone tumors, they may help to distinguish primary bone tumors from metastatic disease, multiple myeloma, or infection.

All patients with a suspicion of a primary bone tumor should have a complete blood count with platelets performed. Increases in specific marrow cell derivatives may help to diagnose patients with myeloproliferative disorders, whereas, pancytopenia may suggest marrow replacement caused by certain myeloproliferative or metastatic diseases. Careful attention to patients with thrombocytopenia, anemia, and/or leukopenia may be necessary before biopsies, either open or CT-directed, can be performed. The erythrocyte sedimentation rate can be elevated in a broad variety of tumors, and as a rule, is nonspecific. However, it rarely exceeds 100 except in infections or tumors such as Ewing's sarcoma/primitive neuroectodermal tumor (PNET) and certain myeloproliferative disorders.

Additional blood studies should be guided by the differential diagnosis that is generated after initial history, physical exam and radiographic tests. Apart from their diagnostic importance, certain laboratory tests may be required before more thorough radiographic tests can be performed. For example, a prothrombin time/partial thromboplastin time is generally required on all patients undergoing a CT-directed biopsy. Similarly a baseline creatinine/blood urea nitrogen is necessary before angiography. As diagnostic tools, laboratory tests can be extremely helpful, such as the use of serum and urine protein electrophoresis. The presence of a monoclonal spike is considered nearly pathopneumonic for multiple myeloma. Similarly, elevated prostate-specific antigen, and α-fetoprotein are considered to be suggestive of metastatic disease, and help to localize the origin of the metastatic tumor.

Evaluation of cerebrospinal fluid (CSF) can provide important information when guided by clinical suspicion. Not only can CSF provide cells for cytological diagnosis in tumors that invade the dura, but also changes in CSF glucose, protein, and leukocytes may help to identify infectious processes and/or spinal cord compression.

2.5. STAGING

In general, staging systems attempt to predict outcome among patients with benign and malignant tumors using clinical variables such as the histological grade of the tumor, local behavior, and metastatic spread. In bone and soft tissue sarcomas, staging systems have also been designed as a preoperative aide, helping to define the surgical margins needed for optimal local control.

For benign tumors of bone, the Enneking system is widely used and divides tumors into one of three categories: (1) inactive, (2) active, and (3) aggressive (12). The underlying clinical diagnosis, as well as the reaction of local bone to the tumor generally predicts the biological behavior and natural history of the disease process. Although benign lesions rarely metastasize, a few notable exceptions exist and deserve special consideration. Giant-cell tumor and chondroblastoma have a demonstrable capacity to metastasize (13–16) and, therefore, radiographic evaluation of the chest should be performed at diagnosis to screen for patients with distant disease.

To address malignant bone lesions, Enneking developed a surgical staging system based on the grade of the tumor, intra-/extra-compartmental status, and metastatic disease (17). Modifications of the classic Enneking staging system are currently being considered, including the American Joint Committee on Cancer system that is premised on grade and tumor size. Additionally, Hart et al. (18) have proposed a unique staging system for tumors of the spine based on a lesion's location and local extension. The vertebral body is divided into 12 sectors similar to a clock-face, and the tumor location is plotted according to this grid. Furthermore, five layers are described, beginning with the paraspinal soft tissues peripherally to the intradural space centrally. The system is primarily descriptive, and can therefore be applied to both benign and malignant tumors. Initial testing of this system on giant cell tumors of the spine suggest higher rates of local recurrence in lesions that extend into both anterior and posterior elements, although these differences were not statistically significant (18).

For malignant tumors, staging studies typically include a chest radiograph, chest CT, bone scan, and sufficient imaging studies of the primary tumor to identify its extent both within and outside the bone with confidence.

2.6. BIOPSY

If clinical, radiographic, and laboratory examinations do not lead to a definitive diagnosis, a biopsy should be performed in order to provide tissue for pathological evaluation. This is generally required in most cases, either before or concurrent with

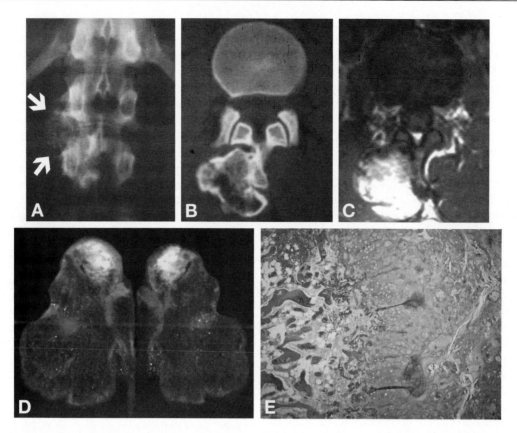

Fig. 1. A 21-yr-old male with a long history of a right paraspinal mass that recently became painful with heavy lifting. (**A**) Anteroposterior radiograph of the lumbar spine reveals a mass in the right paraspinous region that is calcified.(**B**) Axial computed tomography images demonstrate that the mass is continuous with the spinous process and that the marrow space flows into the mass. (**C**) Magnetic resonance axial image redemonstrates the mass and strongly suggests that it is an osteochondroma, although a clear cartilage cap is not evident. After resection of the lesion, (**D**) shows the gross specimen. The mass is multilobulated and does have a cartilage cap that is not pathologically thickened. (**E**) Hematoxylin and eosin (H&E) stain of the lesion at the junction of the cartilage cap and the underlying bone.

definitive surgical treatment. All diagnostic and staging examinations should be performed before biopsy, because surgery can alter the appearance of the tumor on subsequent studies. The biopsy must also be planned and performed with great care so as not to compromise later resection of the tumor.

Perhaps the most common method of biopsy in the spine is CT-directed biopsy. Although this technique may be useful in a number of tumors, there are some notable exceptions. Specifically, lesions that are predominantly osteoblastic, such osteoid osteoma or osteoblastic osteosarcoma, may not be penetrable using the biopsy needle. Also, in the case of small lesions, it may be difficult to obtain sufficient tissue for definitive diagnosis using CT-directed biopsy techniques.

Open biopsies are rarely needed for cases of spine tumors, but must be considered when CT-directed biopsy is not feasible, or after previous attempts have failed to provide diagnostic tissue. Longitudinal incisions should be used in order to facilitate excision of the biopsy tract during later resection. Minimizing tissue dissection will also help to preserve normal tissue architecture and prevent the formation of large hematomas. Hematomas, and/or seromas, that develop after biopsy result in dissemination of tumor cells beyond the region of the biopsy, especially if tissue planes have been developed during

the approach. Because the hematoma is considered a contaminated space, it must be excised *en bloc* with the primary tumor, often complicating later reconstruction and closure.

In selected cases, clinical suspicion may be high for a specific neoplastic entity, such as giant cell tumor or osteoblastoma. In these cases, biopsy can be performed at the same time as surgical resection, with the biopsy being used to confirm the suspected diagnosis before proceeding with definitive treatment. In general, if there is any disagreement between initial clinical suspicion and the frozen biopsy specimen, then it is preferable to perform a staged procedure, waiting for formal pathological confirmation.

3. TUMOR-LIKE LESIONS OF THE SPINE
3.1. OSTEOCHONDROMA

Osteochondromas of the spine account for less than 10% of all osteochondromata, and are rarely symptomatic *(19–21)* (Fig 1). They are not tumors, but separated portions of the growth plate that lag behind the growing bone. They continue to grow until their growth plate of origin closes *(21)*. They are, therefore, slow-growing masses that are typically painless, but can be associated with mechanical symptoms. As a whole, osteochondromas are usually diagnosed before the end of growth, but those involving the spine are often discovered later, often after trauma has rendered them symptomatic. Osteochondromas can occur as isolated events, or, can be part of multiple hereditary exostosis. Both manifestations of osteochondromas are more common in males than females *(19,22)*.

Gross histology is often all that is required for diagnosis. Osteochondromas are bony outgrowths from the underlying bone, covered by a thick cartilage cap. The marrow space of the underlying bone typically flows into and is continuous with the marrow space of the osteochondroma, helping to distinguish them from osteomas. This feature can often be observed on radiographs and/or CT scans, making diagnosis relatively easy.

Treatment typically consists of observation, with surgical resection restricted to those cases where the osteochondroma causes disabling mechanical and/or radicular symptoms. Recurrence after resection is low, and occurs when incomplete resections are performed. Fewer than 20 cases of cord compression from osteochondroma have been reported, and most were located in the cervical spine *(23)*. In a series of 16 such cases, 88% had good neurological recovery after resection, and no recurrences were reported *(23)*. Malignant transformation of osteochondromas into chondrosarcoma has been reported, and is most common in patients with multiple hereditary exostoses *(24)*. When this occurs, these lesions tend to be relatively low-grade tumors *(25)* that respond well to wide resection.

3.2. EOSINOPHILIC GRANULOMA

Eosinophilic granuloma (EG), also known as histiocytosis X or Langerhans' cell histiocytosis, represents a benign, self-limiting process that usually causes focal areas of well-demarcated bone resorption. The underlying etiology of this disorder is unknown. It characteristically afflicts individuals during their first two decades of life, and has a 2:1 predilection for males *(26)*. Although the spine is involved in 10 to 15% of cases *(1)*, the most commonly affected bones are typically the skull and flat bones of the pelvis, rib cage, and shoulder girdle. Within the spine, EG is most commonly localized to the vertebral body, resulting in collapse that can be observed on lateral radiographs such as the classic *vertebra plana*. Biopsy is usually necessary in cases of solitary lesions where the diagnosis is not evident. When biopsy confirms the diagnosis, curettage is usually the only indicated treatment. In cases of multifocal disease where biopsy is considered unnecessary, the lesions can be followed and most will resolve spontaneously *(27,28)*. Surgical intervention is indicated only in those cases of documented progression or where there is significant instability/deformity caused by the lesion. In lesions that are not amenable to surgical resection, low dose radiation therapy has been shown to be effective *(29)*.

In approx 10% of cases in a series by Schajowicz et al. *(30)*, EG was part of a larger symptom complex, notably Hand-Schüller-Christian (9%) and Letterer-Siwe (1.2%) diseases. In Hand-Schüller-Christian disease, the lesions are mulifocal and are associated with diabetes insipidus and exophthalmos *(31,32)*. Letterer-Siwe disease, the more acute form, is characterized by numerous small lesions involving nearly all bones with severe systemic symptoms such as fever, lymphadenopathy, and anemia *(32)*. Although Hand-Schüller-Christian disease is not generally fatal, Letterer-Siwe disease can cause death.

3.3. PAGET'S DISEASE

Paget's Disease is a metabolic disorder that occurs when the balance between osteoclast-mediated bone resorption and osteoblast-mediated bone formation is disrupted, resulting in bony pain and deformity *(33)*. The precise etiology of Paget's Disease is unclear. It predominantly afflicts individuals of northern European descent, and typically begins after the age of 50. Although Paget's Disease is an extremely common disorder (some studies have suggested that it occurs in up to 3% of the elderly population *[34]*), it is asymptomatic in approximately two-thirds of patients. Paget's Disease can be restricted to a single bone or it can be multifocal. It involves the lumbar and thoracic spine in 60 and 45% of cases, respectively *(35)*.

Paget's Disease is characterized by three distinct phases *(33)*, each of which can exist concurrently in different locations of the same bone. The first phase is characterized by bone resorption, during which osteoclasts resorb bone out of proportion to the bone's capacity to remodel. Radiographically, this phase appears as a radiolucency, and generally occurs early in the disease process. This stage is followed by an osteoblastic phase during which new bone formation predominates, however, the newly formed bone is not laid down in response to mechanical stresses, and, therefore, is more disorganized woven bone. Finally, the last phase is the so-called "burnt out" phase during which bone turn-over decreases, but the new bone is grossly thickened with a characteristic coarse trabecular appearance to the bone. The resulting hypertrophic bone often leads to nerve entrapment syndromes and deformity. Histologically, pagetoid bone is characterized by thick trabeculae that encroach on the marrow space and are remarkable for cement lines. The disjointed remodeling which occurs also leads to bone that is more susceptible to fracture. Treatment relies on medical management using bis-phosphonates, calcitonin, and other osteoclast inhibitors *(36)*. Surgery is indicated for pathological fractures and nerve entrapment.

A small cohort of patients with Paget's disease will develop a secondary sarcoma, an especially aggressive form of osteosarcoma that forms in pagetoid bone *(37)*. The high grade of these tumors, coupled with the more limited range of chemotherapeutic agents that can be administered to this age group, results in a 5-yr survival that is less than 10%. In every other respect, it is treated like high-grade osteosarcoma of the spine.

3.4. FIBROUS DYSPLASIA

In 1938, Lichtenstein *(38)* described fibrous dysplasia as a polyostotic disease. Shortly after in 1942 *(39)*, however, he recognized that both monostotic and polyostotic forms of the disease exist. Despite its recognition for over half a century, the etiology of fibrous dysplasia remains largely unknown, and no effective treatments have been developed to combat it. It is usually diagnosed during childhood, and demonstrates no significant gender predilection. Histologically, fibrous dysplasia is characterized by fibroblastic replacement of the marrow space, and trabecular seams that are composed of immature reactive bone in the shape of "chinese characters" (Fig. 2). The monostotic form accounts for 20% of cases, and typically follows a more benign course *(40,41)*. It is extremely rare in the spine, but 22 cases have been described in the literature, distrib-

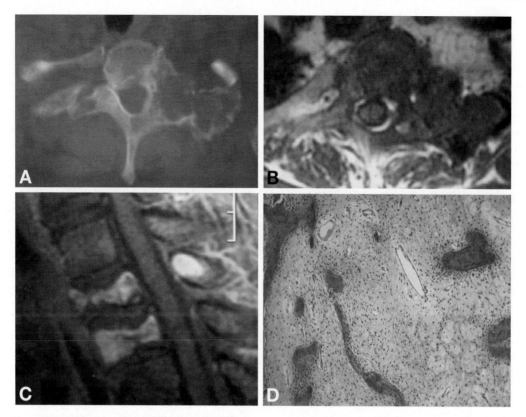

Fig. 2. A 41-yr-old male with history of neck and radicular arm pain. Initial radiographs provided inadequate visualization of the cervico-thoracic junction. (**A**) An axial computed tomography (CT) scan was obtained which demonstrated a left-sided eccentric lesion involving the pedicle of T_1, which was further imaged on magnetic resonance (**B,C**). A CT-directed biopsy was performed which yielded a pathologic specimen, (**D**), with fibrous replacement of the marrow and irregular bone spicules rimmed with osteoblasts most consistent with fibrous dysplasia. The patient underwent a C7–T1 corpectomy with C6–T2 strut instrumented fusion.

uted nearly equally throughout the cervical, thoracic, and lumbar spine *(40)*. Polyostotic fibrous dysplasia, although less common overall, accounts for the majority of cases involving the spine. The polyostotic form most often occurs in the setting of systemic endocrine abnormalities, such as hyperparathyroidism *(42)* and Cushing's Syndrome *(43)* or with McCune-Albright Syndrome *(44)*, which is characterized by pigmented cutaneous lesions and precocious puberty.

Treatment is largely supportive, with surgery reserved only for those cases where pathological fracture leads to unacceptable deformity and/or neurological compromise. Simple curettage has a high rate of recurrence, even when combined with local adjuvant therapy, and complete resection is often extremely difficult in the spine *(45)*. Therefore, close surveillance is important. Malignant transformation in either of the two forms of fibrous dysplasia is extremely rare, occurring in less than 1% of cases *(46)*.

3.5. ANEURYSMAL BONE CYST

Spinal involvement occurs in 10 to 30% of cases of aneurysmal bone cysts, making it one of the most commonly affected areas of the body *(47,48)* (Fig 3). When it occurs in the spine, it preferentially affects the thoraco-lumbar region and localizes to the posterior elements in 60% of cases *(47)*. Although aneurysmal bone may occur at any age, they most commonly occur during the first two decades of life, and are slightly more com-

mon in females *(48)*. Somewhat unique to aneurysmal bone cysts is their ability to involve adjacent vertebral segments, often as many as three in a row *(1)*.

Histologically, aneurysmal bone cysts are composed of multiple blood-filled chambers, each lined by a unique pseudo-endothelium. The cellular portion of the tumor is characterized by numerous giant cells in a background of spindle-shaped stromal cells. Although aneurysmal bone cysts generally contain cystic spaces, up to 7% are what is known as "solid aneurysmal bone cysts," and this variant is more frequent in the spine *(49)*. Radiographically, aneurysmal bone cysts cause cortical expansion and thinning, and internally, have a characteristic "bubbly" appearance created by the multiple cavernous chambers of the cyst. Large cysts can be easily detected on plain films, but smaller cysts may be missed. MRI is, perhaps, the most diagnostic imaging modality for aneurysmal bone cysts in that it demonstrates the multiple cysts within the lesion. Furthermore, the old areas of hemorrhage within each chamber separate into two phases, creating the nearly pathomneumonic "fluid–fluid" levels.

In the treament of aneurysmal bone cysts, removal of the lesion is typically accomplished by curettage, as opposed to marginal resection, given the technical difficulties involved with large resections in the spine. Local recurrence after curettage has been estimated at between 13 and 30%, and most of

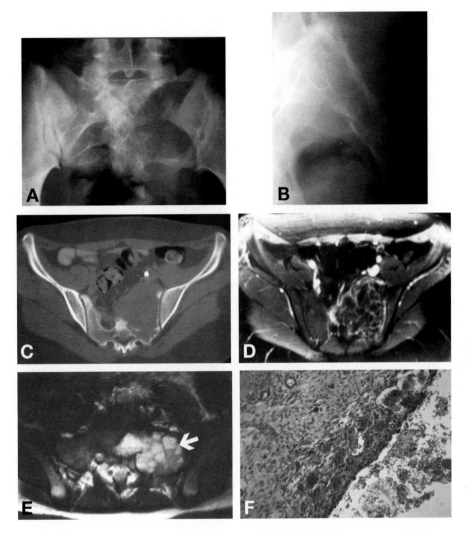

Fig. 3. A 16-yr-old female with 6-mo history of left hip pain associated with occasional numbness along the posterior aspect of the left leg. (**A,B**) Anteroposterior and lateral radiographs of the sacrum demonstrating a large, radiolucent lesion centered about the sacral ala of S1–S3. (**C**) A computed tomography (CT) scan reveals an expansile lesion with anterior extension that does not violate the sacro-iliac joint. A rim of mineralization, if present, is difficult to visualize on CT scan. (**D,E**) A magnetic resonance provides indicates that the lesion is composed of multiple chambers or cysts, and that "fluid-fluid" levels are present, indicating that the lesion is most likely an aneurysmal bone cyst. Apiration of the lesion produced blood without any malignant cells. An excision and curettage was performed with bone grafting of the resulting defect. The specimen was sent for pathological evaluation. (**F**) It is significant for a thick cyst lining containing numerous giant cells, and empty cystic spaces filled with hemorrhage.

these cases can be treated successfully by a repeat curettage *(48)*. Adjuvant treatments such as radiation therapy and embolization have less clear-cut indications, but may be useful supplemental therapies to reduce the rate of local recurrence *(46,50)*. The rate of malignant transformation is negligible.

4. PRIMARY BENIGN TUMORS OF THE SPINE

4.1. HEMANGIOMA (BENIGN HEMANGIOENDOTHELIOMA)

Although hemangiomas of the spine represent the most common tumor of the spine, they are also the least consequential. At autopsy, 11% of individuals are reported to have hemangiomas *(51)*, however, they rarely cause symptoms and are usually incidental findings on studies obtained for other reasons. Within the spine, the thoracic vertebrae are the most commonly affected

(52). Hemangiomas occur as singular lesions in approximately two-thirds of cases, and are characterized radiographically by vertical trabecular striations ressembling a "honeycomb" that most commonly involve the vertebral body. Plain radiographs alone can be sufficient in those lesions that involve greater than 30–40% of the vertebral body, however, CT/MRI may be more helpful in those lesions that are subtle or small *(53)*.

Neurological symptoms may occur as a result of neural compression caused by cortical expansion or soft tissue extension beyond the vertebral body. Hemangiomas are extremely radiosensitive, and low-dose radiation has been shown to be effective as a treatment for symptomatic lesions *(54,55)*. Similarly, embolization via angiography has been shown to be effective *(56,57)*. In those instances where pathological fracture or deformity result in instability or neurological compromise, surgical resection and stabilization may be indicated.

4.2. OSTEOID OSTEOMA

Osteoid osteoma was first described by Jaffe in *1955 (57)*. It occurs as a cortically based nidus of osteoid-producing cells surrounded by a dense halo of sclerosis, which may be the only radiographic sign at diagnosis. This lesion is usually diagnosed during the first three decades of life, with a peak incidence at age 15, and has a 2:1 male predominance *(58,59)*. Ten to twenty-five percent of all osteoid osteomas occur in the spine, and nearly 70% of painful juvenile scoliotic deformities are associated with osteoid osteoma *(4,60)*. Within the axial skeleton, osteoid osteoma most frequently involves the lumbar spine (59%), followed by the cervical (27%), thoracic (12%), and sacral spine (2%) *(61)*. In each case, it involves the posterior elements in 75% of cases *(59)*. Histologically, the lesion manifests itself as a nidus of highly vascular osteoid-producing spindle cells surrounded by dense sclerotic bone.

Pain is the most common presenting symptom, which is characteristically worse at night, and relieved by non-steroidal anti-inflammatory agents. The majority of scoliotic deformities associated with pain are caused by osteoid osteoma *(4,60)*, underscoring the need to perform a thorough evaluation for this tumor in any patient presenting with this complaint.

On plain radiographs, overlying bony structures often obscure the appearance of osteoid osteoma, making additional imaging studies necessary. The most sensitive study for osteoid osteoma is the bone scan, which targets the rapid bone turnover that is a hallmark of this lesion. Markedly increased uptake of technicium-99 occurs in the area of the lesion, often surrounded by a zone of diminished uptake, creates a distinctive target sign. Although bone scans represent perhaps the most sensitive test for osteoid osteoma, a CT scan is the most specific. Bone windows help to demonstrate the nidus found with osteoid osteoma.

Treatment of this disorder includes both medical and surgical options. Pain associated with osteoid osteoma, as a rule, responds to non-steroidal anti-inflammatory agents. Given the usually self-limited nature of osteoid osteoma, non-steroidal anti-inflammatory drugs (NSAIDs), and observation represent a treatment option. In cases that NSAIDs are either not tolerated or are contra-indicated, or when osteoid osteoma is associated with progressive scoliotic deformties, more aggressive therapies can be considered. Surgical resection involving "burr-down" excision *(62)* or marginal resection may be performed. Resection of the lesions results in reliable pain relief, and nearly all associated scoliotic deformities improved in a recent series of 16 patients *(63)*. Newer treatment modalities have emerged that are less invasive, including both CT-directed percutaneous excision *(64)* or radio-frequency ablation *(65)*. No malignant degeneration of osteoid osteoma have been documented in the literature.

4.3. OSTEOBLASTOMA

Histologically, osteoblastomas are often indistinguishable from osteoid osteoma except for their larger size, but the clinical features and natural history of these two disorders have notable differences (Fig. 4). Like osteoid osteoma, osteoblastoma preferentially affects males by a 2:1 margin and is normally diagnosed early in life *(66–68)*. Spine involvement is even more common in osteoblastoma, accounting for approx 41% of 147 cases reviewed by Marsh *(69)*, and lesions typically localize to the posterior elements in 55% of cases. This tumor has no discernable predilection for particular regions of the spine *(66)*.

The most common presenting symptom in patients with osteoblastoma is focal pain, that is less responsive to NSAIDs than the pain of an osteoid osteoma. The pain is more typically activity-related as opposed to night pain. Cortical expansion can result in impingement of neural elements, causing neurological complaints in nearly 50% of patients *(70)*, which further distinguishes it from osteoid osteoma. Painful scoliotic deformities can also occur in the setting of osteoblastoma, however, they account for a smaller proportion of patients than osteoid osteoma *(4)*.

Radiographically, osteoblastomas are more readily detected on plain radiographs than osteoid osteomas owing to their larger size (>2 cm), and their propensity to cause cortical expansion. The internal characteristics of osteoblastomas can be variable, but ossification is the predominant pattern, consistent with its osteoblastic origin. CT scans with bone windows currently represents the best diagnostic imaging modality for osteoblastoma, especially when combined with myelography for evaluation of neural compression.

Osteoblastoma is a slowly progressive lesion that does not normally respond to conservative management. Surgical resection of the lesion is therefore indicated, however, local recurrences occur in between 10 and 15% of cases, and can be as high as 50% in select high-grade sub-types of osteoblastoma *(66–68)*. Debate exists regarding the adequacy of curettage in the treatment of osteoblastoma, and whether marginal resection results in a lower risk of recurrence. Radiation therapy has not been conclusively shown to be an effective treatment for osteoblastoma *(70)*. Surgical treatment, whether simple curettage or resection, should be planned based on the location of the lesion, concomitant symptoms, and risk of morbidity. Unlike osteoid osteoma, the behavior of osteoblastomas can vary from slow-growing lesions to aggressive subtypes that appear very similar to osteosarcoma. In fact, aggressive osteoblastoma can be easily misdiagnosed as osteosarcoma, or visa versa. Cases of malignant transformation of osteoblastomas have been documented *(71)*, although it is conceivable that the initial lesion was diagnosed incorrectly.

4.4. GIANT CELL TUMOR

Giant cell tumors are borderline malignant tumors that can range in behavior from slow-growing, relatively innocuous tumors to locally aggressive tumors that metastasize. Therein lies many of the challenges underlying the diagnosis and treatment of giant cell tumors involving the spine. As a whole, the spine is a relatively common site of disease for giant cell tumors, comprising between 5 and 10% of all cases of giant cell tumor *(72–75)*. Unlike their appendicular counterparts, however, there is often a significant delay between the onset of symptoms and the diagnosis. Pain and radicular symptoms are the most common presenting complaint, and have often been present for several months before initial contact with a physician.

Spinal giant cell tumors are most commonly diagnosed during the third and fourth decades of life, and are slightly more frequent in women *(73,75)*. Within the axial skeleton, the sacrum is the most common region affected, and lesions are typically

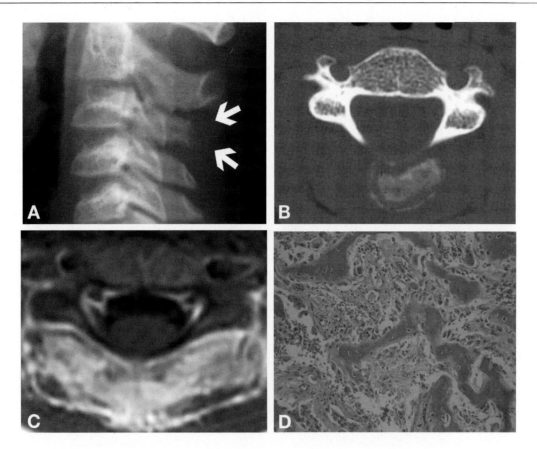

Fig. 4. A 10-yr-old male with neck pain and no neurological complaints. (A) Plain radiographs reveal a subtle radiolucent lesion involving the spinous process of C3. (B) Further imaging with computed tomography provides better visualization of the tumor and reveal intra-lesional ossification. (C) Magnetic resonance confirms that the spinal cord is not compressed by the lesion. Pre-operative imaging and clinical history strongly suggested that the lesion was an osteoblastoma. An *en-bloc* excision of the tumor and lamina of C3 was, therefore, performed. H and E staining of the specimen (D) confirmed the diagnosis of osteoblastoma.

found in the vertebral body. Histologically, giant cell tumors are characterized by numerous giant cells situated in a field of mononuclear cells. Cellular atypia is low to absent. Radiographically, plain films generally demonstrate a well-marginated radiolucent lesion with a variable amount of cortical expansion and local remodeling. Usually, even in the most aggressive case of giant cell tumor, a thin shell of cortical bone will remain at the periphery of the lesion, helping to distinguish it from malignant bone tumors. CT scan and MRI can be extremely helpful adjunctive study, especially if neurological compromise has occurred.

Giant cell tumors involving the spine are typically treated by curettage and local adjuvant therapy. *En-bloc* surgical resection is considered to be the optimal treatment of this disorder and appears to reduce the rate of local recurrence *(76)*. In the spine, the proximity of vital structures to the lesion, as well as the considerable morbidity associated with this approach, has limited the use of *en-bloc* resections in such cases. Embolization for giant cell tumors of the spine has also emerged as a potential new treatment for giant cell tumors, and currently can be used as an adjunct to intra-lesional resection *(77,78)*.

Giant cell tumors of the spine have a considerably worse prognosis than those in the appedicular skeleton, with recurrence rates reaching almost 80% in grade III giant cell tumors *(75)*. Furthermore, metastasis occurs in just under 10% of cases,

and unresectable local recurrences have resulted in patient death. When an isolated metastasis develops, surgical resection is the treatment of choice, given that no systemic therapy is available for the treatment of giant cell tumors of bone.

4.5. CHONDROBLASTOMA

Chondroblastoma of the spine is extremely rare, and publications are mostly limited to case reports (Fig. 5). Still, most cases have been diagnosed during the second to third decade, suggesting that the demographic profile of chondroblastomas involving the spine may parallel that for appendicular cases *(79,80)*. In a recent review of 12 cases by Kurth et al. *(80)*, 50% of chondroblastomas arose in the cervical spine, with the remaining lesions roughly divided evenly between the thoracic and lumbar spine. The most common presenting signs were pain and neurological compromise.

Radiographic evaluation of spinal chondroblastomas generally reveals a well-marginated radiolucent lesion. Internal matrix calcification may be apparent on plain radiographs or CT scan, however, this is not a universal finding in all cases of chondroblastoma. Because of the limited number of cases, it is difficult to define a clear predilection for either the anterior or posterior spinal elements, however, most cases have been reported in the posterior elements. On histology, chondroblastomas are distinguished by polygonal chondroblasts, with a variable

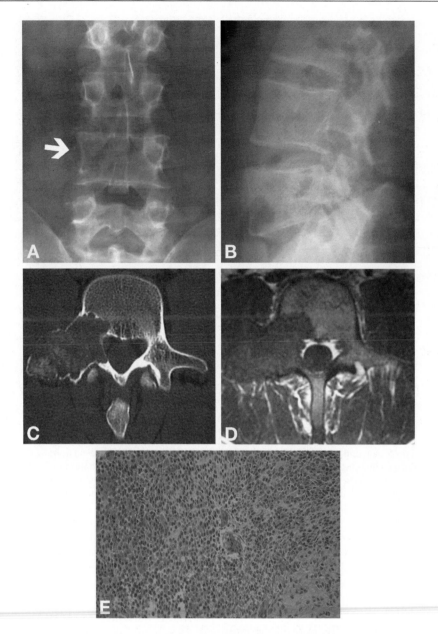

Fig. 5. A 29-yr-old male with a 2-yr history of lower back pain that has slowly become worse. The pain occasionally radiated to the right thigh, however, he did not complain of paresthesias or weakness. (**A,B**) Anteroposterior and lateral radiographs, significant for a classic "winking-owl" sign at the right pedicle of L4. Subsequent computed tomography scan (**C**) reveals an expansile lesion involving the right pedicle and transverse process of L4, containing a limited amount of intra-lesional mineralization. (**D**) Magnetic resonance further demonstrates the extent of the lesion, and suggests that the lesion may be compressing L3 nerve root. No central compression was present. Clinical history and imaging suggested a benign lesion, although a precise diagnosis was not possible. Osteoblastoma was considered to be the most likely diagnosis, therefore, an excision was performed with posterior instrumented L3–L5 fusion. The pathology specimen (**E**) contained polygonal chondroblasts with numerous giant cells, indicating that the lesion was, in reality, chondroblastoma.

amount of eosinophilic cytoplasm and oval nuclei. Chondroblastomas usually contain numerous osteoclast-like giant cells, and matrix calcification, when present, often has a distinctive "chicken-wire" appearance that is a hallmark of this lesion. Cellular atypia can vary from moderate to high, which is thought to reflect its spectrum of behavior from slowly progressive local growth to aggressive local growth and metastatic spread.

Treatment of these lesions consists predominantly of curettage or excision, however, it is not clear whether this treatment is equally effective in the spine, given the limited number of cases. The recurrence rate for chondroblastomas of the spine is, likewise, unclear. Kurth et al. *(80)* report a case of multiple recurrences, the first occurring as late as 7 yr after initial resection. The lack of lengthy follow-up on other case reports, therefore, precludes a more detailed estimation of recurrence after excision of spinal chondroblastomas. Similarly, the rate of metastatic spread and/or malignant transformation is unknown for lesions involving the spine.

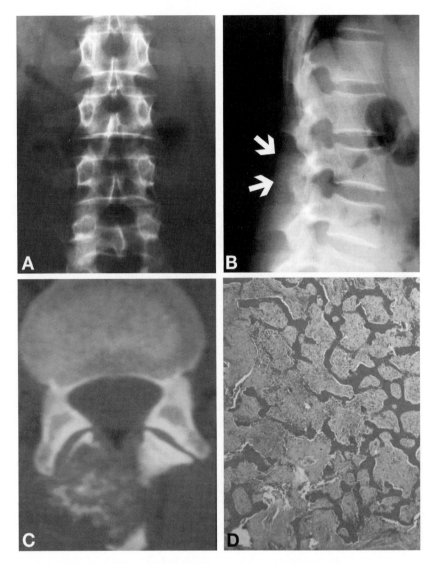

Fig. 6. A 29-yr-old male with a several-year history of mid- to lower back pain. (**A,B**) Anteroposterior and lateral radiographs initially taken demonstrated a subtle, but apparent, radiodensity within the posterior elements of the L3 vertebra. (**C**) A computed tomography scan of the lesion was obtained approx 2 yr later when symptoms failed to resolve, revealing an expansile lesion originating in the spinous process and lamina adjacent to the right facet. The patient was then referred for treatment. Significant intra-lesional mineralization was present, and based on this, the lesion was felt to be most consistent with an osteoblastoma. A marginal resection was performed, and the tissue sent for pathological diagnosis. (**D**) The specimen exhibited abnormal, malignant osteoblasts that stained for vimentin. The cells also demonstrated a permeative pattern resulting in a formal diagnosis of osteosarcoma. The patient was subsequently given chemotherapy, however, developed bilateral pulmonary metastases and eventually succumbed to his disease.

5. PRIMARY MALIGNANT TUMORS OF THE SPINE

5.1. OSTEOSARCOMA

Osteosarcoma of the spine carries with it an especially bleak prognosis *(81,82)*. Although lesions tend to be diagnosed earlier in the spine owing to neurological compression early in the tumor's course, prognosis is often compromised by technical difficulties in achieving a wide resection during surgical resection (Fig. 6).

Osteosarcoma of the spine accounts for approx 2% of all osteosarcomas throughout the body, and 3 to 14% of malignant tumors involving the spine *(81,82)*. Most tumors arise in the lumbosacral region, and involve the vertebral body in up to 90% of cases *(83)*. As an entity, osteosarcoma includes any

malignant spindle tumor that produces osteoid, however, this encompasses a variety of histologic sub-types. Treatment and prognosis are, therefore, dependent on appropriate histologic diagnosis. There is a bimodal distribution in the age of presentation for osteosarcomas involving the spine, with an earlier age group (10–25 yr) representing the more "classic" osteosarcoma, and a second group of individuals over 50 yr presenting with secondary osteosarcomas. When viewed collectively, osteosarcoma of the spine has a generally worse prognosis, and occurs in older age groups when compared to appendicular osteosarcoma *(83)*.

Radiographically, osteosarcomas can range in appearance. The primary lesion can be either radiolucent or radiodense, with prominent periosteal reaction and usually soft tissue extension. The internal characteristics of the lesion demonstrate ossification consistent with its degree of osteoid production. Osteosarcoma of the spine originates at a slightly higher rate in the lumbo-sacral region, and arises eccentrically from the anterior elements in nearly 80 to 90% of cases *(82,83)*. Axial imaging provides better detail on the soft tissue extent of the tumor and, therefore, are critical for preoperative planning.

Numerous histologic sub-types of osteosarcoma exist, designated by its location (central, parosteal, periosteal), grade (low vs high), predominant cell type (osteoblastic, chondroblastic, fibroblastic), or etiology (radiation-induced, Paget's sarcoma). With the exception of low-grade lesions such as parosteal osteosarcomas, these patients receive preoperative chemotherapy followed by surgical resection and usually adjuvant therapy. As with other malignant lesions of the spine, wide resection, or even marginal resections, are often not possible, making radiation therapy and adjuvant chemotherapy necessary to treat the residual disease. Evaluations of the outcome in patients with osteosarcoma of the spine have been hampered by its relative rarity. Most survivors have been described as case reports, and not for the purpose of determining median survival time or 5-yr survival rates. In a recent review of 22 patients, the median survival in cases of spinal osteosarcoma was 23 mo *(84)*. Metastasis at diagnosis, large size, sacral location, and intralesional resections were associated with adverse outcomes *(84)*. Collectively, only three patients were observed to live beyond 6 yr.

5.2. CHONDROSARCOMA

After chordomas, chondrosarcoma is the most common primary malignant tumor of bone in the spine, accounting for approx 7 to 12% of all spine tumors *(85,86)*. Unlike osteosarcoma and Ewing's sarcomas, chondrosarcomas occur later in life, with average age at diagnosis of 45 yr, and are more common in men *(51,87)*. Chondrosarcoma can vary considerably in its behavior, and is generally described according to grades I–III, with each grade corresponding to an increasing tendancy for metastasis and, therefore, a poorer prognosis.

Plain films typically demonstrate a centrally based destructive lesion with calcification. In low-grade chondrosarcoma, the lesion can cause scalloping of the bony cortex or cortical expansion. In high-grade lesion, the tumor can erode through the cortex and form a large extra-osseous mass, also containing diffuse areas of calcification. Although X-rays may be extremely helpful, MRI and/or CT scan provides more detailed information regarding the extent of the tumor both inside and outside the bone of origin. As with all malignant tumors, generally staging studies should also be performed to evaluate for metastatic disease at presentation.

Radiographic diagnosis is generally confirmed through biopsy and pathological evaluation of tissue samples. The grade of the tumor is essential to determine prognosis, and is based primarily on the cellularity of the tumor and pleiomorphism of the tumor cells. Such information is also useful to determine the utility of adjuvant treatments such as radiation therapy.

The treatment of chondrosarcoma is complicated by its lack of response to conventional chemotherapy and/or standard radiation therapy. No clinical trials have demonstrated any survival benefit among patients receiving chemotherapy, and the use of radiation is controversial. This leaves surgical excision as the mainstay of treatment for chondrosarcoma. Not unexpectedly, survival in chondrosarcoma is, therefore, closely associated with adequate excision and uncontaminated margins *(39,88)*. Within the spine, such resections are often unfeasible without significant morbidity, resulting in a poorer prognosis in general for patients with chondrosarcoma of the spine *(85,86,89)*. Median survival in patients with chondrosarcoma of the spine has been estimated to be approx 6 yr. In the chondrosarcoma of the upper cervical spine and skull base, it has been claimed that long-term survival can be increased to approx 90% when surgical resection is combined with proton-photon therapy *(90)*. Proton therapy is especially attractive for the treatment of slow-growing tumors, such as chondrosarcoma and chordoma, and is more sparing of the spinal cord than standard radiation therapy.

5.3. EWING'S SARCOMA (FIG. 7)

Ewing's sarcoma of the spine is a relatively infrequent entity, accounting for only 8% of a series of 402 patients with Ewing's sarcoma reported by Dahlin and Unni *(91)*. It is actually more common for this tumor to metastasize to the spine from other locations, than it is for it to originate there as a primary tumor. Its clinical features are similar to that for all patients with Ewing's Sarcoma, namely it most commonly arises during the second decade of life and affects males more frequently than females *(92,93)*. It is also extremely infrequent in African-American individuals.

The most common presenting symptom among patients with Ewing's sarcoma is pain, most commonly in the sacrococcygeal area. Although cases of Ewing's sarcoma involving the cervical spine exist, they are extremely rare. Osseous findings in Ewing's sarcoma can be extremely subtle. Plain radiographs can, therefore, appear normal, often belying a large soft tissue mass. In this respect, a CT scan or MRI may be far more informative than plain films at defining tumor extent. These imaging studies usually will demonstrate a large mass originating in the vertebral body, with variable amounts of internal mineralization. Laboratory tests such as C-reactive protein and electron spin resonance are often elevated, and can therefore be useful adjuncts for the diagnosis of Ewing's. Histologically, Ewing's sarcomas are composed of sheets of small blue cells, occasionally forming psuedo-rosettes around areas of necrosis. Nearly all Ewing's sarcomas possess a characteristic t11:22 translocation that helps to distinguish it further from other small blue cell tumors.

The treatment of Ewing's sarcoma has varied considerably in the past, however, it is currently treated using a combination of chemotherapy, surgical resection, and radiation therapy, each of which are effective against this tumor individually *(94)*. The use of adjuvant treatments is especially critical given the difficulty of performing wide resection in the spine. The 5-yr survival among a series of 33 patients with Ewing's sarcoma of the vertebral column treated at St. Jude Children's hospital was approx 48% *(95)*. They also found that smaller tumor size at diagnosis and localized disease predicted a better outcome. Although PNET comprises a separate class of tumors, they are

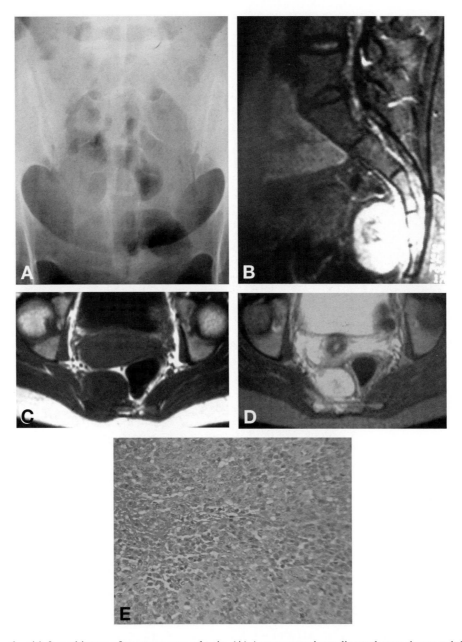

Fig. 7. A 23-yr-old female with 2-mo history of vague coccygeal pain. (A) Anteroposterior radiograph may show a subtle radiolucency in the right inferior aspect of the sacrum. (B–D) Magnetic resonance sagittal and axial images demonstrate a large anterior soft tissue mass originating from the inferior sacrum. (E) A needle biopsy was performed, yielding tissue that was notable for patternless sheets of small blue cells that stained positive for Ewing's specific antigen. Based on a diagnosis of Ewing's sarcoma, she received preoperative chemotherapy, followed by partial sacrectomy and radiation therapy.

closely related to Ewing's tumor both clinically and histologically. Even the t11:22 translocation, the hallmark of Ewing's sarcoma, is a frequent finding in PNET, suggesting that both tumors may represent opposite ends of a single continuum and not completely distinct entities. In every other respect, PNETs are treated much like Ewing's sarcomas, and have a similar prognosis.

5.4 CHORDOMA

Chordomas are the most common primary malignant tumors of the spine, and, unlike the other malignant tumors discussed, they do not normally occur outside of the spine (Fig. 8). They

account for 1 to 4% of all primary bone tumors, and 20% of those arising in the spine (51,96–98). Originating from remnants of the notochord, they typically involve either the sacrococcygeal or spheno-occipital regions of the axial skeleton. The average age at diagnosis is 56, however, they can occur in almost any age group. Sacro-lumbar chordomas have a twofold predilection for males over females (51,97–99).

Clinical presentation is often subtle, with a gradual onset of neurological symptoms, including pain, numbness, motor weakness, and incontinence/constipation. Chordomas are slowly growing lesions and are often quite large when initially

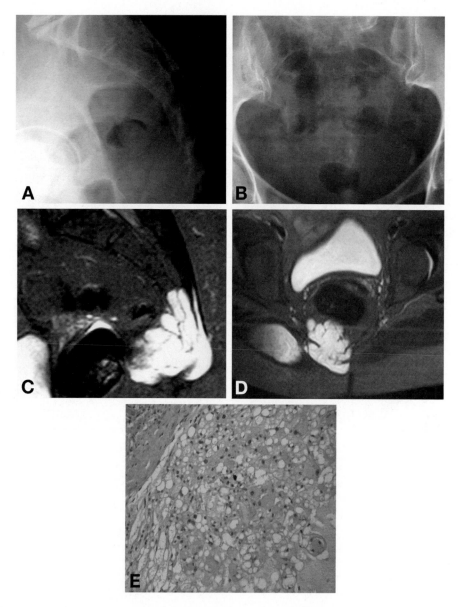

Fig. 8. A 58-yr-old female with vague buttocks' pain, mild constipation, and a mass for 4 mo. (**A,B**) Lateral and anteroposterior radiographs demonstrate a radiolucent lesion involving the right inferior aspect of the sacrum. (**C,D**) Magnetic resonance imaging reveals a multi-lobulated mass extending anterior to the sacrum with high signal on T2-weighted images. Based on these findings, the patient underwent a computed tomography-directed biopsy of the lesion. (**E**) The resulting tissue was notably myxoid, containing chords of multi-vacuolated "physaliphorous" cells. With a diagnosis of chordoma, she underwent a wide resection with partial sacrectomy for treatment.

discovered. When located in the sacrum, the mass usually protrudes anteriorly, thereby preventing the lesion from causing a noticeable external mass.

On radiographic evaluation, the bone from which the tumor arises may demonstrate noticeable changes, but the most impressive feature of chordomas is the large soft tissue mass. Unless a significant amount of internal calcification is present, the soft tissue component can be missed or underestimated on the basis of plain radiographs, and generally requires either a CT scan or MRI for definitive evaluation. On MRI, chordomas are lobulated masses, with a distinctly myxoid, or mucinous, consistency. Because they are generally slow-growing tumors, they are associated with a pseudocapsule.

The histologic appearance of chordomas can very from relatively cellular masses to fluid-filled cysts. Classically, they are composed of chords of physaliphorous cells that are organized into lobules. Because of the variation in their histological appearance, they can be mistaken for myxoid lesions and certain adenocarcinomas.

Similar to chondrosarcoma, chordomas demonstrate a poor response to standard radiotherapy and chemotherapy. Chordomas of the spheno-occipital junction and upper cervical spine have been shown to be responsive to proton therapy (90), especially in men (100). Surgical excision with wide margins, therefore, offers the most reliable means to cure these patients, whether used alone or in combination with adjuvant proton

Table 2
Distribution of Primary Tumors Within the Vertebral Column

	Non-Tumors			Benign Tumors				Malignant Tumors			
	Fibrous Dysplasia	Osteochondroma	Aneurysmal Bone Cyst	Chondroblastoma	Giant Cell Tumor	Osteoblastoma	Osteoid Osteoma	Chondrosarcoma	Chordoma	Ewing's Sarcoma	Osteosarcoma

treatment. The average 10-yr survival among patients with sacral chordomas is 20 to 40% *(99,101)*, usually owing to recurrence and direct spread of the tumor. Clival chordomas have a uniformly worse prognosis, likely because of the technical difficulties in performing wide resection at the spheno-occipital junction *(101)*. The rate of metastasis varies widely in different series, ranging from 10 to 27% for sacral lesions *(99,102)*, however, this rarely represents the cause of death in patients with chordomas.

REFERENCES

1. Weinstein JN, McLain RF. Primary tumors of the spine. Spine 1987; 12:843–851.
2. Masaryk TJ. Neoplastic disease of the spine. Radiol Clin North Am 1991; 29:829–845.
3. Haibach H, Farrell C, Gaines RW. Osteoid osteoma of the spine: surgically correctable cause of painful scoliosis. CMAJ 1986; 135:895–899.
4. Pettine KA, Klassen RA. Osteoid-osteoma and osteoblastoma of the spine. J Bone Joint Surg Am 1986; 68:354–361.
5. Janin Y, Epstein JA, Carras R, Khan A. Osteoid osteomas and osteoblastomas of the spine. Neurosurgery 1981; 8:31–38.
6. Park YK, Ryu KN, Han CS, Bae DK. Multifocal, metachronous giant-cell tumor of the ulna. A case report. J Bone Joint Surg Am 1999; 81:409–413.
7. Kos CB, Taconis WK, Fidler MW, ten Velden JJ. Multifocal giant cell tumors in the spine. A case report. Spine 1997; 22:821–822.
8. Damron TA, Sim FH, Unni KK. Multicentric chondrosarcomas. Clin Orthop 1996:211–219.
9. Enneking WF, Kagan A. The implications of "skip" metastases in osteosarcoma. Clin Orthop 1975:33–41.
10. Enneking WF, Kagan A. "Skip" metastases in osteosarcoma. Cancer 1975; 36:2192–2205.
11. Wuisman P, Enneking WF. Prognosis for patients who have osteosarcoma with skip metastasis. J Bone Joint Surg Am 1990; 72:60–68.
12. Enneking WF. Staging of musculoskeletal tumors. In: F EW, ed. Musculoskeletal tumor surgery. New York, NY: Churchill Livingstone; 1983:87.
13. Kay RM, Eckardt JJ, Seeger LL, Mirra JM, Hak DJ. Pulmonary metastasis of benign giant cell tumor of bone. Six histologically confirmed cases, including one of spontaneous regression. Clin Orthop 1994:219–30.
14. Huvos AG. "Benign" metastasis in giant cell tumor of bone. Hum Pathol 1981; 12:1151.
15. Ramappa AJ, Lee FY, Tang P, Carlson JR, Gebhardt MC, Mankin HJ. Chondroblastoma of bone. J Bone Joint Surg Am 2000; 82A:1140–1145.
16. Birch PJ, Buchanan R, Golding P, Pringle JA. Chondroblastoma of the rib with widespread bone metastases. Histopathology 1994; 25:583–585.
17. Enneking WF, Spanier SS, Goodman MA. A system for the surgical staging of musculoskeletal sarcoma. Clin Orthop 1980:106–120.
18. Hart RA, Boriani S, Biagini R, Currier B, Weinstein JN. A system for surgical staging and management of spine tumors. A clinical outcome study of giant cell tumors of the spine. Spine 1997; 22:1773–1783.
19. Jose Alcaraz Mexia M, Izquierdo Nunez E, Santonja Garriga C, Maria Salgado Salinas R. Osteochondroma of the thoracic spine and scoliosis. Spine 2001; 26:1082–1085.
20. Roblot P, Alcalay M, Cazenave-Roblot F, Levy P, Bontoux D. Osteochondroma of the thoracic spine. Report of a case and review of the literature. Spine 1990; 15:240–243.
21. Albrecht S, Crutchfield JS, SeGall GK. On spinal osteochondromas. J Neurosurg 1992; 77:247–252.
22. Khosla A, Martin DS, Awwad EE. The solitary intraspinal vertebral osteochondroma. An unusual cause of compressive myelopathy: features and literature review. Spine 1999; 24:77–81.

23. Weinstein JN, McLain RF. Tumors of the Spine. In: Rothman RH, Simeone FA, eds. The Spine. Vol. 2. Philadelphia, PA: W. B. Saunders Company; 1992:1279–1318.

24. Willms R, Hartwig CH, Bohm P, Sell S. Malignant transformation of a multiple cartilaginous exostosis–a case report. Int Orthop 1997; 21:133–136.

25. Norman A, Sissons HA. Radiographic hallmarks of peripheral chondrosarcoma. Radiology 1984; 151:589–596.

26. Silberstein MJ, Sundaram M, Akbarnia B, Luisiri A, McGuire M. Eosinophilic granuloma of the spine. Orthopedics 1985; 8:264, 267–74.

27. Nesbit ME, Kieffer S, D'Angio GJ. Reconstitution of vertebral height in histiocytosis X: a long-term follow-up. J Bone Joint Surg Am 1969; 51:1360–1368.

28. Seimon LP. Eosinophil granuloma of the spine. J Pediatr Orthop 1981; 1:371–376.

29. Green NE, Robertson WW, Jr., Kilroy AW. Eosinophilic granuloma of the spine with associated neural deficit. Report of three cases. J Bone Joint Surg Am 1980; 62:1198–1202.

30. Schajowicz F, Slullitel J. Eosinophilic granuloma of bone and its relationship to Hand-Schuller- Christian and Letterer-Siwe syndromes. J Bone Joint Surg Br 1973; 55:545–565.

31. Islinger RB, Kuklo TR, Owens BD, et al. Langerhans' cell histiocytosis in patients older than 21 years. Clin Orthop 2000:231–235.

32. Vogel JM, Vogel P. Idiopathic histiocytosis: a discussion of eosinophilic granuloma, the Hand-Schuller-Christian syndrome, and the Letterer-Siwe syndrome. Semin Hematol 1972; 9:349–369.

33. Singer FR. Paget's Disease of Bone. Topics in Bone and Mineral Disorders. New York, NY: Plenum Medical Book Co; 1977.

34. Altman RD, Bloch DA, Hochberg MC, Murphy WA. Prevalence of pelvic Paget's disease of bone in the United States. J Bone Miner Res 2000; 15:461–465.

35. Meunier PJ, Salson C, Mathieu L, et al. Skeletal distribution and biochemical parameters of Paget's disease. Clin Orthop 1987:37–44.

36. Noor M, Shoback D. Paget's disease of bone: diagnosis and treatment update. Curr Rheumatol Rep 2000; 2:67–73.

37. Moore TE, King AR, Kathol MH, el-Khoury GY, Palmer R, Downey PR. Sarcoma in Paget disease of bone: clinical, radiologic, and pathologic features in 22 cases. AJR Am J Roentgenol 1991; 156:1199–1203.

38. Lichtenstein L. Polyostotic fibrous dysplasia. Arch Surg 1938; 36:874–898.

39. Lichtenstein L, Jaffe HL. Fibrous dysplasia of bone. Arch Pathol 1942; 33:777–816.

40. Chow LT, Griffith J, Chow WH, Kumta SM. Monostotic fibrous dysplasia of the spine: report of a case involving the lumbar transverse process and review of the literature. Arch Orthop Trauma Surg 2000; 120:460–464.

41. Wright JF, Stoker DJ. Fibrous dysplasia of the spine. Clin Radiol 1988; 39:523–527.

42. Hammami MM, al-Zahrani A, Butt A, Vencer LJ, Hussain SS. Primary hyperparathyroidism-associated polyostotic fibrous dysplasia: absence of McCune-Albright syndrome mutations. J Endocrinol Invest 1997; 20:552–558.

43. Danon M, Robboy SJ, Kim S, Scully R, Crawford JD. Cushing syndrome, sexual precocity, and polyostotic fibrous dysplasia (Albright syndrome) in infancy. J Pediatr 1975; 87:917–921.

44. Cohen MM, Jr., Howell RE. Etiology of fibrous dysplasia and McCune-Albright syndrome. Int J Oral Maxillofac Surg 1999; 28:366–371.

45. Nabarro MN, Giblin PE. Monostotic fibrous dysplasia of the thoracic spine. Spine 1994; 19:463–465.

46. Rodenberg J, Jensen OM, Keller J, Nielsen OS, Bunger C, Jurik AG. Fibrous dysplasia of the spine, costae and hemipelvis with sarcomatous transformation. Skeletal Radiol 1996; 25:682–684.

47. Koci TM, Mehringer CM, Yamagata N, Chiang F. Aneurysmal bone cyst of the thoracic spine: evolution after particulate embolization. AJNR Am J Neuroradiol 1995; 16:857–860.

48. Kransdorf MJ, Sweet DE. Aneurysmal bone cyst: concept, controversy, clinical presentation, and imaging. AJR Am J Roentgenol 1995; 164:573–580.

49. Sanerkin NG, Mott MG, Roylance J. An unusual intraosseous lesion with fibroblastic, osteoclastic, osteoblastic, aneurysmal and fibromyxoid elements. "Solid" variant of aneurysmal bone cyst. Cancer 1983; 51:2278–2286.

50. Cory DA, Fritsch SA, Cohen MD, et al. Aneurysmal bone cysts: imaging findings and embolotherapy. AJR Am J Roentgenol 1989; 153:369–373.

51. Huvos AG. Bone Tumors: Diagnosis, Treatment, and Prognosis. Philadelphia, PA: Saunders; 1991.

52. Robbins LR, Fountain EN. Hemangioma of cervical vertebras with spinal cord compression. N Engl J Med 1958; 258:685–687.

53. Healy M, Herz DA, Pearl L. Spinal hemangiomas. Neurosurgery 1983; 13:689–691.

54. Glanzmann C, Rust M, Horst W. [Irradiation therapy of vertebral angiomas: results in 62 patients during the years 1939 to 1975 (author's transl)]. Strahlentherapie 1977; 153:522–525.

55. Faria SL, Schlupp WR, Chiminazzo H, Jr. Radiotherapy in the treatment of vertebral hemangiomas. Int J Radiat Oncol Biol Phys 1985; 11:387–390.

56. Hekster RE, Endtz LJ. Spinal-cord compression caused by vertebral haemangioma relieved by percutaneous catheter embolisation: 15 years later. Neuroradiology 1987; 29:101.

57. Hekster RE, Luyendijk W, Tan TI. Spinal-cord compression caused by vertebral haemangioma relieved by percutaneous catheter embolisation. Neuroradiology 1972; 3:160–164.

58. Greenspan A. Benign bone-forming lesions: osteoma, osteoid osteoma, and osteoblastoma. Clinical, imaging, pathologic, and differential considerations. Skeletal Radiol 1993; 22:485–500.

59. Azouz EM, Kozlowski K, Marton D, Sprague P, Zerhouni A, Asselah F. Osteoid osteoma and osteoblastoma of the spine in children. Report of 22 cases with brief literature review. Pediatr Radiol 1986; 16:25–31.

60. Mehta MH. Pain provoked scoliosis. Observations on the evolution of the deformity. Clin Orthop 1978:58–65.

61. Gamba JL, Martinez S, Apple J, Harrelson JM, Nunley JA. Computed tomography of axial skeletal osteoid osteomas. AJR Am J Roentgenol 1984; 142:769–772.

62. Ward WG, Eckardt JJ, Shayestehfar S, Mirra J, Grogan T, Oppenheim W. Osteoid osteoma diagnosis and management with low morbidity. Clin Orthop 1993:229–235.

63. Ransford AO, Pozo JL, Hutton PA, Kirwan EO. The behaviour pattern of the scoliosis associated with osteoid osteoma or osteoblastoma of the spine. J Bone Joint Surg Br 1984; 66:16–20.

64. Poey C, Clement JL, Baunin C, et al. Percutaneous extraction of an osteoid osteoma of the lumbar spine under CT guidance. J Comput Assist Tomogr 1991; 15:1056–1058.

65. Osti OL, Sebben R. High-frequency radio-wave ablation of osteoid osteoma in the lumbar spine. Eur Spine J 1998; 7:422–425.

66. Kroon HM, Schurmans J. Osteoblastoma: clinical and radiologic findings in 98 new cases. Radiology 1990; 175:783–790.

67. Lucas DR, Unni KK, McLeod RA, O'Connor MI, Sim FH. Osteoblastoma: clinicopathologic study of 306 cases. Hum Pathol 1994; 25:117–134.

68. McLeod RA, Dahlin DC, Beabout JW. The spectrum of osteoblastoma. Am J Roentgenol 1976; 126:321–325.

69. Marsh BW, Bonfiglio M, Brady LP, Enneking WF. Benign osteoblastoma: range of manifestations. J Bone Joint Surg Am 1975; 57:1–9.

70. Sypert GW. Osteoid osteoma and osteoblastoma of the spine. In: Sundaresan N, Schmidek HH, Schiller AL, Rosenthal DI, eds. Tumors of the Spine: Diagnosis and Clinical Management. Vol. 1. Philadelphia, PA: W. B. Saunders Company; 1990:117–127.

71. Mayer L. Malignant degeneration of so-called benign osteoblastoma. Bull Hosp Joint Dis 1967; 28:4–13.

72. Schwimer SR, Bassett LW, Mancuso AA, Mirra JM, Dawson EG. Giant cell tumor of the cervicothoracic spine. AJR Am J Roentgenol 1981; 136:63–67.

73. Smith J, Wixon D, Watson RC. Giant-cell tumor of the sacrum. Clinical and radiologic features in 13 patients. J Can Assoc Radiol 1979; 30:34–39.

74. Bidwell JK, Young JW, Khalluff E. Giant cell tumor of the spine: computed tomography appearance and review of the literature. J Comput Tomogr 1987; 11:307–311.

75. Campanacci M, Boriani S, Giunti A. Giant cell tumors of the spine. In: Sundaresan N, Schmidek HH, Schiller AL, Rosenthal DI, eds. Tumors of the Spine: Diagnosis and Clinical Management. Philadelphia, PA: W. B. Saunders Company; 1990:163–172.

76. Fidler MW. Surgical treatment of giant cell tumours of the thoracic and lumbar spine: report of nine patients. Eur Spine J 2001; 10:69–77.

77. Laus M, Zappoli FA, Malaguti MC, Alfonso C. Intralesional surgery of primary tumors of the anterior cervical column. Chir Organi Mov 1998; 83:43–51.

78. Misasi N, Sadile F. Selective arterial embolization in orthopaedic pathology. Analysis of long-term results. Chir Organi Mov 1991; 76:311–316.

79. Leung LY, Shu SJ, Chan MK, Chan CH. Chondroblastoma of the lumbar vertebra. Skeletal Radiol 2001; 30:710–713.

80. Kurth AA, Warzecha J, Rittmeister M, Schmitt E, Hovy L. Recurrent chondroblastoma of the upper thoracic spine. A case report and review of the literature. Arch Orthop Trauma Surg 2000; 120:544–547.

81. Barwick KW, Huvos AG, Smith J. Primary osteogenic sarcoma of the vertebral column: a clinicopathologic correlation of ten patients. Cancer 1980; 46:595–604.

82. Shives TC, Dahlin DC, Sim FH, Pritchard DJ, Earle JD. Osteosarcoma of the spine. J Bone Joint Surg Am 1986; 68:660–668.

83. Sundaresan N, Schiller AL, Rosenthal DI. Osteosarcoma of the spine. In: Sundaresan N, Schmidek HH, Schiller AL, Rosenthal DI, eds. Tumors of the Spine: Diagnosis and Clinical Management. Philadelphia, PA: W. B. Saunders Company; 1990:128–145.

84. Ozaki T, Flege S, Liljenqvist U, et al. Osteosarcoma of the spine: experience of the Cooperative Osteosarcoma Study Group. Cancer 2002; 94:1069–1077.

85. Hirsh LF, Thanki A, Spector HB. Primary spinal chondrosarcoma with eighteen-year follow-up: case report and literature review. Neurosurgery 1984; 14:747–749.

86. Shives TC, McLeod RA, Unni KK, Schray MF. Chondrosarcoma of the spine. J Bone Joint Surg Am 1989; 71:1158–1165.

87. Aprin H, Riseborough EJ, Hall JE. Chondrosarcoma in children and adolescents. Clin Orthop 1982:226–232.

88. Bergh P, Gunterberg B, Meis-Kindblom JM, Kindblom LG. Prognostic factors and outcome of pelvic, sacral, and spinal chondrosarcomas: a center-based study of 69 cases. Cancer 2001; 91:1201–1212.

89. Camins MB, Duncan AW, Smith J, Marcove RC. Chondrosarcoma of the spine. Spine 1978; 3:202–209.

90. Habrand JL, Schlienger P, Schwartz L, et al. Clinical applications of proton therapy. Experiences and ongoing studies. Radiat Environ Biophys 1995; 34:41–44.

91. Dahlin DC, Unni KK. Bone Tumors: General Aspects and Data on 8,542 Cases. Springfield, IL: Thomas; 1986.

92. Pilepich MV, Vietti TJ, Nesbit ME, et al. Ewing's sarcoma of the vertebral column. Int J Radiat Oncol Biol Phys 1981; 7:27–31.

93. Kornberg M. Primary Ewing's sarcoma of the spine. A review and case report. Spine 1986; 11:54–57.

94. Sharafuddin MJ, Haddad FS, Hitchon PW, Haddad SF, el-Khoury GY. Treatment options in primary Ewing's sarcoma of the spine: report of seven cases and review of the literature. Neurosurgery 1992; 30:610–619.

95. Venkateswaran L, Rodriguez-Galindo C, Merchant TE, Poquette CA, Rao BN, Pappo AS. Primary Ewing tumor of the vertebrae: clinical characteristics, prognostic factors, and outcome. Med Pediatr Oncol 2001; 37:30–35.

96. Eriksson B, Gutenberg B, G. KL. Chordoma. A clinico-pathologic and prognostic study of a Swedish national series. Acta Orthop Scand 1958; 52:49–58.

97. Meyer JE, Lepke RA, Lindfors KK, et al. Chordomas: their CT appearance in the cervical, thoracic and lumbar spine. Radiology 1984; 153:693–696.

98. Bjornsson J, Wold LE, Ebersold MJ, Laws ER. Chordoma of the mobile spine. A clinicopathologic analysis of 40 patients. Cancer 1993; 71:735–740.

99. Sundaresan N. Chordomas. Clin Orthop 1986:135–142.

100. Munzenrider JE, Liebsch NJ. Proton therapy for tumors of the skull base. Strahlenther Onkol 1999; 175:57–63.

101. Sundaresan N, Rosenthal DI, Schiller AL, Krol G. Chordomas. In: Sundaresan N, Schmidek HH, Schiller AL, Rosenthal DI, eds. Tumors of the Spine: Diagnosis and Clinical Management. Philadelphia, PA: W. B. Saunders Company; 1990:192–213.

102. Mindell ER. Chordoma. J Bone Joint Surg Am 1981; 63:501–505.

22 Common Radiotherapy Techniques for Spinal Tumors

MOHAMED A. ELSHAIKH, MD AND ROGER M. MACKLIS, MD

CONTENTS

INTRODUCTION
CLINICAL APPLICATION AND TREATMENT OUTCOME
CONCLUSION
REFERENCES

1. INTRODUCTION

Radiation therapy is an important modality in the management of both primary and metastatic tumors involving the spine and spinal cord. The mesenchymal elements of the spinal column and its contents may give rise to a wide variety of primary tumors. Yet, primary neoplastic lesions of the spine are rare, accounting for roughly 5 to 10% of all skeletal tumors. Metastatic lesions of the spine are far more common *(1)*. True spinal cord neoplasms are relatively rare and typically intradural in location. Radiation therapy has evolved over the past decades to better meet these needs. Better pretreatment imaging studies, megavoltage linear accelerators, and computer-based three-dimensional (3D) treatment planning are all improving radiation dose distributions, thus, decreasing the likelihood of severe acute or late toxicity.

1.1. RADIOBIOLOGICAL CONSIDERATIONS

The spinal cord is a critical dose-limiting structure in the radiotherapeutic treatment of several neoplasms. Treatment of spinal cord tumors with radiation must delicately balance the need to deliver a sufficient dose of radiation to kill the tumor and the need to avoid further injury to the spinal cord. Radiation tolerance of the spinal cord is based on the dose delivered per fraction, total dose, and the volume of tissue treated. The dose per fraction is the most important factor influencing the radiation tolerance of spinal cord *(2,3)*. The radiation tolerance dose that has 5% probability of myelitis within 5 yr from treatment ($TD_{5/5}$) is generally considered to be 5000 cGy for a 5- to 10-cm length of spinal cord, and 4700 cGy for 20 cm of irradiated cord. This tolerance doses was calculated based on 180 to 200 cGy fraction size *(4)*. However, some contemporary experts have suggested that the $TD_{5/5}$ for human spinal cord is actually on the order of 6000 cGy *(5,6)* in the absence of chemotherapy.

From: *Current Clinical Oncology: Cancer in the Spine: Comprehensive Care.*
Edited by: R. F. McLain, K-U. Lewandrowski, M. Markman, R. M. Bukowski,
R. Macklis, and E. C. Benzel © Humana Press, Inc., Totowa, NJ

A University of Florida review of head and neck cancer patients whose cervical cord was incidentally irradiated found a 0.4% incidence of radiation myelitis with total doses between 4501 and 5000 cGy (2 of 471 patients), compared with a 0% incidence with 4001 to 4500 cGy (0 of 514 patients), and a 0% incidence (0 of 75 patients) with doses of more than 5000 cGy *(7)*. A 6% incidence of cervical myelitis was reported in 72 head and neck cancer patients whose cords were treated with at least 5500 cGy with fraction sizes ranged from 150 to 200 cGy. For patients who receive less than 5000 cGy to the cord, the incidence of myelitis was 0% *(8)*.

Though some practitioners believe that the cervical spinal cord is somewhat less sensitive to irradiation, clinical and experimental studies have failed to demonstrate any difference in radio-sensitivity in different segments of the spinal cord *(9)*.

Hyperfractionation is a radiation treatment schedule that exploits the radiobiological principle involving the repair of normal tissues between radiation fractions. Multiple small radiation doses are given on each treatment day, typically a minimum interval of 6 h separates each dose of 120 to 150 cGy per fraction. During the multi-hour interval between radiation doses, the normal tissues undergo repair of the radiation effects. This process of repair of normal tissues allows the safe administration of higher total doses of radiation to most normal tissues like mucosa and skin. However, repair of damage to the spinal cord is slower and experimentally has been shown to require more than 8 h to complete the repair of radiation injury *(10)*. The radiation tolerance of the spinal cord is reduced by 10 to 15% when the interval between radiation fractions is reduced from 24 h to 6 to 8 h *(11)*. Thus, unlike the skin and mucosa, hyperfractionation apparently does not spare the spinal cord from radiation injuries *(10,11)*. There is, therefore, minimal advantage in the use of hyperfractionated radiation schedules to treat spinal cord tumors.

1.2. TECHNIQUE OF EXTERNAL BEAM RADIOTHERAPY FOR SPINAL REGION TUMOR

The most common type of spinal tumor treated with radiotherapy is vertebral body metastatic disease. All patients should undergo formal simulation prior to starting irradiation. The techniques used to treat spinal cord compression with radiation account for the factors of radiation dose and treatment volume. Although a variety of radiation treatment schedules are used, most commonly, 3000 cGy is administered in 10 treatments (300 cGy per treatment) to the area of the spinal disease. Radiobiologically, this is approximately equivalent to administering 3600 to 4000 cGy using conventional 200 cGy/d radiation schedules. A more abbreviated course of radiation is often considered advantageous in patients who are in pain and often have other intervening medical problems (12).

The radiation treatment portal must be defined by information from diagnostic imaging and not solely from clinical presentation. The radiation portal for spinal region tumors is typically 7 to 9 cm wide and is centered at the midline of the spine. Generally, the radiation portal includes the area of spinal cord or cauda equina compression plus a margin of 1 to 2 vertebral bodies above and below the region radiographically involved with metastatic disease (Fig. 1).

Paravertebral extension should be included in the radiation portal when present. All patients with paravertebral tumor should be evaluated with magnetic resonance imaging (MRI) before the administration of radiotherapy to identify potential disease extension along the spinal axis. The decision to include asymptomatic noncontiguous sites of metastatic involvement in the radiation field depends on the extent of disease in the epidural space, associated vertebral collapse, and the potential difficulty that could subsequently be encountered in matching radiation portals.

For primary spinal cord tumors, the treatment field should encompass the radiologically apparent lesion with 3 to 5 cm margin of normal spinal cord both rostrally and caudally. Preoperative sagittal MRI is the most useful study for determining the size and location of the treatment portals. Immobilization devices such as thermoplastic face masks are useful for treatment located in the cervical spine. Whether an associated syrinx (a dilated, fluid-filled intramedullary cavity) should be included in the treatment volume is controversial. At times the syrinx is formed by local mass effect resulting in obstruction of the central canal of the spinal cord; in this situation the syrinx is not a part of the neoplastic process, but instead represents a normal tissue reaction to the nearby tumor's bulk. At other times, the tumor itself may be forming a cystic cavity or syrinx, and the syrinx must be regarded as a part of the malignant process. Clinically distinguishing these situations from one another is difficult. In general, a small syrinx is included in the treatment volume. A syrinx extending for virtually the entire length of the cord need not be completely encompassed by the treatment field unless it is found to be clearly malignant at surgery.

Treatment fields are dependent on the site of involved spinal cord. The cervical spine is usually treated using opposed lateral fields to avoid the oral cavity. For the thoracic spine, a posteroanterior field alone can be used. When treating the lumbar

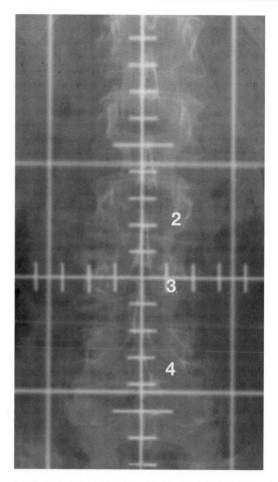

Fig. 1. Example of posteroanterior treatment portal for spinal cord compression at L3 vertebral body.

spine or when the target appears to be midline, a parallel-opposed anteroposterior and posteroanterior beam arrangement may be preferred with equal or nonequal weighting. Wedged pair posterior oblique fields offer the theoretical advantage of decreased morbidity by minimizing the exit dose (Fig. 2). The use of 3D conformal treatment planning with dose-volume histograms has greatly improved the reliability and safety of this technique. Craniospinal irradiation may be employed in the management of seeding tumors such as high-grade ependymoma or medulloblastoma.

Re-irradiation or administration of higher doses of radiation to the spine sometimes requires a specialized technique that ensures that the radiation tolerance of the spinal cord is not exceeded. Examples of these techniques include 3D radiotherapy and intensity-modulated radiation treatment (IMRT). Details about the role of IMRT in spinal neoplasms will be discussed in Chapter 24.

Experimentally, histopathological repair of radiation changes in the spinal cord occurs between 2 and 6 mo; after 6 mo, an approx 40% level of repair is observed (13). The additional radiation that could be safely administered to the spinal cord, though, would generally be less than 50% of the originally prescribed dose, which is usually insufficient to effectively treat recurrent spinal disease. The small potential benefit

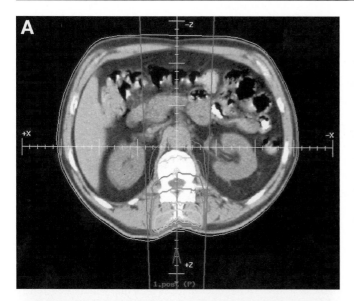

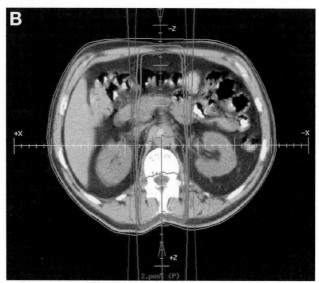

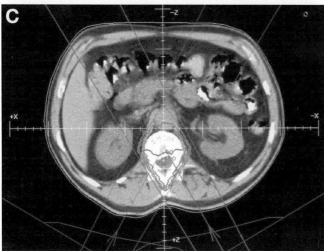

Fig. 2. Examples of radiotherapy treatment planning for spinal region tumors. (**A**) A single posteroanterior field. The axial isodose display reflects a 6 MV photon beam prescribed to a 7 cm depth. (**B**) Paired anteroposterior/posteroanterior using 10 Mev photon beams for tumors approaching medline. The fields are weighted 1:2 anterior-posterior:posterior anterior. (**C**) Paired posterior oblique wedged fields using 10 MeV photon beams and 60° wedges to decrease a high exit dose to the anterior structures with a more conformal radiation dose distribution near the target volume.

in administering an insufficient tumoricidal dose of radiation generally will rarely merit the possible risk of radiation myelopathy. The risk of myelopathy must include factors like the level of pretreatment spinal injury, and the time and dose parameters of the past and currently proposed treatment.

The introduction of 3D treatment planning systems in the late 1990s have enabled radiation oncologists to design highly conformal treatment plans for spinal tumors. Tumor volumes that wrap around the spinal cord are generally difficult to treat. For those institutions that do not have full access to IMRT technology, 3D conformal radiotherapy using a multiple arc technique enables dose escalation to the paraspinal tumors and retreatment of recurrent lesions *(14)*.

2. CLINICAL APPLICATION AND TREATMENT OUTCOME

2.1. SPINAL CORD COMPRESSION AND VERTEBRAL METASTASES

Radiation therapy is a mainstay of treatment of patients with metastatic cancer to the spine. The diagnosis of malignant spinal cord or cauda equina compression is often considered a radiotherapeutic emergency. Corticosteroids have been found

to reduce vasogenic spinal cord edema *(15,16)*, control pains, and improve neurological functions. The dose and form of steroids vary. A dose of 10 to 40 mg of dexamethasone intravenously given immediately, followed by 4 to 10 mg qid, are often used. The lower doses are used for patients with mild pain and, or equivocal signs of myelopathy; the higher doses are used in patients with prominent or rapidly progressive myelopathy. However, in fully ambulatory patients with radiographic but not symptomatic spinal cord compression, radiotherapy can be delivered without steroids *(17)*. In general, the tapering of high-dose steroids is begun within 48 to 72 h after completion of radiotherapy, and the patient is followed closely for signs of steroid-induced complications, such as glucose intolerance and infection.

Early diagnosis is the keystone of all successful cancer therapy. In the case of spinal cord or cauda equina compression, pain represents both the first symptom and a symptom at diagnosis in over 95% *(18,19)*. Pain can be present for days to months before neurological dysfunction evolves. Pain is aggravated by recumbency, and opioid analgesics are frequently required before radiotherapy can be administered in the recumbent position. The prone position may be equally problematic.

A careful neurological assessment is needed to clarify the extent of the disease. All patients who have clinically suspected epidural disease should undergo MRI to the entire spine before radiotherapy *(20)*. This is imperative to accurately define the radiation portal and encompass the entire extent of epidural disease. Findings on the MRI should be correlated with those on bone scan, computed tomography, and plain radiographs to incorporate vertebral and paraspinous metastases adjacent to the area of spinal cord compression.

Spinal cord or cauda equina compression is a potential complication in all patients with documented vertebral metastases. Treatment of symptomatic vertebral metastases is advisable to relieve refractory cancer-related pain and prevent progression of disease that could result in spinal cord or cauda equina compression.

The prognosis of patients undergoing radiotherapy for metastatic epidural spinal cord compression depends on their neurological function at the time treatment begins. In a study of metastatic spine disease with radiographic spinal cord compression but with no clinical signs of myelopathy, Maranzano et al. *(21,22)* found that all patients remained ambulatory following radiation treatment. Patients with neurological signs who are ambulatory at the time of diagnosis usually retain this ability following radiotherapy.

However, only about half of the patients who are paraparetic at presentation regain ambulation, and paraplegic patients rarely are restored to ambulation with radiotherapy *(23)*. Zelefsky et al. reported that 92% of the patients who completed radiation treatment to the spine because of spinal epidural metastasis from prostate carcinoma, experienced pain relief, and 67% had a significant or complete improvement on neurological examination *(24)*.

In newly diagnosed patients with spinal cord compression who underwent surgery first, radiation therapy should be administered after surgery. Unfortunately, there are no good clinical data to document the appropriate waiting period before radiation can begin. Radiation may not only delay skin healing in these patients, but will also delay bone fusion. It is generally recommended to wait 2 to 3 wk after spinal surgery before beginning radiation therapy, unless symptoms or scans show progression.

A statistically significant improvement in functional outcome has been reported with laminectomy and radiotherapy in treatment of epidural spinal cord compression over either modality alone. In lung cancer patients, laminectomy followed by radiotherapy was associated with an improved functional outcome in 82% of patients, as compared to only 45% of patients who were treated with either modality alone *(25)*. Constane et al. reported that 46% of their patients treated with decompressive laminectomy and postoperative radiotherapy had significant neurological improvement compared with 39% of patients treated with radiotherapy alone *(26)*.

A randomized trial comparing laminectomy followed by radiation therapy vs radiotherapy alone in the treatment of spinal epidural metastases showed no significant difference in the effectiveness of treatment in regard to pain relief, improved ambulation, and improved sphincter function *(27)*.

In many situations, there is no universal answer as to what the best management situation should be. Instead, an individual approach should be pursued. Surgical decompression should be considered in (1) patients without a diagnosis, (2) spinal instability, and (3) patients who are neurologically deteriorating, who have been previously irradiated at the site of spinal cord compression. However, the decision-making process must be patient-specific. The results of neurological examination, life expectancy, and co-morbid medical conditions must be carefully taken into account.

2.2. PRIMARY NEOPLASMS OF THE SPINE AND SPINAL CORD

2.2.1. Ependymoma

The favorable location of ependymomas of the cauda equina often permits complete resection. Intramedullary ependymomas often have tissue planes separating the tumor and cord, which facilitate complete resection as well. Postoperative radiotherapy after gross total resection does not appear to be beneficial *(28,29)*. The efficacy of postoperative radiotherapy following incomplete resection of spinal ependymoma is controversial. No randomized studies have been done to evaluate the benefit of radiotherapy in this sitting. However, postoperative radiotherapy has been recommended by many authors after incomplete resection of spinal ependymoma to improve local control *(30–34)*. Although some studies have not found a survival benefit to postoperative radiation treatment in incompletely resected spinal ependymomas, the radiation doses used in these studies were generally less than that which is currently recommended *(35,36)*, and, thus, the results are in doubt. Some authors have suggested close follow-up of patients with incompletely resected low-grade ependymomas using serial MRI scans, reserving postoperative radiotherapy for those patients with rapid tumor growth *(37)*. The 10-yr overall survival rate for patients with primary ependymoma of the spinal cord following surgery and postoperative radiotherapy ranges from 62 to 96% *(38–44)*. The wide range of treatment outcome might be affected by the variability of the extent of surgical resection before radiation therapy.

2.2.2. Astrocytoma

Low-grade astrocytoma and oligodendroglioma are infiltrative and generally lack tissue planes separating the tumor from the cord. Postoperative radiotherapy is recommended for incompletely resected or high-grade lesions *(45–47)*. The effect of radiation therapy on survival is unclear *(48)*. No randomized study has addressed this question. However, a few retrospective studies have suggested a survival benefit to postoperative radiation treatment. In a study from Mayo Clinic *(47)*, patients with diffuse fibrillary astrocytomas who received radiation had a significantly better survival than those who did not. Although there was a trend toward improved survival, radiation therapy did not significantly increase survival in patients with pilocytic astrocytoma. Linstadt et al. *(42)* reported on 12 patients who received postoperative radiotherapy after subtotal resection or biopsy. The 10- and 15-yr disease-free survival was 91 and 74%, respectively. The 5-yr overall survival rate for patients with low-grade astrocytoma of the spinal cord following surgery and postoperative radiotherapy ranges from 60 to 81% *(45,50–52)*.

Most of the studies have not found a dose-response interaction for spinal astrocytomas *(28,39,46,49,50)*. Minehan et al. *(47)*, for example, found no significant difference in survival between patients who received less than 50 vs 50 Gy or more. Because of the great tendency of malignant spinal cord astrocytoma to develop disseminated disease, the 5-yr overall survival rate for patients following surgery and postoperative radiotherapy ranges from 0 to 40% *(28,42,52)*.

2.2.3. Chordoma

Because local recurrence is common with chordoma, radiation therapy is an integral part of the treatment plan. Postoperative radiotherapy is recommended after incomplete surgical resection. Even if the resection margins are negative, recurrence can still occur *(53–55)*, suggesting the routine use of postoperative radiation in this setting. Keisch et al. *(56)* found that patients with lumbosacral tumor treated with surgery and radiation had a longer mean disease-free survival period (6.6 yr) than those treated with surgery alone (4.1 yr) *(p = 0.08)*. Azzarelli et al. *(57)* noted that the two patients in their series who experienced recurrence after radiation therapy did so after 46 and 80 mo, respectively, whereas the median disease-free interval after surgery alone was only 12 mo *(57)*.

The effect of radiation on survival is not clear. Cheitiyawardana *(58)* noted a significant survival benefit when comparing patients who received palliative surgery and low dose radiation (25–30 Gy) vs those who received more radical surgery and higher doses of radiation (30–45 Gy). O'Neill et al. *(53)* also noted a beneficial effect in terms of survival in patients with sacrococcygeal chordomas who underwent subtotal resection and radiotherapy vs subtotal resection alone. On the other hand, other investigators found no significant survival benefits between patients who underwent surgery and radiotherapy and those treated by radical surgery alone *(59,60)*.

There is a clear palliative benefit for radiation treatment in locally advanced or recurrent chordoma *(54,59)*. Fuller and Bloom *(59)*, for example, noted a 96% stabilization or reduction in symptoms in 25 patients who underwent either biopsy or partial resection followed by radiotherapy.

Many authors advocate higher radiation dose (55–70 Gy) for better tumor control *(54,61)*. The clear need for more effective local treatment has resulted in innovative approaches to radiotherapy. Particle beam therapy or IMRT with the potential for dose escalation using highly conformal fields appears to be very promising approaches for patients with chordoma. These modalities will be discussed elsewhere in this book.

2.2.4. Meningioma

Completely resected meningioma generally does not require postoperative irradiation, because the risk of recurrence is only 6% *(62)*. However, subtotally resected meningiomas have a higher risk of local recurrence, and postoperative irradiation is recommended. The recurrence rate after incomplete resection of spinal meningioma ranges from 17 to 100% *(63,64)*. In general, the principles of treatment for intracranial meningiomas should apply.

2.2.5. Multiple Myeloma and Plasmacytoma

Radiation therapy plays an essential role in the management of plasma cell tumors. The role of radiotherapy in myeloma is primarily aimed at palliation or pain relief. Because myeloma is a radio-sensitive tumor, 10 to 20 Gy is usually adequate to alleviate pains. For spinal solitary plasmacytoma, on the other hand, a definitive approach to radiotherapy is employed. In this setting, radiotherapy provides excellent local control, and long-term disease free survival with the recommended dose of 45 to 50 Gy in 25 fractions.

2.2.6. Lymphoma

Lymphomatous involvement of the spine always represents an epidural disease. The treatment for primary epidural non-Hodgkin's lymphoma has generally involved surgery (biopsy for diagnosis or laminectomy for compression) followed by external beam radiotherapy and chemotherapy *(65,66)*.

2.2.7. Eosinophilic Granuloma

Small dose radiotherapy results in excellent local control (71–100%) and pain palliation (93–100%) in patients with eosinophilic granuloma *(67, 68)*. However, postoperative radiotherapy should be reserved for those patients with local recurrence following surgery.

2.3. RADIATION SIDE EFFECTS AND MANAGEMENT

The risk of radiation myelitis is minimal after doses below 4500 cGy delivered in 180 to 200 cGy daily fractions. This risk increases substantially when radiotherapy doses higher than the spinal cord tolerance is given. Radiation induced myelopathy is thought to result from two mechanisms: white matter damage and vasculopathy. White matter damage is associated with diffuse demyelination and swollen axons, which can be focally necrotic and have associated glial reaction. Vascular damage has been shown to be age dependent, and can result in hemorrhage, telangiectasia, and vascular necrosis *(69)*. The two clinical syndromes of radiation-induced spinal cord injuries are as follow:

1. **Transient radiation injury.** This syndrome occurs 2–4 mo following radiotherapy. It usually spontaneously resolves within a few months. Clinically, it is characterized by paresthesia in the extremities. The paresthesia may be evoked or exacerbated by neck flexion (L'Hermitte's sign). Transient demyelination with depletion of the oligodendrocytes is the presumed pathology of this type of spinal cord injury. It could be the first sign of chronic progressive radiation myelopathy, however, it is usually transient, and does not typically progress to delayed radiation myelitis.

2. **Delayed progressive radiation myelopathy.** Most permanent myelopathy occurs approx 1 yr following radiation. Latent period as long as 60 mo or even longer have been reported. The onset is insidious, usually starts with paresthesia of the feet or hands followed by weakness of one or both legs. The symptoms tend to progress steadily, resulting in further sensorimotor disturbances, bowel and bladder dysfunction and paraplegia. The mechanism of radiation induced myelitis is unclear. Theories include intramedullary vascular damage with thrombotic occlusion of the their lumens that progresses to hemorrhagic and white matter necrosis.

There is no known effective treatment for radiation myelitis. Steroids temporarily improve neurological function by decreasing the associated cord edema. The role of hyperbaric oxygen therapy in the treatment or prevention of radiation-induced myelopathy is unclear, with many contradictory results *(70–73)*.

Secondary malignancies, including sarcomas and glioblastoma multiforme have been reported after spinal cord tumor irradiation *(74,75)*. Other side effects can occur depending on the area of the body irradiated and the fields used to treat the tumor.

2.4. RADIOPHARMACEUTICALS IN THE MANAGEMENT OF SPINAL METASTASES

In patients with multiple painful sites, systemic radiopharmaceutical therapy (RPT) has increasingly been recognized as an important contributor to improvement of quality of life. The first report on the use of RPT for the treatment of bone metastases was published by Pecher 60 yr ago *(76)*. Using this modality, all involved osseous sites can be addressed simultaneously with

Table 1
Physical and Clinical Characteristics of Various Radionuclides Commonly Used in Bone Metastases (79,80)

	Physical half-life	β-energy (MeV)	Maximum range in tissue (mm)
Phosphorus[32]	14.3 d	1.71	8.0
Strontium[89]	50.6 d	1.46	6.7
Rhenium1[86]	90.6 h	1.07	4.7
Samarium[153]	46.3 h	0.84	3.4

little long-term toxicity. The theoretical advantages of all targeted RPT lie in the specific localization of the radionuclide at the site of tumor to be treated and the relatively limited distribution of radionuclide at sites of potential limiting toxicity such bone marrow. Most currently available radiopharmaceuticals achieve a therapeutic ratio of approx 10:1 (77).

Historically, ^{32}P was the first radionuclide to be widely used in the treatment of bone metastases with subjective pain improvement in 60 to 80% of patients (78). Because of its side effects with myelosuppression and pancytopenia, ^{32}P has since been replaced by newer, less toxic radionuclides. Table 1 summarizes the physical characteristics of the four most commonly used agents.

The mechanism of uptake for each of the bones seeking radiopharmaceuticals is related to the degree of osteoblastic activity at the site of the metastasis; the selectivity of uptake is related to incorporation within bone rather than within tumor. The complex anatomic relationship between tumor and new bone formation means that the irradiation is delivered to the tumor and the peritumor environment from radionuclide deposited at the bone–tumor interface.

Overall response rates in terms of efficacy of pain palliation ranges from 60 to 80% (81,82). A flare response, associated with a short-lived increase in pain 1 to 2 d after administration, may occur in 10% of patients. The impression gleaned from the literature is that it may predict a good response to the treatment.

Systemic radionuclides may be considered in the following circumstances:

1. In patients with widely metastatic disease, as adjuvant to external beam radiotherapy.
2. When external beam therapy options have been exhausted and normal tissue tolerance has been reached.
3. In patients with life expectancy of at least 3 mo.
4. There is no evidence of imminent epidural cord compression, pathological fracture, or mechanical instability.
5. In patients with good marrow reserve with a white blood cell count of greater than 2500/mm^3 and a platelet count of more than 100,000/mm^3.

3. CONCLUSION

Radiotherapy treatment decisions should be based on a case by case basis considering many factors such as patient age, tumor location and grade, degree of tumor resection, etc. Our treatment recommendation for primary spinal cord tumors in adults is shown in Table 2. With the rarity of spinal cord tumors,

Table 2
Radiotherapeutic Recommendations for Primary Spinal Tumors

Type	Treatment	Total radiation in cGy+
Low grade, complete resection	Observation	—
Low-grade glioma, subtotal resection	Local XRT^a	5040
High-grade astrocytoma	Local XRT	5400
Benign ependymoma, complete resection	Observation	—
Benign ependymoma, subtotal resection	Local XRT	5040
Malignant ependymoma	Craniospinal XRT	5400 (tumor bed dose)
Meningioma, completely resected	Observation	—
Meningioma, subtotal resection	Local XRT	5400
Sacral chordoma	Local XRT	60+

^{a}XRT, megavoltage photon irradiation.
+, Doses are prescribed at 180–200 cGy per fraction, one fraction per day.

prospective studies are difficult to accomplish. One major obstacle to irradiating these tumors to higher doses is the tolerance of normal tissues, particularly the spinal cord. Tumor-specific radiation sensitizers, radioprotectors, and combined modality therapy using radiation with chemotherapy or other molecular therapies are approaches that might be fruitful avenues to pursue. Additionally, radiotherapy dose escalation trials using 3D planning may be helpful, particularly for chordomas and high-grade gliomas.

REFERENCES

1. Dahlin DC, Unni KK. Bone Tumors: General Aspects and Data on 8,542 Cases. Springfield, IL: Charles C. Thomas; 1986.
2. Atkins HL, Tretter P. Time-dose consideration in radiation myelopathy. Acta Radiol Ther Phys Biol 1966; 5:79–94.
3. Wara WM, Philips TL, Sheline GE, et al. Radiation tolerance of the spinal cord. Cancer 1975; 35:1558–1562.
4. Emami B, Lyman J, Brown A, et al. Tolerance of normal tissue to therapeutic irradiation. Int J Radiat Oncol Biol Phys 1991; 21: 109–122.
5. Kim YH, Fayos JV. Radiation tolerance of the cervical spinal cord. Radiology 1981; 139:473–478.
6. Van der Kogel AJ. Retreatment tolerance of the spinal cord. Int J Radiat Oncol Biol Phys 1993; 26:715–717.
7. Marcus RB, Million RR. The incidence of myelitis after irradiation of the cervical spinal cord. Int J Radiat Oncol Biol Phys 1990; 19:3–8.
8. Jeromic B, Djuric L, Mijatovic L. Incidence of radiation myelitis of the cervical spinal cord at doses of 5500 cGy or greater. Cancer 1991; 8:2138–2141.
9. Schulthesiss TE, Stephens LC, Ang KK, Price RE, Peters LJ. Volume effects in Rhesus monkey spinal cord. Int J Radiat Oncl Biol Phys 1994; 9:67–72.
10. Lavey RS, Johnstone AK, Taylor JM, McBride WH. The effect of hyperfractionation on spinal cord response to radiation. Int J Radiat Oncol Biol Phys 1992; 4:68–-686.
11. Ang KK, Jiang GL, Guttenberger, et al. Impact of spinal cord repair kinetics on the practice of altered fractionation schedules. Radiother Oncol 1992; 5:287–294.

12. Janjan, N: Radiotherapeutic management of spinal metastases. J of Pain and Symptom Manage 1995; 1:47–56.

13. Ruifrok ACC, Kleiboer BJ, van der Kogel AJ. Reirradiation tolerance of the immature rat spinal cord. Radiother Oncol 1992; 3:249–256.

14. Pirzkall A, Lohr F, Rhein B, et al. Conformal radiotherapy of challenging paraspinal tumors using multiple arc segment technique. Int J Radiat Oncol Biol Phys 2000;48 :1197–1204.

15. Greenberg HS, Kim JH, Posner JB. Epidural spinal cord compression from metastatic tumor. Results from a new protocol. Ann Neurol 1980; 8:361–366.

16. Ushio Y, Posner R, Posner JB, Shapiro WR. Experimental spinal cord compression by epidural neoplasms. Neurology 1977; 27:422–429.

17. Maranzano E, Latini P, Beneventi S, et al. Radiotherapy without steroids in selected metastatic spinal cord compression patients. A phase II trial. Am J of Clinical Oncol 1996; 19:179–183.

18. Boogerd W, van der Sande JJ. Diagnosis and treatment of spinal cord compression in malignant disease. Cancer Treat Rev1993; 19:129–150.

19. Grant R, Papadopoulous SM, Greenberg HS. Metastatic epidural spinal cord compression. Neur Clin 1991; 9:825–841.

20. Georgy BA, Hasselink JR. MR imaging of spine: recent advances in pulse sequence and special technique. Am J Roentgenol 1994; 162:923–934.

21. Maranzano E, Latini P, Checcaglini F, et al. Radiation therapy in metastatic spinal cord compression–a prospective analysis of 105 patients. Cancer 1991; 67:1311–1317.

22. Maranzano E, Latini P, Checcaglini F, et al. Radiation therapy of spinal cord compression caused by breast cancer: report of a prospective trial. Int J Radiat Oncol Biol Phys 1992; 24:301–306.

23. Gilbert RW, Kim JH, Posner JB. Epidural spinal cord compression from metastatic tumor: diagnosis and treatment. Ann Neurol 1978; 3:40–51.

24. Zelefsky MJ, Scher HI, Krol G, Portenoy RK, Leibel SA, Fuks ZY. Spinal epidural tumor in-patients with prostate cancer. Clinical and radiographic predictors of response to radiation therapy. Cancer 1992; 70:2319–2325.

25. Bach F, Agerlin N, Sorensen JB, et al. Metastatic spinal cord compression secondary to lung cancer. J Clin Oncol 1992; 10:1781–1787.

26. Constans JP, de Divitiis E, Donzelli R, Spaziante R, Meder JF, Haye C. Spinal metastases with neurological manifestations. Review of 600 cases. J Neurosurg 1983; 59:111–118.

27. Young RF, Post EM, King GA. Treatment of spinal epidural metastases: Randomized prospective comparison of laminectomy and radiotherapy. J Neurosurg 1980; 53:741–748.

28. Shirato H, Kamada T, Hida K, et al. The role of radiotherapy in the management of spinal cord glioma. Int J Radiat Oncol Biol Phys 1995; 33:323–328.

29. Epstein FJ, Farmer JP, Freed D. Adult intramedullary spinal cord ependymoma: the results of surgery in 38 patients. J Neurosurg 1993; 79:204–209.

30. Hulshof MCCM, Menten J, Dito JJ, et al. Treatment results in primary intraspinal gliomas. Radioth Oncol 1993; 29:294–300.

31. Di Marco A, Griso C, Pradella R, Campostrini F, Garusi GF. Postoperative management of primary spinal cord ependymoma. Acta Oncol 1988; 27:371–375.

32. Cooper PR. Outcome after operative treatment of intramedullary spinal cord tumors in adults: Intermediate and long-term results in 51 patients. Neurosurgery 1989; 25:855–859.

33. Schwade JG, Wara WM, Sheline GE. Management of primary spinal cord tumors. Int J Radiat Oncol Biol Phys 1978; 4:389–393.

34. Peschel RE, Kapp DS, Cardinale F, Manuelidis EE. Ependymoma of the spinal cord. Int J Radiat Oncol Biol Phys 1983; 9:1093–1096.

35. Sgouros S, Malluci CL, Jackowski A. Spinal ependymoma. The value of postoperative radiotherapy for residual disease control. Br J Neurosurg 1996; 10:559–566.

36. Ferrante L, Mastronardi L, Celli P, Lunardi P, Acqui M, Fortuna A. Intramedullary spinal cord ependymoma: a study of 45 cases with long term follow-up. Acta Neurochir 1992; 119:74–79.

37. Constantini S, Allen J, Epstein F. Pediatric and adult spinal cord tumors. In: Black PM, Loeffler J, eds. Cancer of the nervous system. Cambridge, MA: Blackwell Science; 1997:637–652.

38. Garret PG, Simpson WJK. Ependymomas: results of radiation treatment. Int J Radiat Oncol Biol Phys 1983; 9:1121–1124.

39. Kopelson G, Linggood RM, Kleinman GM, Doucette J, Wang CC. Management of intramedullary spinal cord tumors. Radiology 1980; 135:473–479.

40. Garcia DM. Primary spinal cord tumors treated with surgery and postoperative irradiation. Int J Radiat Oncol Biol Phys 1985; 11:1933–1939.

41. Shaw EG, Evans RG, Scheithauer BW, Ilstrup DM, Earle JD. Radiotherapeutic management of adult intraspinal ependymomas. Int J radiat Oncol Biol Phys 1986; 12:323–327.

42. Linstadt DE, Wara WM, Leibel SA, Gutin PH, Wilson CB, Sheline GE. Postoperative radiotherapy of primary spinal cord tumors. Int J Radiat Oncol Biol Phys 1989; 16:1397–1403.

43. Whitaker SJ, Bessell EM, Ashley SE, Bloom HJ, Bell BA, Brada M. Postoperative radiotherapy in the management of spinal cord ependymoma. J Neurosurg 1991; 74:720–728.

44. Waldron JN, Laperierre NJ, Jaakkimainen L, et al. Spinal cord ependymoma: a retrospective analysis of 59 cases. Int J Radiat Oncol Biol Phys 1993; 27:223–229.

45. Reimer R, Onofrio BM. Astrocytoma of the spinal cord in children and adolescents. J Neurosurg 1985; 63:669–675.

46. Jyothirmayi R, Madhavan J, Nair M, Rajan B. Conservative surgery and radiotherapy in the treatment of spinal cord astrocytoma. J Neurooncol 1997; 33:205–211.

47. Minehan K, Shaw E, Scheithauer B, Davis DL, Onofrio BM. Spinal cord astrocytoma: pathological and treatment considerations. J Neurosurg 1995; 83:590–595.

48. Innocenzi G, Salvati M, Cervoni L, Delfini R, Cantore G. Prognostic factors in intramedullary astrocytomas. Clin Neurol Neurosurg 1997; 99:1–5.

49. Huddart R, Traish D, Ashley S, Moore A, Brada M. Management of spinal astrocytoma with conservative surgery and radiotherapy. Br J Neurosurg 1993; 7:473–481.

50. Sandler HM, Papadopoulos SM, Thornton AF, Ross DA. Spinal cord astrocytoma. Result of therapy. Neurosurgery 1992; 30:490–493.

51. Chun HC, Schmidt-Ullrich RK, Wolfson A, Tercilla OF, Sagerman RH, King GA. External beam radiotherapy for primary spinal cord tumors. J Neurooncol 1990; 9:211–217.

52. Cohen AR, Wisoff JH, Allen JC, Epstein F. Malignant astrocytoma of the spinal cord. J Neurosurg 1989; 70:50–54.

53. O'Neill P, Bell BA, Miller JD, Jacobson I, Guthrie W. Fifty years of experience with chordomas in Southeast Scotland. Neurosurgery 1985; 16:166–170.

54. Rich TA, Schiller A, Suit HD, Mankin HJ. Clinical and pathologic review of 48 cases of chordoma. Cancer 1985; 56:182–187.

55. Thieblemont C, Biron P, Rocher F, et al. Prognostic factors in chordoma: role of postoperative radiotherapy. Eur J Cancer 1995; 31:2255–2259.

56. Keisch ME, Garcia DM, Shibuya RB. Retrospective long-term follow-up analysis in 21 patients with chordomas of various sites treated at a single institution. J Neurosurg 1991; 75:374–377.

57. Azzarelli A, Quagliuolo V, Cerasoli S, et al. Chordomas: natural history and treatment results in 33 cases. J Surg Oncol 1988; 37:185–191.

58. Chetiyawardana AD. Chordoma: results of treatment. Clin Radiol 1984; 35:159–161.

59. Fuller DB, Bloom JG. Radiotherapy for chordoma. Int J Radiat Oncol Biol Phys 1988; 15:331–339.

60. Sundaresan N, Galicich JH, Chu FCH, Huvos AG. Spinal chordoma. J Neurosurg 1979; 50:312–319.

61. Amendola BE, Amendola MA, Oliver E, McClatchey KD. Chordoma: role of radiation therapy. Radiology 1986; 158:839–843.

62. Solero CL, Fornari M, Giombini S, et al. Spinal meningiomas: review of 174 operated cases. Neurosurgery 1989; 25:153–160.

63. Klekamp J, Samii M. Surgical results of spinal meningioma. Acta Neurchir 1996; 65:77–81.

64. Levy WJJr, Bay J, Dohn D. Spinal meningioma. J Neurosurg 1982; 57:804–812.

65. Eeles RA, O'Brien P, Horwich A, Brada M. Non-Hodgkin's lymphoma presenting with extradural spinal cord compression: functional outcome and survival. Br J Cancer 1991; 63:126–129.

66. Raco A, Cervoni L, Salvati M, Delfini R. Primary spinal epidural non-Hodgkin's lymphomas in childhood: a review of 6 cases. Acta Neurochir 1997; 139:526–528.

67. Selch MT, Parker RG. Radiation therapy in the management of Langerhan's cell histiocytosis. Med Pediatr Oncol 1990; 18:97–102.

68. El-Sayed S, Brewin TB. Histiocytosis X: does radiotherapy still have a role? Clin Oncol 1992; 4:27–31.

69. Ruifork ACC, Stephens LC, van der Kogel AJ. Radiation response of the rat cervical spinal cord after irradiation at different ages: tolerance, latency, and pathology. Int J Radiat Oncol Biol Phys 1994; 9:73–79.

70. Luk HK, Baker DG, Fellows CF. Hyperbaric oxygen after radiation and its effect on the production of radiation myelitis. Int J Radiat Oncol Biol Phys 1987; 4:457–459.

71. Poulton TJ and Witcofski RL. Hyperbaric oxygen therapy for radiation myelitis. Undersea Biomed Res 1985; 12:453–458.

72. Feldmeier JJ, Lange JD, Cox SD, Chou LJ, Ciaravino V. Hyperbaric oxygen as prophylaxis or treatment for radiation myelitis. Undersea Hyperb Med 1993; 20:249–255.

73. Calabro F and Jinkins JR: MRI of radiation myelitis: A report of a case treated with hyperbaric oxygen. Eur Radiol 2000; 10:1079–1084.

74. Nadeem SQ, Feun LG, Bruce-Gregorios JH, Green B. Post-radiation sarcoma (malignant fibrous histiocytoma) of the cervical spine following ependymoma. J Neurooncol 1991; 11:263–268.

75. Rappaport ZH, Loven D, Ben-Aharon U. Radiation-induced cerebellar glioblastoma multiforme subsequent to treatment of an astrocytoma of the cervical spinal cord. Neurosurgery 1991; 29:606–608.

76. Pecher C. Biological investigations with radioactive calcium and strontium: preliminary report on the use of radioactive strontium in treatment of metastatic bone cancer. Univ CA Pub Pharmacol 1942; 11:117–149.

77. McEwan AJB. Use of radionuclides for the palliation of bone metastases. Semin Rad Oncol 2000; 10:103–114.

78. Silberstein EB. The treatment of painful osseous metastases with phosphorus 32. Sem Oncol 1993; 20:10–21.

79. Murray T and Hilditch TE. In: Sampson CB, ed. Therapeutic Applications of Radiopharmaceuticals. Text of Radiopharmacy. Theory and Practice, 3rd ed. The Netherlands: Gordon and Breach Science; 1999:369–383.

80. Maisey MN, Britton KE, Coller BD. In: Clinical Nuclear Medicine, 3rd ed. London:Chapman and Hall Medical, 1998.

81. Limouris GS, Shukla SK, Condi-Paphiti A, et al. Palliative therapy using rhenium-186 in painful breast osseous metastases. Anticancer Res 1997; 17:1767–1772.

82. Robinson RG, Preston DF, Schiefelbein M, Baxter KG. Strontium-89 therapy for the palliation of pain due to osseous metastases. JAMA 1995; 274:420–424.

23 Spinal Radiotherapy for the Pediatric Patient

Indications, Special Technical Considerations, and Long-Term Consequences

Adir Ludin, MD

Contents

1. INTRODUCTION

Radiation therapy (RT) in the pediatric population presents challenging dilemmas to the clinician. Some of the pediatric malignancies are treated according to multi-institutional multimodality trials that guide the indications and techniques within specific parameters. Because of the extremely low incidence of primary spinal malignancies, multi-institutional trials have not been implemented. Most experience has been gained through the retrospective single institution review of patient management and outcome. The application of RT as a therapeutic modality in the management of pediatric malignancies has to be carefully evaluated because the potential for long-term consequences in this population is significant. The indications for RT are constantly evolving and in a few instances are controversial.

1.1. MAGNITUDE OF THE PROBLEM

Primary spinal tumors in children are rare. Statistical data is scant, and specific trends are difficult to determine. An analysis of temporal trends in childhood cancer incidence in the United States indicates a 1% average yearly increase in the incidence rates of all neoplasms between 1974 and 1991. Rates increased an average of 2% per year for central nervous system (CNS) tumors. The incidence rate of all CNS tumors in children under 14 yr of age is 28.7 cases per million. The increasing incidence rates were most apparent for children younger than 5 yr *(26)*.

From: *Current Clinical Oncology: Cancer in the Spine: Comprehensive Care.*
Edited by: R. F. McLain, K-U. Lewandrowski, M. Markman, R. M. Bukowski,
R. Macklis, and E. C. Benzel © Humana Press, Inc., Totowa, NJ

Earlier detection may be occurring, but if these trends are an artifact of improvements in diagnostic imaging, flattening of the CNS cancer incidence should be eventually observed.

Rates for all CNS tumors in children under 14 yr are ependymoma 2.4 per million, medulloblastoma 6.5 per million, and astrogial 17.5 per million *(26)*.

Primary intra-medullary tumors are even more rare. The rate of frequency is only 5 to 10% of their intra-cranial counterparts, with an approximate annual incidence of 1 per million children *(35,53)*.

2. PRIMARY INTRAMEDULLARY SPINAL CORD TUMORS

Astrocytomas and ependymomas are the most common types of spinal cord tumors *(35,53)*. Presenting symptoms are pain, motor deficits, gait deterioration, torticollis, and progressive kyphoscoliosis *(9,32)*. Hydrocephalus occurs more frequently than in adults *(32)*.

The management for most intradural tumors is primarily surgical *(35)*. The preferred initial treatment is complete resection *(53)*. Subtotal or total resection should be attempted whenever feasible. This approach achieves histologic diagnosis and in many instances long-term local control *(14,59)*.

Based on the available literature, gross total resection of ependymoma and radical resection of low-grade astrocytoma can be followed by observation *(49)*. In some cases, radical surgery can be performed even in young children *(9)*.

Postoperative RT is indicated in cases of evident residual tumor and when a second surgical procedure is not feasible. Observation without RT can be instituted in cases of incompletely resected pilocytic astrocytoma and in young children in whom delaying radiation until maturity is advisable *(8,21,36,59)*.

Outcomes for ependymomas are better than for low-grade astrocytomas *(31,32)*, with better 5- and 10-yr survival rates for ependymoma (100 and 73%, respectively) than for astrocytoma (58 and 23%, respectively) in one report *(35)*. Gross total removal of ependymomas can be achieved more frequently than astrocytomas *(31,33)*.

The median overall survival for low-grade tumors is 96 mo in the pediatric population *(46)*.

Even patients with disseminated ependymomas and astrocytomas may sometimes achieve long-term progression free survival with cranio-spinal irradiation (CSI) *(46)*. Treatment should be individualized.

2.1. LOW-GRADE SPINAL ASTROCYTOMA

Astrocytomas may be low-grade or high-grade and present at any level of the spinal cord, although the majority of pediatric spinal cord astrocytomas present in the cervical spine and are low-grade *(2,9,14,24,32)*. They are either localized to one area of the cord causing focal widening or involve an extensive portion or entire cord causing holocord widening. They are infiltrative neoplasms and total resection is not generally possible *(31)*. Histology and the time interval between first symptoms and diagnosis are significant prognostic factors on multi-variate analysis *(2)*.

The goal of surgical intervention is to obtain tissue for diagnosis and resect as much as possible without affecting neurological function *(31)*. With the exception of pilocytic astrocytoma, postoperative radiation has been recommended in older series, for all patients with astrocytoma owing to the infiltrative nature of the lesion and frequent incomplete resection *(35)*.

More recent reports suggest that gross total or sub-total resection alone can result in excellent local control and survival rates. In this setting, the benefit of RT is difficult to demonstrate and has no clear influence on survival. Long-term observation with both clinical and radiological review, is acceptable follow-up *(2,31)*. The extent of resection does not influence prognosis or recurrence rates *(24,31,33)*. Favorable outcomes have also been reported after excision of holocord tumors *(5)*.

The recommended dose of RT when indicated is 50 to 55 Gy to a localized area. This dose approaches cord tolerance and must be delivered without unacceptable hot spots in the plan. No dose–response curve has been established *(35)*. Most failures occur locally in the spinal cord, with intracranial failures occurring less frequently *(35)*. Neuraxis dissemination is rare *(18)*.

2.2. HIGH-GRADE SPINAL ASTROCYTOMA

Less than 10% of astrocytomas are high-grade, either anaplastic astrocytomas or glioblastoma multiforme *(32)*. They produce rapid neurological deterioration and are not usually amenable to complete excision. All patients with high-grade tumors undergo surgery at least for diagnostic purposes *(32)*, followed by postoperative RT, which is generally recommended *(33,47)*.

Survival is consistently poor with higher recurrence rates than seen in low-grade tumors *(23)*, and only occasional long-term survivors *(59)*. Median progression-free survival is 10 mo and median overall survival is 13 mo *(31)*. Failures are either local or diffuse. Diffuse failure is ominous, it occurs sooner than local failure, with a median of 2 vs 23 mo, respectively and has a shorter survival, 10 vs 37 mo, respectively *(47)*.

2.3. LOW-GRADE SPINAL EPENDYMOMA

Ependymal tumors arise from the ependymal cells of the cerebral ventricles, central canal of the spinal cord, and cortical rests *(45)*. The primary location of ependymoma is almost equally divided between cranial and spinal. Within the spine, the cervical and lumbar sites are more frequently invaded than the thoracic spine *(22)*.

The majority of intramedullary ependymomas are amenable to complete surgical excision *(43,60)*. Long-term disease-free control of intramedullary ependymomas can be achieved with gross total resection alone *(43)*, resulting in high 5-yr survival rates and low local recurrences *(18,67,76)*. The value of postoperative RT for grossly resected ependymoma is difficult to establish *(33)*.

Encapsulated tumors of the cauda equina or filum terminale are candidates for *en-bloc* resection. Gross total resection should be attempted at the initial surgical intervention, because patients with residual tumor are 5.3 times more likely to suffer eventual dissemination *(60)*. Spinal seeding may occur at the time of failure at the primary site *(74)*.

Postoperative RT is recommended for patients with subtotal resection or biopsy of ependymoma to doses of 40 to 45 Gy or higher if the lesion is extensive *(35)*. Local RT to known low-grade tumor plus margins is effective for control of spinal ependymoma *(22,43,74)*. The majority of failures are at the site of primary disease *(62)*.

The overall survival rate ranges from 20 to 60% *(45)*.

2.4. ANAPLASTIC SPINAL EPENDYMOMA

The incidence of spinal seeding is greater for high-grade tumors and infra-tentorial tumors *(74)*. The risk of meningeal dissemination of intracranial ependymoma is on the order of 5 to 10% *(62)*. Predictive factors for dissemination are histology, proliferation index, and surgical resection. Myxopapillary spinal ependymoma and high-grade intracranial ependymoma have the highest rates of dissemination, while the predominant histology of nondisseminated ependymoma is low-grade. Dissemination usually occurs within 5 yr of surgery *(60)*.

Prophylactic CSI may be beneficial to a small population of patients, though the characteristics of the group are difficult to define *(62)*. It has been proposed for all high-grade ependymomas, and for low-grade ependymomas with evidence of spinal metastasis *(22,63,74)*. CSI is capable of eradicating subclinical spinal metastasis *(22)*. Prophylactic CSI is the standard practice for patients with anaplastic ependymoma, at some institutions *(25)*. The predominant site of relapse is the primary tumor site *(25)*, possibly indicating sterilization of the neuraxis.

The controversial use of CSI has variously been reported to have positive, mixed, or detrimental effect on outcomes. This, with the problem of local failure, limits the indication for CSI to patients with proven dissemination beyond the primary site

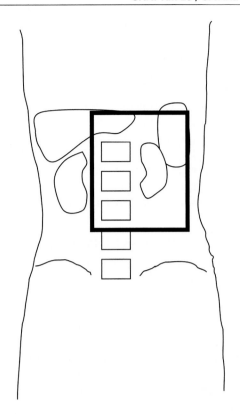

Fig. 1. Schematic example of anterior abdominal field of irradiation. Note the inclusion of the entire width of the vertebral bodies, with a margin.

(45,64). In a multivariate analysis, increased radiation dose to the primary site prolonged overall survival but not CSI (45). Gross total resection at diagnosis improved disease free survival rates, when compared to subtotal resection (45).

Doses used for CSI of anaplastic ependymoma of the posterior fossa are 35 Gy median to the spine, 36.4 Gy median to the brain, and a median conedown dose of 50 Gy to the local field (25).

Given the variable groups who have undergone treatment and the variable result of treatment, the need for CSI can not be substantiated nor refuted conclusively (25).

3. EXTRASPINAL NEOPLASMS

The detailed management of a variety of extradural tumors (i.e., neuroblastoma, rhabdomyosarcoma, Wilms' tumor, and so on) is beyond the scope of this chapter and we will thus address only the elements of management relevant to the spine.

These extradural lesions may extend into the spinal canal by direct growth or through the spinal foramina. However, a common factor in the management of these tumors is that a portion of the spine is included in the radiation field in most of the cases where radiotherapy is indicated (see Fig. 1).

3.1. NEUROBLASTOMA

Surgery alone is adequate therapy for early Pediatric Oncology Group (POG) stage A neuroblastoma demonstrated by a prospective POG study (52).

The optimal management of children, with stage II neuroblastoma has been controversial owing to the generally favorable outcome, regardless of the type of treatment. Neither RT

nor chemotherapy improved the outcome beyond the results obtained with surgery alone. Even patients who received no adjuvant therapy for residual tumor after surgery had a progression free survival equal to that of patients receiving radiation (39).

In a prospective POG study, children with visible residual tumor after surgery could be cured with moderately intensive chemotherapy alone or in combination with surgery (51).

In an important subset of patients, with an intermediate risk prognosis, POG stage C, a randomized prospective study demonstrated that radiotherapy clearly improves disease free survival (59 vs 32%) and overall survival (73 vs 41%) when compared to postoperative chemotherapy alone (4).

Doses used in this study were 30 Gy at 1.5 Gy/Fx for patients over 24 mo of age or 24 Gy for patients between 12 and 24 mo. Then next echelon of lymph nodes were treated with 24 or 18 Gy, respectively (4).

These doses of RT to the spine are in the intermediate range of therapeutic dosing. They are generally well tolerated in the short- and long-term and have a low probability to produce long-term consequences in the spine.

3.2. WILMS' TUMOR

The systematic study of therapy for Wilms' tumor by the National Wilms' Tumor Study (NWTS) has had a major impact on the use of radiotherapy in this disease. The NWTS was created in 1969 with the goal of evaluating treatment strategies for Wilms' tumor. The value of postoperative adjuvant therapy and the reduction of RT doses were systematically studied in successive studies.

The dosage regimens evolved from age based sliding scales with doses between 18 to 40 Gy used in NWTS-1 (12), to replacement of postoperative radiation with 6 mo of chemotherapy in NWTS-2 (11,72), to less intensive regimens for tumors of favorable histology in NWTS-3 (11). The intent of reduction of therapy is to minimize late complications in low risk patients without jeopardizing the good results achieved with more aggressive therapies.

The age-based sliding scale was still used in NWTS-4 for unfavorable histology, while 10.8 Gy was the dose indicated for favorable histology. This was changed in NWTS-5 by the adoption of 10.8 Gy as the therapeutic abdominal dose for Wilms' tumor with favorable or unfavorable histology.

These doses of RT to the spine are in the low range of therapeutic dosing. They are well-tolerated in the short term and are unlikely to produce any detectable long-term consequences in the spine.

3.3. RHABDOMYOSARCOMA

Systematic exploration of the optimal therapy for rhabdomyosarcoma in childhood has been carried out by the Intergroup Rhabdomyosarcoma Study (IRS).

The first IRS determined that there was no evidence that patients derived additional benefit from postoperative radiotherapy for localized tumor after complete excision (40).

Doses of radiation in IRS-2 were defined by the patient's age (>6 yr vs <6 yr) and tumor size (>5 cm vs <5 cm), within a narrow range of 40 to 55 Gy (41).

IRS-3 introduced more complex therapies with earlier initiation of radiation with significantly better outcomes (10).

In the IRS-4, the major radiotherapy randomization is between conventional RT, 50.4 Gy in 24 fractions of 1.8 Gy, and hyper-fractionated RT, 59.4 Gy in 54 fractions of 1.1 Gy twice daily (37).

These doses of RT to the spine are in the high range of therapeutic dosing. They have significant short-term morbidity and are considered to have high likelihood of producing long-term consequences in the spine.

4. NEOPLASMS OF ADJACENT NEURAL STRUCTURES

4.1. MEDULLOBLASTOMA

The definition of medulloblastoma is confined to primitive neuroectodermal tumor of the posterior fossa (13). There are approx 250 children diagnosed with medulloblastoma in the United States annually (19). The 5-yr disease free survival rates are 50 to 65% (13,19,34).

Because of primary site and local infiltration, curative surgical excision is rarely possible. This tumor disseminates malignant cells throughout the sub-arachnoid space via the cerebrospinal fluid (CSF). The incidence of dissemination at diagnosis ranges from 16 to 46% (15). CSI is indicated and required in the management of this disease after surgical treatment (2). No statistical difference was found in the event free survival rates between patients who had gross complete removal vs lesser resections (19).

The generally accepted prescribed doses of RT are: 30 to 36 Gy to the neuraxis and 50 to 56 Gy to the primary site. This has been the subject of intensive research. The goal of CSI is to uniformly deliver the prescribed dose of RT to the entire craniospinal axis with multiple matching fields while protecting the structures outside of the CNS that do not need to be radiated. Please refer to the Subheading 6.

The posterior fossa is the predominant site of failure. The importance of posterior fossa dose has been documented. Patients receiving doses of 50 Gy or more have 5-yr survival rates of 85%, whereas lesser doses have a 38% 5-yr survival rate (69). Local relapse as a component of first failure is a significant problem for patients treated with standard dose radiation, suggesting that the posterior fossa should be treated to doses higher than 56 Gy (48). Isolated spinal cord relapse is rare (15).

In order to decrease the potential for long-term morbidity from radiotherapy for low Chang (6) stage medulloblastomas, the POG and CCSG randomized patients to receive low-dose CSI (23.4 Gy to the neuraxis) vs standard dose CSI (36 Gy to the neuraxis) and 54 Gy to the posterior fossa (71). The protocol was suspended after an increased risk of early recurrence and a lowered 3-yr relapse-free survival was noted (71).

This study was designed to evaluate a patient population not proven at the time to benefit from systemic adjuvant chemotherapy. A previous CCSG study had proven the benefit that chemotherapy provided to patients with advanced Chang stage T3-4 and M1-3 tumors (16,19). The high incidence of extraneural relapse in that study, suggested that the use of chemotherapy should be further explored in this population with early stage M (8). An excess number of total recurrences and recurrences in neuraxis without concomitant posterior fossa recurrence was noted (16).

Encouraging improvements in 5-yr survival were reported with the adjuvant use of three-drug chemotherapy (lomustine, vincristine, and cisplatin) in children with subtotally resected tumors, with infiltration of the brainstem or disseminated disease (54).

Lower doses of radiation to the craniospinal axis (posterior fossa <56 Gy at 1.8 Gy/ Fx, CSI <30 Gy) combined with chemotherapy can substitute for high doses (posterior fossa = 72 Gy at 1 Gy/Fx BID, CSI >30 Gy) without significant differences in relapse rate or survival. Neither dose to the posterior fossa or craniospinal axis was statistically related to recurrence. Failure in the post fossa occurred despite boosts to more than 56 Gy (75).

5. OTHER TUMORS THAT INVOLVE THE SPINE

5.1. DISSEMINATED LOW-GRADE INTRACRANIAL ASTROCYTOMA

Dissemination may occur in low-grade intracranial astrocytomas. These low-grade astrocytomas typically manifest relatively benign growth characteristics, with a favorable long-term response to therapy. Total and subtotal resections yield high long-term survival rates. A small percentage of these low-grade gliomas manifest widespread dissemination either at presentation or later. Spread occurs almost certainly on the basis of CSF dissemination. Operative manipulation and biologic factors may contribute to dissemination. Aggressive treatment of dissemination, including chemotherapy and radiotherapy, either local irradiation or CSI can produce good quality survival (55,56).

5.2. ACUTE LYMPHOBLASTIC LEUKEMIA

The CNS is involved with disease at the time of diagnosis in about 3% of all cases of childhood acute lymphoblastic leukemia (ALL) (7).

Treatment for children with ALL who have CNS disease at diagnosis includes CSI during the consolidation phase of treatment along with systemic chemotherapy (7).

The doses used by CCSG were 24 Gy of cranial irradiation and 12 Gy of spinal irradiation.

Intensive systemic chemotherapy combined with 24 Gy of cranial irradiation and 6 Gy of spinal irradiation with intra-thecal methotrexate provides effective treatment for children with ALL (7).

5.3. EWING'S SARCOMA OF THE CNS

Isolated brain or meningeal disease with Ewing's sarcoma is uncommon. It is infrequently the initial site of relapse. The use of prophylactic CNS treatment with CSI and intra-thecal methotrexate did not alter the subsequent risk of CNS involvement (73).

6. SPECIAL TECHNICAL CONSIDERATIONS

6.1. LIMITED SPINAL IRRADIATION

Radiation to a limited portion of the spine can be achieved with various approaches. The area to be irradiated has to be identified and localized. On plain X-ray films, the vertebral levels can be determined. The depth of the area to be irradiated is determined by lateral films, computed tomography scans, or magnetic resonance imaging (MRI).

The techniques used are, a single posteroanterior (PA) photon beam, a single PA electron beam, a pair of anterior and posterior beams isocentrically placed, a pair of posterior oblique-wedged beams, or other, more complex, non-coplanar arrangements.

6.2. CRANIOSPINAL IRRADIATION

A particular challenge is presented to the radiation oncologist when radiation of the entire cranio-spinal axis is indicated. Multiple fields need to be matched, eliminating gaps between fields ("cold spots") of under irradiated tissue and avoiding field overlaps of high doses ("hot spots").

The radiotherapy technique used for CSI is complex *(27)*. The entire cranio-spinal axis cannot be encompassed in a single radiation field. The treatment should ideally be designed to deliver a uniform dose to the intended target structures, while protecting the uninvolved structures. The most commonly used technique involves administration of cranial radiation with two lateral opposed fields arrayed isocentrically at midplane, matched to one or two PA spinal fields, designed to encompass the entire spinal contents from the upper neck to the distal thecal sac.

Various technical aspects have to be considered when matching these fields. The photon beams have a divergence that can be calculated on the base of the geometrical design of the linear accelerator. The divergence angle can be calculated as Tan^{-1} (0.5 × field length/source to axis distance).

The lateral brain fields are angled with the primary collimator using this formula to match the divergence of the posteroanterior spinal field (*see* Fig. 2).

Similarly, the PA spine field can be angled to match the divergence of the cranial fields by adjusting the couch angle (*see* Fig. 3).

Designing the junction of the fields with this technique yields a geometrically perfect match. When all angle rotations are performed adequately, the dose varies smoothly across the junction without gaps or overdosing *(70)*. The radiation dose at the junction varies with the magnitude of daily setup error. Feathering, or moving the junction by a small, 1 cm distance once a week, increases the uniformity of the dose at the junction, and spreads any potential dose inhomogeneity over a larger spinal length *(30)*, rather than in one spot. This feathering of the junction may be considered as a safety margin but could be superfluous *(70)*.

Establishing the caudal border of the spinal field is equally important. The caudal border of the spinal field has been traditionally established at S2, coinciding with the termination of the spinal sub-arachnoid space. Standard setup with the spinal field ending at S2 may be inadequate in many patients *(27)*. With the use of MRI, the dural sac termination is most frequently seen at S2, however, variability of the caudal dural sac has been found from S1 to S4. Intradural metastatic disease may further extend the dural sac termination distally *(17)*. The lowest termination of the thecal sac can be found below S2 in 9 to 33% of cases, therefore, the lower border of the spinal field has to be individualized according to MRI findings *(17,66)*.

The sub-arachnoid space widens as we move caudally, this has to be considered when selecting the width of the field *(27)*. When designing the lateral cranial blocks, the lateral eye blocks must not block the cribriform plate.

The use of electron beams for irradiation of the spine has been postulated with good patient tolerance *(38)*.

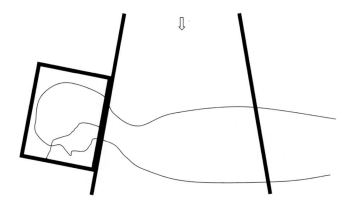

Fig. 2. Schematic lateral diagram of the junction of the lateral cranial and posterior spinal fields.

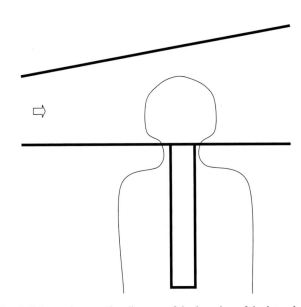

Fig. 3. Schematic posterior diagram of the junction of the lateral cranial and posterior spinal fields.

7. LONG-TERM CONSEQUENCES

Because the late effects of radiotherapy on developing tissues are a cause of major concern for patients and their families, most large clinical trials include a substantive analysis of the long-term impact of radiotherapy on relevant regional tissues.

7.1. SPINAL DEFORMITY

Spinal deformities develop in 22 to 70% of patients after multimodality therapy *(20,23,42,61)*. They include scoliosis, kyphosis, and various combinations of scoliosis, kyphosis, and lordosis *(42)*. The most marked progression of scoliosis occurs during the adolescent growth spurt irrespective of the patient's age at the time of irradiation *(61)*.

The frequency of scoliosis increases as the radiation dose increases. The severity of the scoliosis is also closely related to dosage *(42,50,61)*. Doses of less than 10 Gy are not radiographically detectable *(50)*. Doses of less than 20 Gy are not associated with deformity *(50,57)*, doses between 20 and 30 Gy are associated with scoliosis of less than 20° and doses of more than 30 Gy are associated with scoliosis of more than 20°

(1,50,61). As the length of follow up increases, the severity of the curves increases reflecting the effect of growth in an irradiated spine, with an average of 1° of rate of progression per year *(42)*.

Asymmetrical radiation was associated with more frequent and more severe deformity. However, few children had severe postradiation scoliosis requiring treatment *(42)*.

Radiation changes occur in chondroblasts and the microvasculature of bone. Orthovoltage has a higher differential of energy absorption in bone than megavoltage absorption, which is less dependent on tissue density. This concept has led many to believe that less growth disturbance will be found in megavoltage treated patients. However, the frequency of the changes seen with megavoltage radiation is similar to orthovoltage, though the severity of bony changes is typically less *(28,57)*.

Two periods of extreme sensitivity to radiation are identified: less than 6 yr of age and again at the time of puberty *(23,57,58)*. Marked retardation of vertebral growth can be seen during these periods. Both sitting and standing height have to be measured to detect the full magnitude of the impact. Differences of 2 standard deviations or more, can be found with doses exceeding 35 Gy *(57,58)*.

The most severe changes are seen in patients younger than 2 yr at the time of irradiation *(50,61)*. In children aged 2 to 13 yr and treated with does of 30 Gy, the spine is clinically straight and there are no obvious roentgenological changes 3 to 17 yr after completion of therapy *(1)*.

The magnitude of the loss of stature seems to be correlated to the dose and location of radiation, the stature already achieved at the time of radiation, bilateral femoral head radiation, sex, and predicted adult stature. A predictive model had been described *(68)*.

There is no difference in the ratios of long-term complications of the spine or the organs anterior to the spine when radiation is administered with electron beams compared with photon beams *(23)*.

7.2. ENDOCRINOLOGICAL IMPACT

After CSI, endocrinological deficits can be detected as a result of pituitary dysfunction or peripheral organ failure. Examples are growth hormone deficiency, decreased thyroid stimulating hormone, and hypothyroidism *(13)*. These treatment-related side effects may have major impact on stature and spinal deformity.

7.3. INTELLECTUAL IMPACT

Decreased cognitive function is reported in 36 to 46% of patients undergoing cranial radiation and other CNS therapeutic interventions with intelligence quotient (IQ) decline or need for special schooling *(13,23,71)*.

7.4. SECOND MALIGNANT NEOPLASMS

Second malignant neoplasms are among the most feared complications of pediatric radiotherapy.

The IRS reported that among 1026 long-term survivors treated on IRS-1 and IRS-2 protocols, second malignancies developed in 22 patients, with estimated cumulative incidence of 1.7% at 10 yr *(29)*.

In 2438 patients enrolled in the NWTS, 15 second malignant neoplasms were identified. This number was 8.5 times the expected value, representing a cumulative 10-yr risk of 1% *(3,20)*.

Data from 10 international pediatric centers with nearly 15,000 new patients treated between 1950 and 1970 estimated a cumulative probability of second malignant neoplasm of 3.3% at 20 yr. This represents a 10-fold increase over age adjusted expected rate of cancer. The risk factors cannot be precisely identified, and include radiation, chemotherapy, familial or genetic predisposition, combinations of treatment, and others *(44)*.

Multimodality therapy with high dose radiation and high dose chemotherapy significantly increases the risk of second malignant neoplasms *(1,48,65)*.

8. CONCLUSION

RT has a key role and is an integral part of the management of a wide variety of malignancies in childhood. Improvement in techniques of radiation planning and administration are leading to improved outcomes with decreased short and long-term morbidities.

ACKNOWLEDGMENTS

The author thanks Kelly DeCrane for her assistance in the production of this manuscript.

REFERENCES

1. Bloom HJG, Glees J, Bell J. The treatment and prognosis of medulloblastoma in children. AJR 1969; 105:43–62.
2. Bouffet E, Pierre-Kahn A, Marchal JC, et al. Prognostic factors in pediatric spinal cord astrocytoma. Cancer 1998; 83:2391–2399.
3. Breslow NE, Norkool PA, Olshan A. Second malignant neoplasms in survivors of Wilms' tumor:a report from the National Wilms' tumor study. J Natl Cancer Inst 1998; 80:592–595.
4. Castleberry RP, Kun LE, Shuster JJ, et al. Radiotherapy improves the outlook for patients older than 1 year with POG stage C neuroblastoma.J Clin Oncol 1991; 9:789–795.
5. Chacko AG, Chandy MJ. Favorable outcome after radical excision of a "holocord" astrocytoma. Clin Neurol Neurosurg 2000; 102:240–242.
6. Chang CH, Housepian EM, Herbert C. An operative staging system and a megavoltage radiotherapeutic technique for cerebellar medulloblastoma. J. Neurosurg 1987; 66:80–87.
7. Cherlow JM, Harland S, Steinherz P, et al. CSI for ALL with CNS disease at diagnosis: a report from the CCG. Int J Radiat Oncol Biol Phys 1996; 36:19–27.
8. Chun HC, Schmidt-Ullrich RK, Wolfson A, Tercilla OF, Sagerman RH, King GA.. External beam radiotherapy for spinal cord tumors. J Neurooncol 1990; 9:211–217.
9. Constantini S, Houten J, Miller DC, et al. Intramedullary spinal cord tumors in children under the age of three years. J Neurosurg 1996; 85:1036–1043.
10. Crist W, Gehan EA, Ragab AH, et al: The third IRS. J Clin Oncol 1995; 13:610–630.
11. D'Angio GJ, Breslow N, Beckwith JB, et al. Treatment of Wilms' tumor: results of the third NWTS. Cancer 1989; 64:349–360.
12. D'Angio GJ, Tefft M, Breslow NE, et al. Radiation therapy of Wilms' tumor: results according to dose, field, postoperative timing and histology. Int J Radiat Oncol Biol Phys 1978; 4:769.
13. David KM, Casey ATH, Hayward RD, Harkness WF, Phipps K, Wade AM. Medulloblastoma: is the 5-year survival rate improving? J Neurosurg 1997; 86:13–21.
14. DeSousa AL, Kalsbeck JE, Mealey J, Campbell RL, Hockey A. Intraspinal tumors in children. A review of 81 cases. J Neurosurg 1979; 51:437–445.
15. Deutsch M. Medulloblastoma: staging and treatment outcome. Int J Radiat Oncol Biol Phys 1988; 14:1103–1107.
16. Deutsch M, Thomas PRM, Krischer J, et al. Results of a prospective randomized trail comparing standard dose neuraxis irradiation

(3,600 cGy/20) with reduced neuraxis irradiation (2,340 cGy/13) in patients with low-stage medulloblastoma: a combined Children's Cancer Group-Pediatric Oncology Group Study. Pediatr Neurosurg 1996; 24:167–177.

17. Dunbar S, Barnes P, Tarbell NJ. Radiographic determination of the caudal border of the spinal field in craniospinal irradiation. Int J Radiat Oncol Biol Phys 1993; 26:669–673.

18. Epstein F. Intraaxial tumors of the cervicomedullary junction in children. Pediatr Neurosurg 1987; 7:117.

19. Evans AE, Jenkin RDT, Sposto R, et al. The treatment of medulloblastoma: results of a prospective randomized trial of radiation therapy with and without CCNU, vincristine, and prednisone. J Neurosurg 1990; 72:572–582.

20. Evans AE, Norkool P, Evans I. Late effects for Wilm's tumor. A report from the National Wilms tumor study group. Cancer 1991; 67:331–336.

21. Garcia DM, Marks JE, Latifi HR, Kliefoth AB. Childhood cerebellar astrocytomas: is there a role for postoperative irradiation? Int J Radiat Oncol Biol Phys 1990; 8:815–818.

22. Garrett PG, Simpson WJK. Ependymomas: results of radiation treatment. Int J Radiat Oncol Biol Phys 1983; 9:1121–1124.

23. Gaspar LE, Dawson DJ, Tilley-Gulliford SA, Banerjee P. Medulloblastoma. Long-term follow-up of patients treated with electron irradiation of the spinal field. Radiology 1991; 180:867–870.

24. Goh KY, Velasquez L, Epstein FJ. Pediatric intramedullary spinal cord tumors: is surgery alone engough? Pediatr Neurosurg 1997; 271:34–39.

25. Goldwein JW, Corn BW, Finlay JL, Packer RJ, Rorke LB, Schut L. Is craniospinal irradiation required to cure children with malignant (anaplastic) intracranial ependymomas? Cancer 1991; 67:2766–2771.

26. Gurney JG, Davis S, Severson RK, Fang JY, Ross JA, Robison LL. Trends in cancer incidence among children in the U.S. Cancer 1996; 78:532–541.

27. Halperin BC. Impact of radiation technique upon the outcome of treatment for medulloblastoma. Int J Radiat Oncol Biol Phys 1996; 36:233–239.

28. Heaston DK, Libshitz HI, Chan RC. Skeletal effects of megavoltage irradiation in survivors of Wilm's tumor. AJR 1979; 133:389–395.

29. Heyn R, Haeberlen V, Newton WA, et al. Second malignant neoplasms in children treated for rhabdomyosarcoma. J Clin Oncol 1993; 11:262–270.

30. Holupka EJ, Humm JL, Tarbell NJ, Svensson GK. Effect of set-up error on the dose across the junction of matching cranial-spinal fields in the treatment of medulloblastoma. Int J Radiat Oncol Biol Phys 1993; 27:345–352

31. Houten JK, Cooper PR. Spinal cord astrocytomas: presentation, management and outcome. J Neurooncol 2000; 47:219–224.

32. Houten JK, Weiner HL. Pediatric intramedullary spinal cord tumor: special considerations. J Neurooncol 2000; 473:225–230.

33. Innocenzi G, Raco A, Cantore G, Raimondi AJ. Intrmedullary astrocytomas and ependymomas in the pediatric age group: a retrospective study. Childs Nerv Syst 1996; 12:776–780.

34. Jenkin D, Goddard K, Armstrong D, et al. Posterior fossa medulloblastoma in childhood: treatment results and a proposal for a new staging system. Int J Radiat Oncol Biol Phys 1990; 19:265–274.

35. Kopelson G, Linggood RM, Kleinman GM, Doucette J, Wang CC. Management of intramedullary spinal cord tumors. Radiology 1980; 135:473–479.

36. Linstadt DE, Wara WM, Leibel SA, Gutin PH, Wilson CB, Sheline GE. Postoperative radiotherapy of spinal cord tumors. Int J Radiat Oncol Biol Phys 1989; 16:1397–1403

37. Mandell LR, Ghavimi F, Exelby P, Fuks Z. Preliminary results of alternating combination chemotherapy and hyperfractionated radiotherapy in advanced rhabdomyosarcoma. Int J Radiat Oncol Biol Phys 1988; 15:197–203.

38. Maor MH, Fields RS, Hogstrom KR, van Eys J. Improving the therapeutic ratio of craniospinal irradiation in medulloblastoma. Int J Radiat Oncol Biol Phys 1985; 11:687–697.

39. Matthay KK, Sather HN, Seeger RC, Haase GM, Hammond GD. Excellent outcome of stage II Neuroblastoma is independent of residual disease and radiation therapy. J Clin Oncol 1993; 7:233–244.

40. Maurer HM, Beltangady M, Gehan EA, et al. The IRS-I: A final report. Cancer 1988; 61:209–220.

41. Maurer HM, Gehan EA, Beltangady M, et al. The IRS-II. Cancer 1993; 71: 1904–1922.

42. Mayfield JK, Riseborough EJ, Jaffe N, Nehme ME. Spinal deformity in children treated for neuroblastoma. J Bone Joint Surg Am 1981; 63:183–193.

43. McCormick PC, Torres R, Post KD, Stein BM. Intramedullary ependymoma of the spinal cord. J Neurosurg 1990; 72:523–532.

44. Meadows AT, D'Angio GJ. Incidence of second malignant neoplasms in children: results of an international study. Lancet 1982; 2:1326-1331.

45. Merchant TE, Haida T, Wang M-H, Finlay JL, Leibel SA. Anaplastic ependymoma: treatment of pediatric patients with or without craniospinal radiation therapy. J Neurosurg 1997; 86:943–949.

46. Merchant TE, Kiehna EN, Thompson SJ, Heideman R, Sanford RA, Kun LE. Pediatric low-grade and ependymal spinal cord tumors. Pediatr Neurosurg 2000; 32:30–36.

47. Merchant TE, Nguyen D, Thompson SJ, Reardon DA, Kun LE, Sanford RA. High-grade pediatric spinal cord tumors. Pediatr Neurosurg 2000; 32:1–5.

48. Merchant TE, Wang M-E, Haida T, et al. Medulloblastoma: long-term results for patients treated with definitive radiation therapy during the computed tomography era. Int J Ratiat Oncol Biol Phys 1996; 36:29–35.

49. Nadkarni TD, Rekate HL. Pediatric intramedullary spinal cord tumors. Critical review of the literature. Childs Nerv Syst 1999; 15:17–28.

50. Neuhauser, EBD, Wittenborg MH, Berman CZ, Cohen J. Irradiation effects of roentgen therapy on the growing spine. Radiology 1952; 59:637–650.

51. Nitschke R, Smith EI, Altshuler G, et al. Postoperative treatment of non metastatic visible residual neuroblastoma: a POG study. J Clin Oncol 1991; 9:1181–1188.

52. Nitschke R, Smith EI, Shochat S, et al. Localized Neuroblastoma treated by surgery: a POG study. J Clin Oncol 1988; 6:1271–1279.

53. O'Sullivan C, Jenkin RD, Doherty MA, Hoffman HJ, Greenberg ML. Spinal cord tumors in children: long-term results of combined surgical and radiation treatment. J Neurosurg 1994; 81:507–512.

54. Packer RJ, Sutton LN, Elterman R, et al. Outcome for children with medulloblastoma treated with radiation and cisplatin, CCNU, and vincristine chemotherapy. J Neurosurg 1994; 81:690–698.

55. Pollack IF, Hurtt M, Pang D, Albright AL. Dissemination of low grade intracranial astro-cytomas in children. Cancer 1994; 73:2869–2878.

56. Prados M, Mamelak AN. Metastasizing low grade gliomas in children. Redefining an old disease. Cancer 1994; 73:2671–2673.

57. Probert JC, Parker BR. The effects of radiation therapy on bone growth. Radiology 1975; 114:155–162.

58. Probert JC, Parker BR, Kaplan HS. Growth retardation in children after megavoltage irradiation of the spine. Cancer 1973; 32:634–639.

59. Reimer R, Onofrio BM. Astrocytomas of the spinal cord in children and adolescents. J Neurosurg 1985; 63: 669–675.

60. Rezai AR, Woo HH, Lee M, Cohen H, Zagzag D, Epstein FJ. Disseminated ependymomas of the central nervous system. J Neurosurg 1996; 85:618–624

61. Riseborough EJ, Grabias SL, Burton RI. Skeletal alterations following irradiation for Wilms' tumor. J Bone Joint Surg Am 1976; 58:526–536.

62. Rousseau P, Habrand JL, Ssarrazin D, et al. Treatment of intracranial ependymomas of children: review of a 15-year experience. Int J Radiat Oncol Biol Phys 1994; 28:381–386.

63. Salazar OM. A better understanding of CNS seeding and brighter outlook for postoperatively irradiated patients with ependymomas. Int J Radiat Oncol Biol Phys 1983; 9:1231–1234.

64. Salazar OM, Castro-Vita H, VanHoutte P, Rubin P, Aygun C. Improved survival in cases of intracranial ependymoma after radiation therapy. Late report and recommendations. J. Neurosurg 1983; 59:652–653.

65. Scaradavou A, Heller G, Sklar CA. Second malignant neoplasms in long-term survivors of childhood rhabdomyosarcoma. Cancer 1995; 76:1860–1867.

66. Scharf CB, Paulino AC, Goldberg KN. Determination of the inferior border of the thecal sac using magnetic resonance imaging: implications on radiation therapy treatment planning. Int J Radiat Oncol Biol Phys 1998; 41:621–624.

67. Schiffer D, Chio A, Giordana MT, et al. Histologic prognostic factors in ependymoma. Childs Nerv Syst 1991; 7:177–182.

68. Silber JH, Littman PS, Meadows AT. Stature loss following skeletal irradiation for childhood cancer. J Clin Oncol 1990; 8:304–312.

69. Silverman CL, Simpson JR. Cerebellar medulloblastoma: the importance of posterior fossa dose to survival and patterns of failure. Int J Radiat Oncol Biol Phys 1982; 8:1869–1876.

70. Tatcher M, Glicksman AS. Field matching considerations in craniospinal irradiation. Int J Radiat Oncol Biol Phys 1989; 17:865–869.

71. Thomas PRM, Deutsch M, Mulhern, R, et al. Reduced dose neuraxis irradiation in low stage medulloblastoma: the POG and CCG study. SIPO XXVII meeting-abstracts. Med Pediatr Oncol 1995; 25: 277–287.

72. Thomas PRM, Tefft M, Farewell VT, Norkool P, Storer B, D'Angio GJ. Abdominal relapses in irradiated second NWTS patients. J Clin Oncol 1984; 2:1098–1101.

73. Trigg ME, Makuch R, Glaubiger D. Actuarial risk of isolated CNS involvement in Ewing's sarcoma following prophylactic cranial irradiation and intrathecal methotrexate. Int J Radiat Oncol Biol Phys 1985; 11:699–702.

74. Vanuytsel LJ, Bessell EM, Ashley SE, Bloom HJ, Brada M. Intracranial ependymoma: long-term results of a policy of surgery and radiotherapy. Int J Radiat Oncol Biol Phys 1992; 23:313–319.

75. Wara WM, Le QT, Sneed PK, et al. Pattern of recurrence of medulloblastoma after low-dose craniospinal radiotherapy. Int J Radiat Oncol Biol Phys 1994; 30:551–556.

76. Whitaker SJ, Bessel EM, Ashley SE, et al. Postoperative radiotherapy in the management of spinal cord ependymoma. J Neurosurg 1991; 74:720–728.

24 Conformal Radiotherapy for Spinal Lesions

R<small>ICHARD</small> L. C<small>ROWNOVER</small>, MD, PhD

C<small>ONTENTS</small>

I<small>NTRODUCTION</small>
P<small>HYSICAL</small> G<small>RADIENTS</small>
B<small>IOLOGICAL</small> G<small>RADIENTS</small>
C<small>ONFORMAL</small> T<small>ECHNIQUES</small>
R<small>EFERENCES</small>

1. INTRODUCTION

In the spine, as elsewhere, conventional doses and treatment schedules in radiotherapy have been titrated to the clinical tolerance of normal tissues. Protracted treatment courses delivered over several weeks, "fractionated schedules," are a radiobiological compromise employed to permit normal tissue repair between multiple small doses of radiation with the goal of reducing morbid late effects of treatment. Radiotherapy is widely used because this approach is often successful in dealing with microscopic disease or particularly radio-sensitive tumors, however, for bulky disease or radio-resistant tumors, sterilizing tumoricidal doses may never be reached owing to limitations imposed by nearby critical structures such as the spinal cord.

Conformal radiotherapy, in which the high-dose region is shaped to fit the target lesion and the incidental dose to adjacent normal tissues is limited, can be employed in strategies that vary depending on the clinical situation. When treating lesions with an established effective dose, conformal techniques can permit reduction of dose to adjacent tissues with a resultant decrease in acute and late morbidity. In cases where tumors have not been reliably controlled by conventional doses, the localized dose applied to the tumor can be increased, or "escalated," to a higher total, whereas doses nearby are held constant to maintain normal-tissue effects at the level, which was considered acceptable previously. Both approaches would represent an improvement in therapeutic ratio for radiotherapy. In some situations, both goals can be accomplished simultaneously.

Before pursuing the holy grail of highly conformal radiotherapy, it is important to acknowledge two points. First, if treatments are tightly localized, then the target volume must be drawn accurately to avoid geographic misses and ablative damage to normal structures. Reviewing target volumes with diagnostic radiologists and surgeons is prudent. Second, it is possible to reduce the treatment volume by excluding areas that would have been "incidentally" treated by conventional techniques and subsequently discover that those areas become sites of failure, that is, they were actually important therapeutic targets that were not previously appreciated as such. For instance, there might be microscopic tracking along nerves or ill-defined routes of nodal drainage that have always been covered by standard beam arrangements. Without careful attention it would be quite easy to conduct an unintentional "clinical trial" demonstrating an increase in marginal misses.

2. PHYSICAL GRADIENTS

Conventional radiation treatments are delivered through a small number of beams: typically one to four. With these techniques, dose is prescribed to a crude volume encompassing the target. When a small number of beams are used, each beam carries a significant fraction of the dose and a biologically meaningful amount of tissue damage occurs along the path of each beam (Fig. 1). The rate of change in dose fall-off at the edge of a treatment plan is known as the "dose-gradient." A "steep gradient" would indicate that the delivered dose decreases sharply at the edge of a treatment plan, conversely, a "shallow gradient" means that the dose gradually rolls off over a significant distance. Conventional external-beam treatments have shallow gradients, often delivering substantial doses even several centimeters from the intended target.

In conformal treatments, a large number of convergent beams are directed at a target so that no single beam carries much of the radiation dose. In this situation, very little damage is done to tissues as an individual beam traverses the body, but at the point where the beams intersect a very high, localized dose of radiation is delivered. By clever positioning and weighting of the beams, the high-dose region can be shaped to match the target lesion "like a glove." This can be accomplished in a variety of ways such as an array of fixed isocentric beams,

From: *Current Clinical Oncology: Cancer in the Spine: Comprehensive Care.*
Edited by: R. F. McLain, K-U. Lewandrowski, M. Markman, R. M. Bukowski,
R. Macklis, and E. C. Benzel © Humana Press, Inc., Totowa, NJ

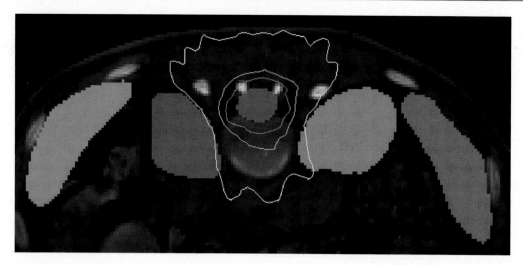

Fig. 1. Intensity-modulated radiotherapy isodose distribution used to avoid the kidneys during conformal radiotherapy of a recurrent ependymoma. The prescription isodose line is circular and encompasses the spinal canal. Tissues outside the larger isodose line, which abuts the kidneys, received less than 20% of the prescribed dose.

rotational arcs, or multiple noncoplanar beams. Radiosurgery represents the extreme situation in which a large number of beams are used to almost completely exclude normal tissues from the treatment volume so that a large ablative dose of radiation can be delivered in a single fraction.

Radiosurgery, first with the γ-knife and subsequently with modified linear accelerators, has gradually gained credibility as an alternative to surgery for entire classes of patients. A confluence of recent developments in computer science, medical imaging, and robotics has contributed to a new generation of radiation treatment devices capable of delivering dose distributions comparable or even superior to those achievable with implants—non-invasively and to surgically inaccessible sites. It should be acknowledged that the pioneers of radiosurgery and the entrepreneurs who drive the ongoing development of conformal radiotherapy platforms are almost exclusively neurosurgeons who bypassed the dogmas of their more conservative colleagues in radiation oncology. In recent years, radiation oncologists have collaborated in developing expanded applications beyond the central nervous system where knowledge of routes of tumor spread and normal tissue tolerance for a variety of organs becomes important.

With the exception of isocentric "shot placement," treatment planning with large numbers of beams was not feasible before the advent of inexpensive high-performance computers capable of "inverse treatment planning." Traditional treatment planning proceeds "forward" in the sense that a human operator (dosimetrist, medical physicist, or physician) designs a set of treatment fields which are all in one plane for geometric simplicity, then calculates the resultant dose distribution and makes small modifications as needed until an acceptable plan is generated. The forward approach has been carried to its practical limit with three-dimensional conformal radiotherapy, in which the target volume is delineated on an imaging study such as a computed tomography (CT) or magnetic resonance imaging scan, then "beams-eye views" are generated for up to a dozen noncoplanar beams. In each beams-eye view, shaping blocks

are drawn to make the beam fit the tumor cross-section as projected from that particular direction. As the name suggests, "inverse planning" proceeds in reverse order; the physician supplies information about what the final plan should look like in terms of desired dose to the target and dose limitations for other structures, then software searches for a beam arrangement that would achieve the desired goals. Inverse planning is frequently compared to the method of image reconstruction using CT scanners; instead of interpreting CT beam data to generate an image, the desired "picture," in this case the requested dose distribution, is known and the beams to produce it are back-calculated.

Intensity-modulated radiotherapy (IMRT) is a simple concept. When a beam-modifying metal wedge is placed in the path of a radiation beam it causes the intensity of the beam to vary from one area to another by attenuating the beam more where the metal is thicker and less where the metal is thinner; the metal wedge modulates the intensity of the beam across its profile. Varying the intensity across a beam profile can improve dose homogeneity, minimizing hot and cold spots when treating a part of the body that varies in thickness such as the breast or neck. This simplest case is so trivial that the term IMRT would not be used to describe it, though the core principles are relevant.

More complex intensity modulation can be accomplished using a multi-leaf collimator, which consists of a number of parallel metal fingers positioned to move in and out of a treatment beam under computer control to produce intricate variations in a beam's intensity profile. With multiple shaped intensity modulated beams dose can be shaped to fit targets that are highly irregular or even concave. Physical dose-gradients of commercially available IMRT systems are generally not adequate for radiosurgery, but fractionated conformal radiotherapy is finding many applications. In the spine, lesions have been treated with doughnut shaped plans, which leave a cold region in the spinal canal virtually untouched. The isodose plan shown in Fig. 1 was used to spare the kidneys of a young woman during fractionated treatment of a recurrent ependymoma.

A serious limitation of inverse treatment planning is determining when a plan is "good enough." Objective tools for quantitative comparison of plans are lacking, presently, such decisions are still based on the physician's subjective interpretation. The calculations that have been used for many years in radiotherapy are only "adequate" for conventional techniques, radiation oncologists are trained to be skeptical of dose calculations where dissimilar tissues are abutting or where air cavities are present. In conformal treatments, the calculation algorithms must be more subtle, appropriately accounting for variations in tissue density and "second-order" physical effects that were beyond the computational scope of prior software. Sophisticated Monte Carlo calculation techniques, developed by national weapons laboratories, are now appearing in treatment planning systems; the resulting "correct" dose-calculations must be evaluated carefully by clinicians because the calculated values cannot be compared directly with historical experience. This represents another place where unintentional, and potentially harmful, clinical trials could occur.

When low energy orthovoltage machines and Cobalt sources were used for external beam treatments, extensive moist desquamation was observed frequently. This is because the dose was greatest at the body surface so that delivering dose to a deep tumor required giving high doses to the skin. Treatments became more tolerable with the introduction of high-energy linear accelerators (LINACs), which provide relative "skin sparing." For these devices, the energy deposition is higher inside the body than at the surface because of a "build up" phenomenon, which can be pictured as a growing wave that starts from the point where the beam first encounters the body. Beyond the build up region, the wave dissipates exponentially as energy is gradually lost to the tissue. For multiple beams, there is no great gain from using higher energies because the surface dose is so widely distributed; hair loss and dermal erythema associated with conformal treatments are minimal and only seen in the area directly overlying a superficially located tumor. This means that a modified Cobalt machine could be used to deliver highly conformal state-of-the-art radiotherapy — good news for parts of the world where the cost and maintenance requirements of a LINAC are prohibitive.

The final point regarding physical dose is that in reaching a target, even a lightly weighted radiation beam must pass through tissue and deposit some energy along the path. A subtle cost of conformal treatments is that numerous low-dose beams may actually deposit a larger "integral dose," or total distributed dose, to the body than a small number of conventional beams. Distributing dose at low levels over large volumes of the body has raised concerns of induced malignancies in the future, this issue is of particular importance in pediatric patients. Caution must also be used to avoid "dose dumping" into particularly sensitive tissues, such as the lungs, where a widely distributed low-dose of radiation may have functional significance.

3. BIOLOGICAL GRADIENTS

Because dose fall-off at the edge of a radiosurgical treatment volume is not perfectly sharp, a few millimeters separation between the target lesion and critical structures has been a typical requirement for consideration of radiosurgery in the brain.

Attention has been shown for structures, such as the optic chiasm, brain stem, speech areas, and sensorimotor strip, where induced deficits would have a significant negative impact on quality of life, this appropriately conservative approach has resulted in a low incidence of complications that obscure the true dose–response relationships. Common sense dictates that all lesions in or near the spinal cord should also be managed cautiously.

Even with sophisticated delivery and treatment planning systems, when a lesion is located in extensive contact with a critical structure, it may be impossible to achieve a physical dose gradient that sharply discriminates between the target and adjacent tissue. In these cases, the biological gradient can be improved by use of fractionation. When small doses of radiation are delivered to a tissue each day, significant repair has time to occur between doses, which reduces the cumulative damage, the amount of repair between fractions increases rapidly as the size of the daily dose is decreased.

As an illustrative example of how fractionation can help localize radiation effects, suppose that a 1.5-cm metastatic adenocarcinoma in the spine has epidural extension within 2 mm of the spinal cord. Based on historical results with similar tumors in the brain, a reasonable objective would be to deliver a minimum of 24 Gy in a single fraction to the entire tumor. A radiosurgical plan is developed that has a high peaking dose inside the tumor and covers the entire lesion with at least 24 Gy, however, it is found that even with best planning efforts, a portion of the spinal cord will still receive 14 Gy, which would exceed the nominal tolerance dose of 8 Gy in a single fraction. An unattractive option would be to reduce the dose to that portion of the tumor that is immediately adjacent to the cord knowing that this will compromise the probability of durable tumor control, instead, fractionated schedules are explored as an alternate approach. The linear-quadratic model developed by Fowler (1) can provide some guidance in comparing schedules, but still requires skilled clinical judgement as a "sanity check" on the results. If the total dose is divided over 5 d, then the daily cord dose falls from 14 to 2.8 Gy. Calculations based on reasonable assumptions regarding tumor kinetics and rates of normal-tissue repair, reveal that the biological impact on the cord would be reduced by approximately two-thirds even though the physical dose delivered to the cord is still 14 Gy. For comparison, a common palliative regimen used "safely" for spinal cord compression is 20 Gy in five fractions of 4 Gy daily, demonstrating that the calculation is consistent with clinical experience. Because the daily doses to the tumor remain quite large, 8 Gy or more each day, there is minimal reduction in efficacy for tumor control, if a larger number of fractions were required, then the total physical dose might have to be increased.

4. CONFORMAL TECHNIQUES

The earliest way of delivering localized treatments was "by treating from the inside out" with implanted radioactive sources: a technique that is formally known as "brachytherapy." Years of clinical experience with these techniques have demonstrated the efficacy of localized high-dose radiation treatments even in dealing with bulky tumors. From brachytherapy,

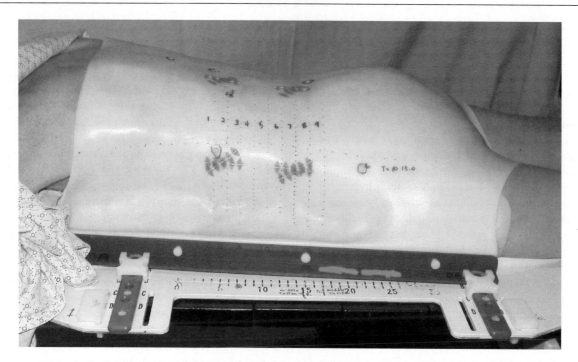

Fig. 2. Aquaplast body mold for immobilization during fractionated conformal radiotherapy of the spine.

much has been learned about the doses required to consistently sterilize tumors and the optimal target volumes at risk of tumor involvement, these insights provide guidance for initial trials with newer conformal technologies. With the exception of cervix and prostate implants, brachytherapy is practiced in only a few specialized centers because implant techniques require special skills in the physician and medical physicist. General application of brachytherapy is also hampered by results that are markedly user-dependent.

Brachytherapy is not commonly employed in the spine, but there are scattered reports from tertiary-care centers. In 1987, a report from University of California at San Francisco described treatment of a chordoma in the upper cervical spine that was recurrent following intensive external beam radiotherapy that had delivered 60 Gy to the cervical cord. A platinum foil was shaped to the cord and positioned in the epidural space before placement of an array of permanent I-125 sources to deliver an additional 50 Gy (2). No neurological injury resulted and the patient died of unrelated causes 19 mo later without evidence of disease. More recently, physicians at the University of Arizona described use of a gold foil to shield the thoracic cord when managing a chondrosarcoma recurrent after resection and postoperative external-beam radiotherapy that had delivered 45 Gy to the cord. The gold foil was shaped to enclose the thecal sac and nerve root sleeves before placement of permanent I-125 sources. Those authors report that an additional 120 Gy was delivered, whereas the cord received only 1% of the implant dose. Tumor had not recurred at the time of the report 18 mo following implant (3). A recent report from the University of Arizona describes 26 patients with malignant tumors compressing the spinal cord who were treated with paraspinal brachytherapy as an adjunct to surgical decompression and resection of tumor. Strings of I-125 seeds were placed with

careful attention to avoid direct contact with neural tissue. Twenty-two of the sites also received external beam radiotherapy (EBRT). No adverse effects were observed and 2-yr local control was 82.6%. Notably, all four local recurrences happened in patients whose tumors had progressed following EBRT (4).

IMRT was initially used to treat tumors in the brain or head/neck region where immobilization was relatively easy to accomplish. It has now been generalized to many other sites in the body. To treat spinal lesions, we have used an aquaplast mold encompassing approximately one-third of the patient's body centered on the treatment site (Fig. 2). The mold locks down to the edges of the treatment table and also snaps down to the table between the patient's legs. Alignment tattoos are placed on the patient's skin where they can be visualized through holes punched in the immobilization device. We have used this arrangement to deliver conventional schedules of radiation to well-defined targets within the vertebral bodies or spinal canal at all levels of the spine: cervical, thoracic, lumbar, and sacral. Particularly in the thoracic region, we have been selective in applying this technique only to relatively thin patients. With a snugly fitting body mold, respiratory motions are directed primarily toward the diaphragm and have not hampered accurate delivery of conservatively designed treatment plans. When we applied the same immobilization technique to dynamic radiosurgery with the CyberKnife®, position confirmation of fiducials in the lumbar spine taken at approx 1-min intervals during two treatments showed anatomic displacements that were consistently less than 2 mm. A group at the University of Heidelberg described a more elaborate non-invasive fixation device for extracranial stereotactic radiotherapy (5). In their system a body cast/head mask combination enclosed the head and extended to the mid-thigh level. During treatments, the body cast was rigidly attached to a stereotactic body frame. Based on five patients treated to sites in the thoracic and lumbar spine, they estimated that the overall accuracy "can be safely estimated to be ≤3.6 mm." These techniques are adequate for fractionated treatments, but are too imprecise for ablative radiosurgical dosing unless target tracking is employed.

Radiosurgery in the brain using a frame attached to the skull is only precise to within a couple of millimeters. As previously noted, anatomic flexibility and internal motions of the body introduce additional uncertainty in dose delivery for spinal lesions. In an attempt to circumvent these problems, an invasive technique was developed to immobilize a segment of the spine for radiosurgery (6,7). This approach involves exposing the spinous processes of vertebral bodies immediately above and below the target level, which are then clamped to a rigid external frame. From phantom measurements a localization accuracy of 1.4 mm was reported. Nine patients with recurrent tumors in the spinal column have been treated with this pioneering invasive approach. Acute toxicity has been minor and three patients evaluable at 1 yr show tumor control at the treated site.

A non-invasive radiosurgical platform is available at a small number of sites in the United States and Japan. The CyberKnife consists of a robotic manipulator wielding a compact linear accelerator. As with other radiosurgical platforms, numerous convergent beams are used to produce a highly conformal dose distribution. What is unique about the CyberKnife is that before delivery of each beam, a pair of orthogonal diagnostic radiographs are obtained and from these stereoscopic views the current location of the target can be deduced rapidly and precisely. This is accomplished by triangulation from several small metal fiducials that are implanted in the spine under local anesthesia or directly from image correlations based on skeletal anatomy. The robotic manipulator quickly adjusts the position of the radiation source to produce idealized geometry that conforms to the original prescription. Researchers at Stanford published initial results treating spinal lesions with the CyberKnife (8). They described 16 patients treated with doses of 11 to 25 Gy delivered in one to five fractions. No acute toxicity was reported. The paper from Stanford indicates "alignment of the treatment dose with the target volume within ± 1 mm…" (8). At the Cleveland Clinic, a modification of this approach has been used to treat the spine, and also to successfully track and treat moving tumors in the lung.

Therapeutic proton beams have fundamentally different physical properties than photon beams and deposit energy in a pattern that is quite distinctive. Proton beams have a sharp peak in energy deposition at depth in tissue, which is followed by an abrupt drop. This exotic pattern can be exploited to deliver very high doses abutting critical structures. Unfortunately, proton machines are prohibitively expensive and only two facilities are open in the United States.

4.1. CLINICAL SITUATIONS WARRANTING USE OF CONFORMAL TECHNIQUES

For non-infiltrative well-visualized lesions, where the effective dose and necessary target volume are both well established, one generally wants to limit the exposure of sensitive normal tissues to a subclinical level in which optimal repair of cellular damage is possible. We have used this strategy to treat eight ependymomas in three patients. All three patients were surgical failures. Conventional schedules of approx 54 in 2-Gy daily doses were delivered to the spinal canal with 2-cm craniocaudal margins on the visualized tumor. Care was taken to ensure that the spinal canal was covered homogeneously without significant "hot spots" in the treatment plan. Doses to structures at the level of the tumor to be treated, such as the kidneys in a patient with lumbar lesions, were tightly constrained. Six of the eight lesions were controlled at 2 yr. The two recurrent lesions were in one patient and they have recently been treated again using radiosurgery. Longitudinally infiltrating astrocytic tumors arising in the cord may also be amenable to this approach using generous margins.

Many benign lesions would seem perfect targets for radiosurgical techniques because they are not infiltrative, they are easily visualized radiographically, and their slow proliferation obviates the need for fractionation, however, enthusiasm for ablative treatment of these lesions is tempered by realization that collateral radiation damage contributing to late morbidity may have many years to express itself clinically. In and around the brain, radiosurgery has shown clinical efficacy for meningiomas, schwannomas, ependymomas, glomus tumors, and arteriovenous malformations. There is no reason to presume that similar treatments should be less effective for lesions of identical histology located in the spine. Chordomas and chondrosarcomas are good examples of tumors that are not adequately controlled by doses in the upper range of what can be delivered safely with conventional techniques. The most successful outcomes in the axial skeleton have been reported for mixed photon/proton therapy following maximal debulking (9,10). It remains to be established whether dose escalation with highly conformal techniques will prove as effective as protons. If conformal radiotherapy is undertaken, the strategy is to hold the peripheral dose at conventionally accepted tolerance levels, while delivering a high-peaking central dose to the tumor or resection bed. We have used this strategy for patients who were rendered ineligible for proton therapy protocols owing to interventions before consultation at our institution. Patients with newly diagnosed chordomas and chondrosarcomas should be informed of proton results before definitive treatment is initiated. This is particularly important because the surgical techniques employed may be altered by anticipation of postoperative proton therapy. Osteosarcoma is another histology that may benefit from dose-escalation strategies.

Patients with symptomatic progression of metastatic disease in the spine after radiotherapy should be evaluated for surgery. Interstitial implant in conjunction with surgery may be beneficial for selected patients. If they are not surgical candidates because of their poor prognosis or intercurrent conditions, then cautious re-irradiation may represent the only therapeutic option. Assuming that the original course of radiotherapy delivered a typical dose of 30 Gy, then in a context of diffusely progressive disease, where life expectancy is severely limited, a gentle additional palliative course of 20 Gy in 10 fractions, employing conventional techniques, may provide relief of pain until the end of life. Such end-of-life situations do not generally warrant the resources required for highly conformal treatments. Patients with a localized recurrence who are expected to live at least several months, present a more serious challenge. The palliative regimen previously described would have little chance of providing long-term control of disease, but would create a significant risk of delayed damage to the spinal cord. Designing a high-dose plan, which encompasses the metastatic lesion or entire vertebral body but relatively spares the spinal cord, may permit delivery of therapeutically meaningful doses. The strategy here would be to design a plan that provides a sharp separation between the vertebral body and spinal canal, then prescribe the dose as aggressively as permitted by residual cord tolerance. Calculating residual tolerance does not have a well-defined algorithm, it depends on the original treatment schedule and also the interval since prior treatment. In definitive situations which warrant aggressive treatment, conventional cord doses may be pushed to 54 Gy rather than the frequently used limiting value of 45 Gy. When preparing for re-irradiation, the use of 54 in 2 Gy divided doses as the limiting value, with the important caveat that prior surgical manipulations or drug therapy, may have lowered the threshold for cord damage. Using the spinal canal as proxy for the cord itself provides a reassuring margin of prescribing safety.

REFERENCES

1. Fowler JF. The linear-quadratic formula and progress in fractionated radiotherapy. Br J Radiol 1989; 62:679–694.
2. Gutin PH, Leibel SA, Hosobuchi Y, et al. Brachytherapy of recurrent tumors of the skull base and spine with iodine-125 sources. Neurosurgery 1987; 20:938–945.
3. Hamilton AJ, Lulu B, Baldassarre S, Wai CC, Cassady RJ. The use of gold foil wrapping for radiation protection of the spinal cord for recurrent tumor therapy. Int J Radiat Oncol Biol Phys 1995; 32:507–511.
4. Rogers L, Theodore N, Dickman C, et al. Surgery and permanent I-125 seed paraspinal brachytherapy for malignant tumors with spinal cord compression. Int J Radiat Oncol Biol Phys 2002; 54;503–513.
5. Lohr F, Debus J, Frank C, et al. Noninvasive patient fixation for extracranial stereotactic radiotherapy. Int J Radiat Oncol Biol Phys 1999; 45:521–527.
6. Hamilton AJ, Lulu BA, Fosmire H, Stea B, Cassady JR. Preliminary clinical experience with linear accelerator-based spinal stereotactic radiosurgery. Neurosurgery 1995; 36:311–319.
7. Hamilton AJ, Lulu BA, Fosmire H, Gossett L. LINAC-based spinal stereotactic radiosurgery. Stereotact Funct Neurosurg 1996; 66:1–9.
8. Ryu, SI, Chang SD, Kim DH, et al. Image-guided hypo-fractionated stereotactic radiosurgery to spinal lesions. Neurosurgery 2000; 49:838–846.
9. Hug EB, Fitzek MM, Liebsch NJ, Munzenrider JE. Locally challenging osteo- and chondrogenic tumors of the axial skeleton: results of combined proton and photon radiation therapy using three-dimensional treatment planning. Int J Radiat Oncol Biol Phys 1995; 31:467–476.
10. Hug EB, Laredo LN, Slater JD, et al. Proton radiation therapy for chordomas and chondrosarcomas of the skull base. J Neurosurg 1999; 91:432–439.

25 Photon- and Proton-Beam Radiotherapy in the Treatment of Spine Tumors

THOMAS F. DELANEY, MD, MICHAEL J. HARRIS, MD,
FRANCIS J. HORNICEK, MD, PhD, AND ROBERT F. MCLAIN, MD

CONTENTS

1. INTRODUCTION

Over the last 30 yr, the treatment of primary and metastatic tumors of the cervical, thoracic, and lumbar spine has evolved dramatically. In the case of primary tumors of the spine, advances in neoadjuvant treatments and instrumentation techniques have offered patients with previously inoperable disease new options with reasonable chances of cure. When the overall morbidity of radical resection makes it a poor treatment option, radiation therapy can be combined with more conservative surgical procedures or can be used in lieu of surgery for palliation, or even cure in some instances. With new advances in radiotherapy techniques, greater doses of radiation (often tumorocidal doses) can be administered to the majority of tumor volume with fewer effects on the surrounding structures and, most particularly, minimal risk to the spinal cord. It is imperative for the clinician and surgeon to be familiar with these new techniques so that the care of their patients can be optimized, with the highest potential for long-term survival and reduced morbidity.

This chapter is divided into two sections. The first reviews photon radiotherapy techniques used to treat specific primary malignancies, metastatic deposits, and aggressive benign tumors of the spine. The second section is devoted to proton therapy. This chapter serves as an overview of external radiotherapy techniques used in the treatment of primary tumors and metastatic deposits in the cervical, thoracic, and lumbar spine. In addition, a list of references is provided for the clinician who wishes to further investigate these techniques and their applications.

2. RADIOTHERAPY FOR SARCOMAS OF THE SPINE AND PARASPINAL SOFT TISSUES

There is emerging information in a number of recent reports on the importance of gross total resections of sarcomas of the spine, in contrast to piecemeal resections or biopsy alone. These tumors are more frequently being treated like those of the extremities. Surgery is best performed by oncological surgeons with specialty expertise in the spine. Because of the difficulty of achieving microscopically negative margins, radiation therapy can have an important role in providing durable local control in these patients and should be administered at the time of initial treatment in patients with positive margins. The experience in extremity sarcomas, the most common anatomic site for these lesions, is that the combination of radiation therapy and limb-preserving surgery has produced high rates of local control. When adjacent normal tissue tolerance has permitted, radiation therapy doses have been 60 Gy or more when close or positive surgical margins are encountered. Indeed, local control is improved, in the setting of positive margins, with doses of more than 64 Gy (1,2). For unresected sarcomas, there appears to be a similar advantage for doses above 63 Gy (3). These doses have been difficult to achieve in the past in lesions in close proximity to the spinal cord, which is at risk for radiation-induced transverse myelitis at doses of 50 Gy or more. New radiation techniques have made it possible to deliver tumoricidal doses of this magnitude to lesions in or near the axial spine.

Advances in external radiation treatment planning and delivery have made it possible to more closely shape the radiation dose distribution around the tumor and spare normal tissue using "conformal radiotherapy." This refers to a variety of techniques that aim to closely contour the radiation dose around the tumor, limit dose to surrounding normal tissue, with the dual

From: *Current Clinical Oncology: Cancer in the Spine: Comprehensive Care.*
Edited by: R. F. McLain, K-U. Lewandrowski, M. Markman, R. M. Bukowski,
R. Macklis, and E. C. Benzel © Humana Press, Inc., Totowa, NJ

benefits of improving local tumor control and reducing normal tissue complications. These conformal radiotherapy techniques include proton or charged particle radiation therapy, three-dimensional (3D) conformal photon radiation therapy, and intensity-modulated radiation therapy (*see* Chapter 24). The techniques all use computed tomography (CT) and or magnetic resonance imaging (MRI) images of the tumor and adjacent normal tissue acquired with the patient in a reproducible position (often by immobilization with a thermoplastic cast) and referenced in space to reproducible landmarks on or in the patient or cast. These images are then transferred to a 3D radiotherapy treatment-planning computer where the desired tumor volume target and critical normal structures are outlined by the radiation oncologist *(4,5)*. Beam trajectories or radio-isotope source placement can then be planned to maximize dose to the tumor and optimally spare critical normal tissues, which, in the case of lesions in the spine, will be the spinal cord or cauda, equina, and depending on the anatomic level, can also include brain, cranial nerves, optic chiasm, parotid glands, heart, esophagus, lungs, kidneys, liver, and bowel.

The use of 3D conformal photon radiation therapy (3DCRT) has now become common practice in most centers. Using beam's eye viewing of volumes defined on a treatment planning CT scan, beam directions and beam shapes can be selected to conform to the shape of the projected target and minimize dose to critical normal structures. Despite its appellation, it can be difficult to conform the beam around certain 3D structures such as the spinal cord. Intensity-modulated radiation therapy (IMRT) uses modifications in the intensity of the beam across the irradiated fields to enhance the capability of conforming dose distributions in 3D *(6)*. Dosimetric comparisons of 3DCRT plans with IMRT plans indicate that IMRT can yield significantly better dose distributions in some situations at the expense of additional time and resources.

New technologies are being developed that should significantly reduce the time needed to plan, implement, and verify these treatments. Practitioners have begun to apply IMRT to treatment of spinal and paraspinal tumors. Patients undergo a CT-myelogram immobilized in the radiation therapy treatment position for radiation therapy treatment planning. Alternatively, an MRI obtained in the treatment position can be used for image fusion with the radiation therapy planning CT for localization of the spinal cord and tumor delineation. The spinal cord can be localized with high precision and spared from excessive dose, while delivering high doses to the tumor bed. Daily orthogonal imaging of the patient is obtained to confirm accuracy of treatment set-up before dose delivery each day. This kind of dose distribution is not achievable with conventional radiotherapy *(6a)*.

Our preference has been to employ moderate dose external beam radiation therapy (20–45 Gy) before resection to reduce the risk of tumor seeding at the time of surgery, followed by additional intra-operative and postoperative radiation therapy as dictated by surgical findings and pathological resection margin status.

Intra-operative radiation therapy can be employed to increase radiation dose to the dura in situations in which tumor is resected off of the dura. Orthovoltage or electron beam radiation delivered via sterile cones or radioisotope brachytherapy are two technical means of achieving appropriate intra-operative dose delivery. A group from Memorial Sloan Kettering Cancer Center reported 3-yr local control in 43% of 49 patients with paraspinal tumors implanted for a variety of nonlung cancer histologies, 26 of whom had sarcomas *(7)*. No cases of radiation myelitis were reported. There are dosimetric limitations with the currently available temporary iridium-192 applicators which deliver higher than optimal doses to the spinal cord and with permanent iodine-125 implants, which may be difficult to align in an optimal,) permanent, geometric array. Therefore, we have developed new Yttrium-90 radioisotope applicators to allow for temporary, intra-operative placement of a plaque on the dura to deliver very high doses (generally 10 Gy) to the dural surface with low energy electrons with minimal dose to the spinal cord in approx 10 min (Fig. 1) *(8)*.

2.1. METASTATIC DISEASE

In general, the indications for external beam radiation are pain without instability, deformity, or significant epidural spinal cord or cauda equina compression. The most successful predictor of outcome of patients treated for metastatic disease to the spine causing spinal cord compression is the patient's neurological status at the time of treatment.

Results from a recent randomized study suggest that the use of radical decompressive surgery with radiotherapy allows patients with a single site of cord compression from metastatic solid tumors (excluding lymphomas, leukemias, germ-cell tumors) to retain the ability to walk longer (median 126 vs 35 d) or regain ambulation more frequently (56 vs 19%) than radiotherapy alone *(9)*.

Radiotherapy is usually delivered to the spine with lateral fields to the cervical spine, posterior fields to the thoracic spine, weighted posterior/anterior fields for the lumbosacral spine, occasionally with the addition of lateral fields for lesions below the level of the kidneys. Dose schedules of 30 Gy in 10 fractions or 40 Gy in 20 fractions are frequently used. Katagiri et al. recently examined the results of nonsurgical treatment for spinal metastases *(10)*. Between 1990 and 1995, 101 patients with spinal metastases were treated with radiation therapy and/or chemotherapy without surgical intervention and had follow-up for more than 24 mo. Neurological status, pain relief, functional improvement, and cumulative survival rate were assessed. Of the total treated, 67 patients (66%) were evaluated as being neurologically stable or improved after treatment. Pain relief was achieved in 67%, and 64% showed functional improvement. Primary lesion responsiveness to nonsurgical therapy influenced the survival, neurological recovery, pain control, and function. They considered lymphoma, prostate cancer, breast cancer, multiple myeloma, and ovarian cancer as responsive tumors; indeed, 87% of such patients maintained or regained useful motor function compared to only 49% of patients with non-small cell cancer, hepato-cellular carcinoma, gastric, colon cancer, and other histologies that were considered nonresponsive. Neurological findings before therapy were useful in predicting ambulatory status after treatment. Nonsurgical treatment was often successful when primary tumors were

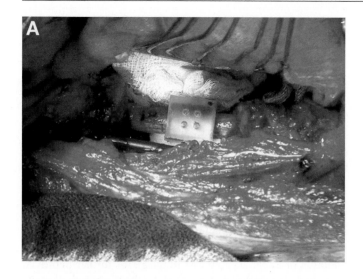

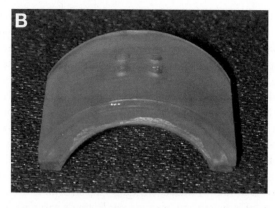

Fig. 1. (**A**) Yttrium-90 dural plaque in place at time of resection of spine sarcoma. (**B**) Yttrium-90 dural plaque. (Reproduced with permission from ref. 8.)

responsive to radiation therapy and/or chemotherapy. This was seen even when neurological deficits were found, particularly for lesions in the lumbar spine. Spinal metastases of less responsive tumors, unless patients were neurologically intact, responded less well to therapy. Most of the patients who were successfully treated enjoyed relief lasting nearly until death. Their functional ability was limited by general debility, rather than by local tumor regrowth.

2.2. PLASMACYTOMA

The primary spinal lesion in patients with solitary plasmacytoma of bone (SBP) can be controlled in the great majority of patients with radiation therapy (11,12). A recent review of the experience at the M. D. Anderson Cancer Center reported local control of tumor in 55 of 57 patients (96%) with a median radiation dose of 50 Gy, with all patients receiving at least 30 Gy (13). Median survival was 11 yr. No significant acute or late toxicity was seen. However, 51% of the patients ultimately went on to develop multiple myeloma. These results were similar to those reported earlier in smaller series. In the M.D. Anderson series, among those 11 patients with disappearance of myeloma protein, only 2 developed multiple myeloma, in contrast to progression in 57% of patients with persistent protein peak. Interestingly, seven of eight patients whose disease was staged by plain radiographs went on to develop myeloma, compared to only one of seven staged with MRI (13). Four of twelve patients evaluated for presumed solitary plasmacytoma had other medullary involvement detected elsewhere in the spine by MRI. This finding emphasizes the greater sensitivity of MRI in delineating occult intramedullary disease away from a presumed solitary bone plasmacytoma. With the increasing use of MRI in these patients, it is likely that diagnosis of solitary bone plasmacytoma will become less common, as more of these patients will be found at initial staging to have multiple myeloma. The fraction of patients with SBP who are cured, however, will likely increase, as MRI staging will exclude more patients who already have multiple myeloma.

2.3. PRIMARY LYMPHOMA OF BONE

The Massachusetts General Hospital reported its experience in the management of 37 patients with primary bone lymphoma treated with combined modality therapy (CMT) (14). Two pa-

tients were treated with complete resection of the tumor, while 35 patients underwent radiation therapy with a median total dose of 54 Gy (range 38.35–66.5). All patients received combination chemotherapy, which contained doxorubicin in 33 cases. Actuarial disease-free survival (DFS) at 5 and 10 yr was 78 and 73%, respectively, while overall survival (OS) was 91 and 87%, respectively. No local failures were seen. Pathological fracture at presentation influenced DFS (p = 0.005) and OS (p =0.017) adversely. OS was compromised in patients older than 60 yr (p = 0.059) and DFS in patients with pelvic primaries (p = 0.015). CMT was associated with improved DFS (p = 0.0008) and OS (p = 0.0001) compared to historical controls treated with local measures only. Ten patients (27%) developed complications, usually in weight-bearing bones, requiring orthopedic procedures following completion of therapy at a median of 25.5 mo (range 4–228). A recent report from the Netherlands confirmed the favorable outcome of treatment in these patients (15). Combined modality therapy seems to be superior to localized treatment alone in other reports as well (16,17). Although combined modality treatment is favored in adults, there is emerging evidence from a recent Pediatric Oncology Group study that these lesions can be managed with chemotherapy alone in pediatric patients (18). Recently, 2-fluoro-2-deoxy-D-glucose (FDG) positron emission tomography (PET) has been shown to be suitable for identifying osseous involvement in malignant lymphoma with a high positive predictive value with greater sensitivity and specificity than bone scintigraphy (19).

2.4. EWING'S SARCOMA OF BONE

Because of the difficulties associated with resection of these lesions when they occur in the spine, including the problems in securing negative surgical margins and the possibility of interrupting or delaying critical chemotherapy, these lesions are generally being treated with chemotherapy and radiotherapy. Radiotherapy doses in the range of 50 Gy are used, respecting spinal cord tolerance. Axial location remains a poor prognostic feature.

The Mayo Clinic reported that the local recurrence rate in the extremities with radiation alone was between 15 and 20% (20). In their series, there was a 3.5% incidence of the disease in the spine. The 5-yr survival rate with spinal disease was 33% and the local recurrence rate was 50%. Large reported series of patients with Ewing's sarcoma of the spine are not available; however, the effectiveness of surgical resection along with adjuvant treatment was supported by a report of four patients with primitive neuroectodermal tumor or extra-skeletal Ewing's sarcoma of the spine *(21)*. All of the patients were treated with multi-agent chemotherapy and radiation. However, the only patient that remained alive at the time of publication also underwent wide surgical excision of the lesion and stem cell transplantation. These numbers are similar for disease that is treated in the pelvis with radiation alone. In the pelvis (as in the spine), it is often not possible to remove the tumor with negative margins without sacrificing vital structures. Because the doses that have been used to treat Ewing's sarcoma in the spine and the pelvis in the past have been limited by less sophisticated radiation therapy techniques, there is some enthusiasm that IMRT or protons will improve the treatment outcome in these sites with less normal tissue morbidity than either of these older radiotherapy techniques or surgery *(22)*. As previously noted, there may be a role for combining surgery with radiotherapy and chemotherapy in selected cases.

2.5. GIANT CELL TUMOR

Treatment of giant cell tumor of bone generally involves wide resection of the lesion in aggressive tumors or curettage with or without bone-grafting or the use of cement in those tumors with less bone destruction. Radiation therapy has been used for patients who cannot be operated on for medical reasons, who have a tumor that is technically difficult to resect, or have recurrent tumors. A recent retrospective survey of 20 patients who had giant cell tumor of bone and were managed with a single course of megavoltage radiation (40–70 Gy), documented that the tumor had not progressed in 17 of the 20 patients after a median duration of follow-up of 9.3 yr *(23)*. Thus, the actuarial 10-yr rate for lack of progression was 85%. Local regrowth was evident in 1 patient, who had received radiation alone, and in 2 of the 13 patients who had been managed with partial resection and radiation. Operative treatment was successful in the three patients in whom the radiation treatment had failed. They concluded that giant cell tumor of bone was effectively treated with megavoltage radiation in twenty patients in whom operative resection would have been difficult or was not feasible. The rate of tumors that did not progress with this regimen of radiation was similar to that reported by investigators from several other centers *(24,25)*. Furthermore, these results closely rival those obtained with modern curettage procedures. Malignant sarcomatous transformation was not observed, although the authors emphasized that longer duration of follow-up of a larger group of patients would be necessary to provide a better estimate of the risk of malignant transformation.

3. PROTON-BEAM RADIOTHERAPY

Radiation therapy can be a very effective modality for management of tumors involving the spine and paraspinal soft tissues. It has become the primary local therapy for responsive tumors such as lymphoma, solitary plasmacytoma/multiple myeloma, and Ewing's sarcoma. It can provide effective palliation for metastatic disease. For spinal chondrosarcomas, osteosarcomas and chordomas, as well as the soft tissue sarcomas of the paraspinal soft tissues, surgical resection is being complemented by increasingly sophisticated, high-precision radiation therapy techniques that should improve the outcome for patients with these challenging tumors. One such high-precision modality is proton-beam therapy, which allows increased radiation dose to the tumor bed while limiting radiation exposure to uninvolved tissues *(26)*.

The advantages of bringing improved technology into the radiation therapy clinic have been amply demonstrated over the years. The adoption of megavoltage cobalt units moved the maximum dose from the skin surface which had been the case with 250 kVp and lower energy ortholvotage machines to a depth of 4 mm. Radiation therapy doses were no longer limited by the acute skin reaction but could be increased to match the much greater radiation tolerance of the deeper structures. The adoption of linear accelerators in the 1970s further improved the achievable dose distribution, as did the use of radiotherapy treatment simulators to plan treatment and the use of individually shaped portals. The adoption of brachytherapy and intra-operative radiotherapy improved dose distribution and clinical results at a variety of clinical sites including sarcomas. Most recently, the availability of computer based treatment planning with modern imaging technologies (CT, MRI, PET) have, like the earlier technical improvements previously noted, enhanced the ability of the radiation oncologist to deliver radiation to the tumor while minimizing normal tissue dose. Therefore, there is confidence that the smaller treatment volumes, the reduction of normal tissue dose and volume irradiated, and the increase in dose to the tumor target achievable with protons will, like these earlier technological advances, result in clinical gains in cancer therapy.

The rationale for the use of protons (or other charged particles) rather than photons (which have traditionally been used for radiation therapy) is the superior dose distribution which can be achieved with protons. Protons and other charged particles deposit energy in tissue through multiple interactions with electrons in the atoms of cells, although a small fraction of energy is transferred to tissue through collisions with the nuclei of atoms. The energy loss per unit path length is relatively small and constant until near the end of the proton range where the residual energy is lost over a short distance, resulting in a steep rise in the absorbed dose (energy absorbed per unit mass). This portion of the particle track, where energy is rapidly lost over a short distance, is known as the Bragg peak. The initial low-dose region in the depth–dose curve, before the Bragg peak, is referred to as the plateau of the dose distribution and is about 30% of the Bragg peak maximum dose. The Bragg peak is too narrow for practical clinical applications. For the irradiation of most tumors, the beam energy is modulated in order to achieve a uniform dose over a significant volume. This is accomplished by superimposing several Bragg peaks of descending energies (ranges) and weights to create a region of uniform dose over the depth of the target; these extended regions of uniform dose are called "spread-out Bragg peaks" (SOBP). The depth–dose curve for a proton beam modulated to achieve a 10-cm SOBP is shown in Fig. 2. For comparison, Fig. 2 also shows the depth–dose curve for 15 MV photons, a beam commonly used to treat deep-seated tumors. For illustration, a tumor is indicated in the

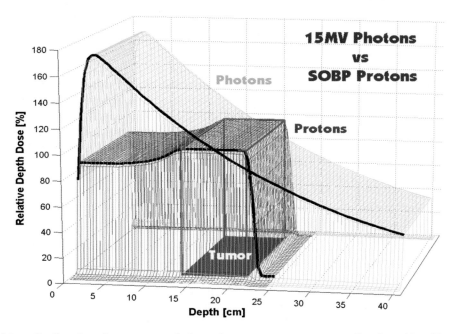

Fig. 2. Comparison of dose distributuions for a proton and photon beam to treat a tumor extending from 13 to 23 cm deep to skin surface. Although protons haqve a slightly higher skin dose than photons, their dose distribution is otherwise more favorable, with less dose to normal tissue in front of the tumor and no exit dose to normal tissue.

region between 13 and 23 cm in depth. The red lines represent an "ideal" dose distribution that covers the tumor. The proton dose distribution is characterized by a relatively low dose region in normal tissue proximal to the tumor, a uniform high dose region in the tumor, and zero dose beyond the tumor. If proton beam alignments are chosen that place a desired normal tissue beyond the range of the beam, it will be effectively spared from any significant radiation dose.

By contrast, the photon dose distribution is characterized by a maximum dose in normal tissue proximal to the tumor, a lower and non-uniform dose in the tumor, and significant dose to normal tissues and organs beyond the tumor. Photon beams, however, have a lower dose in the entrance (build-up) region and will therefore have more skin sparing than proton beams. If multiple beams are used to treat a particular tumor, effective skin sparing can also be achieved with protons. The lateral penumbra is comparable for protons and photons at depths up to about 10 cm; however, owing to multiple scattering, the proton penumbra will be larger at deeper depths.

The proton dose advantage is purely physical; there is no predicted biological advantage to proton over photons.

For many of the early proton machines, the energy of the beam (which dictated the depth of the Bragg peak) was only of sufficient energy to treat superficial lesions (i.e., those of the eye) or intermediate depth lesions (i.e., the base of the skull) (27,28). Few of the machines had the energy to treat all sites in the body. Because of these technical factors and the interests of the involved physicians, the clinical sites that had initially received the most interest were uveal melanomas in the eye and base of skull sarcomas. The major emphasis for proton therapy clinical research initially was dose escalation for tumors for which local control with conventional radiotherapy was poor, initially including base of skull tumors and locally advanced

prostate cancer and more recently hepatocellular carcinoma and non-small cell lung cancer (41). Increasingly, there is interest in protocols aimed at morbidity reduction in those tumor sites in which tumor control with photons is good. Many pediatric tumors fall into this category (31,32). It should be emphasized that dose escalation and morbidity reduction are not mutually exclusive when using protons and that the opportunity for both may be present in any given patient.

As discussed previously, proton therapy provides a means to reduce the irradiated (treated) volume and therefore decrease both the volume of irradiated normal tissues and organs and the total radiation dose that they receive. This may increase the tolerance of the patient to radiation and allow for higher doses to be delivered to the target volume, thus, achieving a higher tumor control probability (TCP) (33). Furthermore, with proton beams, higher TCPs may be achieved without increasing the incidence or severity of treatment-related morbidity. Additionally, the more conformal treatment volumes of proton therapy should result in a reduced frequency and severity of co-morbidity between radiation and chemotherapy, thus, allowing for improved treatment compliance and increased treatment intensity (34,35).

Improvements of dose distributions may result in reductions in treatment morbidity and improvements in quality of life. Radiation therapy alone, or in combination with surgery and/or chemotherapy, has been effective in the treatment of a broad range of solid tumors. In some tumor sites, high rates of local control have been achieved with modern radiation therapy techniques (36). However, there remains a challenge to reduce the treatment-related complications currently associated with radiation therapy and the co-morbidity resulting from the combination of radiation and chemotherapy (34). Superior dose distributions, which permit the delivery of high tumor doses while reducing or eliminating the dose delivered to normal tissues and organs, offer a significant potential for the reduction of treatment morbidity *(37)*. Pediatric tumors have a higher cure rate in general, however, the late effects of radiation in children are more pronounced because developing tissues are being irradiated. Proton radiation should maintain the high cure rates of photon therapy while decreasing the morbidity seen in photon treatments *(30–32)*.

3.1. SARCOMAS OF THE SKULL BASE

Treatment of patients with sarcomas of the skull base is difficult and complex because of the proximity of the brain stem and the base of the brain. These factors have limited both surgical approaches and treatment with conventional radiation therapy. The rapid fall off of dose at the end of the range of the proton beam was judged to be particularly suitable for treatment of these tumors. Indeed, the physical advantage of proton allowed for very significant dose escalation for these patients. Rosenberg et al. reported the actuarial 5- and 10-yr actuarial local control rates for 200 patients treated at Massachusetts General Hospital/Harvard Cyclotron Laboratory *(38)*. Chondrosarcomas of the base of the skull who received a median dose of 72.1 cobalt gray equivalent (CGE) in 38 fractions had 5- and 10-yr actuarial rates of 99 and 98%, respectively. Although it is sometimes stated that chondrosarocomas are not sensitive to radiation therapy, these results would clearly contradict that assertion. Interestingly, patients with chordomas of the skull base treated to a similar median dose of 68.9 CGE did significantly worse with actuarial local control rates of 59 and 44% at 5 and 10 yr, respectively. Similar results were reported by Hug et al. from Loma Linda, who noted local control in 92% of patients with chondrosarcoma and 76% of patients with chordomas. They reported symptomatic grade 3–4 toxicities in 5% of patients *(36)*. These results are substantially better than those achievable with series in which patients with chondrosarcomas and chordomas of the skull base were treated with photons to a median dose of 55 Gy in which the estimated local control was only 36%.

These treatments can be given with acceptable toxicity to the brain and optic structures in view of the major morbidity and mortality, which accompany uncontrolled tumor growth.

3.2. SARCOMAS OF THE SPINE AND PARASPINAL TISSUES

Radiotherapy for treatment of tumors of the spine and paraspinal soft tissues is constrained by the radiation tolerance of the spinal cord which is generally quoted at 45 Gy, owing to the proximity of the spinal cord. This dose is well below that necessary to reliably control most sarcomas, which require doses of approx 60 Gy for sublinical microscopic disease, 66 Gy for microscopically positive margins, and in excess of 70 Gy for gross residual disease. Therefore, proton radiotherapy, with its ability to spare adjacent tissues, offers advantages for treatment of tumors in this location. Isacsson et al. compared conformal radiotherapy treatment plans with photons and protons for patients with cervical Ewing's sarcoma *(33)*. Even when delivered as only the final 20% of the treatment as boost to treat the gross disease, they noted a 5% improvement in local control for a comparable predicted risk of spinal cord injury.

Hug et al. presented results on combined photon/proton treatment of 47 patients with osteo- and chondrogenic tumors of the axial skeleton *(36)*. Radiation was delivered postoperatively in 23 patients, pre- and postoperatively in 17, and as sole treatment in 7 patients. Mean radiation doses of 73.9 CGE, 69.8 CGE, and 61.8 CGE were delivered to group 1 (20 patients with recurrent/primary chordoma or chondrosarcoma), group 2 (15 patients with osteogenic sarcomas) and group 3 (12 patients with giant cell tumors, osteo- or chondroblastomas) respectively. Five-year actuarial local control and survival for patients with chondrosarcoma was 100 and 100% and with chordoma was 53 and 50%, respectively. Actuarial 5-yr local control for patients with osteosarcoma was 59%. The 5-yr actuarial local control and survival for the group 3 patients were 76 and 87%. Overall, improved local control was noted for primary vs recurrent tumors, gross total resection, and target doses greater than 77 CGE. Similar results have been presented in 52 patients with spinal and paraspinal tumors treated with charged-particle therapy at the University of California Lawrence Berkley Laboratory *(36a)*. Local control was obtained in 58% of previously untreated patients with 3-yr survival of 61%.

3.3 EWING'S SARCOMA

Management problems for Ewing's sarcomas are complex owing to: (1) the critical importance of the normal structures in the vicinity of the tumor; and (2) the frequent finding that surgical resection margins are positive or close. For truncal and retroperitoneal sites, surgical resection and radiation are limited by the proximity of the tumor to critical organs such as liver, kidney, bowel, and great vessels. Local failure rates are often greater than 50%. Highly localized dose distributions offer the possibility of increasing local control, as well as decreasing late effects. Smith et al. performed comparative treatment planning comparing intensity modulated photons with intensity modulated protons for a patient with a pelvic Ewing's sarcoma and noted sparing of the intestine, rectum, bladder, and femoral head in the proton plan compared with the photon plan *(36b)*. These results demonstrate a significant potential for reduction of treatment morbidity for the proton plan as compared to the photon plan. In addition to less acute morbidity to bowel and marrow during concurrent chemoradiation, one would anticipate a reduction in late, radiation induced tumors, a problem with conventional photon radiotherapy for these patients *(39)*.

3.4. COMPARATIVE TREATMENT PLANS

The use of 3DCRT has now become common practice in sophisticated radiation oncology departments around the world. Using beam's eye viewing of volumes defined on a treatment planning CT scan, beam directions and beam shapes can be selected to conform to the shape of the projected target and minimize dose to critical normal structures. In spite of its appellation, it can be difficult to conform the beam around certain 3D structures, such as the spinal cord. IMRT uses modifications in the intensity of the beam across the irradiated fields to enhance the capability of conforming dose distributions in 3D. Dosimetric comparisons of 3DCRT plans with IMRT plans indicate that IMRT can yield significantly better dose distributions in some situations; although planning and treatment require more time and resources. New technologies are being developed that should significantly reduce the time needed to plan, implement, and verify these treatments. The proton beam can also be modulated in similar fashion and is expected to offer additional advantages, especially decreased radiation dosages to normal surrounding tissues (29,35).

In general, it is possible to deliver prescribed tumor doses in a uniform manner using either protons or photons. If, for a given target dose, protons deliver significantly less integral dose to normal tissues and organs, this provides an opportunity for dose escalation while keeping the normal tissue complication probability (NTCP) comparable to those produced by photon irradiation. On the other hand, if local control is satisfactory but NTCPs are high, as in many pediatric cancers, then less integral dose should produce fewer treatment-related complications. Also, reduced integral dose will lead to less co-morbidity when chemotherapy and radiation therapy are combined, thus, to better treatment compliance and the potential for increased treatment intensity.

Improvements in dose distributions (better dose localization) have the potential for increased rates of local control and disease-free survival and decreased early and late effects of radiation treatment. Better dose distributions may also lead to decreased co-morbidity of radiation and chemotherapy treatments and, thus, better treatment compliance and/or increased treatment intensity. This is especially important in the era of multimodality treatments where chemotherapy plus radiation is used for treatment in many disease sites, such as large high-grade extremity soft-tissue sarcomas and head and neck cancers. Highly localized dose distributions may make it possible to retreat patients who have failed locally and have been treated to tolerance with previous therapy.

The tools used to achieve highly localized dose distributions have included conformal external beam photons and electrons, brachytherapy, intra-operative therapy, CT and MRI coupled with 3D treatment planning, multi-leaf collimators, intensity modulation, and heavy-charged particles, in particular protons. In recent times, many of these techniques have been combined to achieve extremely conformal dose distributions (e.g., high-energy photon beams, used with modern imaging, inverse treatment planning, multi-leaf collimators, and intensity modulation). However, there are physical limits to further significant improvements in dose localization using photon beams. These limits are governed by the inherent physical nature of photon interactions in tissue. Exponential depth dose curves, common to all photon beams, result in at least three undesirable conditions when treating deep-seated tumors. For any given photon beam, the maximum dose will occur in normal tissue proximal to a deep-seated target and the depth dose across the target will be nonuniform. In addition, significant dose will be delivered to normal tissues and organs distal to the tumor. These limitations can be mitigated in part by use of multi-port therapy, however, these characteristics often lead to compromises between target dose and dose to normal critical tissues and organs.

Proton beams lead to fewer such compromises because they have none of the limitations of photon beams previously described. In addition, in modern proton therapy facilities with isocentric gantries and beam-scanning capabilities, protons can be delivered with intensity modulation techniques and, thus,

maintain their advantages over photons, even when the most advanced techniques are used. Therefore, based on physical principles, beam for beam and technique for technique, proton beams will always deliver a more localized dose distribution. The question is, will those improved dose distributions provide substantial improvements in treatment outcomes?

Based on the physical nature of protons, the excellent clinical results obtained so far and the treatment planning comparisons shown by several investigators, in comparison to photons, proton therapy has the potential to improve clinical outcomes (33). Reviews of the clinical results of proton therapy by Spiro et al. (40) and DeLaney et al. (41) describe impressive results from several proton therapy centers. However, with the exception of two clinical trials for prostate cancer conducted jointly by Massachusetts General Hospital and Loma Linda University Medical Center, few prospective, randomized trials have been carried out. The primary reasons for this are: there are few proton therapy facilities, most existing facilities have had limitations in capacity and energy, and few facilities have modern delivery systems including isocentric gantries and beam scanning capabilities. Therefore, even though more than 39,000 patients have been treated with protons worldwide, only a few hundred have been treated in prospective, randomized clinical trails.

However, this situation is rapidly changing. There are now approx 20 facilities treating patients with proton beams with about 10 more being built or under serious planning. Many of the new facilities will be hospital-based with the capacity of treating large numbers of patients. For example, the Northeast Proton Therapy Center on the Massachusetts General Hospital campus in Boston will have the capacity to treat more than 1000 patients per year. It will be necessary to conduct prospective, randomized clinical trials in a large number of disease sites in order to quantify the improvements in clinical outcomes with protons.

REFERENCES

1. Zagars GK, Ballo MT. Significance of dose in postoperative radiotherapy for soft tissue sarcoma. Int J Radiat Oncol Biol Phys 2003; 56:473–481.
2. Kepka L, Suit HD, Goldberg SI, et al. Radiation therapy for control of soft tissue sarcomas resected with positive margins. Connective Tissue Oncology Society Meeting, Montreal, Canada, November, 2004.
3. DeLaney T, Kepka L, Goldberg S, Suit H. Results of radiation therapy for unresected soft tissue sarcomas. ESTRO meeting, Amsterdam, October 2004.
4. Goitein M, Abrams M. Multidimensional treatment planning: Beam's eye view, back projection, and projection through CT sections. Int J Radiat Oncol Biol Phys 1983; 9:789–797.
5. Goitein M, Abrams M. Multi-dimensional treatment planning I. Delineation of anatomy. Int J Radiat Oncol Biol Phys 1983; 9: 777–787.
6. Convery DJ, Rosenbloom ME. The generation of intensity-modulated fields for conformal radiotherrapy by dynamic collimation. Phys Med Biol 1992; 37:1359–1374.
6a. Yamada Y, Lovelock DM, Yenice KM, et al. Multifractionated image-guided and stereotactic intensity-modulated radiotherapy of paraspinal tumors: a preliminary reprot. Int J Radiat Oncol Biol Phys 2005; 62:53–61.
7. Armstrong JG, Fass DE, Bains M, et al. Paraspinal tumors: techniques and results of brachytherapy. Int J Radiat Oncol Biol Phys 1991; 20:787–790.

8. DeLaney TF, Chen GT, Mauceri TC, et al. Intraoperative dural irradiation by customized Iridium-192 and Yttrium-90 brachytherapy plaques. Int J Radiat Oncol Biol Phys. 2003; 57:239–45.

9. Regine WF, Tibbs PA, Young A, et al. Metastatic spinal cord compression: a randomized trial of direct decompressive surgical resection plus radiotherapy vs. radiotherapy alone. Int J Radiat Oncol Biol Phys 2004; 57:S125.

10. Katagiri H, Takahashi M, Inagaki J, et al. Clinical results of nonsurgical treatment for spinal metastases. Int J Radiat Oncol Biol Phys 1998; 42:1127–1132.

11. McLain RF, Weinstein JN. Solitary plasmacytomas of the spine: Report of 84 Cases. J Spinal Disord 1989; 2:69–74.

12. Poor MM, Hitchon PW, Riggs CE Jr. Solitary spinal plasmacytomas: management and outcome. J Spinal Disord. 1988; 1:295–300.

13. Liebross RH, Ha CS, Cox JD, Weber D, Delasalle K, Alexanian R. Solitary bone plasmacytoma: outcome and prognostic factors following radiotherapy. Int J Radiat Oncol Biol Phys 1998; 41:1063–1067.

14. Fidias P, Spiro I, Sobczak ML, et al. Long-term results of combined modality therapy in primary bone lymphomas. Int J Radiat Oncol Biol Phys 1999; 45:1213–1218.

15. Heyning FH, Hogendoorn PC, Kramer MH, et al. Primary non-Hodgkin's lymphoma of bone: a clinicopathological investigation of 60 cases. Leukemia 1999; 13:2094–2098.

16. Baar J, Burkes RL, Gospodarowicz M. Primary non-Hodgkin's lymphoma of bone. Semin Oncol 1999; 26:270–275.

17. Christie DR, Barton MB, Bryant G, et al. Osteolymphoma (primary bone lymphoma): an Australian review of 70 cases. Australasian Radiation Oncology Lymphoma Group (AROLG). Aust N Z J Med 1999; 29:214–219.

18. Suryanarayan K, Shuster JJ, Donaldson SS, Hutchison RE, Murphy SB, Link MP. Treatment of localized primary non-Hodgkin's lymphoma of bone in children: a Pediatric Oncology Group study. J Clin Oncol 1999; 17:456–459.

19. Moog F, Kotzerke J, Reske SN. FDG PET can replace bone scintigraphy in primary staging of malignant lymphoma. J Nucl Med 1999; 40:1407–1413.

20. O'Connor MI, Pritchard DJ. Ewing's sarcoma. Prognostic factors, disease control, and the reemerging role of surgical treatment. Clin Orthop 1991; 262:78–87.

21. Harimaya K, Oda Y, Matsuda S, Tanaka K, Chuman H, Iwamoto Y. Primitive neuroectodermal tumor and extraskeletal Ewing sarcoma arising primarily around the spinal column: report of four cases and a review of the literature. Spine 2003; 28:E408–E412.

22. Bacci G, Ferrari S, Bertoni F, et al. Prognostic factors in nonmetastatic Ewing's sarcoma of bone treated with adjuvant chemotherapy: analysis of 359 patients at the Istituto Ortopedico Rizzoli. J Clin Oncol 2000; 18:4–11.

23. Chakravarti A, Spiro IJ, Hug EB, Mankin HJ, Efird JT, Suit HD. Megavoltage radiation therapy for axial and inoperable giant-cell tumor of bone. J Bone Joint Surg Am 1999; 81:1566–1573.

24. Bell RS, Harwood AR, Goodman SR, Fornasier VL. Supervoltage radiotherapy in the treatment of difficult giant cell tumors of bone. Clin Orthop 1983; 174:208–216.

25. Khan DC, Malhotra S, Stevens RE, Steinfeld AD. Radiotherapy for the treatment of giant cell tumor of the spine: a report of six cases and review of the literature. Cancer Invest 1999; 17:110–113.

26. Miller DW. A review of proton beam radiation therapy. Med Phys 1995; 22:1943–1954.

27. Miralbell R, Cella L, Weber D, Lomax A. Optimizing radiotherapy of orbital and paraorbital tumors: intensity-modulated X-ray beams vs. intensity-modulated proton beams. Int J Radiat Oncol Biol Phys 2000; 47:1111–1119.

28. Austin-Seymour M, Munzenrider J, Goitein M, et al. Fractionated proton radiation therapy of chordoma and low grade chondrosarcoma of the base of skull. J Neurosurg 1989; 70:13–17.

29. Lomax AJ, Bortfeld T, Goitein G, et al. A treatment planning intercomparison of proton and intensity modulated photon radiotherapy. Radiother Oncol 1999; 51:257–271.

30. Lin R, Hug EB, Schaefer RA, Miller DW, Slater JM, Slater JD. Conformal proton radiation therapy of the posterior fossa: a study comparing protons with three-dimensional planned photons in limiting dose to auditory structures. Int J Radiat Oncol Biol Phys 2000; 48:1219–1226.

31. Mirabell R, Lomax A, Bortfeld T, Rouzand M, Carrie C. Potential role of proton therapy in the treatment of pediatric medulloblastoma/primitive neruo-ectodermal tumors: reduction of the supratentorial target volume. Int J Radiat Oncol Biol Phys 1997; 38:477–484.

32. Mirabell R, Lomax A, Russo M. Potential role of proton therapy in the treatment of pediatric medulloblastoma/primitive neuro-ectodermal tumors: spinal theca irradiation. Int J Radiat Oncol Biol Phys 1997; 38:805–811.

33. Isacsson U, Hagberg H, Johansson KA, Montelius A, Jung B, Glimelius B. Potential advantages of protons over conventional radiation beams for paraspinal tumors. Radiother Oncol 1997; 45:63–70.

34. Zurlo A, Lomax A, Hoess A, et al. The role of proton therapy in the treatment of large irradiation volumes: A comparative planning study of pancreataic and biliary tumors. Int J Radiat Oncol Biol Phys 2000; 48:277–288.

35. Lomax AJ, Boehringer T, Coray A, et al. Intensity modulated proton therapy: A clinical example. Med Phys 2001; 28:317–324.

36. Hug EB, Fitzek MM, Liebsch NJ, Munzenrider JE. Locally challenging osteo- and chondrogenic tumors of the axial skeleton: results of combined proton and photon radiation therapy using three-dimensional treatment planning. Int J Radiat Oncol Biol Phys 1995; 31:467–476.

36a. Nowakowski VA, Castro JR, Petti PL, et al. Charged particle radiotherapy of paraspinal tumors. Int J Radiat Oncol Biol Phys 1992; 22:295–303.

36b. Smith AR, Loeffler JS, Suit HD. The potential for proton beam therapy to improve clinical outcomes: comparisons of proton and x-ray treatment plans for the purpose of tumor dose escalation and/or reduction of treatment-related mobidity. Int J Radiat Oncol Biol Phys 2000; 48:338.

37. Glimelius B, Isacsson U, Blomquist E, Grusell E, Jung B, Montelius A. Potential gains using high-energy protons for therapy of malignant tumors. Acta Oncologica 1999; 38:137–145.

38. Rosenberg AE, Nielsen GP, Keel SB, et al. Chondrosarcoma of the base of the skull: a clinicopathologic study of 200 cases with emphasis on its distinction from chordoma. Am J Surg Pathol 1999; 23:1370–1378.

39. Kuttesch JF Jr, Wexler LH, Marcus RB, et al. Second malignancies after Ewing's sarcoma: radiation dose-dependency of secondary sarcomas. J Clin Oncol 1996; 14:2818–2825.

40. Spiro IJ, Smith AR, Lomax A, Loeffler JS: Proton beam radiation therapy. In: DeVita VT, Hellman S, Rosenberg SA eds. Cancer: Principles and Practice of Oncology. Philadelphia, PA: Lippincott Williams and Wilkins; 2001:3229–3235.

41. DeLaney TF, Smith AR, Lomax A, Adams J, Loeffler JS. Proton Beam Radiation Therapy. Principles and Practice of Oncology Updates 2003; 17:1–10.

26 Spinal Metastasis

Indications for Surgery

IAIN H. KALFAS, MD

1. INTRODUCTION

Each year approx 1.37 million new cases of cancer are diagnosed in the United States. It is estimated that approx 563,700 of these new cases will die from their disease *(1)*. Despite significant advances in the overall management of cancer in the past decades, the major cause of death in most cases remains metastatic disease and its complications. The three most common sites for metastasis are the lungs, liver, and skeletal system. The spine is the most common site for skeletal metastasis. Based on autopsy studies, approx 5 to 30% of patients with cancer will develop spinal metastasis, with 20% of these patients developing epidural compression *(2–7)*.

The management of spinal metastasis has evolved over the past several decades. Currently, radiotherapy, chemotherapy, and a variety of surgical options constitute the primary treatment options available for patients with spinal metastasis. This chapter focuses on the indications for surgery in these patients.

2. EPIDEMIOLOGY

Metastatic tumors are the most common tumors affecting the spine. The most common primary sites of origin for a spinal metastasis are breast, lung, prostate, and the hematopoietic system. In most clinical series these primary sites alone account for 50–66% of all metastasis to the spine. However, approx 10% of patients with symptomatic spinal metastasis present without a known primary site *(8)*.

Although the lumbar spine represents the most common site for spinal metastasis, approx 70% of symptomatic lesions involve the thoracic spine, 15% involve the lumbosacral spine, and 15%

involve the cervical spine. The majority of these tumors occur in the extradural space with most originating within the vertebral body. Approximately 5% of spinal metastatic tumors are intradural and extramedullary, whereas 3% are localized to the intramedullary space (Fig. 1) *(9)*.

The route of spread to the spine has been demonstrated by Batson *(10)*, who noted that during periods of increased intra-abdominal/intrathoracic pressure, the abdominopelvic organs are drained preferentially via the valveless vertebral venous plexi. This is the primary mechanism of spread by which tumors of the abdominal and pelvic organs embolize to the vertebrae. Spinal metastasis may also develop as a result of local spread of tumor, such as is the case with the local spread of rectal carcinoma to the sacrum. The vertebrae, with their rich vascular network and cancellous bone interstices, offer a fertile ground for implantation of tumor cells. This preferential affinity for bone tissue by tumor cells has been termed "osteotropism" *(6)*.

3. CLINICAL PRESENTATION

Approximately 90 to 95% of patients with spinal metastasis present with pain as their chief complaint *(5,8,11–16)*. The pain may have been present for a period of several weeks to a year, with a mean duration of 8 wk. The pain may be axial, radicular, or referred. A smaller percentage of patients may present with neurological deficits including sensory, motor, bowel, or bladder dysfunction. In all patients with cancer who present with back pain, neck pain, or symptoms of spinal cord compression, the working diagnosis should be spinal metastasis until proven otherwise.

The natural history of untreated spinal metastasis is generally one of relentless progression towards paralysis as well as

From: *Current Clinical Oncology: Cancer in the Spine: Comprehensive Care.*
Edited by: R. F. McLain, K-U. Lewandrowski, M. Markman, R. M. Bukowski,
R. Macklis, and E. C. Benzel © Humana Press, Inc., Totowa, NJ

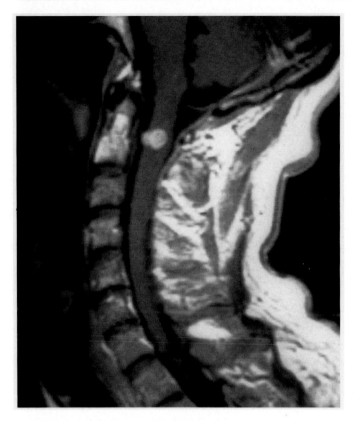

Fig. 1. Sagittal magnetic resonance imaging demonstrating an intramedullary metastatic melanoma at the C2 level.

loss of bowel and bladder function. Early diagnosis in these patients is critical because the results of treatment are dependent, to a large extent, on the neurological status of the patient immediately before treatment. Advances in neuroradiological imaging have greatly facilitated the ability to make an early and accurate diagnosis in many of these patients.

The prognosis of these patients is directly related to three factors: the biology of the tumor, the pretreatment neurological status, and the treatment given (17–19). Identifying the location and extent of the spinal metastasis and initiating treatment before the loss of ambulatory function is the primary goal in these patients. However, some patients may present with the rapid onset of neurological deficit necessitating urgent surgical decompression without the benefit of a full clinical and radiological assessment. This early surgery is generally associated with a greater morbidity and less than optimal results (20). Every effort should be made to stabilize the patient with conservative measures in order to allow for the proper planning of the any needed surgical approach.

4. CONSERVATIVE MANAGEMENT

The management of spinal metastasis continues to evolve. Current treatment options include chemotherapy, radiation therapy, surgery, or a combination of these options. Although many metastatic tumor types respond very well to radiation therapy and chemotherapy, others do not. The wide variety of tumor types, sites of location, degrees of neurological involvement, and overall extent of disease necessitate that each patient

have an individualized treatment plan. Developing this individualized plan requires a thorough understanding of all conservative and available surgical options.

Chemotherapy typically involves the use of steroids to reduce the vasogenic edema that can affect the spinal cord in these patients. In addition to reducing tumor related edema, steroids can also act as an oncolytic agent to diminish the mass of some tumors (i.e., lymphomas or neuroblastomas) (21,22). However, the use of high-dose steroids can also result in the development of peptic ulcers, glucose intolerance, and poor wound healing. Therefore, when steroids are used, a gastric mucosal protecting agent is also administered and the serum glucose is closely monitored.

Radiation therapy is often considered the primary option for treating most cases of spinal metastasis (8,18,22–24). The reasons for this include the fact that most cases occur in the setting of widespread systemic disease with an estimated life expectancy of only a few months. Approximately 50% of the patients treated with radiation therapy can be expected to achieve pain palliation and neurological improvement with the median duration of response lasting 3 to 6 mo. Patients with radio-sensitive tumors and those who are ambulatory when radiation therapy begins are more likely to remain ambulatory after treatment.

Radiation therapy techniques typically use a single posterior portal with one or two vertebral margins. This can result in unequal radiation dosage particularly for anteriorly located tumors. Most standard fractionation techniques use a course of 3000 cGy given in 10 fractions over 2 wk. Smaller daily dose rates may allow a higher total dose to be given.

Because a majority of patients with spinal metastasis are initially evaluated by an oncologist or neurologist, it is not uncommon for virtually all of these patients to be referred for radiation therapy without surgical consultation. This can lead to the inappropriate use of radiation therapy as the initial management option in a large number of patients. The most common setting for this is in the patient with spinal instability secondary to vertebral body collapse or progressive spinal kyphosis (Fig. 2). In this setting, a higher degree of local control can be achieved by using radiation therapy postoperatively to eradicate microscopic residual tumor (25).

5. SURGICAL MANAGEMENT

The surgical management of spinal metastasis has also gone through an extensive evolution over the last several decades. The earlier surgical management option for this condition was a laminectomy. The indiscriminate use of laminectomy, however, resulted in overall poor outcome and a high rate of complications (26). Numerous studies subsequently demonstrated that the combined use of laminectomy and radiation therapy had no demonstrable advantage over laminectomy alone (11,26,27). This subsequently led to a reduced utilization of surgery for the management of these patients.

In 1978, Kakulas et al. (28) studied the pathological anatomy of the spinal metastasis finding tumor destruction of the vertebral body in the majority of specimens examined. The vertebral body collapse was noted to be generally asymmetrical with the anterior border of the vertebrae compressed more than the

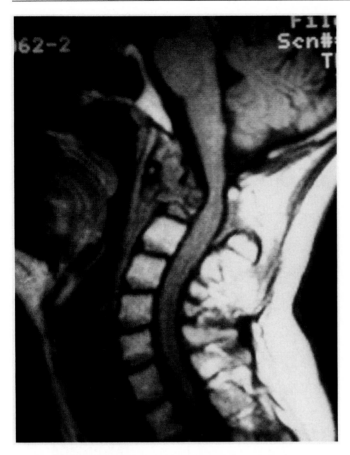

Fig. 2. Sagittal magnetic resonance imaging demonstrating metastatic involvement of C2 vertebrae with collapse and anterior angulation.

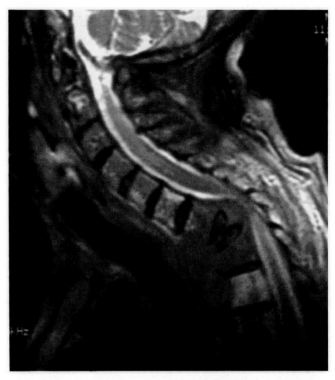

Fig. 3. Sagittal magnetic resonance imaging demonstrating significant collapse and kyphosis at C7–T2 owing to extensive metastatic disease. A posterior decompressive procedure is contraindicated in this patient.

posterior elements. This resulted in an angulation of the spine that produced a maximal impact on the ventral spinal cord *(28)*. This led to the conclusion that, in a majority of patients with spinal metastasis, laminectomy alone was an inappropriate surgical option (Fig. 3).

Several studies have assessed the clinical outcome of patients undergoing laminectomy for metastatic disease. Wright *(29)* noted that laminectomy in patients with anterior column involvement produced only half as many favorable results when compared to laminectomy in patients with no ventral involvement. Brice and McKissock *(30)* noted that none of the 26 patient with anterior column involvement in their series had neurological improvement following laminectomy. Findlay *(31)* reported that patients with vertebral collapse generally have a reduced prospect for preserving or regaining ambulation and an increased risk of neurological deterioration and postoperative spinal instability. The word "laminectomy" unfortunately became synonymous with all forms of surgery, resulting in the widespread use of radiation therapy in these patients regardless of their clinical status or the nature of the compression.

These anatomic observations, as well as improvements in surgical approach and spinal fixation options, subsequently led to the increased use of anterior approaches for spinal metastasis. In 1985, Siegal et al. *(3)* reported a prospective series evaluating the effects of ventral spinal surgery for metastasis. A

vertebrectomy was performed for patients with lesions ventral to the spinal cord and a laminectomy was performed for patients with lesions dorsal to the spinal cord. Surgical patients were compared with a second group treated with radiation therapy alone. Only 30% of patients treated with radiation therapy alone retained or regained ambulation, compared to 40% of the laminectomy patients and 80% of the vertebrectomy patients. The operative mortality was similar for both surgical approaches, but postoperative complications were more common in the laminectomy group, usually because of poor wound healing following radiation therapy *(3)*.

Several surgical strategies are currently available for the management of spinal metastasis. An in-depth discussion of these strategies is beyond the scope of this chapter. In general, surgical options vary according to the type of tumor, the overall prognosis of the patient, the clinical status of the patient, the location of the tumor, the sensitivity to radiation therapy, and the presence or absence of spinal instability. Surgical approach options include percutaneous biopsy, laminectomy, corpectomy with reconstruction, a posterolateral approach, or a combination of these options (Fig. 4). Each of these surgical approach options is frequently combined with a variety of spinal instrumentation options.

In a select group of patients, an *en-bloc* resection may be feasible, however, most tumors are removed through a less aggressive intralesional approach. The proximity of these tumors to neural and vascular structures limits the ability to obtain sufficient tumor margins during resection (Fig. 5). Furthermore, the

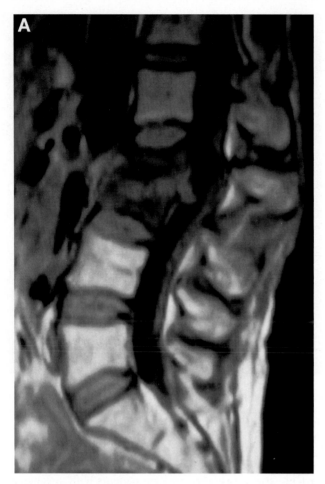 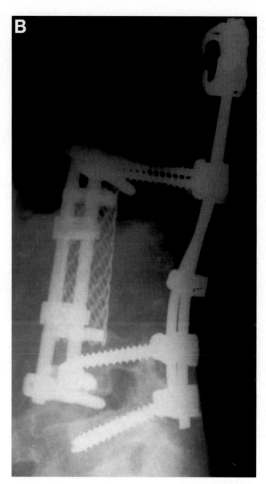

Fig. 4. **(A)** Sagittal magnetic resonance imaging demonstrating metastatic tumor at L2–L3 with significant loss of anterior column support. **(B)** Lateral radiograph following L2–L3 corpectomy with anterior and posterior fixation.

general condition and overall prognosis of these patients frequently makes the *en-bloc* approach unrealistic and prone to a significant surgical morbidity.

In most patients with pathologies other than metastasis, neural compression and spinal instability would lead to an aggressive surgical intervention with early decompression and stabilization. However, the shortened life span of patients with metastasis coupled with "quality-of-life" issues necessitates the use of a different set of criteria be used to assess the need for surgery. Although decompression and stabilization may preserve or restore neurological function and ease the pain of segmental instability, they do not prolong life from an oncological standpoint and may actually cause undue morbidity and mortality. These facts lead to a specialized set of indications for surgery in the patient with spinal metastasis.

6. SURGICAL INDICATIONS

As surgical options for the management of spinal metastasis have evolved so have the indications for surgery in these patients. It is important to have a clear rationale for surgery and to base the selected procedure on the expected goals of therapy as well as the location of the tumor and the overall prognosis of the patient. In general, indications for surgery include (1) establishing a tissue diagnosis when a needle biopsy is unsuccessful

or contraindicated, (2) failure of radiation therapy (radio-resistant tumors) or progression of neurological deterioration during or following radiation therapy, (3) spinal instability owing to vertebral collapse or progressive spinal deformity, and (4) epidural compression secondary to bone fragments from a vertebral fracture. Although these indications are relatively easy to identify, they need to be adjusted according to a variety of clinical, radiographic, and anatomic factors that may be affecting the individual patient with the spinal metastatic lesion.

Tokuhashi et al. *(32)* proposed a scoring system using six parameters: (1) general condition of the patient, (2) number of extraspinal bone metastasis, (3) number of vertebral metastasis, (4) metastasis to internal organs, (5) the primary tumor site, and (6) the severity of the neurological deficits. Each parameter is given a score of 0 to 2 points with a maximum of 12. Aggressive surgery was recommended for patients having a score of 9 or more and palliative surgery reserved for patients with scores of 5 or less *(32)*. Although this approach may simplify the decision making in these patients, the real difficulty lies with those patients who have and indeterminate prognosis.

When a radiographic and clinical evaluation of the patient fails to identify the type of tumor affecting the patient, a needle or trocar biopsy can be attempted typically with the use of computed tomography guidance. For many patients with spinal

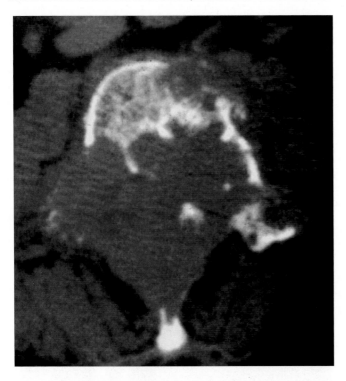

Fig. 5. Axial computed tomography image demonstrating extensive metastatic involvement of lumbar vertebrae with extension into the epidural space. Epidural tumor extension limits the option for *en-bloc* tumor resection.

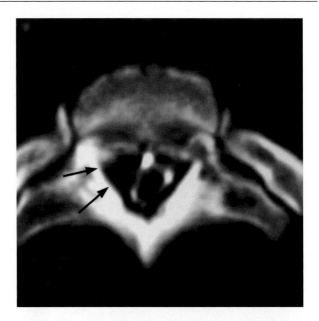

Fig. 6. Axial computed tomography/myelography image demonstrating a metastatic tumor at the T2 level. The tumor is only in the epidural space. An open biopsy, as opposed to a needle biopsy, is indicated.

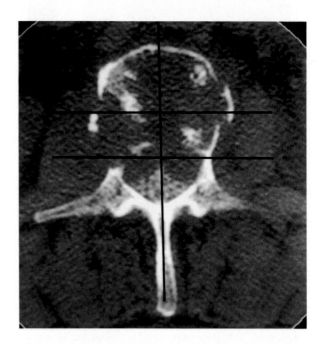

Fig. 7. Axial computed tomography image with schematic overlay demonstrating a method for determining spinal instability in a patient with spinal metastasis. The axial plane of the involve vertebrae is divided into six zones. Lytic destruction of three or more of these zones indicates spinal instability.

metastasis, this may be the only procedure required. Not infrequently, however, the ventral or epidural location of a metastatic lesion may preclude this percutaneous procedure or the biopsy obtained may be of insufficient quality and amount to establish a diagnosis necessitating an open surgical biopsy (Fig. 6). This open biopsy approach is frequently combined with a more definitive decompressive procedure with or without stabilization.

Surgery is also indicated in patients with radio-resistant tumors and in patients whose neurological deficits continue to progress during or following radiation treatments. A frequent scenario is that of a patient undergoing radiation treatments in the setting of spinal instability. Because it can frequently be difficult for even a spinal surgeon to identify and quantify spinal instability, it is not unusual for a neurologist or oncologist to begin radiotherapy in this setting.

Unfortunately, in the metastatic spine, there is little consensus on what constitutes instability except in the obvious cases of fracture-dislocation, vertebral translation, or significant kyphosis.

Kostuik and Weinstein *(34)* attempted to base stability in the setting of spinal metastasis using the three-column model originally proposed by Denis *(33)* for thoracolumbar trauma. For spinal metastasis, each of the three components of the spinal column (anterior, middle, and posterior) are divided into two halves creating a total of six zones. They proposed that spinal instability in the setting of tumor existed if three or more of these zones in the axial plane were destroyed by tumor *(34)* (Fig. 7).

Siegal et al. *(19)* proposed a number of criteria that contributed to spinal instability in the setting of metastasis. These criteria included: (1) anterior and middle-column involvement or more than 50% collapse of vertebral body height, (2) middle- and posterior-column involvement or shearing deformity, (3) three-column involvement, (4) involvement of same column in two or more adjacent vertebrae, and (5) iatrogenic,

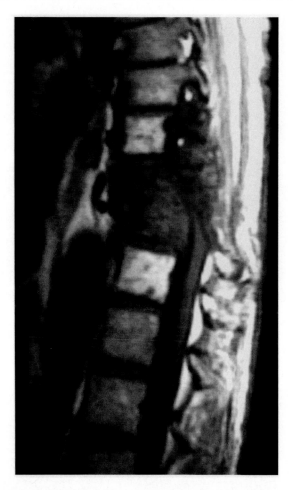

Fig. 8. Sagittal magnetic resonance imaging demonstrating anterior and posterior column involvement of the mid-thoracic spine. A combined anterior and posterior reconstruction is indicated.

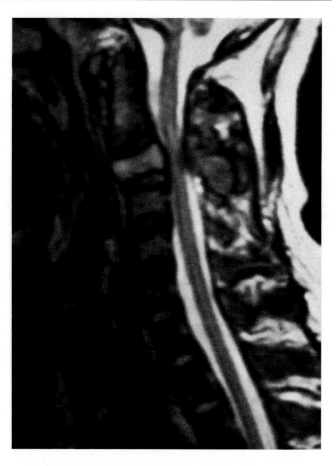

Fig. 9. Sagittal magnetic resonance imaging demonstrating metastatic involvement of C3 vertebrae with expansion of posterior vertebral bony cortex into the epidural space. Compression of the neural elements by bone will not respond to radiation therapy.

which includes laminectomy in the setting of anterior and/or middle column disease or resection of more than 50% of vertebral body *(19)*.

Harms *(35)* suggested that the spine be considered as a mobile two-column structure with an anterior articulation through the intervertebral disc and a posterior articulation through the facet joints. The spinal column is viewed as a load-sharing system with 80 to 90% of the axial load passing through the anterior column and the remaining load through the posterior column. Although most tumors affect the anterior and middle columns, ventral reconstruction alone may not be sufficient to restore torsional stability or tensile strength if the dorsal elements are also involved (Fig. 8). This requires a combined anterior and posterior reconstruction *(35)*.

Surgery is also indicated when epidural compression in a patient with a significant or progressive neurological deficit related primarily to bone compression. This is the case with a tumor-related vertebral body fracture or deformity. Although epidural compression secondary to tumor mass frequently responds to radiation therapy, bone compression does not *(14)* (Fig. 9).

7. CONCLUSION

The management of a patient with spinal metastasis is frequently a challenging task. Although conservative management is appropriate for a majority of these patients, surgical options continue to evolve playing a greater role in treating this problem. The indications for surgery in this patient population are varied and at times complex. The specific indications previously outlined need to be tailored to the individual patient. The risks and benefits of a surgical approach should be balanced with the patient's overall condition and prognosis, and the goals and expectations for surgery should be realistic.

REFERENCES

1. American Cancer Society. Cancer Facts and Figures. 2004. Available from: www.cancer.org/docroot/pro/content/pro_1_1_Cancer_Statistics_2004_presentation.asp. Accessed August 30, 2005.
2. Barron KD, Hirano A, Araki S, Terry RD. Experiences with metastatic neoplasm involving spinal cord. Neurology 1959; 9:91–106.
3. Siegal T, Siegal T. Surgical decompression of anterior and posterior malignant epidural tumours compressing the spinal cord: a prospective study. Neurosurgery 1985; 17:424–432.
4. Sundaresan N, Degiancinto GV, Hughes JEO. Surgical treatment of spinal metastasis. Clin Neurosurg 1986; 33:503–522.

5. Sundaresan N, Krol G, Digiancinto GV, et al. Metastatic tumors of the spine. In: Sundaresan N, Schmidek HH, Schiller AL, et al., eds. Tumors of the Spine. Diagnosis and Clinical Management. Philadelphia, PA: WB Saunders; 1990:279–304.

6. Sundaresan N, Krol G, Hughes JEO, et al. Tumors of the spine: diagnosis and management. In: Tindall GT, Cooper PR, Barrow DL, eds. The Practice of Neurosurgery. Baltimore, MD: Williams and Wilkins; 1996:1303–1322.

7. Wong DA, Fornasier VL, MacNab I. Spinal metastases: the obvious, the occult and the imposters. Spine 1990; 15:1–4.

8. Maranzano E, Latini P, Checcaglini F, et al. Radiation therapy in metastatic spinal cord compression. A prospective analysis of 105 consecutive patients. Cancer 1991; 67;1311–1317.

9. Perrin RG, McBroom RJ. Surgical treatment for spinal metastasis: the posterolateral approach. In: Sundaresan N, Schmidek HH, Schiller AL et al., eds. Tumors of the Spine: Diagnosis and Clinical Management. Philadelphia, PA: WB Saunders; 1990:305–315.

10. Batson OV. The role of the vertebral veins in metastatic processes. Ann Intern Med 1942; 16:38–45.

11. Black P. Spinal metastasis: current status and recommended guidelines for management. Neurosurgery 1979; 5:726–746.

12. Byrne TN: Spinal cord compression from epidural metastasis. N Engl J Med 1992; 327:614–619.

13. Chow TSF, McCutcheon IE. The surgical treatment of metastatic tumours within the intradural extramedullary compartment. J Neurosurg 1996; 85:225–230.

14. Harrington KD. Metastatic disease of the spine. J Bone Joint Surg (Am) 1986; 68:1110–1115.

15. Kostuik JP, Errico TJ, Gleason TF, Errico CC. Spinal stabilization of vertebral column tumors. Spine 1988; 13:250–256.

16. Sundaresan N, Galicich JH, Lane JM, Bains MS, McCormack P. Treatment of epidural neoplastic cord compression by vertebral body resection and stabilization. J Neurosurg 1985; 63:676–684.

17. Bach F, Larsen BH, Rohde K, et al. Metastatic spinal cord compression. Occurrence, symptoms, clinical presentations and prognosis in 398 patients with spinal cord compression. Acta Neurochir 1990; 107:37–43.

18. Kim RY, Spencer SA, Meredith RF, et al. Extradural spinal cord compression: analysis of factors determining functional prognosis-prospective study. Radiology 1990; 176:279–282.

19. Siegal T, Siegal T. Current consideration in the management of neoplastic spinal cord compression. Spine 1989; 14:223–228.

20. Turnbull ADM, Starnes HF. Surgical Emergencies in the Cancer Patient. Chicago, IL: Year Book Medical Publishers; 1987.

21. Murovic j, Sundaresan N. Pediatric spinal axis tumors. Neurosurg Clin North Am 1992; 3:947–958.

22. Posner JB, Howieson J, Cvitkovic E. "Disappearing" spinal cord compression: oncolytic effect of gluococorticoids (and other chemotherapeutic agents) on epidural metastasis. Ann Neurol 1977; 2:409–413.

23. Jeremic B, Grujicic D, Cirovic V, Djuric L, Mijatovic L. Radiotherapy of metastatic spinal cord compression. Acta Oncol 1991; 30:985–986.

24. Tomita T, Galicich JH, Sundaresan N. Radiation therapy for spinal epidural metastasis with complete block. Acta Radiol Oncol 1983; 22:135–143.

25. Sundaresan N, Digiancinto GV, Hughes JEO, Cafferty M, Vallejo A. Treatment of neoplastic spinal cord compression: results of a prospective study. Neurosurgery 1991; 29:645–650.

26. Findlay GFG. Adverse effects of the management of malignant spinal cord compression. J Neurol Neurosurg Psychiatry 1984; 47:761–768.

27. Gilbert RW, Kim JH, Posner JB. Epidural spinal cord compression from metastatic tumour: diagnosis and treatment. Ann Neurol 1978; 3:40–51.

28. Kakulas BA, Harper GC, Shibasaki K, Bedbrook GM. Vertebral metastases and spinal cord compression. Clin Exp Neurol 1978; 15:98–114.

29. Wright RL. Malignant tumours in the spinal extradural space: results of surgical treatment. Ann Surg 1963; 157:227–231.

30. Brice J, McKissock W. Surgical treatment of malignant extradural spinal tumours. Br Med J. 1965; 1:1339–1342.

31. Findlay GFG. The role of vertebral body collapse in the management of malignant spinal cord compression. J Neurol Neurosurg Psychiatry 1987; 50:151–154.

32. Tokuhashi Y, Matsuzaki H, Toriyama S, Kawano H, Ohsaka S. Scoring system for the preoperative evaluation of metastatic spine tumor prognosis. Spine 1990; 15:1110–1113.

33. Denis F. Spinal instability as defined by the three-column spine concept in acute spinal trauma. Clin Orthop 1984; 189:65–76.

34. Kostuik JP, Weinstein JN. Differential diagnosis and surgical treatment of metastatic spine tumors. In: Frymoyer JW, ed. The Adult Spine: Principles and Practice. New York, NY: Raven Press; 1991:861–888.

35. Harms J. Screw-threaded rod system in spinal fusion surgery. Spine State Art Rev 1992; 6.

27 Biopsy

Principles and Approaches

PAUL PARK, MD, FRANK LAMARCA, MD, AND ROBERT F. MCLAIN, MD

CONTENTS

1. GOALS OF BIOPSY

The primary goal of biopsy is to obtain adequate tissue for histopathological diagnosis with minimal amount of trauma *(1)*. In patients with a known primary tumor, biopsy is often used to confirm metastatic disease or to obtain tissue for hormonal evaluation *(2)* Without a history of malignancy, the appropriately performed biopsy plays a crucial role in the diagnosis and subsequent management process. Conversely, a poorly planned biopsy can result in misdiagnosis, complications, and adversely limit potential treatment options.

2. STAGING

Biopsy is the last step in the diagnostic process known as staging, which is the practice of classifying a tumor with respect to its anatomical extent and histological differentiation *(3)*. Proper staging optimizes the surgeon's ability to plan an operation most appropriate for the specific tumor type. In the staging process, the patient who presents with a lesion suspicious for tumor undergoes a thorough clinical exam followed by appropriate laboratory and radiographic studies before biopsy. Laboratory testing typically consists of a complete blood count, electrolytes, serum creatinine, blood urea nitrogen, calcium, alkaline phosphatase, total protein and serum protein electrophoresis, serum transferrin, and assays for tumor antigens, such as the prostatic specific antigen and carcinoembryonic antigen

(2). Radiographic studies include plain roentgenograms of the spine in addition to computed tomography (CT) and/or magnetic resonance imaging, which more clearly delineates the anatomical location and structure of the suspected tumor. Another study to consider is the technetium bone scan, which is very sensitive to the presence of metastases to the spine *(4,5)*. Proper prebiopsy staging narrows the differential diagnosis, helps define the extent of the tumor, and provides confidence in the frozen section analysis so that definitive surgery can be accomplished, in specific situations, at the time of an open biopsy *(6)*. Conversely, early biopsy before a complete radiographic evaluation can alter the anatomical characteristics of the tumor and thereby limit the ability to narrow the differential diagnosis and determine the anatomical extent of the tumor.

3. BIOPSY PLANNING

After thorough prebiopsy staging, there are several factors to consider when planning the biopsy. Particularly for primary malignant bone tumors, the institution where the patient undergoes the biopsy is an important consideration. Studies have shown that misdiagnoses, complications, and adverse outcomes were more common if the biopsy was performed at a referring institution rather than the treating institution *(1,7)*. Although uncertain as to the cause for this discrepancy, relatively less experience in dealing with primary bone tumors as well as lack of ability to perform accurate diagnostic studies, definitive surgery, and adjunctive treatment, were hypothesized factors. Another important step before biopsy involves consultation with the pathologist who will be analyzing the specimens *(8,9)*.

From: *Current Clinical Oncology: Cancer in the Spine: Comprehensive Care.*
Edited by: R. F. McLain, K-U. Lewandrowski, M. Markman, R. M. Bukowski,
R. Macklis, and E. C. Benzel © Humana Press, Inc., Totowa, NJ

The pathologist should be experienced with metastatic and primary bone neoplasms. In addition, findings of the prebiopsy staging with the resultant differential diagnosis should be conveyed to the pathologist so that in potentially difficult diagnostic cases, adequate preparations (i.e., specialized techniques such as immunofluorescence) can be made (3,6,10). Planning the biopsy is often given little thought, however, proper placement of the biopsy is crucial. An appropriately planned biopsy site must be capable of being removed *en bloc* with a malignant neoplasm (6). If the biopsy is referred to a radiologist, the planned site and trajectory should be confirmed so that an improper tract is not made (10).

4. BIOPSY TECHNIQUE

After selecting an appropriate biopsy site, the options for biopsy technique can be divided into two main categories: open and closed. Historically, open biopsy was the most common method and has the main advantages of providing relatively large tissue samples for analysis and a lower possibility for a sampling error (6,11). Disadvantages to open biopsy include the risk for operative hematoma, tumor spillage, infection, pathological fracture, and requirement for a general anesthetic. Open techniques consist of the incisional and excisional biopsy. Most open biopsies are incisional primarily because they result in less local tumor spillage than excisional biopsies (6). Excisional biopsies are considered only for small or benign tumors, cases in which the diagnosis is fairly certain or when the tumor is located in an expendable anatomic site. Guidelines for open biopsy of musculoskeletal tumors are applicable to spine tumors and include the following (3,6,12,13): (1) a biopsy tract that is amenable to removal *en bloc* during the subsequent definitive surgery is used. (2) The most direct route to the tumor is chosen in order to avoid crossing multiple tissue planes. There is minimal disruption of adjacent compartments or neurovascular structures. If inadvertent violation of adjacent compartments occurs, contaminated structures are removed with the tumor. (3) An adequate sample is taken from the periphery of the tumor because this area is often the most viable and representative. Frozen section analysis is performed to ascertain that representative tissue is obtained. Samples for culture are also sent. (4) A bloodless operative field is optimal to avoid postoperative hematoma and consequent tumor spillage. Methylmethacrylate can be used to obtain hemostasis at bony biopsy sites. (5) If a drain is used, its point of entry into the skin is made along the path of the planned incision so that the presumably contaminated drain tract can be excised with the malignant tumor during the subsequent surgery.

Fine needles for aspiration and bone trephines are the predominant instruments utilized in closed biopsy (9,14–17). Typically, lytic lesions are amenable to fine-needle aspiration techniques, whereas sclerotic lesions will require use of a bone trephine. A variety of bone trephines are available including the Craig, Ackerman, and Jamshidi needles (18–20). These trephines are designed to obtain a core of tissue from bone without distorting its architecture so that optimal histopathological analysis can be performed. Advantages of closed over open biopsy include the potential to avoid surgery, earlier institution of radiotherapy, ability to obtain tissue from deeper areas in the lesion, decreased risk of pathological fracture, use of local rather than general anesthesia, cost savings, and rapid differentiation of primary from metastatic lesions (11,17,18, 21,22). The main drawbacks of closed biopsy are decreased diagnostic accuracy and a greater potential for a sampling error. The technical aspects of closed biopsy vary and are based on the location of the tumor. Proper prebiopsy radiographic evaluation will assist in determining the optimal method. A lateral or anterolateral approach is amenable for a lesion in the cervical spine except at C2 or C3 where a transpedicular approach is safer (22–24). In the thoracolumbar spine, the posterolateral or transpedicular approach is employed (9,11,18,22,25). The posterolateral approach has been the most commonly used technique particularly with extraosseous lesions extending into the paraspinal region. For lesions confined within the vertebral body, the transpedicular approach appears to be a safer alternative with decreased risks for pulmonary or nerve root injury (11,26).

5. RELATIVE INDICATIONS

In general, closed biopsy should be considered the technique of choice because of its relatively high diagnostic accuracy, decreased morbidity, and cost. An open biopsy is typically reserved for cases in which closed biopsy has failed or when a primary bone tumor is suspected based on prebiopsy staging (11,27). In addition, open biopsy may be considered in tumors that appear to be highly vascular, such as renal cell (26). Anatomic limitations can also influence biopsy choice. Owing to the smaller vertebra and closer proximity of the lung and pleura, closed biopsy of the upper thoracic spine involves increased risk and as a consequence open biopsy should be considered (28,29). Patients with significant spinal deformity may also benefit from open biopsy (27).

6. DIAGNOSTIC ACCURACY

Open biopsy is considered to have the highest diagnostic accuracy because relatively large amounts of tissue can be obtained (11,27). Since the advent of closed biopsy, reported diagnostic accuracy has ranged widely from 21 to 100% (8,9, 14–17,22,24,30–33). In recent years, however, overall diagnostic rates have been much higher. Presently, fluoroscopic guidance appears to be nearly as effective as CT guidance with reports of 77.5 to 89% diagnostic accuracy (4,16,32). In comparison, reported CT-guided diagnostic rates range from 71 to 100% (17,22,31,33). CT guidance is of particular use when the lesion is small, deep-seated, or visible by bone scan, but not by plain X-ray (22,31). The primary advantage of fluoroscopic guidance, in contrast, is the ability to assess needle positioning in real-time (27,29). In addition to image guidance, the type of lesion may influence diagnostic accuracy. In one study of 75 patients, diagnostic accuracy appeared to be higher (96%) for metastatic disease than in primary bone tumors (82%) (8). Larger bore needles (internal diameter ≥2 mm) are also associated with higher diagnostic accuracy when obtaining core tissue samples owing to the decreased likelihood of crush artifact (15,33). Another potential factor impacting diagnostic

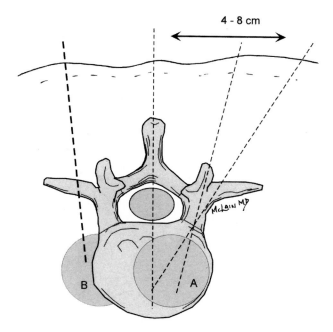

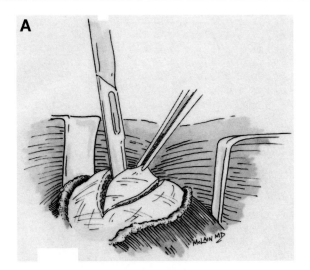

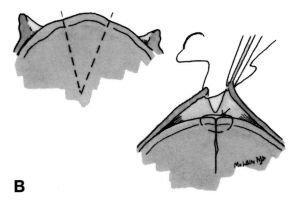

Fig. 1. Percutaneous biopsy approaches. For intravertebral lesions (**A**), a transpedicular approach offers the best chance of obtaining diagnostic tissue without contaminating the field. The approach may be performed through a minimal open incision, or through a percutaneous stab wound technique. If the lesion provides a paraspinous soft-tissue mass (**B**), this may be biopsied directly under fluoroscopic or computed tomography guidance.

Fig. 2. Open incisional biopsy. (**A**) Technique is important to obtaining adequate tissue without risking tumor spread. The outer capsule is exposed and bleeding controlled before taking the biopsy. (**B**) Once an adequate biopsy is taken, using a sharp scalpel to limit crush or cautery artifacts, the capsule is closed tightly to prevent hematoma formation.

accuracy is the region of the spine biopsied. Specifically, closed biopsy of thoracic lesions has been associated with lower rates of diagnosis *(31)*. This decreased accuracy was attributed to difficulties with access to thoracic spine lesions even with CT-guidance. Finally, the assistance of an experienced pathologist cannot be over emphasized in obtaining an accurate diagnosis *(8,21)*.

7. CONTRAINDICATIONS

Any type of bleeding disorder is typically considered an absolute contraindication to open or closed biopsy. More relative contraindications to closed biopsy include tumors that appear to be highly vascular as well as densely sclerotic lesions because of the potential of slippage of the needle *(4,30)*.

8. TECHNIQUES

Needle biopsy is typically performed from a posterolateral approach, aiming for the pedicle, vertebral body, or a recognized paraspinous mass. Access to the vertebral body is gained through a transpedicular approach to minimize the risk of spreading tumor into the paraspinous soft tissues along the needle tract. If a primary spine malignancy is strongly suspected, the needle path must be closer to the midline so that it can be excised during the definitive excision.

The needle placement most often used starts with a stab wound 4 to 8 cm off the midline at the level of the involved vertebra (Fig. 1). To access a vertebral body lesion, the needle is directed to the junction of the transverse process and the lateral facet margin, then driven through the cortex into the

lateral aspect of the pedicle. From this point the needle can be passed directly into the tumor mass, or a guidewire placed and a sheath placed to allow passage of a Craig Needle biopsy trochar, capable of harvesting larger pieces of ossified tissue.

Open, incisional techniques vary with the location of the tumor and the complexity of the definitive incision. If incisional biopsy is planned as a confirmatory step just before excision, the definitive incision can be initiated and developed up to the point that the tumor capsule is clearly defined and vascular control established (Fig. 2). An elliptical incision through the capsule will provide a section of tumor tissue including the capsule and the leading margin of the tumor. The capsule can then be closed while frozen section confirms the diagnosis. If the primary lesion is confirmed, a wide excision can be completed. If a benign or metastatic lesion is identified, a less destructive, marginal or intralesional excision may be adequate.

If an incisional biopsy is performed well in advance of the final resection, the approach must minimize soft-tissue contamination and not expose tissues that cannot later be excised. If a paraspinous incision is used, it will have to be incorporated

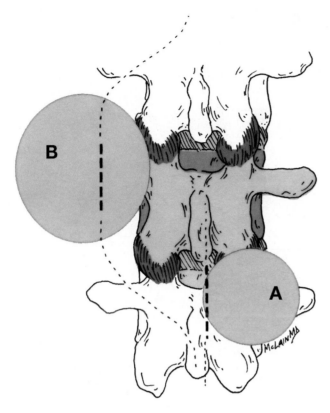

Fig. 3. Posterior incisions. To obtain a wide margin in a primary sarcoma excision, the biopsy tract must be excised with the tumor. (**A**) Paramedian tumors may be biopsied through a midline approach. (**B**) Large, eccentric masses may be biopsied through a paramedian incision. The curvilinear incision for the final excision also allows the surgeon to create flaps that provide access to a larger field without undue tissue tension.

into a curvilinear (Sedon-type) incision, so that the entire tract is removed with the final specimen (Fig. 3).

9. COMPLICATIONS

The major complications of open biopsy can be generalized to those expected for spine surgery including the risks of anesthesia, infection, bleeding, and injury to the spinal cord or nerve roots. Complications associated with closed biopsy vary depending on the region biopsied. In the cervical spine, the potential risks include airway compromise and vascular injury *(8,24)*. In the thoracolumbar spine, the most common risks are pulmonary injury (pneumothorax), nerve root injury, bleeding, and infection *(4,9,11,16,17,27,29,32,33)*. Less commonly observed are injuries involving the spinal cord and great vessels *(34)*. Overall, reported complication rates from closed biopsy range from 0 to 20% with the majority noting no significant complications *(4,14,17,21,22,25–27,29,30,34)*. Factors impacting complication rates for closed biopsy include the approach utilized and the size of the needle used for biopsy. Generally, smaller needles are associated with decreased risk *(4,11)*. For thoracolumbar lesions, a transpedicular approach appears to minimize the risk for pulmonary and nerve root injury *(11,26,32)*.

10. CONCLUSION

The biopsy is typically a crucial part of the diagnostic evaluation for the patient presenting with a possible spine tumor. Biopsy, however, should be the last step in the diagnostic process known as staging. Proper prebiopsy staging followed by appropriate biopsy planning and technique will optimize the subsequent management process.

REFERENCES

1. Mankin H, Mankin CJ, Simon MA. The hazards of the biopsy, revisited. J Bone Joint Surg 1996; 78:656–663.
2. Asdourian P. Metastatic Disease of the Spine. In: Bridwell K, DeWald RL, eds. The Textbook of Spinal Surgery. Philadelphia, PA: Lippincott-Raven; 1997:2007–2050.
3. Peabody T, Gibbs CP, Simon MA. Evaluation and Staging of Musculoskeletal Neoplasms. J Bone Joint Surg 1998; 80:1204–1218.
4. Stoker D, Kissin CM. Percutaneous vertebral biopsy: a review of 135 cases. Clin Radiol 1985; 36:569–577.
5. Colman L, Porter BA, Redmond J, et al. Early diagnosis of spinal metastases by CT and MR studies. J Comput Assist Tomogr 1988; 12:423–426.
6. Simon M. Biopsy of musculoskeletal tumors. J Bone Joint Surg 1982 ;64:1253–1257.
7. Mankin H, Lange TA, Spanier SS. The hazards of biopsy in patients with malignant primary bone and soft-tissue tumors. J Bone Joint 1982; 64:1121–1127.
8. Kattapuram S, Khurana JS, Rosenthal DI. Percutaneous needle biopsy of the spine. Spine 1992; 17:561–564.
9. Ottolenghi C. Aspiration biopsy of the spine. J Bone Joint Surg 1969; 51:1531–1544.
10. Springfield D, Rosenberg A. Biopsy: complicated and risky. J Bone Joint Surg 1996; 78:639–643.
11. Stringham D, Hadjipavlou A, Dzioba RB, Lander P. Percutaneous transpedicular biopsy of the spine. Spine 1994; 19:1985–1991.
12. Bickels J, Jelinek J, Shmookler B, Malawer M. Biopsy of musculoskeletal tumors. In: Malawer M, Sugarbaker PH, eds. Musculoskeletal Cancer Surgery. Dordrecht/Boston/London: Kluwer Academic Publishers; 2001:37–45.
13. Levine A, Crandall DG. Treatment of primary malignant tumors of the spine and sacrum. In: Bridwell K, DeWald RL, eds. The Textbook of Spinal Surgery. Philadelphia, PA: Lippincott-Raven; 1997:1984–1987.
14. Moore T, Meyers MH, Patzakis MJ, Terry R, Harvey PJ. Closed biopsy of musculoskeletal lesions. J Bone Joint Surg 1979; 61:375–380.
15. Fyfe I, Henry APJ, Mulholland RC. Closed vertebral biopsy. J Bone Joint Surg 1983; 65:140–143.
16. Laredo J, Bard M. Thoracic spine: percutaneous trephine biopsy. Radiology 1986; 160:485–489.
17. Ghelman B, Lospinuso MF, Levine DB, O'Leary PF, Burke SW. Percutaneous computed-tomography-guided biopsy of the thoracic and lumbar spine. Spine 1990; 16:736–739.
18. Ackermann W. Application of the trephine for bone biopsy. JAMA 1963; 184:11–17.
19. Jamshidi K, Swaim WR. Bone marrow biopsy with unaltered architecture: a new biopsy device. J Lab Clin Med 1971; 77:335–342.
20. Craig F. Vertebral body biopsy. J Bone Joint Surg 1956; 38:93–102.
21. DeSantos L, Murray JA, Ayala AG. The value of percutaneous needle biopsy in the management of primary bone tumors. Cancer 1979; 43:735–744.
22. Babu N, Titus VTK, Chittaranjan S, Abraham G, Prem H, Korula RJ. Computed tomographically guided biopsy of the spine. Spine 1994; 19:2436–2442.
23. Tampieri D, Weill A, Melanson D, Ethier R. Percutaneous aspiration biopsy in cervical spine lytic lesions. Neuroradiology 1991; 33:43–47.
24. Brugieres P, Gaston A, Voisin MC, Ricolfi F, Chakir N. CT-guided percutaneous biopsy of the cervical spine: a series of 12 cases. Neuroradiology 1992; 34:358–360.

25. Renfrew D, Whitten CG, Wiese JA, El-Khoury GY, Harris KG. CT-guided percutaneous transpedicular biopsy of the spine. Radiology 1991; 180:574–576.

26. Jelinek J, Kransdorf MJ, Gray R, Aboulafia AJ, Malawer MM. Percutaneous transpedicular biopsy of vertebral body lesions. Spine 1996; 21:2035–2040.

27. Hadjipavlou A, Kontakis GM, Gaitanis JN, Katonis PG, Lander P, Crow WN. Effectiveness and pitfalls of percutaneous transpedicle biopsy of the spine. Clin Orthop and Relat Res 2003; 411:54–60.

28. Fazzi U, Waddell G. Semi-open needle biopsy of the upper thoracic spine. Spine 1994; 19:1395–1396.

29. Metzger C, Johnson DW, Donaldson WF. Percutaneous biopsy in the anterior thoracic spine. Spine 1993; 18:374–378.

30. Bender C, Berquist TH, Wold LE. Imaging-assisted percutaneous biopsy of the thoracic spine. Mayo Clin Proc 1986; 61:942–950.

31. Kornblum M, Wesolowski DP, Fischgrund JS, Herkowitz HN. Computed tomography-guided biopsy of the spine. Spine 1998; 23:81–85.

32. Pierot L, Boulin A. Percutaneous biopsy of the thoracic and lumbar spine: transpedicular approach under fluoroscopic guidance. AJNR Am J Neuroradiol 1999; 20:23–25.

33. Yaffe D, Greenberg G, Leitner J, Gipstein R, Shapiro M, Bachar GN. CT-guided percutaneous biopsy of thoracic and lumbar spine: a new coaxial technique. AJNR Am J Neuroradiol 2003; 24:21112113.

34. Donaldson W, Johnson DW. Percutaneous biopsy of the thoracic spine. Neurosurg Clin N Am 1996; 7:135–144.

28 Problem-Based Decision Making

MICHAEL P. STEINMETZ, MD, ANIS O. MEKHAIL, MD,
AND EDWARD C. BENZEL, MD

CONTENTS

1. INTRODUCTION

1.1. PROBLEM-BASED DECISION MAKING VS EVIDENCE-BASED DECISION MAKING

The surgical decision-making process is an art form. No single strategy always works, and even the most inadequate of strategies will work occasionally. The decision-making process involves the assimilation of prior experience of others (e.g., by a learned assessment of the literature), and an in-depth knowledge and awareness of the application of biomechanical and anatomical factors and principles (1).

Although problem-based decision making is based on the foundations of evidence and logic, it should not be confused with evidence-based decision making. Sackett (2) defines evidence-based medicine as "the conscientious, explicit, and judicious use of the current best evidence in making decisions about the care of individual patients." There are inherent flaws if only an evidence-based strategy is considered for the decision-making process. First, statistical manipulation can be used to portray clinical variables, problems, and solutions in a deceptive manner. Second, data is often insufficient to make relevant decisions that are based on objective and statistically significant data alone. Third, evidence-based methodology is based on "large population" assessments that do not effectively consider all subpopulations. Essentially, the literature suffers from selection bias, i.e., data is often selectively presented. For example, if a study generated "undesirable" results (to the author[s]), the author would not submit the data for publication in the literature. On the other hand, desirable results would be submitted for publication. Errors of logic (see Subheading 3.1.2.) may then be made from a strict adherence to evidence-based decision making. Many of the problems associated with

From: *Current Clinical Oncology: Cancer in the Spine: Comprehensive Care.*
Edited by: R. F. McLain, K-U. Lewandrowski, M. Markman, R. M. Bukowski,
R. Macklis, and E. C. Benzel © Humana Press, Inc., Totowa, NJ

an evidence-based methodology approach to decision making may be overcome by utilizing a "common sense" approach to the careful assessment of the "evidence." Problem-based decision making utilizes this "common sense" approach. It is, therefore, logic-based. However, the evidence must not be ignored. Both are necessary components of the clinical decision-making process. One provides the foundation of knowledge (evidence-based), and the other provides the rational thought required to fill the "gaps" in our knowledge (problem-based). Sackett (2) also acknowledges this. He states, "Good doctors use both individual clinical expertise and the best available external evidence, and neither alone is enough. Without clinical expertise, practice risks become tyrannized by evidence, because even excellent external evidence may be inapplicable to or inappropriate for an individual patient. Without current best evidence, practice risks rapidly become out of date, to the detriment of patients" (2).

1.2. REGIONAL VARIATIONS

There exists a significant discrepancy in the rates of spinal surgery, region to region. This may be, in part, a manifestation of clinical decision-making errors or differences in style. A proportion of these errors may be avoided when the patient is involved in the decision-making process.

The rates of spine surgery vary sixfold across geographic regions, and the rates of spinal fusion vary 10-fold (3). The region-specific rates of spinal fusion are haphazard (i.e., there may be a region with very high rates of spinal fusion immediately adjacent to one with a very low rate). This pattern suggests that the variability stems from physicians' practice and decision-making styles rather than the characteristics of the population (3), thus, underscoring the need to standardize the decision-making process.

Shared decision making is the process of giving patients informed choices about their treatment based on current best

Table 1
Decision-Making Errors

A. Errors of consideration
   1. Errors of omission
   2. Errors of logic
   3. Errors of obscurity
B. Error of prioritization

evidence, as opposed to informed consent *(3)* It utilizes both problem-based and evidence-based data to educate patients. Deyo et al. *(4)* reported significantly decreased rates of lumbar spine disk surgery when patients were assigned to watch a video regarding the choice between surgical and nonsurgical therapies. Conversely, when patients watched a video regarding surgery for spinal stenosis, they were somewhat more likely to choose surgery *(4)* Shared decision making may be the first step in the standardization process. The next steps involve error reduction strategies.

2. ERRORS IN THE DECISION-MAKING PROCESS

Before we are able to describe the process, a discussion of error is appropriate. Most capable clinicians, when faced with a complex decision involving multiple variables, can make "strategic" errors during the decision-making process. These errors are of two types: (1) errors of consideration and (2) errors of prioritization (Table 1). Both errors of consideration and of prioritization are commonly and innocently made. Most have no ill effect. Nevertheless, when these errors are made, the variables that compose the clinical problem or clinical dilemma at hand (except in situations involving errors of obscurity) were, simply stated, inappropriately or inaccurately processed.

2.1. ERRORS OF CONSIDERATION

When multiple familiar variables (i.e., variables that are evident to the clinician) affect the decision-making process, one or more of these variables may be omitted by not being considered (errors of omission) or they may be inappropriately considered (errors of logic). In a study of 69 cervical spine injury patients, 56% suffered a pitfall of management, 17 pitfalls were owing to an error in surgical decision making *(5)*. During the treatment process, some variables are unknown to the physician. An example of this is a patient with occult pancreatic cancer who is being considered for an elective spine deformity correction operation. These variables are "obscure," and the resultant error is one of obscurity. These types of errors are usually not the "fault" of the clinician, therefore they are unequivocally not below the standard of care.

2.2. ERRORS OF PRIORITIZATION

As previously stated, most complex problems are comprised of several components. To solve these problems, the overall problem should be divided into components and assigned a priority. A surgeon may consider all variables appropriately, but if they are not considered in an orderly manner, a suboptimal result may ensue. Almost always, one component of the overall problem takes precedence over another. This is the primary component, and it is the most important component of the operation or treatment strategy. It, in turn, dictates the need for

and the type of procedure that comprises the secondary component, and so on. Usually, spinal decompression is the primary component of a complex operation. The decompression component of the overall operation may destabilize the spine, thus, altering the choice of the secondary component of the procedure, the stabilization component. Therefore, the prioritization of the components of the treatment strategy and the solution order is vital. Such a prioritization process helps ensure that neural decompression, as well as the acquisition of spinal stability, is safely achieved. It also solidifies in the surgeon's mind the relative importance of each component of the operation and promotes rational decision making.

3. EXAMPLES OF DECISION-MAKING ERRORS

It is instructional to consider examples of each of the aforementioned decision-making errors, the three types of errors of consideration and errors of prioritization (Table 1).

3.1. ERRORS OF CONSIDERATION
3.1.1. Errors of Omission

Errors of omission usually occur because the clinician did not appropriately consider a "familiar variable" during the decision-making process. The most prevalent reason for this is the near-infinite amount of information available to the clinician during this process. For example, nonunion (pseudoarthrosis) may result if one does not consider critical, relevant variables (e.g., diabetes, osteoporosis, tobacco abuse).

3.1.2. Errors of Logic

Errors of logic occur because the clinician fails to strictly apply the principles of logic to the clinical problem at hand. However, one person's logic is not necessarily that of the next. A clinical algorithm may be chosen on the basis of bias, clinical experience, and others. The logic used is also based on these variables and understandings. A given process (algorithm), however, may be logical to some, but illogical to others. It is, therefore, emphasized that logic is relative.

3.1.3. Errors of Obscurity

To not consider a variable that is unbeknownst to the clinician is not only understandable, it is usually acceptable. It is impossible to consider an unfamiliar variable. Therefore, no further discussion on this topic is necessary, except for the need for appropriate emphasis placed on knowledge base acquisition. The greater the knowledge base, the less likely the occurrence of an error of obscurity. In other words, knowledge base acquisition minimizes the incidence of unfamiliar variables.

3.2. ERRORS OF PRIORITIZATION

To consider all variables, but to apply them in an order that is considered illogical or inappropriate, is not uncommon. A clinician may determine all the relevant clinical variables affecting a pathological process, however, if these variables are not considered in an orderly manner, a suboptimal result may ensue. For example, to consider spinal deformity correction before considering neural decompression may result in an increased neurological deficit.

4. THE PROCESS

The problem-based decision-making process is a strategy that involves (1) the separation of complex problems or dilem-

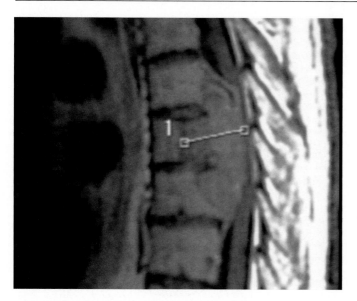

Fig. 1. Sagittal magnetic resonance imaging of the thoracic spine. A ventral T8–T10 process is observed.

Table 2
Hypothetic Prioritized Component Problem List

1. Neural decompression
2. Axial load-bearing capability
3. Prevention and/or correction of spinal deformity

mas into their component parts, (2) the prioritization of the component parts, and (3) the orderly solution of each portion of the overall problem posed by each of the component parts in order to methodically solve the overall problem. Problem-based decision making can make a seemingly "impossible" problem "solvable."

A patient with a ventral T8 through T10 pathological process may serve as an example (Fig. 1). The patient is a 40-yr-old male. He is a smoker with no other co-morbidities. The differential diagnosis includes metastasis, primary spinal tumor, and infection. A metastatic work-up (chest computed tomography [CT], abdominal CT, and so on) is negative and there are no other signs of infection (fever, elevated white blood cell count or sedimentation rate).

Establishing the diagnosis is the first goal. This clinical decision-making goal is not always achieved. In fact, it may not be necessary to establish a diagnosis at all costs. Clinical confidence regarding the diagnosis must be considered. In a patient with known metastatic cancer, the clinician may confidently assume that the lesion is a metastatic tumor. On the other hand, a patient with a similar lesion without the diagnosis of a primary malignant tumor may not engender the same degree of confidence regarding the etiology of the lesion. Therefore, "confidence" is relative. In our patient example, one cannot confidently determine the etiology of the lesion. Therefore, an aggressive search for the diagnosis is warranted. This may be accomplished via CT-guided needle biopsy or an open procedure.

A CT-guided needle biopsy of the lesion revealed chordoma. A treatment strategy can then be formulated. One must first consider if the problem is best addressed surgically, or by a non-operative strategy. Consideration should also be given to the potential for cure. Is this pathological process one that may be cured with surgery or some other non-surgical strategy?

In this clinical example, a surgical strategy is chosen. It is felt that cure is likely if a complete resection (*en bloc*) is obtained. In

order to achieve a complete resection, a complete spondylectomy of T8 through T10 is planned. It is felt that the patient is a "good" candidate for such an aggressive approach. Such an approach provides the best chance for a cure. This plan is discussed with the patient and family. The patient's fears, desires, and expectations should also be included in this discussion, and in the ultimate decision.

Ultimately, the surgical strategy should be broken down into its component parts, the component parts prioritized, and each solved sequentially (Table 2). Neural decompression assumes first priority. This is so in this, and in most cases, because the priorities of neurologic function are usually the highest priority of any spine operation (1). The need for neural decompression also dictates the surgical approach to the pathology. As a general rule of thumb, ventral lesions should be approached ventrally, and dorsal lesions should be approached dorsally (1). The majority of spinal metastasis involve the vertebral body (6), therefore, optimal decompression is often from a ventral approach. This is not feasible in all patients. For example, a patient's poor medical condition may preclude a transthoracic approach to a thoracic spine lesion. A dorsal or dorsolateral approach or a transpedicular or lateral extracavitary approach, may be employed instead. In our example, a spondylectomy of T8 through T10 is planned. This encompasses a 360° bony removal. It is felt best to approach this via a bilateral lateral extracavitary approach. This will allow *en bloc* tumor resection (360°) and neural element decompression (Fig. 2).

After the type of decompression has been determined, consideration should next be given to the axial load-bearing capability of the spine (Table 2). A thoracolumbar fracture may serve as an instructive example here. McCormack et al. (7) demonstrated that with a thoracolumbar burst fracture, if there were multiple fracture fragments with significant space between them (dispersion of fragments), it is unlikely that this vertebral body will ever effectively bear an axial load (Fig. 3). In this situation, the ventral column should be reconstructed, i.e., with a strut graft, or a cage.

The aforementioned data from the trauma literature may be extrapolated to tumor surgery. If a tumor has destroyed a vertebral body, the vertebral body may not be able to effectively bear an axial load. Reconstruction of the ventral column is biomechanically and clinically appropriate in this situation. The axial-load bearing capability may be iatrogenically reduced as well. After vertebrectomy, the ventral column will usually be rendered incompetent, and reconstruction made necessary. This may be accomplished through strut graft placement, a cage, or a chest tube filled with polymethylmethalcrylate. If a vertebrectomy is not performed, one must decide if the tumor laden vertebral body is stable enough to bear an axial load. One

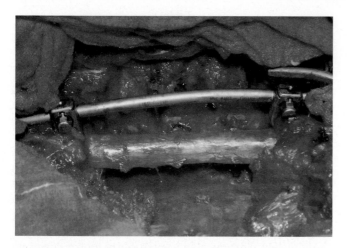

Fig. 2. Spondylectomy of T8–T10 has been completed. There is complete (360°) decompression of the spinal cord.

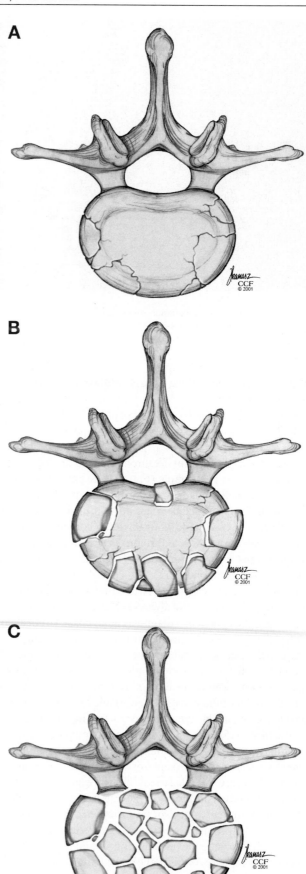

may consider dorsal implant placement in this situation. If such is chosen, a long moment arm construct should be employed. If short segment dorsal instrumentation is used without ventral column reconstruction, instrumentation failure and a resultant spinal instability may occur. If this component of the overall procedure is ignored and the ventral column not supported, progressive spinal deformity leading to neurological deficit may occur.

After a three-level spondylectomy, the ventral column must be reconstructed. In this case, a titanium cage filled with iliac crest autograft was placed in the vertebrectomy defect. This restored the weight-bearing capacity of the ventral column and will aid in the prevention of postoperative kyphosis. Bone graft was chosen over bone cement because of the good chance of long survival.

Next, consideration is given to deformity correction and progression (Table 2). Every effort should be used to re-align the spine to prevent further deformity progression. The risk for deformity progression may be from the original spinal pathology or because of the iatrogenic instability from tumor resection and decompression. Deformity is usually corrected and progression is prevented with the placement of spinal instrumentation. Implants may be placed ventrally, dorsally, or via a combined ventral and dorsal approach. One must consider the amount of instability present and the forces required to correct and prevent further deformity progression. In certain circumstances "more is better" and consideration should be given to a 360° (combined ventral and dorsal) operation.

Fig. 3. *(opposite page)* Schematic of a burst fracture demonstrating: **(A)** few fracture fragments with no dispersion of the fragments, **(B)** more fragments compared to **A** with some dispersion of the fragments, and **(C)** many fracture fragments with significant space between the fragments (wide dispersion of fragments). The fractures depicted in **A** and **B** may be effective at bearing an axial load and may be treated with external bracing. It is unlikely that the vertebral body in **C** will be effective at bearing an axial load, either at this time or in the future. In this situation, the ventral column should be reconstructed.

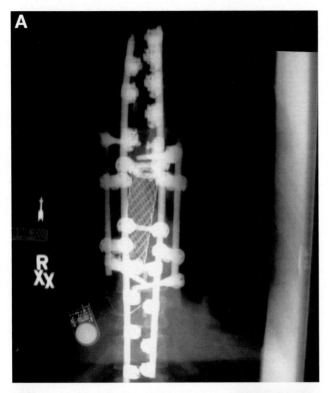

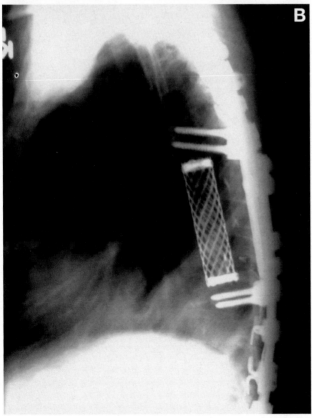

In cases such as complete spondylectomy, a "more is better" strategy is best employed. In the case presented here, a cage filled with autograft was placed ventrally. A ventral screw and rod construct was also fashioned bilaterally. Considering the extent of iatrogenic instability present in this case, a long moment arm dorsal construct was also placed. An "out-rigger" was fashioned to bilaterally connect the ventral to the dorsal components of the implant (Fig. 4).

5. CONCLUSIONS

Complex problems may be effectively, efficiently, and safely solved if the problem-based decision-making process is employed. The patient should be included in this shared decision-making process. An orderly solution of each of the components of the overall problem is optimal. Consideration should be given to the possible errors that may occur. Using the aforementioned approach, and combining it with evidence gained from the literature, forms the basis of problem-based methodology. Utilizing this strategy, the seemingly "impossible" problem truly becomes "solvable."

REFERENCES

1. Benzel EC. Biomechanics of Spine Stabilization. Chicago, IL: American Association of Neurological Surgeons; 2001.
2. Sackett D. Evidence-based medicine . Spine 1998; 10:1085–1086.
3. Lurie JD, Weinstein JN. Shared decision-making and the orthopaedic workforce. Clin Orthop 2001; 385:68–75.4.   Deyo RA, Cherkin DC, Weinstein J, Howe J, Ciol M, Mulley AG Jr. Involving patients in clinical decisions: Impact of an interactive video program on outcomes and use of back surgery. Med Care 2000; 38:959–969.
5. Rao S, Vadani KM, Jamieson K, Schildhauer T. Pitfalls in the surgical management of cervical spine injuries. Eur Spine J 1996; 5:153–160.
6. Perrin RG, McBroom RJ. Anterior versus posterior decompression for symptomatic spinal metastasis. Can J Neurol Sci 1987; 14:75–80.
7. McCormack T, Karaikovic E, Gaines RW. The load sharing classification of spine fractures. Spine 1994; 19:1741–1744.

Fig. 4. (**A,B**) Postoperative AP and lateral radiograph. A cage has been placed ventrally. Also placed ventrally is a bilateral screw/rod construct. The ventral construct has been connected to the dorsal construct via "out-riggers."

29 Spinal Cord and Nerve Root Decompression

KEITH R. LODHIA, MD, MS, PAUL PARK, MD,
AND GREGORY P. GRAZIANO, MD

CONTENTS

1. INTRODUCTION

Tumors of the vertebral column include both primary and metastatic lesions. These tumors can cause significant morbidity consisting of lesional pain and pain from deformity. Compression of the spinal cord and spinal nerve roots can also cause radicular pain as well as neurologial deterioration including sensory deficits, weakness, paralysis, and/or sexual/bowel/ bladder dysfunction. In cases of metastatic lesions, the spine is the most common region of osseous involvement (1). Metastatic vertebral spine lesions can result in pathological fractures or have significant epidural tumor involvement, both of which can lead to neurological deterioration (2). Mortality and morbidity can be significant in malignant tumors and overall treatment is best addressed by a multidisciplinary approach.

Classically, surgery for most malignant spinal tumors consisted of simple posterior element decompression with tumor debulking or excision, if possible, with or without radiation therapy. Alternatively radiation therapy alone has been employed without surgical intervention as the results of decompression and adjuvant radiation and that of radiation alone were historically comparable (3,4). Urgent laminectomy has been performed for decompression in those patients with tumor causing acute spinal cord compression, however, the window of efficacy is generally considered to be within 24 to 36 h of neurological decline (5). Decompressive laminectomy, however, does not address deformity correction or prevention and rarely attends to disease of the anterior vertebral column in an adequate fashion. This is important because the majority of metastatic lesions involve the richly vascular vertebral body and are rarely found exclusively in the posterior bony elements (6).

More recently, in patients with isolated primary and metastatic disease of the vertebral column, a more aggressive approach to surgical management has been employed (7,8). Patients with isolated disease usually have a more favorable prognosis and better long-term survival than those patients with diffuse spinal involvement (8). This has lead to operations for decompression and spinal column reconstruction being performed early, before radiation therapy. This adjuvant approach is rational as spinal radiation before surgical spine management appears to be associated with increased wound complications (9). Surgical management of these isolated lesions often involve both anterior and posterior approaches to address gross total tumor removal, neural element decompression, and restoration of spinal stability (10–14). Circumferential decompressive operations may lead to longer periods of ambulation ability, decreased pain, as well as prolonged bowel and bladder control when compared with radiation therapy alone (10,15).

Primary tumors of the vertebral column include a variety of malignant and benign conditions. Tumors including multiple myeloma and neoplastic-like lesions such as aneurysmal bone cysts and hemangiomas can present either as mass lesions or pathological fractures requiring decompressive operations in conjunction with spinal reconstruction and fusion (7,16). Other primary malignant vertebral tumors, such as osteoblastoma, can have significant epidural extension necessitating decompression of the epidural space in addition to vertebral lesional excision (17).

Intrinsic tumors of the spinal cord, while rare, can cause pain and present with neurological involvement. The majority of intramedullary lesions consist of ependymomas, astrocytomas, and hemangioblastomas. On rare occasions metastatic disease

From: Current Clinical Oncology: Cancer in the Spine: Comprehensive Care.
Edited by: R. F. McLain, K-U. Lewandrowski, M. Markman, R. M. Bukowski,
R. Macklis, and E. C. Benzel © Humana Press, Inc., Totowa, NJ

can be found intrinsic to the spinal cord, but metastatic lesions to the spinal cord usually present as purely extradural masses. Decompression of intramedullary tumors is performed typically by laminectomy followed by midline myelotomy and microsurgical tumor excision (18,19). In general, posterior spinal fusion is not necessary in these cases, although, in the pediatric population postlaminectomy kyphosis after spinal cord tumors occurs in up to 50% of patients (20,21). Consequently, instrumented posterior spinal fusion or laminoplasty may be indicated in the young population especially if a preexisting deformity or malalignment of the spinal column exists before a laminectomy (16,22).

2. SURGICAL TREATMENT OF TUMORS OF THE OCCIPITOCERVICAL JUNCTION

Tumors of the craniocervical junction are uncommon and can include both primary lesions, such as meningiomas, giant cell tumors, schwannomas, and chordomas, and, very rarely, metastatic disease (23,24). Like the subaxial spine, metastases will frequently involve the anterior elements of the atlas and axis. This can make total resection of atlantoaxial tumors difficult. Unlike other regions of the spine, however, spinal cord decompression and adequate pain relief can often be obtained from a posterior decompression and fusion without the need for an anterior approach (24,25). Obviously isolated posterior approaches can make it difficult for a complete tumor resection, usually demanding adjuvant therapy. Palliative therapy using occipitocervical instrumentation for immobilization without the necessity for bony fusion can be an alternative in patients with metastatic involvement of C1–C2 and a limited life span (26).

2.1. ANTERIOR APPROACHES TO THE CRANIOCERVICAL JUNCTION

Similar to other areas of the spine, neoplastic disease of the upper cervical spine often involves the anterior elements. The odontoid process and anterior portions of C1–C2 can often best be approached transorally (27,28). Following transoral dens resection, the cavity can be reconstructed using allograft or autograft bone. The use of cancellous autograft and a titanium mesh cage can also be used for reconstruction (29). Given the degree of spinal instability produced by anterior procedures, augmention with posterior occipitocervical instrumentation is often performed. The addition of posterior occipitocervical instrumentation can reduce the necessity of using a rigid halo fixation device and the associated morbidity of such devices.

An anterolateral approach has also been described for tumor resection of an aneurysmal bone cyst isolated to the lateral mass of the atlas and not involving the axis (30). This approach allows removal of the ventral tumor involvement as well as resection of more lateral elements that are often not possible with a transoral approach (31).

2.2. POSTERIOR APPROACHES TO THE CRANIOCERVICAL JUNCTION

Although tumor debulking of anterior midline located lesions of the craniocervical junction can be done using the transoral approach, more lateral lesions require additional strategic approaches. The posterolateral/far lateral approach to the cervical spine has been used successfully to address tumors of the foramen magnum and upper cervical spine region (32). Unlike the anterolateral approach, the far lateral approach allows for a larger exposure and for mobilization of the vertebral artery if necessary (i.e., "extreme" lateral approach).

Many tumor decompressive and debulking operations of the craniocervical junction require simultaneous instrumented fusion owing to instability from the lesional pathology or from the destabilizing nature of the tumor decompression procedure. Posteriorly, various methods of atlantoaxial instrumentation and fusion have been described (33–37). One of the most common techniques of C1–C2 fusion is the transarticular screw fixation method described by Magerl (34). This method has a high arthodesis rate, although aberrant vertebral artery anatomy limits using this technique in all patients. Alternatively, Harms et al. (33) has recently introduced the use of C1 lateral mass and C2 pedicle screws connected by rods as another means of rigid fixation. Moreover, in cases where the anatomy precludes placement of axis pedicle screws, the lamina of the axis has also been used as an alternative fixation point (38). Biomechanically, the atlantoaxial polyaxial screw method of Harms and Magerl C1–C2 transarticular screw fixation appear equal with regards to load-bearing and movement resistance, both being superior to posterior sublaminar wiring techniques (39–42). Clinically, the screw fixation methods result in higher fusion rates than posterior wiring techniques used alone (43–45). In addition, the rigid internal fixation techniques have obviated the necessity for rigid external/halo immobilization postoperatively. Ultimately the type of instrumentation used to facilitate spinal arthrodesis in the occipitocervical region needs to be addressed on a case-by-case basis and will vary depending on the bony and vertebral artery anatomy as well as the involvement of the tumor and its effects on hardware placement.

3. SURGICAL TREATMENT OF TUMORS OF THE SUBAXIAL CERVICAL SPINE

3.1. POSTERIOR APPROACHES

Laminectomy has been a standard approach for decompression of the subaxial cervical spine and can be done quickly and safely in most cases of acute spinal cord compression. In cases involving patients with high risk for operative morbidity, this approach may be preferred for gaining rapid neural element decompression. Moreover, the posterior approach is often ideal in cases of benign primary extramedullary dumbbell tumors of the cervical spine (46). Cervical decompressive laminectomy, however, can lead to kyphosis postoperatively, even in cases without pre-existing deformity. The rate of kyphosis following laminectomy may be even more pronounced in patients with anterior disease involvement of the spine. Because of this propensity, posterior cervical fusion often needs to be done in conjunction with a decompressive laminectomy in patients with a reversal of the normal cervical lordotic curve or with gross cervical spine deformity. For patients with significant deformity, including vertebral body collapse, an anterior approach may be necessary and possibly preferred, especially if long-term patient survival is expected. Correction of a severe kyphotic deformity may ultimately be best addressed with a combined approach.

3.2. ANTERIOR APPROACHES

Anterior approaches to the subaxial cervical spine are familiar to most spine surgeons. The standard anterior spine approach first described by Smith et al. *(47)* and Cloward *(48)* is performed via a transverse skin incision or alternatively, an incision along the anterior sternocleidomastoid border and allows access to the prevertebral region. This approach to the cervical spine typically addresses pathology at the C2–C7 vertebral levels but can occasionally provide access further caudally to T2. Cervical corpectomy and anterior diskectomy can be used to remove anterior vertebral body tumor and combined with an allograft or autograft bone strut graft, can be used to reconstruct the region and reduce cervical kyphosis *(49)*. Metal alloy mesh cages with bone grafting are also an effective alternative strut graft *(50–52)*. Additionally, polymethylmethacrylate has been used successfully for vertebral body reconstruction in patients with a limited lifespan in whom reconstruction and immediate stabilization, not spinal fusion, are the primary goals *(53–55)*. The anterior approach also has been used in this region of the spine for ventrally located extramedullary and intramedullary spinal cord tumors *(56,57)*.

Anterior instrumentation is frequently used for additional construct stability. The most commonly used hardware is an anterior plate but additional instrumentation used after a corpectomy for tumor includes the telescopic plate spacer or titanium cages *(58)*. These instruments may help augment spinal fusion rate and the addition of anterior plating also protects from anterior graft dislodgment *(59,60)*. Anterior stabilizing hardware also may negate the need for postoperative rigid cervical fixation. Because the majority of malignant tumors of the cervical spine are anteriorly based within the vertebral corpus, anterior approaches for decompression of neural elements and vertebral reconstruction are often ideal.

More recently, combined anterior and posterior approaches of the cervical spine have been employed for tumor resection, reconstruction, and spinal fusion *(61–63)*. The combined approach can be performed either as a staged procedure or in one operative setting *(63)*. Overall fusion rates using the combined approach in the cervical spine appear superior to the anterior approach alone *(64)*. Some relative indications for a combined approach include severe kyphotic deformity or instability, circumferential or three-column tumor involvement, and isolated local disease that can be addressed by vertebrectomy *(61)*. Poor bone quality with osteopenia, prior local irradiation, or other factors that may lead to a decreased fusion rate, may also lead to choosing a combined anterior-posterior approach. The combined procedure, however, adds additional surgical risks to the patient and may add to increased overall cost of treatment.

4. SURGICAL TREATMENT OF TUMORS OF THE CERVICOTHORACIC JUNCTION

Tumors of the cervicothoracic junction are often difficult entities to deal with surgically. The complex regional anatomy can cause difficulty in surgical exposure and can add to the morbidity of operating in this region. Because of these difficulties, various disciplines such as spine surgery, thoracic surgery, and head and neck surgery have contributed to surgical progress in this area.

Tumors of the cervicothoracic region account for 15% of patients with spine tumors *(65)*. Pain, neurological symptoms, and kyphosis can develop from tumors in the cervicothoracic junction and treatment should address these symptoms. Numerous approaches have been employed to gain access to tumors of this region.

4.1. ANTERIOR APPROACHES

A standard Smith-Robinson anterior neck approach to the lower cervical and upper thoracic spine, staying above the sternum, can gain caudal exposure to the vertebral body of T2 *(66,67)*. This approach is familiar to neurosurgical and orthopedic spine surgeons, but the operating space obtained can be limited. Further caudal exposure is usually limited by the manubrium sterni. Lateral exposure is also limited by this approach. Consequently, more lateral lesions such as nerve sheath tumors may best be approached posteriorly *(68)*.

A limited proximal sternotomy in addition to the standard anterior cervical approach can be used to gain additional caudal spine exposure. Modifications of this technique with a transverse incision limb allows for a manubriotomy without total sternotomy *(69)*. Others have used an endoscope to allow for anterior exposure and visualization of the cervicothoracic junction without the need for a sternotomy *(70)*. A proximal sternotomy can also be supplemented by an anterolateral thoracotomy creating a "trap door" to expose the cervicothoracic spine ventrally *(71)*. This technique that combines an anterior neck incision with a partial median sternotomy and anterolateral thoracotomy has been referred to as the "hemi-clamshell" approach *(72)*.

Transclavicular anterior approaches to the cervicothoracic junction have also been employed to approach more lateral spine lesions such as those extending near the lung apex *(73)*. By dividing the clavicle, exposure of the subclavian vessels and brachial plexus trunks can be obtained allowing access to the lateral cervicothoracic region. Others have used similar approaches anteriorly with mobilization of the medial clavicle along with part of the manubrium sternum rotated toward a sternocleidomastoid flap *(74)*. When approaching the spine via the transclavicular route, it should be noted that injury to the sternoclavicular joint or clavicular nonunion can be a source of morbidity in addition to the more obvious risks of neurovascular injury.

Reconstruction of the cavity after cervicothoracic corpectomy for tumor can be accomplished using various strut grafts. These may include: mesh cages, iliac crest autograft/allograft, fibular allograft, or methylmethacrylate/Steinmann pin constructs *(65)*.

4.2. POSTERIOR APPROACHES

Decompressive laminectomy for spinal cord compression caused by tumor in the cervicothoracic region is the most straightforward surgical approach to address acute neural injury. Several additional posterior approaches for tumor of the cervicothoracic spine can be done in conjunction with a laminectomy, if necessary, for further tumor removal or reconstruction. These procedures may allow ventral decompression or circumferential decompression in a single operative setting.

Transpedicular approaches do allow limited access to the ipsilateral vertebral body, but offer limited exposure and can put the spinal cord at risk for injury with inadvertent cord manipulation. A costotransversectomy approach can be employed for lesions throughout the thoracic region including the cervicothoracic junction. This involves removal of the proximal rib head and transverse process in addition to removal of the pedicle to access the lateral vertebral body. A major drawback to this approach is the lack of exposure to the floor of the canal and to the anterior most portions of the vertebral body. This may lead to an incomplete decompression of the thecal sac and subtotal resection of the anterior portions of tumor. The addition of an endoscope used in conjunction with the transpedicular approaches may aid in the extent of tumor resection including improved visualization of the canal floor *(75,76)*.

The lateral extracavitary approach to the vertebral body is a more lateral variation of the costotransversectomy technique and involves a more extensive rib resection to gain better exposure of the vertebral body *(77,78)*. This technique allows excellent visualization of the vertebral body and floor of the spinal canal and can allow for a near complete corpectomy unlike the various costotransversectomy techniques. The lateral extracavitary approach can be used for certain high thoracic lesions to access the entire vertebral body, but the medial border of the scapula above T3 often impedes using this approach at the cervicothoracic junction. Positioning of the arm to rotate the scapula laterally, however, may allow adequate access. Lesions at T1 and T2 may best be approached by unilateral or bilateral (if near complete vertebrectomy is desired) costotransversectomy, as the scapula will be less likely to inhibit this approach. An additional modification of the lateral extracavitary approach has also been described *(79)*. The lateral parascapular extrapleural approach allows for lateral mobilization of the parascapular muscles toward the scapula, thus aiding in the lateral exposure of the superior most thoracic vertebrae.

All of the extended posterior techniques mentioned allow access to both the anterior and posterior elements of the spine in a single setting. The posterolateral approaches allow the surgeon to perform reconstruction of the anterior elements in addition to posterior instrumentation through the same incision. Single approaches may be preferred in patients who are too ill to undergo a rigorous combined anterior and posterior decompression and reconstruction procedure *(14,80,81)*. For isolated spine disease that is extensive or circumferential, a single posterior or anterior approach may not suffice. In such cases, complete removal of tumor may involve staged approaches utilizing both posterior and anterior decompression to achieve total vertebrectomy *(82)*.

After posterior decompressive approaches, the development of post-procedure kyphosis may be especially pronounced given the unique transition from lordosis to kyphosis at the cervicothoracic junction. Posterior instrumented fusion using various plates or screw-rod combinations is frequently employed to avoid this progressive deformity in cases of posterior decompressive laminectomies. The obvious instability created surgically with the more extensive posterior vertebrectomy

approaches necessitates instrumented spinal fusion in most cases. This is often performed using a series of cervical lateral mass screws and thoracic pedicle screws/hooks joined by a rod construct. Although lateral mass screws are commonly used throughout most of the subaxial cervical spine, this is not the usual case at the C7 vertebrae where pedicle screws are preferred given its unique anatomy *(66,83)*. Pedicle screws can be placed at C7 because the pedicles are typically quite large compared to the more rudimentary lateral masses at this level.

If a vertebral corpectomy is included at the cervicothoracic junction, additional anterior reconstruction with a strut graft is needed. In addition to the strut grafts previously mentioned for anterior corpectomy defects, rib autograft harvested during the lateral extracavitary or other lateral approaches can be used for ventral spine reconstruction of the high thoracic region.

5. SURGICAL TREATMENTS OF TUMORS OF THE THORACOLUMBAR SPINE

Tumors of the thoracolumbar spine are not uncommon and can be primary as well as metastatic in origin. Metastatic tumors of the spine are most commonly found in the thoracic region of the spine *(6)*. The surgical treatment of tumors of this region remains an ongoing challenge. Improved survival of patients with spine metastases has allowed surgery to play an increasing role in the total care of these patients. Although medical and radiation therapies are employed as mainstay therapy for spine tumors, surgery remains an option in patients with metastatic tumors that are radio-resistant, for spinal instability, neurological decline, and for refractory pain *(59)*. The main goal of surgery in patients with malignant spine tumors continues to be focused on improvement in their quality of life.

5.1. ANTERIOR APPROACHES

The thoracolumbar spine spans the region from the thorax to the pelvis. Because of this, various approaches and anatomic considerations need to be addressed in accessing the spine anteriorly. For simplicity sake, all approaches that are not approached in the dorsal midline or involving a paraspinal approach will be considered "anterior" approaches.

The classic approach for gaining access to thoracic vertebral lesions involves a thoracotomy. Because of the propensity of tumors to invade the vertebral corpus, the anterior approach to this region seems logical. Posterolateral thoracotomy usually can gain ready access to the vertebral bodies of the thoracic spine from T3 to T10. This anterior approach also allows for significant deformity correction in cases where restoration of alignment secondary to pathological fractures of the thoracic spine is necessary. Additionally pain relief and relief of neurological deficits may be superior using anterior decompression of neural elements rather than a decompressive laminectomy approach *(12,84–86)*. In cases with anterior epidural cord compression and vertebral body involvement, thoracotomy may be preferred to the posterior route *(84)*. However, lesions in the upper thoracic region, above T4, may be more difficult to approach with a thoracotomy given the proximity of the aortic arch and great vessels of the thorax. In cases such as these a right-sided thoracotomy or posterior approach may be the preferred route. Thoracotomies can also entail significant pain postoperatively and accompanying tube thoracostomy drainage. The need to deflate a lung intra-operatively may not be tolerated in patients with preexisting poor pulmonary function.

Laparotomies or combination thoracotomy and laparotomy incision may be necessary to access the thoracolumbar junction and the lower lumbar spine. A laparotomy can generally reach lesions from L1 to the sacrum while a combined thoracoabdominal approach is needed to reach lesions at T11 and T12. The drawbacks can include significant postoperative ileus and a prolonged hospital stay. As opposed to a transperitoneal approach, a retroperitoneal laparotomy approach may be better tolerated from a gastrointestinal standpoint and has a low complication rate (87). By avoiding the peritoneal cavity the abdominal viscera are less likely to be injured and one can avoid having to deal with difficult adhesions in patients who have had prior abdominal surgery.

Various laparoscopic or anterior endoscopic approaches to the lumbar spine have been routinely used recently (88–90). The use of anterior endoscopy in tumor decompression and reconstruction operations, however, is limited because of the smaller window of exposure obtained. The limited exposure can make it difficult to mobilize the great vessels and to obtain adequate exposure for a full corpectomy. Despite this, with improvements in equipment and techniques, tumors of the lumbar region may be managed in the future with endoscopic approaches.

Thoracoscopic approaches to the thoracic spine have been used successfully for spine surgery decompression and reconstruction with a low complication rate (91). Thoracoscopy has also been used for spinal cord decompression and vertebral body reconstruction in cases of metastatic thoracic spine tumors (92). Combined thoracoscopic surgery and posterior surgical approaches have also been used in dealing with benign dumbbell tumors (93,94). The use of the thoracoscopic approaches is limited by the small working portals, which make dealing with long construct operations difficult. The use of thoracoscopy for complex spine surgery also is noted to have a steep initial learning curve (91).

Reconstructing the anterior thoracolumbar spine after anterior decompressive surgery is similar to that of the cervical spine. Allograft or autograft bone with or without anterior instrumentation can be used, as well as titanium mesh cages or other spacer devices (95–97). As previously mentioned with regard to the cervical spine, various forms of polymethylmethacrylate grafts can also be used as a vertebral body replacement in the thoracolumbar spine in those patients with a limited lifespan who require immediate reconstruction after anterior vertebral body resection (98).

5.2. POSTERIOR APPROACHES

Decompressive laminectomy remains the easiest and quickest technique for spinal cord decompression of the thoracolumbar spine. This may be the preferred treatment in acute neurological decline in patients with a spinal column mass. This method, however, does not address anterior disease removal. Laminectomy, therefore, can be done in conjunction with a posterolateral approach to better address the ventral pathology. In debilitated terminal patients with spinal tumor, some have advocated a hemilaminectomy and transpedicular decompression of anterior spine disease without further stabilization, instrumentation, or reconstruction to improve their quality of life (80). Procedures such as a costotransversectomy or lateral extracavitary approach can allow access to the vertebral body as well as the posterior elements of the thoracolumbar spine. These approaches allow for a more complete resection of tumor and access to anterior and posterior columns for reconstruction in patients with benign tumors or those with better short-term prognosis (99). The transpedicular or costotransversectomy approach may also be augmented with the use of an endoscope posteriorly to better visualize the decompression of the canal (75,76). Compared with the anterior approaches to the thoracolumbar spine, costotransversectomy may be better suited for patients with poor pulmonary function and for those with lesions of the upper thoracic spine. The rate of complications for costotransversectomy do not appear to be any different than for that of thoracotomy (81). The lateral extracavitary approach has been used for tumor decompression and spine reconstruction as mentioned previously. This technique provides ideal exposure of the posterior bony elements as well as the anterior vertebral column from T3 to L4 and with modifications to S1 (77). Tumor extension more anteriorly going into the body cavity may, however, necessitate an anterior surgical approach. Other variations for vertebrectomy involve modifications of these posteriolateral approaches which are ideal for decompressing and reconstructing the spine anteriorly and posteriorly via a single approach (100,101).

Some authors have advocated complete *en-bloc* spondylectomy for isolated primary and metastatic spine tumors (102–103). This may be useful in tumors that involve all three columns of the spine. The goal in this case is not only improvement of pain and functional status but also theoretical improvement in local tumor control and recurrence. Unfortunately, using the Tomita spondylectomy approach the results of recurrent tumor were still non-ideal (104). Rather than removing tumor in a piecemeal fashion as is the case in performing a spondylectomy from a single posterior approach, some authors recommend a combined technique. By combining an anterior and posterior approach for complete spondylectomy the tumor recurrence rate may be lower than via a single approach (13). Overall it appears that total spondylectomy approaches, as a whole, are best used in cases of isolated spine disease and in non-debilitated patients who can tolerate this procedure.

6. CONCLUSION

Decompression and resection of tumors of the spine has evolved from simple decompressive laminectomies for neural element decompression and palliation to more complex surgical procedures that may allow improvement in pain and life expectancy. The goals of a given operation and the location and extent of the tumor will dictate the surgical approach used. Over the years, innovative techniques and approaches have been developed to address tumors of the spine. These advances have allowed radical tumor removal in select cases and for the correction of the unstable spine. Improved instrumentation and use of biomechanically sound principles has lead to improved arthrodesis rates following spinal surgery for tumor. Continued improvement in survival rates for patients with isolated malignant spine tumors has likewise prompted the adoption of more extensive surgical therapy to help treat these patients. Newer advances in minimally invasive spinal procedures will improve the care of patients with spinal tumors and have broader use in the future.

REFERENCES

1. Gokaslan ZL. Spine surgery for cancer. Curr Opin Oncol 1996; 8:178–181.
2. Klimo K, Kestle JRW, Schmidt MH. Treatment of metastatic spinal epidural disease: a review of the literature. Neurosurg Focus 2003; 15:1–9.
3. Gilbert RW, Kim JH, Posner JB. Epidural spinal cord compression from metastatic tumor: diagnosis and treatment. Ann Neurol 1978; 3:40–51.
4. Young RF, Post EM, King GA. Treatment of spinal epidural metastases. Randomized prospective comparison of laminectomy and radiotherapy. J Neurosurg 1980; 53:741–748.
5. Dahlbeck S, Kagan AR. Spinal cord compression, infection, and unknown primary cancers. Am J Clin Oncol 2001; 24:315–318.
6. Ratliff JK, Cooper PR. Metastatic spine tumors. South Med J 2004; 97:246–253.
7. Durr HR, Wegener B, Krodel A, Muller PE, Jansson V, Refior HJ. Multiple myeloma: surgery of the spine: retrospective analysis of 27 patients. Spine 2002; 27:320–324.
8. Sundaresan N, Rothman A, Manhart K, Kelliher K. Surgery for solitary metastases of the spine: rationale and results of treatment. Spine 2002; 27:1802–1806.
9. Ghogawala Z, Mansfield FL, Borges LF. Spinal radiation before surgical decompression adversely affects outcomes of surgery for symptomatic metastatic spinal cord compression. Spine 2001; 26:818–824.
10. Gokaslan ZL, York JE, Walsh GL, et al. Transthoracic vertebrectomy for metastatic spinal tumors. J Neurosurg 1998; 89:599–609.
11. Cooper PR, Errico TJ, Martin R, Crawford B, DiBartolo T. A systematic approach to spinal reconstruction after anterior decompression for neoplastic disease of the thoracic and lumbar spine. Neurosurgery 1993; 32:1–8.
12. Walsh GL, Gokaslan ZL, McCutcheon IE, et al. Anterior approaches to the thoracic spine in patients with cancer: indications and results. Ann Thorac Surg 1997; 64:1611–1618.
13. Fourney DR, Abi-Said D, Rhines LD, et al. Simultaneous anterior-posterior approach to the thoracic and lumbar spine for the radical resection of tumors followed by reconstruction and stabilization. J Neurosurg 2001; 94:232–244.
14. Yao KC, Boriani S, Gokaslan ZL, Sundaresan N. En bloc spondylectomy for spinal metastases: a review of techniques. Neurosurg Focus 2003; 15:1–5.
15. Regine WF, Tibbs PA, Young A, et al. Metastatic spinal cord compression: a randomized trial of direct decompressive surgical resection plus radiotherapy vs. radiotherapy alone. Int J Radiat Oncol Biol Phys 2003; 57:S125.
16. Parikh SN, Crawford AH. Orthopaedic implications in the management of pediatric vertebral and spinal cord tumors: a retrospective review. Spine 2003; 28:2390–2396.
17. Raskas DS, Graziano GP, Herzenberg JE, Heidelberger KP, Hensinger RN. Osteoid osteoma and osteoblastoma of the spine. J Spinal Disord 1992; 5:204–211.
18. Jallo GI, Kothbauer KF, Epstein FJ. Intrinsic spinal cord tumor resection. Neurosurgery 2001; 49:1124–1128.
19. Roonprapunt C, Silvera VM, Setton A, Freed D, Epstein FJ, Jallo GI. Surgical management of isolated hemangioblastomas of the spinal cord. Neurosurgery 2001; 49:321–327.
20. Lonstein JE. Post-laminectomy kyphosis. Clin Orthop 1977:93–100.
21. Otsuka NY, Hey L, Hall JE. Postlaminectomy and postirradiation kyphosis in children and adolescents. Clin Orthop 1998:189–194.
22. Freiberg AA, Graziano GP, Loder RT, Hensinger RN. Metastatic vertebral disease in children. J Pediatr Orthop 1993; 13:148–153.
23. York JE, Gokaslan ZL. Craniocervical junction neoplastic conditions. Seminars in Neurosurgery 2002:145–150.
24. Bilsky MH, Shannon FJ, Sheppard S, Prabhu V, Boland PJ. Diagnosis and management of a metastatic tumor in the atlantoaxial spine. Spine 2002; 27:1062–1069.
25. Phillips E, Levine AM. Metastatic lesions of the upper cervical spine. Spine 1989; 14:1071–1077.
26. Schaeren S, Jeanneret B. Occipitocervical Instrumentation. Tech Orthop 2002; 17:287–295.
27. Crockard HA. Anterior approaches to lesions of the upper cervical spine. Clin Neurosurg 1988; 34:389–416.
28. Schmelzle R, Harms J. [Craniocervical junction–diseases, diagnostic application of imaging procedures, surgical technics]. Fortschr Kiefer Gesichtschir 1987; 32:206–208.
29. Sar C, Eralp L. Transoral resection and reconstruction for primary osteogenic sarcoma of the second cervical vertebra. Spine 2001; 26:1936–1941.
30. Bongioanni F, Assadurian E, Polivka M, George B. Aneurysmal bone cyst of the atlas: operative removal through an anterolateral approach. A case report. J Bone Joint Surg Am 1996; 78:1574–1547.
31. McAfee PC, Bohlman HH, Riley LH Jr., Robinson RA, Southwick WO, Nachlas NE. The anterior retropharyngeal approach to the upper part of the cervical spine. J Bone Joint Surg Am 1987; 69:1371–1383.
32. Kratimenos GP, Crockard HA. The far lateral approach for ventrally placed foramen magnum and upper cervical spine tumours. Br J Neurosurg 1993; 7:129–140.
33. Harms J, Melcher RP. Posterior C1-C2 fusion with polyaxial screw and rod fixation. Spine 2001; 26:2467–2471.
34. Magerl F, Seemann PS. Stable posterior fusion of the atlas and axis by transarticular screw fixation. New York, NY: Springer-Verlag; 1986.
35. Brooks AL, Jenkins EB. Atlanto-axial arthrodesis by the wedge compression method. J Bone Joint Surg Am 1978; 60:279–284.
36. Simmons E. Alternatives in the surgical stabilization for the upper cervical spine. In: Tator CH, ed. Early Management of Acute Spinal Cord Injury. New York, NY: Raven; 1982:393–434.
37. Sonntag VKH, Dickman CA. Posterior atlantoaxial wiring techniques. In: Dickman CA, Spetzler RF, Sonntag VKH, eds. Surgery of the Craniovertebral Junction. New York, NY: Thieme; 1997:783–794.
38. Wright N. Posterior C2 Fixation Using Bilateral, Crossing C2 Laminar Screws. J Spinal Disord 2004; 17:158–162.
39. Melcher RP, Puttlitz CM, Kleinstueck FS, Lotz JC, Harms J, Bradford DS. Biomechanical testing of posterior atlantoaxial fixation techniques. Spine 2002; 27:2435–2440.
40. Henriques T, Cunningham BW, Olerud C, et al. Biomechanical comparison of five different atlantoaxial posterior fixation techniques. Spine 2000; 25:2877–2883.
41. Dickman CA, Crawford NR, Paramore CG. Biomechanical characteristics of C1-2 cable fixations. J Neurosurg 1996; 85:316–322.
42. Puttlitz CM, Melcher RP, Kleinstueck FS, Harms J, Bradford DS, Lotz JC. Stability analysis of craniovertebral junction fixation techniques. J Bone Joint Surg Am 2004; 86:561–568.
43. Coyne TJ, Fehlings MG, Wallace MC, Bernstein M, Tator CH. C1-C2 posterior cervical fusion: long-term evaluation of results and efficacy. Neurosurgery 1995; 37:688–692.
44. Dickman CA, Sonntag VK. Surgical management of atlantoaxial nonunions. J Neurosurg 1995; 83:248–253.
45. Stillerman CB, Wilson JA. Atlanto-axial stabilization with posterior transarticular screw fixation: technical description and report of 22 cases. Neurosurgery 1993; 32:948–954.
46. Asazuma T, Toyama Y, Maruiwa H, Fujimura Y, Hirabayashi K. Surgical strategy for cervical dumbbell tumors based on a three-dimensional classification. Spine 2004; 29:E10–E144.
47. Robinson RA, Smith GW. Anterolateral cervical disc removal and interbody fusion for cervical disc syndrome. Bull John Hopkins Hosp 1955; 96:223–224.

48. Cloward RB. The anterior approach for removal of ruptured cervical disks. J Neurosurg 1958; 15:602–617.

49. Eleraky MA, Llanos C, Sonntag VK. Cervical corpectomy: report of 185 cases and review of the literature. J Neurosurg 1999; 90:35–41.

50. Narotam PK, Pauley SM, McGinn GJ. Titanium mesh cages for cervical spine stabilization after corpectomy: a clinical and radiological study. J Neurosurg 2003; 99:172–180.

51. Dorai Z, Morgan H, Coimbra C. Titanium cage reconstruction after cervical corpectomy. J Neurosurg 2003; 99:3–7.

52. Majd ME, Vadhva M, Holt RT. Anterior cervical reconstruction using titanium cages with anterior plating. Spine 1999; 24:1604–1610.

53. DeWald RL, Bridwell KH, Prodromas C, Rodts MF. Reconstructive spinal surgery as palliation for metastatic malignancies of the spine. Spine 1985; 10:21–26.

54. Miller DJ, Lang FF, Walsh GL, Abi-Said D, Wildrick DM, Gokaslan ZL. Coaxial double-lumen methylmethacrylate reconstruction in the anterior cervical and upper thoracic spine after tumor resection. J Neurosurg 2000; 92:181–190.

55. Liu JK, Apfelbaum RI, Chiles BW, Schmidt MH. Cervical spinal metastasis: anterior reconstruction and stabilization techniques after tumor resection. Neurosurg Focus 2003; 15:1–7.

56. Pluta RM, Iuliano B, DeVroom HL, Nguyen T, Oldfield EH. Comparison of anterior and posterior surgical approaches in the treatment of ventral spinal hemangioblastomas in patients with von Hippel-Lindau disease. J Neurosurg 2003; 98:117–124.

57. O'Toole JE, McCormick PC. Midline ventral intradural schwannoma of the cervical spinal cord resected via anterior corpectomy with reconstruction: technical case report and review of the literature. Neurosurgery 2003; 52:1482–1485.

58. Coumans JV, Marchek CP, Henderson FC. Use of the telescopic plate spacer in treatment of cervical and cervicothoracic spine tumors. Neurosurgery 2002; 51:417–424.

59. Walker MP, Yaszemski MJ, Kim CW, Talac R, Currier BL. Metastatic Disease of the Spine: Evaluation and Treatment. Clin Orthop 2003; 1:S165–S175.

60. Brown JA, Havel P, Ebraheim N, Greenblatt SH, Jackson WT. Cervical stabilization by plate and bone fusion. Spine 1988; 13:236–240.

61. Sundaresan N, Steinberger AA, Moore F, et al. Indications and results of combined anterior-posterior approaches for spine tumor surgery. J Neurosurg 1996; 85:438–446.

62. McAfee PC, Bohlman HH. One-stage anterior cervical decompression and posterior stabilization with circumferential arthrodesis. A study of twenty-four patients who had a traumatic or a neoplastic lesion. J Bone Joint Surg Am 1989; 71:78–88.

63. McAfee PC, Bohlman HH, Ducker TB, Zeidman SM, Goldstein JA. One-stage anterior cervical decompression and posterior stabilization. A study of one hundred patients with a minimum of two years of follow-up. J Bone Joint Surg Am 1995; 77:1791–1800.

64. Schultz KD Jr, McLaughlin MR, Haid RW Jr, Comey CH, Rodts GE Jr, Alexander J. Single-stage anterior-posterior decompression and stabilization for complex cervical spine disorders. J Neurosurg 2000; 93:214–221.

65. Le H, Balabhadra R, Park J. Surgical treatment of tumors involving the cervicothoracic junction. Neurosurg Focus 2003; 15:1–7.

66. Bellabarba C, Nemecek AN, Chapman JR. Management of Injuries to the Cervicothoracic Junction. Tech Orthop 2002; 17:355–364.

67. Fielding JW, Stillwell WT. Anterior cervical approach to the upper thoracic spine. Spine 1976; 1:158–161.

68. Gieger M, Roth PA, Wu JK. The anterior cervical approach to the cervicothoracic junction. Neurosurgery 1995; 37:704–709.

69. Luk KD, Cheung KM, Leong JC. Anterior approach to the cervicothoracic junction by unilateral or bilateral manubriotomy. A report of five cases. J Bone Joint Surg Am 2002; 84:1013–1017.

70. Le Huec JC, Lesprit E, Guibaud JP, Gangnet N, Aunoble S. Minimally invasive endoscopic approach to the cervicothoracic junction for vertebral metastases: report of two cases. Eur Spine J 2001; 10:421–426.

71. Nazzaro JM, Arbit E, Burt M. "Trap door" exposure of the cervicothoracic junction. Technical note. J Neurosurg 1994; 80:338–341.

72. Korst RJ, Burt ME. Cervicothoracic tumors: results of resection by the "hemi-clamshell" approach. J Thorac Cardiovasc Surg 1998; 115:286–294.

73. Kubo T, Nakamura H, Yamano Y. Transclavicular approach for a large dumbbell tumor in the cervicothoracic junction. J Spinal Disord 2001; 14:79–83.

74. Birch R, Bonney G, Marshall RW. A surgical approach to the cervicothoracic spine. J Bone Joint Surg Br 1990; 72:904–907.

75. McLain RF, Lieberman IH. Endoscopic approaches to metastatic thoracic disease. Spine 2000; 25:1855–1858.

76. McLain RF. Endoscopically assisted decompression for metastatic thoracic neoplasms. Spine 1998; 23:1130–1135.

77. Wolfla CE, Maiman DJ. Lateral extracavitary approach. Tech Neurosurg 2003; 8.

78. Larson SJ, Holst RA, Hemmy DC, Sances A Jr. Lateral extracavitary approach to traumatic lesions of the thoracic and lumbar spine. J Neurosurg 1976; 45:628–637.

79. Fessler RG, Dietze DD Jr, Millan MM, Peace D. Lateral parascapular extrapleural approach to the upper thoracic spine. J Neurosurg 1991; 75:349–355.

80. Weller SJ, Rossitch E Jr. Unilateral posterolateral decompression without stabilization for neurological palliation of symptomatic spinal metastasis in debilitated patients. J Neurosurg 1995; 82:739–744.

81. Wiggins GC, Mirza S, Bellabarba C, et al. Perioperative complications with costotransversectomy and anterior approaches to thoracic and thoracolumbar tumors. Neurosurg Focus 2001; 11:1–9.

82. Mazel Ch, Grunenwald D, Laudrin P, Marmorat JL. Radical excision in the management of thoracic and cervicothoracic tumors involving the spine: results in a series of 36 cases. Spine 2003; 28:782–792.

83. Mazel C, Hoffmann E, Antonietti P, Grunenwald D, Henry M, Williams J. Posterior cervicothoracic instrumentation in spine Tumors. Spine 2004; 29:1246–1253.

84. Siegal T. Surgical decompression of anterior and posterior malignant epidural tumors compressing the spinal cord: a prospective study. Neurosurgery 1985; 17:424–432.

85. Siegal T, Tiqva P. Vertebral body resection for epidural compression by malignant tumors. Results of forty-seven consecutive operative procedures. J Bone Joint Surg Am 1985; 67:375–382.

86. Sundaresan N, Galicich JH, Lane JM, Bains MS, McCormack P. Treatment of neoplastic epidural cord compression by vertebral body resection and stabilization. J Neurosurg 1985; 63:676–684.

87. Bianchi C, Ballard JL, Abou-Zamzam AM, Teruya TH, Abu-Assal ML. Anterior retroperitoneal lumbosacral spine exposure: operative technique and results. Ann Vasc Surg 2003; 17:137–142.

88. Bergey DL, Villavicencio AT, Goldstein T, Regan JJ. Endoscopic lateral transpsoas approach to the lumbar spine. Spine 2004; 29:1681–1688.

89. Regan JJ, Guyer RD. Endoscopic techniques in spinal surgery. Clin Orthop 1997:122–139.

90. Onimus M, Papin P, Gangloff S. Extraperitoneal approach to the lumbar spine with video assistance. Spine 1996; 21:2491–2494.

91. Khoo LT, Beisse R, Potulski M. Thoracoscopic-assisted treatment of thoracic and lumbar fractures: a series of 371 consecutive cases. Neurosurgery 2002; 51:104–117.

92. McAfee PC, Regan JR, Fedder IL, Mack MJ, Geis WP. Anterior thoracic corpectomy for spinal cord decompression performed endoscopically. Surg Laparosc Endosc 1995; 5:339–348.

93. Konno S, Yabuki S, Kinoshita T, Kikuchi S. Combined laminectomy and thoracoscopic resection of dumbbell-type thoracic cord tumor. Spine 2001; 26:E130–E134.

94. Citow JS, Macdonald RL, Ferguson MK. Combined laminectomy and thoracoscopic resection of a dumbbell neurofibroma: technical case report. Neurosurgery 1999; 45:1263–1265.

95. Dvorak MF, Kwon BK, Fisher CG, Eiserloh HL 3rd, Boyd M, Wing PC. Effectiveness of titanium mesh cylindrical cages in anterior column reconstruction after thoracic and lumbar vertebral body resection. Spine 2003; 28:902–908.

96. Buttermann GR, Glazer PA, Bradford DS. The use of bone allografts in the spine. Clin Orthop 1996:75–85.

97. Cotler HB, Cotler JM, Stoloff A, et al. The use of autografts for vertebral body replacement of the thoracic and lumbar spine. Spine 1985; 10:748–756.

98. Errico TJ, Cooper PR. A new method of thoracic and lumbar body replacement for spinal tumors: technical note. Neurosurgery 1993; 32:678–680.

99. McCormick PC. Surgical management of dumbbell and paraspinal tumors of the thoracic and lumbar spine. Neurosurgery 1996; 38: 67–74.

100. Akeyson EW, McCutcheon IE. Single-stage posterior vertebrectomy and replacement combined with posterior instrumentation for spinal metastasis. J Neurosurg 1996; 85:211–220.

101. Bilsky MH, Boland P, Lis E, Raizer JJ, Healey JH. Single-stage posterolateral transpedicle approach for spondylectomy, epidural decompression, and circumferential fusion of spinal metastases. Spine 2000; 25:2240–2249.

102. Tomita K, Kawahara N, Baba H, Tomita K, Kawahara N, Baba H. Total en bloc spondylectomy for solitary spinal metastases. Int Orthop 1994; 18:291–298.

103. Tomita K, Kawahara N, Baba H, Tsuchiya H, Fujita T, Toribatake Y. Total en bloc spondylectomy. A new surgical technique for primary malignant vertebral tumors. Spine 1997; 22:324–333.

104. Sakaura H, Hosono N, Mukai Y, Ishii T, Yonenobu K, Yoshikawa H. Outcome of total en bloc spondylectomy for solitary metastasis of the thoracolumbar spine. J Spinal Disord Tech 2004; 17:297–300.

30 Metastatic Disease of the Cervical Spine

Ashley R. Poynton, MD, FRCSI, FRCS, Mark H. Bilsky, MD,
Federico P. Girardi, MD, Patrick J. Boland, MD,
and Frank P. Cammisa, Jr., MD, FRCS

Contents

1. INTRODUCTION

Metastatic spine tumors occur in 5 to 10% of all cancer patients (1–9). Cervical spine involvement is relatively uncommon, accounting for less than 10% of all spinal metastases (6,7,9,10). The most prevalent tumors are lung, breast, prostate, kidney, and thyroid (2,3,11–13). Most patients presenting with cervical spine tumors generally have extra-cervical and extra-spinal sites of disease at presentation (6). Radiation therapy, surgery, or a combination, are the primary treatment modalities for cervical spine tumors. Treatment decisions are based primarily on the segmental level of cervical spine involvement, radio-sensitivity of the tumor, presence of mechanical instability, and prior treatment.

Advances in imaging and the early diagnosis and treatment of symptomatic cervical spine metastases have improved patient outcomes (14). The prospects of quadriplegia and respiratory arrest resulting from metastases make effective treatment of spinal cord compression and instability perhaps even more compelling than in patients who present with thoracic and lumbar spine tumors. Operative considerations unique to the cervical spine include management of the vertebral artery, tumor extension into the brachial plexus, and difficult ventral approaches for the high cervical spine and cervicothoracic junction.

In this chapter, the assessment and management of the atlanto-axial and subaxial cervical spine are discussed separately. These two regions are different with regard to definition of instability, risk of neurological dysfunction, and management strategies.

2. CLINICAL PRESENTATION

Pain is the predominant symptom of cervical spine metastases (6,15,16), although asymptomatic metastases are often identified by screening (7). Pain may be biological, mechanical, or both (14,16). Biological pain is nocturnal or early morning pain that probably results from inflammatory mediators secreted by the tumor. Early recognition of this pain and definitive treatment of the tumor with radiation or operation may prevent mechanical compromise and neurological dysfunction. Significant mechanical pain or movement-related pain heralds the loss of structural integrity of the vertebral column, either from bony erosion by the tumor process or pathological fracture. Commonly, patients with cervical spine tumor experience referred pain to the trapezius muscles, shoulder, and interscapular regions, which may reflect mild instability.

Neurological involvement presents with radiculopathy, myelopathy or myeloradiculopathy. The incidence of neurological deficits in metastases to the lower cervical spine has been reported to be as high as 25 to 35% (17–22), whereas the incidence of neurological deficits attributable to upper cervical metastases is less (0–22%) (17–19,23–25). Some studies have reported the incidence of neurological involvement between 40 and 70% when radicular symptoms are included (18,20). Associated motor, sensory, or reflex deficits may also occur. Ambulatory status at presentation has significant prognostic implications and is dependent on primary tumor type (26). Autonomic dysfunction, such as urinary retention, resulting from cervical spine disease is an end-stage neurological finding and signifies poor prognosis for recovery (27). Lower cranial nerve dysfunction signifies disease involving the base of skull.

From: *Current Clinical Oncology: Cancer in the Spine: Comprehensive Care.*
Edited by: R. F. McLain, K-U. Lewandrowski, M. Markman, R. M. Bukowski,
R. Macklis, and E. C. Benzel © Humana Press, Inc., Totowa, NJ

3. PATIENT EVALUATION

The initial evaluation of any patient presenting with cervical spine or associated radicular pain and/or neurological dysfunction must commence with a thorough history and physical examination. In many cases the primary tumor is evident from the history.

Plain cervical spine radiography is a useful first line investigation. However, a normal appearing plain radiograph in no way rules out metastatic disease. Up to 60% of patients with spinal metastatic disease may have normal plain radiographs, because 50% demineralization is required before a lytic lesion can be identified (28,29). Plain radiographs are useful in assessing cervical spine alignment and deformity, presence of pathological fractures, and stability.

Magnetic resonance imaging (MRI) is the modality of choice in assessing spinal metastatic disease. It is the most sensitive and specific modality for detecting spinal metastases and is excellent for assessing the entire spine for bone, epidural, and paraspinal involvement. The extent and degree of spinal cord compression is readily appreciated with MRI. The identification of intramedullary spinal cord signal changes is another advantage of MRI and this may be prognostically useful (30). Leptomeningeal metastatic disease may be seen with contrast-enhanced MRI (31).

Computed tomography (CT) quantifies the degree of lytic bone destruction and helps differentiate osteoblastic from osteolytic metastases. The degree of bony retropulsion secondary to a pathological fracture can also be clearly identified. CT is not a good screening tool for metastatic disease and may fail to identify metastatic deposits in up to 52% of cases (32). Myelogram is useful in patients with contraindications to MRI (e.g., pacemaker) or in those who have spinal implants. MRI should be attempted in patients with spinal implants before subjecting them to a myelogram, because the majority of cervical instrumentation systems are MRI compatible (i.e., titanium) and tumor recurrence can be readily visualized.

Nuclear medicine tests may be helpful in patient assessment. MRI has largely replaced bone scintigraphy for spinal assessment. The relative lack of specificity compared to MRI limits its role in spinal assessment (33). In patients without a known primary cancer, bone scan may help identify a more readily accessible site for biopsy (e.g., rib) than the cervical spine. Conversely, 18-fluoro-2-deoxy-D-glucose positron emission tomography (PET) may be useful in assessing the presence of tumor suggested by MRI scans. Equivocal MRI scans that show hypointense marrow signal changes on T1-weighted images may be further evaluated with PET to help determine whether the changes are the result of tumor, degenerative changes, or osteoporosis (34).

4. MANAGEMENT

The primary treatment modalities for cervical spine metastases are radiation therapy and surgery. The treatment decisions differ between the atlanto-axial and subaxial spine and are considered separately. Cytotoxic chemotherapy, hormones, and immunotherapy play a more limited role. Two of the most commonly used chemotherapy agents, steroids and bisphos-phonates, are used for palliation and not specifically for tumor treatment. Steroids are used to treat patients with epidural spinal cord compression and to alleviate biological pain, while definitive therapy is undertaken. Bisphosphonates (e.g., pamidronate), which inhibit osteoclast activity, may be used in patients with tumor infiltration to prevent fracture. In large prospective, randomized trials for breast carcinoma and multiple myeloma (35–38), pamidronate has been shown to significantly reduce skeletal events (i.e., symptomatic fractures).

4.1. ATLANTO-AXIAL SPINE

Patients with atlanto-axial tumor present with biological pain, but also generally have significant mechanical pain in flexion and extension. The majority of patients additionally have a component of lateral rotation pain that helps distinguish atlanto-axial pain from subaxial spine tumor. This mechanical pain, although severe, is usually not indicative of instability requiring an operation. Given the wide mid-sagittal diameter of the spinal canal at C1–C2, the vast majority of patients are neurologically intact, including many of those with significant fracture dislocations (17–19,23–25). Neurological injury, when it occurs, usually results from fracture dislocation and, less frequently, from epidural tumor compression. The widespread use of MRI for tumor screening of the spine and early immobilization with an external orthosis has markedly reduced the number of patients presenting with significant neurological deficits, including severe quadraparesis (23).

Neutral lateral cervical spine radigraphs are used to evaluate fracture subluxations of the atlanto-axial spine for displacement and angulation. Review of the literature confirms that patients with normal spinal alignment or minimal fracture subluxations respond to hard collar immobilization and radiation therapy (17,23,25,39). Patients with odontoid fractures with less than 5 mm displacement, or C2 involvement with less than 11° angulation and 3.5 mm subluxation between C2 and C3 (Hangman's fracture, Francis grade 4), generally respond to non-operative therapy, as assessed by resolution of mechanical neck pain, lack of deformity progression, and ability to wean from the hard collar (39). The tumor histology, radio-sensitivity of the tumor, and extent of bone infiltration, as seen on MRI, do not seem to impact on the response to radiation therapy or subsequent need for an operation (39). Osteolytic tumors often results in destruction of the C2 body, odontoid, and/or facet joints. Despite extensive destruction, the majority of patients with normal alignment or minimal subluxation respond to non-operative therapy (39). Presumably, these patients develop a fibrous union and occasionally show re-ossification (e.g., multiple myeloma).

Operation is reserved for patients with fracture subluxations greater than 5 mm at C1/C2 or 3.5 mm subluxation and greater than 11° angulation at C2/C3 (Hangman's fracture, Francis grade 4). Other surgical indications include patients who have undergone prior radiation to overlapping ports, unknown diagnosis, and patients who progress following radiation. The latter indication includes patients with persistent neck pain and new fracture subluxations.

4.1.1. Surgical Strategies

The vast majority of patients requiring operation for atlanto-axial metastatic spine tumors can be managed with dorsal fixation *(25,39–41)*. Rarely is ventral decompression indicated or necessary. Preoperative spinal fracture reduction may be attempted with awake traction, however, patients can often be re-aligned intra-operatively with a wake-up test performed to assess neurological function.

The levels of fixation depend on the ability to reduce the fracture subluxation and the integrity the dorsal elements of C1 and C2. Occipitocervical fusion is indicated if there is destruction of the C1 dorsal arch and/or C2 dorsal elements, involvement of the C1 lateral masses and/or occipital condyles, or irreducible C1/C2 subluxation. If a fracture cannot be adequately reduced, a C1 laminectomy to decompress the spinal cord is performed and the construct extended to the occiput. Isolated C1/C2 stabilization is indicated when disease is confined to the odontoid process and ventral arch of C1. Additionally, atlanto-axial alignment should be achieved before placing instrumentation. In most cases in which there is tumor in the C2 vertebral body it is advisable to instrument to C3, or beyond if there is subaxial disease.

A variety of techniques have been developed for occipitocervical, C1/C2, and C1–C3 stabilization. Historically, Luque rectangles with sublaminar wires were used to achieve occipito-cervical fusion *(20)*. More recently, lateral mass plate systems have been developed that permit the contouring either plates or rods to the occiput (e.g., Summit system, Johnson and Johnson, Depuy-Acromed, Boston, MA) (Fig. 1). C1/2 stabilization can be achieved using wiring techniques *(42)* or cervical sublaminar clamp systems. The authors have used the Apofix sublaminar hook-rod system (Medtronic Sofamor Danek, Memphis, TN) with great success in providing durable, rigid fixation in the metastatic cancer population *(39)* (Fig. 2). For long fixation in the cervical spine, lateral mass plates may provide a rigid construct that allows the termination of the construct below the occiput (Fig. 3). The use of C1/C2 transarticular screws is often contraindicated owing to the degree of bony destruction, but C2 pedicle screws are often possible if there is no pedicle destruction. Most modern instrumentation systems do not require reinforcement with polymethyl methacrylate (PMMA) *(20)*, as has been previously reported.

Ventral decompression may be indicated to decompress significant ventral tumor causing persistent spinal cord compression and to establish a diagnosis in the absence of a more accessible tumor biopsy. A transoral approach provides exposure to the ventral arch of C1, odontoid process, and body of C2 *(41,43–45)*. Lateral resection of tumor is limited through this approach. If more lateral or additional subaxial spine exposure is required, one option is to use a retropharyngeal approach as described by McAfee *(46)*. The retropharyngeal approach, to the upper cervical spine has a lower risk of infection than the transoral approach. It also provides exposure of the entire cervical spine from clivus to cervicothoracic junction and is particularly useful if disease in the body of C3 requires ventral resection and reconstruction. The retropharyngeal approach, however, requires detailed knowledge of head and neck surgical anatomy and should not be attempted by surgeons unfamiliar with this region. Ventral reconstruction options include, autograft or allograft strut grafts, cages, PMMA, plates, and vertebral body prosthesis.

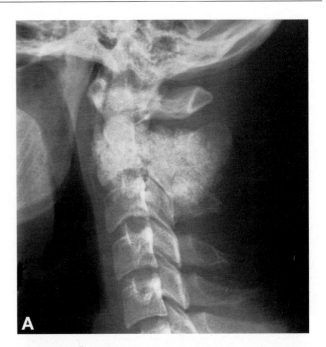

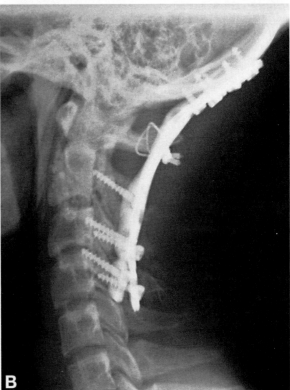

Fig. 1. A 20-yr-old male presented with osteogenic sarcoma of the right femur with extension into the popliteal fossa. He underwent neoadjuvant chemotherapy followed by resection and Finn knee reconstruction. More than 3 yr later, he presented with severe neck pain in flexion, extension, and lateral rotation. Plain radiographs (**A**) showed metastatic osteogenic sarcoma. The patient underwent four cycles of salvage chemotherapy with complete resolution of his pain. Surgery was undertaken in an attempt to achieve local tumor control. He underwent C2 laminectomy, lateral mass resection C1 and C2, and posterior fixation using lateral mass plates contoured to the occiput (**B**). Postoperatively he received 6000 cGy intensity-modulated radiation therapy. At the time of death, more than 3 yr later, he had no evidence of local recurrence or neck pain.

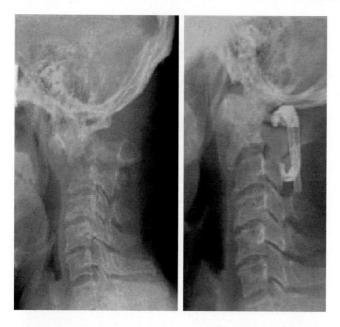

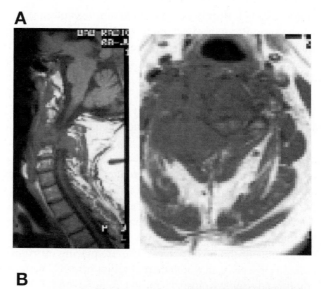

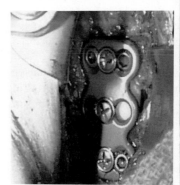
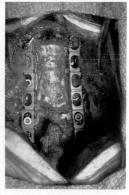

Fig, 2. Patient with no prior history of malignancy presented with severe neck pain. Systemic work-up was unrevealing. Plain radiographs (**A**) showed significant fracture subluxation. The patient underwent C1 to C3 fixation with sublaminar hook-rod system. She was subsequently diagnosed with lymphoma and has received local radiation therapy and systemic chemotherapy.

Sjöström et al. *(24)* reported a series of six patients with pathological odontoid fractures treated with ventral decompression and stabilization *(24)*. A Southwick-Robinson approach was used to access the ventral aspects of C2 and C3. The metastatic deposit was resected where possible. Reconstruction consisted of two 3.5-mm screws from the caudel end-plate of C2 into the dens. The cavity from the tumor resection was filled with PMMA and the construct further reinforced by a ventral C2–C3 plate. Additional dorsal C1–C3 fixation was performed in two patients. There were no fixation failures with a median survival of 27 mo. The same author reported a series of 12 upper cervical spine metastases in a subsequent paper. Nine of these had pathological odontoid fractures and were treated in a similar fashion previously described. Fixation failed in three due to local progression of disease.

4.2. SUBAXIAL CERVICAL SPINE

Metastatic disease of the subaxial cervical spine is more common than that of the atlanto-axial spine. As with atlanto-axial tumors, the majority of patients can be managed with

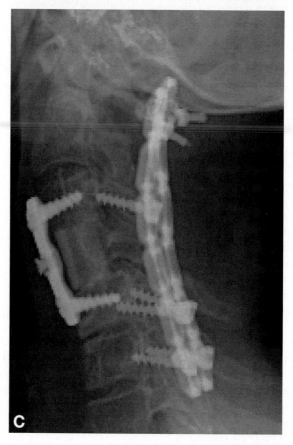

Fig. 3. A 62-yr-old woman with known history of lymphoma presented with severe neck pain. Magnetic resonance imaging (**A**) showed C3 vertebral body destruction and right C3–C4 lateral mass destruction. Owing to the subaxial instability, the patient underwent a C3 vertebrectomy and ventral reconstruction using fibula allograft and an ventral plate. (**B**) Intraoperative photograph. (**C**) Plain radiographs. During the same operation, she underwent a C3 and C4 laminectomy and facet resection, followed by dorsal segmental fixation with lateral mass plates, using a sublaminar wire at C1 for fixation. She subsequently underwent radiation therapy and has been without evidence of local recurrence for more than 3 yr.

radiation therapy, but there are distinct differences between their presentation and management. In contrast to the atlanto-axial spine, mechanical instability pain resulting from a compression or burst fracture is generally an indication for surgery. Further, lytic destruction of the vertebral body and concomitant dorsal element tumor virtually always results in instability pain and requires surgical intervention. Conversely, while models have been proposed to define or predict spinal instability (47), many patients who have vertebral body fractures have no instability pain and do not require immediate operation. A second difference between regions of the cervical spine reflects the etiology of myelopathy or radiculopathy. In the subaxial spine, these result from epidural tumor compression, rather than the fracture subluxations seen in the atlanto-axial spine.

4.2.1. Surgical Strategies

Subaxial spine tumors arising from the vertebral body should be addressed with a ventral approach and vertebral body resection (17–22). Kyphotic deformities may be reduced pre-operatively in an awake patient using skull traction, however, fixed deformities can often be readily reduced intra-operatively following tumor decompression. The Smith-Robinson approach (48) provides excellent exposure from C3 to C7 and usually T1 can be reached. High cervical approaches (e.g., C3 corpectomy) may require specialized services of the head and neck team to avoid trauma to the superior laryngeal and hypoglossal nerves.

A number of approaches to the cervicothoracic junction have been described. The trap door or hemiclamshell approach includes a dissection along the ventral border of the sternocleidomastoid muscle, extending down the sternum and across the fourth interspace (49). It is more easily accomplished from the right to avoid operating over the aortic arch, but carries a higher risk of recurrent laryngeal stretch injury. More recently for limited resections extending to T2, the authors have begun to use a ventral sternocleidomastoid incision and manubrial osteotomy, which provides excellent exposure (50) (Fig. 4). Both of these approaches are surprisingly well tolerated. Cervicothoracic junction vertebral body metastases, as high as C7, may also be addressed via a dorsolateral transpedicular approach (51).

The technique of ventral decompression in the subaxial cervical spine is relatively straightforward. All tumor-infiltrated vertebral bodies should be identified and resected. Tumor decompression includes resection of the posterior longitudinal ligament to identify a normal dural plane. Once the midline dura mater has been identified, the nerve roots can be dissected as far as the brachial plexus. Tumor can often be skeletonized from the vertebral arteries. Pre-operative balloon occlusion or at a minimum an MRI showing patency of the contralateral vertebral artery and/or circle of Willis is important before intra-operative dissection of the vertebral artery, in case sacrifice becomes necessary. On rare occasions, the vertebral artery may be infiltrated with tumor, precluding aggressive dissection. Another important pre-operative consideration is that of vocal cord function. Recurrent laryngeal nerve palsy may occur secondary to tumor infiltration. This should be identified using fiber optic laryngoscopy, and if a unilateral palsy is noted, the operative approach should be on the same side.

As with the atlanto-axial spine reconstruction, fixation of the subaxial spine should provide sufficient stability to allow the patient to be managed with minimal external support postoperatively. The use of halo vests is not well-tolerated in this patient group and has not been used in our institutions for patients with metastatic tumor. Ventral reconstruction techniques have evolved over the years. PMMA combined with a variety of instrumentation (27,52) including Kirchner wires (53), Steinmann pins (53), Harrington (54), and Knodt rods (55) have been used with some success. As a stand-alone method of stabilization, this may not be sufficient and a significant failure rate has been reported (56). Loosening and failure of fixation appears to be the most common reason (56) as PMMA alone offers poor resistance to hyperextension and rotation (52,57).

The use of rigid internal plate fixation for cervical spine stabilization has become more commonplace in the management of degenerative and traumatic conditions of the cervical spine (58–60). This method of fixation is also effective following decompression for cervical spinal metastatic disease (18,20,61). When using this method, it is imperative that the vertebral bodies used for screw fixation are free of tumor. An interbody strut is required in addition to plate fixation. Autograft iliac crest or fibula may be used. However, in this group of patients with limited life expectancy, the additional donor site morbidity makes this choice less desirable. Allograft iliac crest or fibular struts are extremely useful in this regard (Fig. 3). However, if the patient is to receive postoperative radiotherapy there is a higher risk of pseudoarthrosis. Other options include titanium mesh implants packed with bone graft.

The decision to combine a ventral subaxial decompression with a dorsal procedure must be given careful consideration in all cases. In cases where resection of more than one vertebral body is required, supplemental dorsal instrumentation is warranted to ensure stability (19,62–64). Ventral reconstruction alone in these cases may fail, particularly where there is residual disease as is the situation in the majority of these cases (19,62,63). Circumferential epidural metastases often necessitate combined ventral and dorsal decompression and stabilization. A ventral decompression alone may not be sufficient to adequately decompress the spinal cord. Additional dorsal decompression achieves this, but dorsal instrumentation should be used for stability. A combined procedure is indicated in the presence of dorsal element destruction. When this occurs, it is usually associated with ventral disease at the same level and there is often a translational deformity present in addition to the usual kyphosis. Finally, in cases where life expectancy is likely to be more than 1 yr, it may be prudent to perform a combined procedure, even for single level ventral metastatic disease, because local progression of disease is likely to occur and may lead to failure of ventral fixation.

Lateral mass instrumentation systems provide excellent fixation in cases where early postoperative mobilization is preferable. The use of dorsal wiring techniques, often supplemented by PMMA, has been widespread in the past. This technique is inferior to lateral mass fixation systems and usually requires external immobilization postoperatively (20). Lateral mass fixation has now superseded wiring techniques in patients with

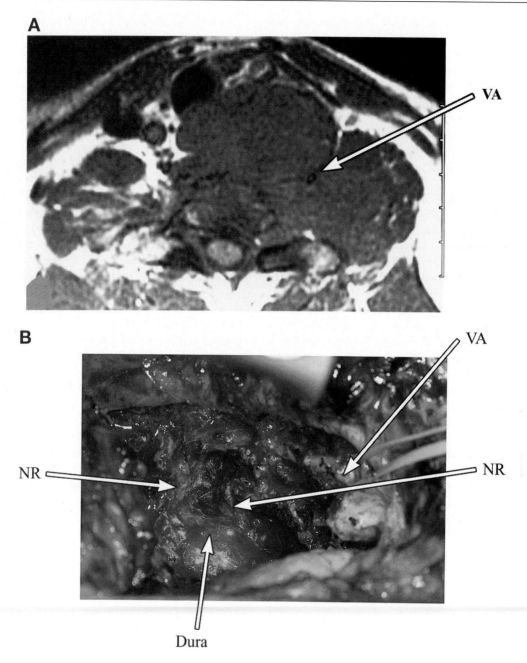

Fig. 4. A 57-yr-old patient with metastatic chordoma to C7 and T1 with a large ventral spinal mass **(A)**. Patient was approached via a left dissection ventral to the sternocleidomastoid muscle and manubrium osteotomy, without a hemiclamshell extension. **(B)** Intra-operative picture: the vertebral artery was identified at its origin and tumor was readily dissected. An intralesional resection of the vertebral body was then accomplished with dissection of the nerve roots (C8 and T1) following removal of the posterior longitudinal ligament. **(C,D** *[opposite page]*) Anterior/posterior plain radiographs and lateral computed tomography scan. Ventral reconstruction was accomplished with autologous iliac crest graft. A posterior approach was then taken to resect the C7 facet and dissect tumor from the C8 and T1 nerve roots. Dorsal segmental fixation over the cervicothoracic junction was accomplished with a lateral mass plate-rod system. NR, nerve root; VA, vertebral artery.

sub-axial metastatic disease *(20)*. Hard or soft collar immobilization is generally sufficient.

A large proportion of patients who require surgery for cervical spine metastases undergo pre-operative radiotherapy or chemotherapy. Those who have not usually do so postoperatively. Concern arises with regard to bone graft incorporation. Animal studies suggest that preoperative radiation has little effect on strut graft incorporation *(65,66)* Postoperative radia-

tion may have a more detrimental effect and it is recommended that it is delayed for 3 to 6 wk *(65)*.

REFERENCES

1. Brihaye J, Ectors P, Lemort M, Va Houtte P. The management of spinal epidural metastases. Adv Tech Stand Neurosurg 1998; 16:121–176.
2. Barron KD, Hirano A, Araki S. Experiences with metastatic neoplasms involving the spinal cord. Neurology 1959; 9:91–106.

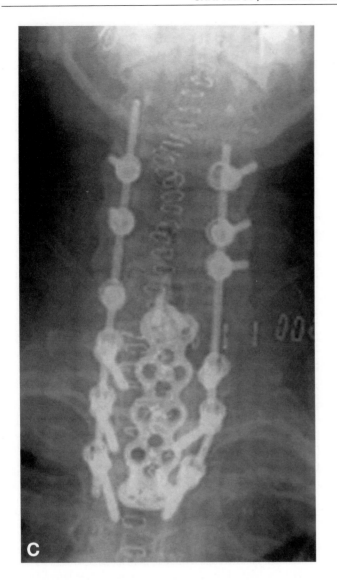

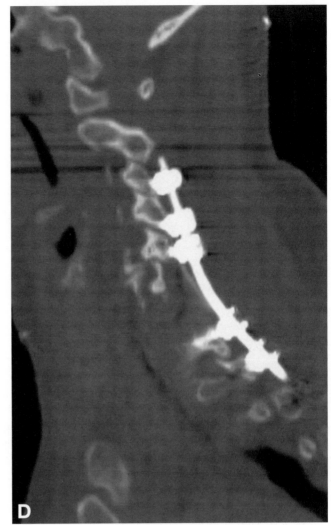

3. Constans J, de Divitiis E, Donzelli R, Spaziante R, Meder JF, Haye C. Spinal metastases with neurological manifestations. Review of 600 cases. J Neurosurg 1983; 59:111–118.

4. Hammerberg K. Surgical treatment of metastatic spine disease. Spine 1992; 17:1148–1153.

5. Nottebaert M, vonHochsetter A, Exner G, Schreiber A. Metastatic carcinoma of the spine. Int Orthop 1987; 11:345–348.

6. Rao S, Babini K, Schildhauer T, Borges M. Metastatic malignancy of the cervical spine. A nonoperative history. Spine 1992; 17:407–412.

7. Schaberg J, Gainor B. A profile of metastatic carcinoma of the spine. Spine 1985; 10:19–20.

8. Walsh GL, Gokaslan ZL, McCutcheon IE, et al. Anterior approaches to the thoracic spine in patients with cancer: indications and results. Ann Thorac Surg 1997; 64:1611–1618.

9. Kleinman W, Kiernan H, Michelsen W. Metastatic cancer of the spinal column. Clin Orthop 1978; 126:166–173.

10. Perrin R, McBroom R, Perrin R. Metastatic tumors of the cervical spine. Clin Neurosurg 1991; 37:740–755. 11.   Boland PJ, Lane JM. Sundaresan N. Metastatic disease of the spine. Clin Orthop 1982; 169:95–102.

12. Sim F. Diagnosis and Management of Metastatic Bone Disease. A Multidisciplinary Approach. New York, NY: Raven; 1988.

13. Tolli T, Cammisa F, Lane J, Martin T. Metastatic disease of the spine. In: Wiesel S, Boden S, eds. Seminars in Spine Surgery. Vol 7. Philadelphia, PA: WB Saunders; 1995:277–287.

14. Bilsky MH, Lis E, Raizer J, Lee H, Boland P. The diagnosis and treatment of metastatic spinal tumor. Oncologist 1999; 4:459–469.

15. Asdourian PL, Mardjetko S, Rauschning W, Johnsson H Jr, Hammerberg KW, DeWald RL. An evaluation of spinal deformity in metastatic breast cancer. J Spinal Disord 1990; 3:119.

16. Asdourian P. Metastatic disease of the spine. In Bridwell K (ed). The Textbook of Spinal Surgery. Ed 2. Philadelphia, PA: Lippincott-Raven Publishers; 1997:2007–2050.

17. Jenis GL, Dunn EJ, An HS. Metastatic disease of the cervical spine. A review. Clin Orthop 1999; 359:89–103.

18. Atanasiu J, Badatcheff F, Pidhorz L. Metastatic lesions of the cervical spine. Spine 1993; 18:1279–1284.

19. Jonsson B, Jonsson H Jr, Karlstrom G, Sjostrom L. Surgery of cervical spine metastases a retrospective study. Eur Spine J 1994; 3:76–83.

20. Marchesi DG, Boos N, Aebi M. Surgical treatment of tumors of the cervical spine and first two thoracic vertebrae. J Spinal Disord 1993; 6:489–496.

21. Matsui H, Tatezaki S, Tsuji H. Ceramic vertebral body replacement for metastatic spine tumors. J Spinal Disord 1994; 7:248–254.

22. Solini A, Orsini G, Broggi S. Metal cementless prosthesis for vertebral body replacement of metastatic malignant disease of the cervical spine. J Spinal Disord 1989; 2:254–262.

23. Nakamura M, Toyama Y, Suzuki N, Fujimura Y. Metastases to the upper cervical spine. J Spinal Disord 1996; 9:195–201.

24. Sjostrom L, Olerud S, Karlstrom G, Hamberg M, Jonsson H. Anterior stabilization of pathologic dens fractures. Acta Orthop Scand. 1990; 61:391–393.

25. Sundaresan N, Galicich JH, Lane JM, Greenberg HS. Treatment of odontoid fractures in cancer patients. J Neurosurg 1981; 54:187–192.

26. Barron KD, Hirano A, Araki S, Terry RD. Experiences with metastatic neoplasms involving the spinal cord. Neurology 1959; 9:91–106.

27. Sherk H, Nolan J, Mooar P. Treatment of tumors of the cervical spine. Clin Orthop 1988; 233:163–167.

28. Chabot M, Herkowitz H. Spine tumors: patient evaluation. In: Weisel S, ed. Seminars in Spine Surgery. Vol 7. Philadelphia, PA: WB Saunders; 1995:260–268.

29. Silverberg E, Lubera J. Cancer statistics. 1988. Cancer 1998; 381: 5–22.

30. Wada E, Ohmura M, Yonenobu K. Intramedullary changes of the spinal cord in cervical spondylotic myelopathy. Spine 1995; 20:2226–2232.

31. Moulopoulos LA, Kumar AJ, Leeds N. A second look at unenhanced spinal magnetic resonance imaging of malignant leptomeningeal disease. Clin Imaging 1997; 21:252–259.

32. Avrahami E, Tadmor R, Kaplinsky N. The role of T2-weighted gradient echo in MRI demonstration of spinal multiple myeloma. Spine 1993; 18:1812–1818.

33. Frank JA, Ling A, Patronas NJ et al. Detection of malignant bone tumors: MR imaging vs scintigraphy. Am J Radiol 1990; 155:1043–1048.

34. Dehdashti F, Siegal BA, Griffeth LK, et al. Benign versus malignant intraosseous lesions: discrimination by means of PET with 2-[F-18] Fluoro-2-Deoxy-D-Glucose. Radiology 1996; 200:243–247.

35. Ferpos E, Palermos J, Tsionos K, et al. Effect of pamidronate administration on markers of bone turnover and activity in multiple myeloma. Eur J Haematol 2000; 65:331–336.

36. Hortobagyi GN, Theriault RL, Lipton A, et al. Long-term prevention of skeletal complications of metastatic breast carcinoma with pamidronate. J Clin Oncol 1998; 16:2038–2044.

37. Lipton A, Theriault RL, Hortobagyi GN, et al. Pamidronate prevents skeletal complications and is effective palliative treatment in women with breast cancer and osteolytic bone metastases: long-term follow-up of two randomized, placebo controlled trials. Cancer 2000; 88:1082–1090.

38. Theriault RL, Lipton A, Hortobagyi GN, et al. Pamidronate reduces skeletal morbidity in women with advanced breast cancer and lytic bone lesions: a randomized, placebo-controlled trial. J Clin Oncol 1999; 17:846–895.

39. Bilsky MH, Shannon FJ, Sheppard S, Prabhu V, Boland PJ. Diagnosis and management of metastatic tumor to the atlanto-axial spine. Spine, (In Press).

40. Phillips E, Levine AM: Metastatic lesions of the upper cervical spine. Spine 1989; 14:1071–1077.

41. Piper JG, Menezes AH. Management strategies for tumors of the axis vertebra. J Neurosurg 1996; 84:543–551.

42. Sherk H, Snyder B. Posterior fusions of the upper cervical spine: indications, techniques and prognosis. Orthop Clin North Am 1978; 9:1091–1099.

43. Fang H, Ong G. Direct anterior approach to the upper cervical spine. J Bone Joint Surg 1962; 44A:1588–1604.

44. Hadley MN, Spetzler RF, Sonntag VKH. The transoral approach to the superior cervical spine. A review of 53 cases of extradural cervicomedullary compression. J Neurosurg 1972; 36:16–23.

45. Menezes AH, Traynelis VC. Gantz BJ. Surgical approaches to the craniovertebral junction. Clin Neurosurg 1994; 41:187–203.

46. McAfee P, Bohlman H, Riley L Jr, Robinson RA, Southwick WO, Nachlas NE.. The anterior retropharyngeal approach to the upper part of the cervical spine. J Bone Joint Surg 1987; 69:1371–1383.

47. Kostuik JP, Errico TJ, Gleason TF, Errico CC. Spinal stabilization of vertebral column tumors. Spine 1988; 13:250–256.

48. Robinson R, Riley L. Techniques of exposure and fusion of the cervical spine. Clin Orthop 1995; 109:78–84.

49. Nazzaro JM, Arbit E, Burt M. "Trap door" exposure to the cervicothoracic junction. Technical notes. J Neurosurg 1994; 80:338–341.

50. Darling GE, McBroom R, Perrin R. Modified anterior approach to the cervicothoracoc junction. Spine 1995; 20:1519–1521.

51. Bilsky MH, Boland P, Lis E, Raizer J, Healey JH. Single-stage posterolateral transpedicular approach for spondylectomy, epidural decompression and circumferential fusion of spinal metastases. Spine 2000; 25:2240–2249.

52. Dunn EJ. The role of methylmethacrylate in the stabilization and replacement of tumors of the cervical spine: a project of the Cervical Spine Research Society. Spine 1977; 2:15–24.

53. Rao S, Davis R. Cervical Spine Metastases. In: Clark C, ed. The Cervical Spine. The Cervical Spine Research Society. Philadelphia, PA: Lippincott-Raven; 1998:603–619.

54. Harrington K. The use of methylmethacrylate for vertebral-body replacement and anterior stabilization of pathological fracture-dislocations of the spine due to metastatic malignant disease. J Bone Joint Surg 1981; 63:36–46.

55. Siegal T, Tiqva P, Siegel T. Vertebral body resection for epidural compression by malignant tumors. Results of forty-seven consecutive procedures. J Bone Joint Surg 1985; 67:375–382.

56. McAfee P, Bohlman H, Ducker T, Eismont F. Failure of stabilization of the spine with methylmethacrylate. A retrospective analysis of twenty-four cases. J Bone Joint Surg 1986; 65:1145–1157.

57. Clarke CR, Kegi KJ, Panjabi MM. Methylmethacrylate stabilization of the cervical spine. J Bone Joint surg 1984; 66:40–46.

58. Aebi M, Zuber K, Marchesi D. Treatment of cervical spine injuries with anterior plating. Indications techniques and results. Spine 1991; 16:S38–S45.

59. Jonsson H, Cesarini K, Petren-Mallmin M, Raushning W. Locking screw-plate fixation of cervical spine fractures with and without ancillary posterior plating. Arch Orthop Trauma Surg 1991; 111:1–12.

60. Mann D, Bruner B, Keene J, Levin A. Anterior plating of unstable cervical spine fractures. Paraplegia 1990; 28:564–572.

61. Hall D, Webb J. Anterior plate fixation in spine tumor surgery. Spine 1991; 16:S80–S83.

62. McAfee PC, Bohlman HH. One-stage anterior cervical decompression and posterior stabilization with arthrodesis. A study of twenty-four patients who had a traumatic or neoplastic lesion. J Bone Joint Surg 1989; 71:78–88.

63. Perrin RG, McBroom RJ. Anterior versus posterior decompression for symptomatic spinal metastasis. Can J Neurol Sci 1987; 14:75–80.

64. Vaccaro AR, Falatyn SP, Scuderi GJ, et al. Early failure of long segment anterior cervical plate fixation. J Spinal Disord 1998; 11:410–415.

65. Bouchard J, Koka A, Bensauan M, Stevenson S, Emery S. Effect of irradiation on posterior spinal fusions. A rabbit model. Spine 1994; 19:1836–1841.

66. Emery S, Brazinski M, Koka A, Bensusan JS, Stevenson S. The biological and biomechanical effects of irradiation on anterior spinal bone grafts in a canine model. J Bone Joint Surg 1994; 76:540–548.

31 Metastatic Disease of the Thoracolumbar Spine

L. BRETT BABAT, MD AND ROBERT F. MCLAIN, MD

CONTENTS

1. INTRODUCTION

Metastases are the neoplasms most commonly seen by both orthopaedic and neurosurgeons, and the spine is the site most frequently involved (9,20). At autopsy, more than 70% of patients who die of cancer have vertebral metastases (23). Although nearly all malignancies may metastasize to bone, carcinoma of breast and bronchogenic origin, lymphoma, and multiple myeloma account for half of all spinal metastases (4,11,12,20,35,38,51).

The clinical behavior of the primary tumor determines the importance of metastatic disease; more aggressive, less treatable primaries frequently kill patients before spinal metastases become clinically relevant. However, as medical and adjuvant treatments improve, cancer patients are surviving longer, and the effects of metastatic disease on quality of life, including independence and pain, must be considered. Technology has made it possible to perform aggressive surgery with less morbidity, and improved spinal instrumentation allows early postoperative mobilization. The majority of patients with metastatic spinal tumors are best treated non-operatively, with radiation therapy (RT) and chemotherapy. However, surgical treatment can significantly improve patient comfort, function, and survival.

2. GOALS OF SURGICAL TREATMENT

Surgical intervention is indicated when more conservative therapy fails to control tumor progression, particularly in cases of mechanical instability or impending instability, neurologi-

cal compromise, or intractable pain. Surgery may also provide a diagnosis when the primary remains unknown after systemic workup and fine-needle aspiration. In cases where bony destruction and collapse have already occurred, especially with resulting bony impingement on the spinal cord, surgery provides the only method of redress.

For patients with metastatic disease, it is generally not the role of the spine surgeon to try to "cure" the patient, though solitary metastases of less aggressive primaries may be so treated. Rather, the goal ought to be to help maximize quality of life, as many patients with metastatic disease may survive for years. In simple terms, the surgeon seeks to relieve pain and to improve function, or at least to prevent further deterioration. More specifically, at the end of surgery, the neural elements should be free of impingement, the risk of symptom recurrence should be minimized, and the spine should be stable, with sagittal balance secured. To that end, there are three phases of surgery to consider: resection, decompression, and stabilization.

3. OPTIONS

3.1. MARGINS OF RESECTION

As in all musculoskeletal surgery, appropriate treatment is predicated on careful pre-operative planning. A clear understanding of the location and extent of the tumor is essential. Although anatomic compartments are difficult to define around the spine, natural planes of dissection do exist.

Weinstein (47) divided the vertebral body into four zones, I–IV, with tumor extension described A–C: intra-osseous, extraosseous, and distant spread (Fig. 1). Although this schema is intended to describe primary spine tumors, the zones and

From: *Current Clinical Oncology: Cancer in the Spine: Comprehensive Care.*
Edited by: R. F. McLain, K-U. Lewandrowski, M. Markman, R. M. Bukowski,
R. Macklis, and E. C. Benzel © Humana Press, Inc., Totowa, NJ

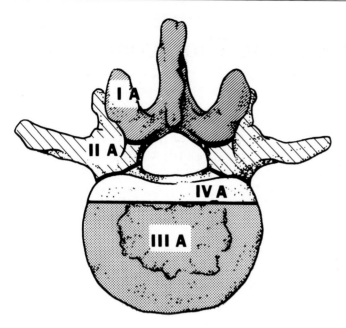

Fig. 1. Zones of resection. Four zones, defined to describe tumor extension within the vertebral body, permit careful planning for excision of focal metastases as well.

extensions remain useful concepts in the discussion of metastatic disease. Zone IA indicates the spinous process, inferior facet, and pars. Zone IIA includes the superior facet, transverse process, and pedicle. Zone IIIA is the anterior 75% of the body, and zone IVA is the posterior 25% body, including the posterior cortex directly anterior to the spinal canal and neural elements. Zones I–IVB describe extraosseous extension of tumor from the corresponding areas of the vertebra. As the vast majority of spinal metastases occur in the vertebral body, most patients will have tumor involving zones III and IV.

In the case of an isolated metastasis, especially when long-term survival is reasonably expected, obtaining the widest possible margin may profoundly affect patient outcome. In their series of spinal metastases, Sundaresan et al. *(43)* showed that resection of all gross tumor led to a median survival of longer than 2 yr, compared with historic median survival times of 6 mo with less aggressive procedures. Tomita et al. *(44)* treated 28 patients with favorable prognostic indicators with *en-bloc* vertebrectomy, yielding a mean survival of 38.2 mo, and successful local control in 93%. In contrast, Hosono *(22)* reported a local recurrence rate of 24% after anterior decompression, although it is unclear from that report whether the resections were marginal or intralesional. Isolated metastases from less imminently lethal tumors, mainly breast, colon, prostate, and kidney, should be managed like primary tumors of the spine. Wide resection may be possible for lesions in zones IA–IIIA, and, by removing the surrounding compartments, IVA lesions may likewise be widely resected. Wide margins are frequently not feasible in type B lesions, as important vascular and neural structures adjacent to the tumor cannot be resected. In these cases, a marginal resection is likely at best, and intralesional resection is frequently all that is possible.

When there are metastases to multiple organs, wide resection of spinal tumors becomes less important to the overall prognosis. Nonetheless, the surgeon should make every reasonable effort to remove as much of the tumor as possible, as complete resection can extend life and improve its quality *(43)*.

3.2. DECOMPRESSION VS STABILIZATION

In addition to directly compromising neural elements, spinal tumors produce pain and neurological deficits through fracture and instability. Pathological fractures occur along a continuum. At one end, resorption of bone may itself be painful, especially when osteopenia is sufficient for microfractures to occur. At the other end of the spectrum, gross failure of vertebral bodies leads to compression fractures, or even low-energy burst-type fractures with canal compromise. Local destruction may lead to painful instability and deformity, which, especially in the thoracic spine, may injure the neural elements.

3.2.1. Neurologically Intact

For patients with painful instability, but no neurological deficits, the goal is to stabilize the spine, both to relieve pain and to prevent neurological compromise.

In radiosensitive tumors, stabilization should be established with posterior instrumentation, with little or no effort given to decompression. Tumor growth may then be controlled with subsequent irradiation. Radio-resistant tumors need surgical treatment that is more aggressive, and resection and stabilization should be performed together. This may entail either combined anterior and posterior approaches, or a posterolateral approach. In either case, stabilization is necessary both anteriorly and posteriorly, to reestablish sagittal balance and posterior tension band function.

Those patients with a stable spine, but in whom the tumor has caused significant bony destruction, with impending collapse, present a more difficult decision. An impending pathological fracture does not itself require prophylactic stabilization. A compressed vertebra may continue to bear load, and may not produce instability or neurological compromise *(21)*. However, in the thoracic spine, canal compromise is likely to produce a significant and often irreversible neural deficit. Here, destruction of more than 50% of the body or significant pedicle involvement warrants prophylactic treatment *(11)*, either by surgical stabilization, or possibly by a minimally invasive technique, such as kyphoplasty or vertebroplasty *(34)*.

In the lumbar spine, with its more capacious and forgiving canal, a more conservative approach is reasonable. Radiosensitive tumors, even those compromising greater than 50% of the body, may be irradiated successfully. If collapse does occur, operative stabilization and decompression, if warranted, may be performed. Radio-resistant tumors should be stabilized when they significantly compromise two columns of the spine, as destruction of both the anterior and middle column will lead to instability *(10,50)*.

3.2.2. Neurologically Compromised

Involvement of the neural elements changes treatment focus. Decompression is necessary to relieve pain and to prevent progressive deterioration. Neurological function may be improved by decompression, especially for patients with slowly progressive deficits treated early. Radio-sensitive tumors causing gradually progressive neural compromise may be treated with radiation, assuming no associated instability. If the deficit progresses rapidly, or if the tumor is radio-resistant, the cord and roots must be decompressed directly. When neural compromise is secondary to bony impingement from vertebral collapse or instability, surgery becomes the only effective means of addressing the problem.

3.3. SELECTING A SURGICAL APPROACH: OPTIONS

3.3.1. Posterior

Posterior approaches, long the mainstay of spinal tumor surgery, are now used only in highly selected cases. This is because most spinal metastases involve the anterior elements, zones III and IV. In these patients, laminectomy provides no benefit beyond radiation alone. An uncontrolled, retrospective review by Nicholls et al. (36) demonstrated neurological improvement in only 24% of 38 patients who underwent laminectomy. Furthermore, although Constans et al. (7) obtained some improvement combining radiotherapy with laminectomy, Gilbert et al. (15) found laminectomy to be of no benefit beyond radiotherapy alone. Decompressive laminectomy does not allow access to tumor or bone fragments anterior to the cord, and posterior surgery may lead to or exacerbate kyphosis. The resulting increased compression in these already compromised patients may be neurologically devastating.

In a review of 746 cases in the literature, McLain and Weinstein (31) noted only 38% of posteriorly decompressed patients had a satisfactory neurological outcome. Furthermore, the improvements were weighted toward those patients with less deficit pre-operatively. More recently, however, Bauer (2) demonstrated significant neurological improvement with a more aggressive posterior approach, including drilling of both pedicles and removal of anterior tumor or bone fragments, combined with segmental stabilization. In this prospective study of 67 patients, 76% had meaningful neurological improvement, and the majority maintained this improvement until death or 1-yr follow-up. Wide posterior decompression and stabilization was recommended for patients with visceral or brain metastases, for those with significant cardiovascular or pulmonary disease, and for those with multiple spinal metastases. By preventing kyphosis, rigid segmental stabilization seems to maintain the benefits of even the less than maximal decompression achieved with a posterior approach. Shimizu et al. (39) noted neurological improvement in 9 of 11 patients with multiple spinal metastases. After laminectomy, these patients were stabilized with Luque rods, sublaminar wires, and methylmethacrylate. However, neurological improvement was maintained for less than 6 mo in 45% of these cases.

3.3.2. Anterior

Most metastatic spinal disease involves the anterior elements. In response to the poor outcome associated with laminectomy, surgeons began to approach spinal metastases anteriorly. Harrington (18) reported significant neurological improvement in 68% of patients approached anteriorly. Of the 38 patients with metastases to the thoracic or lumbar spine, 66% improved one or more Frankel grades, and 38% of patients improved two or more grades. Similarly, Fidler (13) reported neurological improvement in 14 of 15 patients who presented with a deficit, and pain was relieved in all but one patient.

Siegal and Siegal (42) reported the results of 47 consecutive anterior approaches for epidural compression by metastatic disease. Seventy-four percent of the 35 patients who were nonambulatory preoperatively regained the ability to walk, 86% of the 22 patients incontinent of bowel and bladder regained control, 61% of the 45 patients who were in unremitting pain had complete resolution, and an additional 31% had partial relief. The same group (41) presented a prospective study of anterior and posterior resection, based on location of compression: lesions in the body were approached anteriorly, and those in the posterior elements were treated by laminectomy. Those who did not fit their surgical indications received radiotherapy. In this last group, only 30% gained or retained the ability to ambulate. In the laminectomy group, 34% of pre-operative nonambulators gained that ability, and 47% had improved continence. In the vertebrectomy group, 75% of nonambulators were able to walk postoperatively, and 87% regained continence. Although pain reduction results are not available for the laminectomy and radiation groups, 54% of anteriorly approached patients had complete resolution of pain, and another 34% had an improvement.

In their review of the literature, McLain and Weinstein (31) found 427 cases of anterior decompression for which there was objective neurological grading. Seventy-nine percent of these had significant improvement, and 77% were able to ambulate independently, with intact bowel and bladder function. Because of such success, especially compared to laminectomy, the anterior approach to spinal metastases has largely become the gold standard for spinal decompression when surgical treatment proves necessary.

3.3.3. Posterolateral

Many patients require both anterior and posterior decompression, or anterior decompression with both anterior and posterior instrumentation. Others may have comorbidities that make them poor candidates for anterior surgery. To avoid subjecting the former patients to both anterior and posterior approaches, and to minimize risk to the latter, some have advocated the posterolateral approach (3,33,48).

In the thoracic spine, the posterolateral approach is essentially a transpedicular resection in combination with a 3- to 4-cm costotransversectomy. In the lumbar spine, the transpedicular approach is augmented with resection of the medial aspect of the transverse process. Curved and reverse angle curettes are then used for tumor resection anteriorly. Anterior reconstruction is performed through the same approach, utilizing either methyl methacrylate sometimes augmented with Steinmann pins or a variation thereof, or using a mesh cage with cement or bone graft. Resection through this approach is always intralesional.

Initially, the results with posterolateral approaches were disappointing. Dewald et al. (11) reported that only one of five patients regained the ability to walk, and survival was less than 6 mo. Bridwell et al. (5) were disappointed by their inability to resect the tumor as adequately as they could through an anterior approach, though they did note that 60% of their neurocom-promised patients improved postoperatively. Overby and Rothman (37) treated 11 non-ambulatory patients.

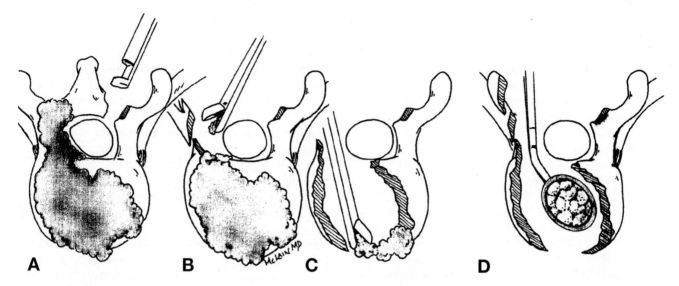

Fig. 2. Posterolateral decompression technique. **(A)** Decompression begins with a laminectomy approach providing wide exposure to the spinal canal and reducing pressure on the spinal cord. **(B)** The pedicle and proximal rib are removed on the side of most severe involvement. **(C)** Currettes and pituitary rongeurs remove tumor from within the bone, creating a cavity. **(D)** A cage or bone strut can be placed into the cavity to restore anterior spinal support.

Although 82% of them improved neurologically, only 64% became ambulatory. Bilsky et al. *(3)* reported on a series of 25 patients, of whom 9 had a pre-operative deficit. Only five (56%) of these patients improved neurologically and three patients (12%) worsened one or more Frankel grades.

Recently, there have been more encouraging reports. Muhlbauer et al. *(33)* reported that 82% of their patients improved neurologically and 70% of non-ambulators were able to walk postoperatively, though most required a cane or walker. In this approach, decompression is carried out by removing the pedicle and posterior-lateral cortex of the vertebral body (Fig. 2) and removing the tumor tissue within the body piece by piece. The tumor or bone that may be compressing the spinal cord is collapsed into the vertebral body defect, using a reverse curette and taking care not to compress or manipulate the spinal cord. The surgeon removes as much tumor as can be seen from the posterolateral corner, and may use a dental mirror to see further medially. Inevitably, some tumor is left behind, usually directly anterior to the cord. McLain *(29)* reported a promising modification of the approach, utilizing an endoscope to illuminate and visualize the body anterior to the cord, without requiring manipulation of the cord (Fig. 3). In 2001, McLain *(30)* reported a pilot series of nine consecutive patients, all of whom retained or regained normal strength and function. Pre-operatively, six patients were Frankel B, C, or D; all improved to grade E postoperatively. All nine patients maintained normal sensation, bladder and bowel function, and independent ambulation until terminal care or last follow-up, at 3 to 36 mo. Importantly, there was a dramatic reduction in both intensive care unit an in-patient days, compared to open thoracotomy.

4. SELECTING AN APPROACH: SPECIFIC INDICATIONS

When selecting the approach, neural decompression, tumor resection, and subsequent spinal stabilization must all be con-

sidered. Patient co-morbidities, tumor dissemination, and surgeon's experience must be considered. It is of paramount importance to consider the biomechanical effect of the resection, as the reconstruction that follows must re-establish stability.

4.1. ZONE I AND II LESIONS: THE POSTERIOR ELEMENTS

Rarely is metastatic disease confined to the posterior elements *(24)*. However, these unusual Zone I lesions should be approached through a posterior incision sufficient to allow resection of any soft tissue mass. Posterior stabilization with segmental instrumentation should be part of the procedure, even in the rare decompression that itself does not produce instability, as local recurrence may well lead to instability. Furthermore, for patients likely to survive longer than 6 to 12 mo, fusion should be attempted. Although this may be difficult to attain in a previously irradiated tissue bed, or in a patient undergoing chemotherapy, instrumentation without fusion has a limited, unpredictable life expectancy, which might be briefer that that of the patient *(22)*. In the thoracolumbar region, multilevel laminectomies may result in progressive kyphosis. In the lower lumbar spine, resection of a total of one facet at any single level may lead to spondylolisthesis *(1)*.

For patients with an isolated metastasis, especially when the primary tumor bears a relatively good prognosis, wide excision should be attempted. Although sacrificing a thoracic nerve root is not neurologically devastating, ligation of the associated segmental artery may prove dangerous in the lower thoracic watershed region. A pre-operative angiogram should facilitate this decision. Sacrifice of a lumbar root is less acceptable.

Zone II lesions should be approached posterolaterally. Again, it is rare for spinal metastases to be strictly posterior, but in these cases, anterior surgery is not needed. A posterolateral approach enables the surgeon to access the contralateral lamina as well as the junction of the pedicle and body on the involved side, making wide excision possible for isolated IIA lesions.

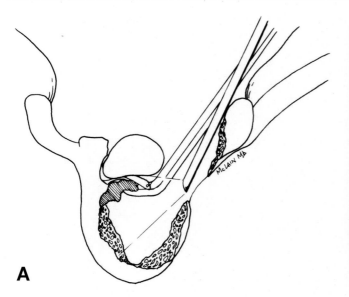

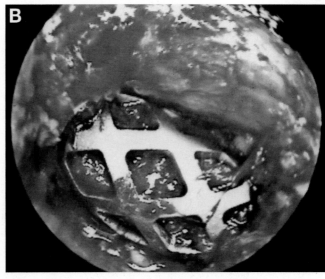

Fig. 3. **(A)** A 70°-angled endoscope provides light and magnification while searching the volar surface of the spinal cord for residual tumor. **(B)** The image through the scope shows the regions of the vertebral body and cord shielded from the traditional approach.

Generally, however, neural compression is caused by extension from the soft-tissue component of B tumors. In these cases, wide excision is not possible without removing a segment of the dura. Marginal or intralesional resection is therefore the only acceptable option.

In the case of a posterior tumor sufficient to compromise stability without causing a neural deficit, local control may be obtained through radiotherapy in many cases. If the tumor is radiosensitive, surgeons should remove enough tumor to ensure that inflammation caused by RT does not precipitate cord compression. If the tumor is not radiosensitive, a full resection should still be performed. The exposure necessary to stabilize the spine should provide all the necessary access to the tumor. If the lesion is radio-resistant and is not removed, it may grow to compromise the neural elements, and a second surgery in an unhealthy patient would be needed.

4.2. ZONE III AND IV LESIONS: THE VERTEBRAL BODY

In general, lesions anterior of the vertebral body are best decompressed by an anterior approach *(13,19,26,29,40,41)*. True zone III lesions should not actually compromise neurological function. To do so, the tumor would have to involve zone IV, or a pathological fracture with bony retropulsion would have to occur. Either of these conditions would then represent a zone IV lesion. Barring an isolated lesion with a good prognosis for survival that would warrant a wide resection, the primary indication for surgery in a metastasis isolated to zone III would be impending instability or intractable pain, and decompression would not be needed. In these cases, local control may be obtained by marginal resection through an anterior approach, with cage or strut graft reconstruction, followed by RT.

Patients more commonly require the attention of the spine surgeon when there is cord compromise. Again, isolated metastases to these zone IV lesions, if they are of favorable tissue type, should be widely excised when possible. This necessi-

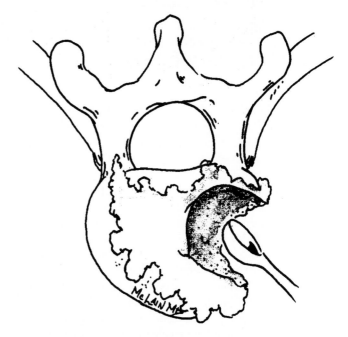

Fig. 4. Anterior curettage of a metastatic lesion.

tates a combined anterior and posterior approach, to free the body from the posterior elements, so reconstruction is needed both anteriorly and posteriorly.

The majority of zone IV lesions occur in patients with disseminated disease or otherwise poor prognosis and have most successfully been approached anteriorly. When possible, a marginal resection should be performed, but an intralesional resection is often all that is attainable (Fig. 4). However, there are situations where the endoscopically assisted posterolateral approach, which is always intralesional, can obtain adequate decompression and full anterior column recontruction with reduced surgical morbidity. This is particularly true for thoracic metasases above T5, where anterior access is difficult at

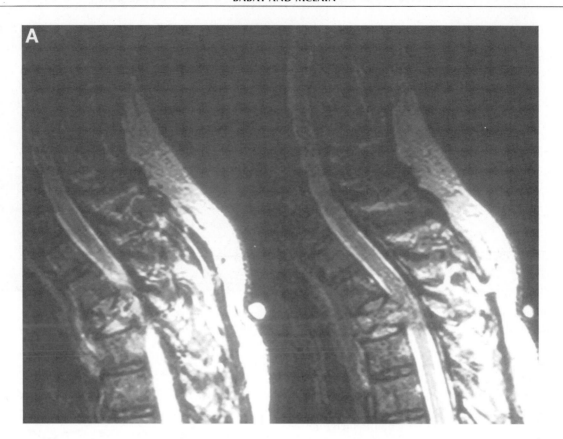

best. Scapular retraction, sternotomy, or splitting of the clavicle is required to gain access to T2 or T3 lesions, and the great vessels are difficult to mobilize at this level. The endoscopic posterolateral approach may actually provide for a more thorough resection and decompression in these cases. Additionally, patients with compromised pulmonary function from parenchymal involvement or previous lung resection may not tolerate a transthoracic or thoracoscopic anterior approach (Fig. 5).

4.3. COMBINED LESIONS

Metastatic lesions may compromise the cord both anteriorly and posteriorly. Even when anterior decompression would itself provide relief, a posterior approach will be needed to ensure that the posterior structures can withstand tensile and shearing forces—a competent tension band. Otherwise, these patients with compromised anterior elements are likely to subside into kyphosis or lysthese. A combined anterior and posterior approach is needed. The decision to pursue a formal anterior/posterior combined resection and reconstruction has to be based on an expected survival benefit and improved quality of life. This is often unlikely in metastic disease.

5. SPECIFIC CONSIDERATIONS

5.1. TUMOR TYPE AND BEHAVIOR

Although essentially all malignancies may metastasize to the spine, breast, bronchogenic, prostate, and lymphoreticular tumors account for 60% of spinal metastases requiring treatment. Because spinal metastases from breast, prostate, and renal tumors appear early in the disease, patients frequently live long enough that spinal metastases must be addressed. Patients with pulmonary primaries or multiple myeloma often die soon after

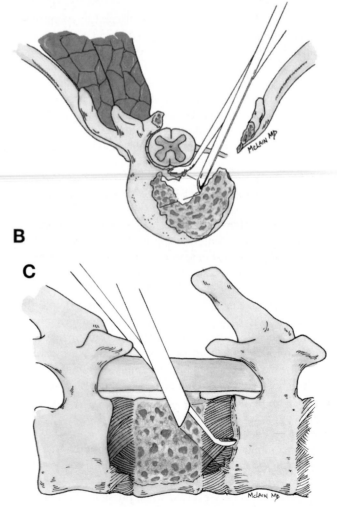

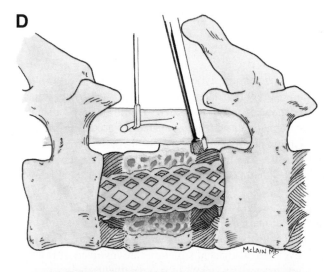

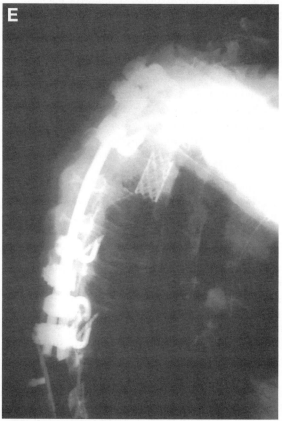

Fig. 5. Endoscopically assisted approach to upper thoracic metastases. **(A, opposite page)** Magnetic resonance imaging demonstrates metastatic lesion of the T3 vertebral body, a notoriously difficult level to reach through any anterior method. **(B, opposite page)** Endoscopic view during video-assisted posterolateral corpectomy allows removal of all of the tumor, anterior to cord. **(C, opposite page)** Complete corpectomy and preparation of endplates for reconstruction. **(D)** The nerve root is retracted, and a cage is placed posterolaterally to restore anterior column support. **(E)** Postoperative lateral radiograph. The patient had complete recovery of cord function and ambulation, and relief of pain for the remainder of his life.

the appearance of spinal metastases and frequently do not need more than palliative treatment for their spinal tumors.

Furthermore, multiple myeloma, lymphoma, and prostatic carcinoma tend to be quite radiosensitive, and radiotherapy frequently yields excellent results in these patients, limiting the need for surgery *(6,31,45)*. Although breast carcinoma metastases are also frequently radio-sensitive, as many as 30% of patients do not improve clinically with radiation alone *(16,45)*. Typically, renal tumors prove radio-resistant, as do many gastrointestinal carcinomas. The latter tend to metastasize to the liver and lungs before the spine, overshadowing the importance of osseous metastases. However, with increasing longevity, the need to treat spinal metastases from colorectal and gastrointestinal tumors is increasing.

Because renal tumors tend to metastasize early in the disease and respond poorly to radiation, patients with spinal metastases frequently need surgical intervention. It is important to remember that these tumors are extraordinarily vascular. Most surgeons will order an angiogram and ask their radiology colleagues to embolize them 24 to 48 h before surgery can result in catastrophic hemorrhage.

5.2. SAGITTAL BALANCE

At the end of the reconstructive procedure, spinal stability and balance must be restored. In addition to preventing further kyphosis or spondylolisthesis, pre-existing deformity must be addressed. While both hyperkyphosis of the thoracic spine and lumbar "flat back" (hypolordosis) are unacceptable, the thoracolumbar junction is the area of greatest concern. It is in this transitional area that kyphosis is most likely to occur, with resulting pain, and, frequently, neurological injury. Several reconstructive methods can be employed to address this problem.

Non-segmental instrumentation is sufficient to stabilize the spine after limited laminectomy. However, when more than the posterior column is involved with disease, these constructs tend to fail, either by pulling loose or breaking. Segmental stabilization distributes forces widely over the spinal column with good results *(29,33,39,49)*. These constructs resist bending moments in thoracic tumors, allow for rotational correction, and, with the cantilevering effect of pedicle screws, better maintain axial alignment, even in the face of reduced anterior support. Pedicle instrumentation depends, however, on bone quality, especially in anteriorly deficient constructs. Screw bending failure can be expected when a deficient anterior column is not reconstructed.

Anterior constructs allow for alternative or additional support of sagittal balance. Patients with isolated lesions and long-term survival potential may be reconstructed with autograft. Large, multilevel defects present more of a challenge, and may be supported with bone- or cement-filled titanium mesh cages. Rigid reconstruction locking plates, placed anterolaterally, provide compression and fixation across the graft. Alternatively, Steinmann pins, or a variation thereof, may be used as "rebar" imbedded in methyl methacrylate to improve the cement's resistance to shearing forces and its fixation to the spine. Non-biological cement constructs have a finite life. These should be reinforced with bony fusion for patients likely to survive longer than 4 to 6 mo.

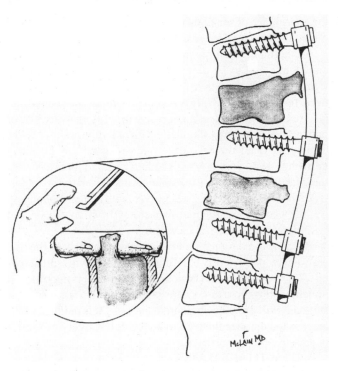

Fig. 6. Wide decompression through a classic laminectomy approach can be successful for patients with multilevel disease. Segmental spinal instrumentation, using hooks and screws at multiple fixation points, can stabilize the spine and resist the collapse into kyphosis that makes laminectomy without fusion a poor choice.

5.3. MULTILEVEL DISEASE

Because of the extensive nature of the resection and subsequent reconstruction, anterior surgery may be impractical for patients with extensive spinal metastases. This includes those whose anterior lesions compromise more than two adjacent levels, or whose metastases involve non-contiguous vertebrae. After exhausting all non-surgical options, an aggressive posterior decompression with segmental instrumentation is a reasonable choice (Fig. 6). Shimizu et al. *(39)* noted neurological improvement in 82% of patients with multiple metastases so treated, and no patient's status worsened. Hammerberg *(17)* approached patients with more then two involved levels posteriorly, including bilateral transpedicular resection, and those with only one or two involved bodies anteriorly. He noted neurological improvement in 12 of 17 (70%) patients posteriorly decompressed and instrumented, and 8 of 10 who underwent an anterior procedure. Segmental instrumentation plays a pivotal role in the success of these cases.

5.4. CHEST WALL INVOLVEMENT

It is not uncommon for spinal metastases to involve the adjacent rib head and costovertebral angle *(8)*. Although resection is certainly possible through a traditional transthoracic approach, it must be remembered that the rib resected for the approach is generally one or two levels above the involved vertebra. Although it is possible to make the approach through the involved rib, access to higher thoracic levels is severely curtailed. This may make both resection of the proximal extent of the tumor and reconstruction difficult. More than one rib may need to be resected. Another option is the posterolateral

approach. Resection of the rib head and its articulation with the vertebra is a routine part of the procedure.

5.5. INVOLVEMENT OF VITAL STRUCTURES

Although IIIA lesions can be marginally or widely resected throughout the spine, type B lesions, those with soft tissue extension, may not be addressed as easily. Invasion of adjacent vital structures may necessitate an intralesional resection. Again, for patients with disseminated disease, the primary concerns are to adequately decompress involved neural elements and to ensure stability. Resection of the tumor is secondary, and an intralesional resection may be all that is reasonably undertaken.

Patients with isolated metastases from treatable primaries, and occasional patients with local recurrence of a previously resected colon or renal primary, are best served by wide resection, even when adjacent structures are involved. It is not uncommon to sacrifice an involved sympathetic chain, or even an involved nerve root. When more vital structures are involved, it is important to have a surgeon from the appropriate subspecialty involved (e.g., thoracic, vascular, or general surgery). This team approach should be arranged before surgery, while planning the case, to ensure appropriate positioning, approach, and surgeon availability. It must be remembered that, for patients with disseminated disease, the risk and recovery required for a major vascular reconstruction may outweigh the benefits of such an aggressive approach.

6. CONTRAINDICATIONS

For patients with anterior pathology, not only is laminectomy no better than radiotherapy, but it may be overtly harmful. Blind manipulation of the cord to decompress anteriorly carries a high risk of additional neurological injury *(28)*, and, if retropulsed vertebral fragments cannot be removed, the compression will not be relieved. By compromising the posterior structures, aggressive posterior decompression can lead to progressive kyphosis and increased cord compression, especially in the face of an incompetent anterior column.

Patients with poor pulmonary function are poor candidates for a transthoracic approach. This includes those with severe chronic obstructive pulmonary disease, which is common in the lung cancer population. Parenchymal tumor compromises function, as does previous lung resection. These patients may well be better served by forgoing an anterior approach in lieu of an endoscopically assisted posterolateral approach. The need to take down the diaphragm for a thoracolumbar exposure may similarly compromise these patients. It is advisable to test baseline pulmonary function pre-operatively.

The posterolateral approach should not be employed for patients with solitary metastases and a good prognosis, unless the tumor is radiosensitive and other comorbidities preclude the use of the transthoracic approach. The posterolateral approach is almost always intralesional. Patients with isolated metastases and an otherwise good prognosis should be offered wide resection whenever possible.

7. COMPLICATIONS

Sundaresan et al. *(43)* have reported complication rates as high as 48% following tumor excision. They found the complication rate to be statistically higher for patients over age 65, in those who have had prior treatment, and in the presence of parapareses. Nonetheless, neurological deterioration is on the order of 5% or less (25,43,46).

The risk of complications is highest in previously irradiated patients, whose tissues are fragile and poorly vascularized. Poor wound healing is by far the most common problem in this population, with most large series reporting wound breakdown in 5 to 20% of these patients (2,5,43). Furthermore, irradiated vessels become friable, and minor intra-operative dissection may cause severe hemorrhage that is difficult to control. To lessen these risks, surgeons might be afforded the opportunity to consult before patients are irradiated.

Unless a wide excision is accomplished, local recurrence may be anticipated in nearly all patients, should they live long enough. The risk of local recurrence is greater in patients who live longer, with local recurrence in up to 41% of thyroid cancer patients. Radio-resistant tumors are also more likely to recur, and rates as high as 50% have been reported in renal cancer (22). This underscores the importance of obtaining the best possible margins in those patients with a prognosis of long-term survival or whose tumor is not radio-sensitive.

Bleeding is always a risk in surgery, but much more so in tumor surgery, where it may be difficult to control. In addition to being hypervascular, tumors around the spine frequently involve large vessels, and the exposures necessary put these structures at further risk. Pre-operative embolization and careful dissection help to limit this risk.

Failure of the reconstruction is another problem. McAfee et al. (27) treated 24 patients referred for failure of fixation that had relied on methyl methacrylate. Only five of these instances occurred when it was used anteriorly, but all of these were patients treated for tumor. None of these constructs was reinforced with posterior instrumentation. Segmental instrumentation, together with appropriate anterior reconstruction, can last for the duration of the patient's life, even in the absence of a fusion. The highest rates of failure are seen in strictly posterior and posterolateral resections for tumors involving the anterior structures, without anterior reconstruction. Even in these cases, failure rates are relatively low; Bridwell (5) noted loosening in 1 of 25 patients, Bauer (2) in 6% of 67 patients.

All surgery for spinal metastases incurs the risks associated with the chosen approach. Excessive retraction may injure the liver or spleen in right- or left-sided lumbar and thoracolumbar approaches, respectively. The position of the retractors must be checked frequently, and the assistant should know what structures lay behind the retractors. Although pneumothorax is always encountered after the transthoracic approach, it may also result from retropleural, posterolateral, and even strictly posterior approaches about the thoracic spine. If ventilation becomes difficult or if oxygen saturation decreases during surgery, pneumothorax must be suspected. Even if there are no clinical signs, a postoperative X-ray should be obtained to ensure there is not a small but expanding pneumothorax.

Because of its proximity, anterior approaches to the lower lumbar spine result in injury to the sympathetic chain in a small number of patients. Superior hypogastric plexus damage dur-

ing anterior approach to the lumbosacral junction may result in retrograde ejaculation in some men, especially those who are older or who have peripheral vascular disease, not uncommon in the metastatic tumor population. Careful handling of the prevertebral tissues, especially subperiosteal dissection, helps to minimize this risk.

8. SUMMARY

Because progress has been made in the treatment of cancer, more patients are surviving long enough for spinal metastases to become clinically important. Concomitant, advances in surgical technique and instrumentation have improved survival and neurological outcome after spinal surgery. Appropriate surgical treatment of these individuals can significantly improve their length and quality of life.

REFERENCES

1. Abumi K, Panjabi MM, Kramer KM, Duranceau J, Oxland T, Crisco JJ. Biolmechanical evaluation of lumbar spinal stability after graded facetectomy. Spine 1990; 15:1142–1147.
2. Bauer HC. Posterior decompression and stabilization for spinal metastases: analysis of sixty-seven consecutive patients. J Bone Joint Surg 1997; 79:514–523.
3. Bilsky MH, Boland P, Lis E, Raizer JJ, Healey JH.. Single stage posterolateral transpedicle approach for spondylectomy, epidural decompression, and circumferential fusion of spinal metastases. Spine 2000; 25:2240–2250.
4. Black P. Spinal metastasis: current status and recommended guidelines for management. Neurosurgery 1979; 5:726–746.
5. Bridwell KH, Jenny AB, Saul T, Rich KM, Grubb RL. Posterior segmental spinal instrumentation (PSSI) with posterolateral decompression and debulking for metastatic thoracic and lumbar spine disease: limitations of the technique. Spine 1988; 13:1383–1394.
6. Bruckman, JE, and Bloomer, WD. Management of spinal cord compression. Semin Oncol 1978; 5:135–140.
7. Constans JP, De Divitiis E, Donzelli R, Spaziante R, Meder JF, Haye C. Spinal metastasis with neurological manifestations: review of 600 cases. J Neurosurg 1983; 59:111–118.
8. Cybulski GR, Stone JL, Opesanmi O. Spinal cord decompression via a modified costotransversectomy approach combined with posterior instrumentation for management of metastatic neoplasms of the thoracic spine. Surg Neurol 1991; 35:280–285.
9. Dahlin DC. Bone Tumors: General Aspects and Data on 6221 Cases. 3rd ed. Springfield, IL: Charles C Thomas; 1978.
10. Denis F. The three column spine and its significance in the classification of acute thoracolumbar spine injuries. Spine 1983; 8:817–831.
11. Dewald RL, Bridwell KH, Prodromas C, Rodts MF. Reconstructive spinal surgery as palliation for metastatic malignancies of the spine. Spine 1985; 10:21–26.
12. Drury AB, Palmer PH, Highman WJ. Carcinomatous metastases to the vertebral bodies. J Clin Pathol 1964; 17:448–460.
13. Fidler MW. Anterior decompression and stabilisation of metastatic spinal fractures. J Bone Joint Surg 1986; 68:83–90.
14. Flynn JC, Price CT. Sexual complications of anterior fusion of the lumbar spine. Spine 1984; 9:489–492.
15. Gilbert RW, Kim JH, Posner JB. Epidural spinal cord compression from metastatic tumor: diagnosis and treatment. Annals Neurol 1978; 3:40–51.
16. Greenberg HS, Kim JH, Posner JB. Epidural spinal cord compression from metastatic tumor. Ann Neurol 1980; 8:361–366.
17. Hammerberg KW. Surgical treatment of metastatic spine disease. Spine 1992; 17:1148–1153.
18. Harrington KD. Current concept review. Metastatic disease of the spine. J Bone Joint Surg 1986; 68:1110–1115.

19. Harrington KD. Anterior decompression and stabilization of the spine as a treatment for vertebral collapse and spinal cord compression from metastatic malignancy. Clin Orthop 1988; 233:177–197.

20. Harrington KD. Metastatic diseases of the spine. In: Harrington, KD ed. Orthopaedic Management of Metastatic Bone Disease. St. Louis, MO: CV Mosby; 1988:309–383.

21. Hipp JA, Springfield DS, Hayes WC. Predicting pathologic fracture risk in the management of metastatic bone defects. Clin Orthop 1995; 312:120–135.

22. Hosono N, Yonenobu K, Fuji T, Ebara S, Yamashita K, Ono K. Orthopaedic management of spinal metastases. Clin Orthop 1995; 312:148–159.

23. Jaffe HL. Tumors and Tumorous Conditions of the Bone and Joints. Philadelphia, PA: Lea and Febiger; 1958.

24. Klekamp J, Samii H. Surgical results for spinal metastases. Acta Neurochir (Wein) 1998; 140:957–967.

25. Kostuik JP, Errico TJ, Gleason TF, Errico CC. Spinal stabilization of vertebral column tumors. Spine 1988; 13:250–256.

26. Manabe S, Tateishi A, Abe M, Ohno T. Surgical treatment of metastatic tumors of the spine. Spine 1989; 14:41–47.

27. McAfee PC, Bohlman HH, Ducker T, Eismont FJ. Failure of stabilization of the spine with methylmethacrylate: a retrospective review of twenty-four cases. J Bone Joint Surg 1986; 68:1145–1157.

28. Martin NS, Williamson J. The role of surgery in the treatment of malignant tumors of the spine. J Bone Joint Surg 1970; 52:227–237.

29. McLain RF. Endoscopically assisted decompression for metastatic thoracic neoplasms. Spine 1998; 23:1130–1135.

30. McLain RF. Spinal cord decompression: an endoscopically assisted approach for metastatic tumors. Spinal Cord 2001; 39:482–487.

31. McLain RF, Weinstein JN. Tumors of the spine. In: Herkowitz HN, Garfin SR, Balderston RA, et al. eds. Rothman-Simeone: The Spine. Philadelphia, PA: WB Saunders; 1999:1171–1206.

32. Millburn L, Hibbs GC, Hendrickson FR. Treatment of spinal cord compression from metastatic carcinoma. Cancer 1968; 21:447–452.

33. Muhlbauer M, Pfister W, Eyb R, et al. Noncontiguous spinal metastases and plasmacytomas should be operated on through a single posterior midline approach, and circumferential decompression should be performed with individual reconstruction. Acta Neurochiurgica (Wien) 2000; 142:1219–1230.

34. Murphy KJ, Deramond H. Percutaneous vertebroplasty in benign and malignant disease. Neur Imag Clin 2000; 10:535–545.

35. Nather A, Bose K. The results of decompression of cord or cauda equina compression from metastatic extradural tumors. Clin Orthop 1982; 169:103–108.

36. Nicholls PJ, Jarecky TW. The value of posterior decompression by laminectomy for malignant tumors of the spine. Clin Orthop 1985; 201:210–213.

37. Overby MC, Rothman AS. Anterolateral decompression for metastatic epidural spinal cord tumors: results of a modified costotransversectomy approach. J Neurosurg 1985; 62:344–348.

38. Perrin RG, McBroom RJ. Anterior vs. posterior decompression for symptomatic spinal metastasis. Can J Neurol Sci 1987; 14:75–80.

39. Shimizu, K, Shikata, J, Iida, H, Iwasaki R, Yoshikawa J, Yamamuro T. Posterior decompression and stabilization for multiple metastatic tumors of the spine. Spine 1992; 17:1400–1404.

40. Siegal T, Siegal T, Robin G, Lubetzki-Korn I, Fuks Z. Anterior decompression of the spine for metastatic epidural cord compression: A promising avenue of therapy? Ann Neurol 1982; 11:28–34.

41. Siegal T, Siegal T. Surgical decompression of anterior and posterior malignant epidural tumors compressing the spinal cord: a prospective study. Neurosurg 1985; 17:424–431.

42. Siegal T, Tiqva P, Siegal T. Vertebral body resection for epidural compression by malignant tumors: results of forty-seven consecutive operative procedures. J Bone Joint Surg 1985; 67:375–382.

43. Sundaresan N, Sachdev VP, Holland JF, et al. Surgical treatment of spinal cord compression from epidural metastasis. J Clin Oncol 1995; 13:2330–2335.

44. Tomita K, Kawahara,N, Kobayashi T, Yoshida A, Murakami H, Akamaru T. Surgical strategey for spinal metastases. Spine 2001; 26:298–306.

45. Tomita T, Galicich JH, and Sundaresan N. Radiation therapy for spinal epidural metastases with complete block. Acta Radiol Oncol 1983; 22:135–143.

46. Weigel B, Maghsudi M, Neumann C, Kretschmer R, Muller FJ, Nerlich M. Surgical management of symptomatic spinal metastases: postoperative outcome and quality of life. Spine 1999; 24:2240–2246.

47. Weinstein JN. Surgical approach to spine tumors. Orthopaedics 1989; 12:897–905.

48. Weinstein JN, McLain RF. Primary tumors of the spine. Spine 1987; 12:843–851.

49. West JL. Posterior instrumentation for reconstruction in spine tumors. Sem Spine Surg 2000; 12:38–41.

50. White AA, Panjabi MM. Surgical constructs employing methylmethacrylate. In: White AA, Panjabi MM, eds. Clinical Biomechanics of the Spine. Philadelphia, PA: JB Lippincott; 1978:423–431.

51. Young RF, Post EM, King GA. Treatment of spinal epidural metastases. J Neurosurg 1980; 53:741–748.

32 Complex Lumbosacral Resection and Reconstruction Procedure

DARYL R. FOURNEY, MD, FRCSC AND ZIYA L. GOKASLAN, MD, FACS

CONTENTS

1. INTRODUCTION

Surgical resection, reconstruction, and internal fixation of the spine are often indicated in the management of patients with lumbosacral neoplasms. Because of the complex anatomy of this region, aggressive resections are technically demanding and often involve long operative times and significant blood loss. Some wide resections may require the purposeful sacrifice of nerve roots, with inherent functional consequences for the patient. In addition, the unique biomechanical features of the lumbosacral junction, combined with the destructive nature of neoplastic processes and the resection of such disease, present a challenging problem in terms of spinal reconstruction and stabilization. The purpose of this chapter is to review the important anatomic, biomechanical, and functional considerations of this region; to provide a step-by-step description of techniques for the resection of lumbosacral tumors; and to describe current methods of spinopelvic reconstruction and stabilization. Although the differential diagnosis of lumbosacral lesions is broad and includes inflammatory conditions as well as a variety of developmental abnormalities and cysts, the discussion here is limited to the management of neoplastic disease.

2. ANATOMICAL AND BIOMECHANICAL CONSIDERATIONS

The lumbosacral junction is a unique region of the spinal column because it is a transition zone in which the mobile lower lumbar segments meet the highly immobile sacrum and pelvis. Several factors contribute to unique load-bearing characteris-

tics within this region. One of these is that the lumbosacral junction is exposed to the largest loads borne by any area of the spine. In addition, although it has a greater range of motion than any thoracic or lumbar level in the sagittal (flexion-extension) plane, the lumbosacral junction has a very limited range of motion in the axial plane, as well as with rotation and lateral bending.

Because of the normal lordotic curvature of the lumbar spine, the lumbosacral intervertebral disk possesses a steep angle with respect to the horizontal. The lumbar spine therefore has a tendency to slip forward on the sacrum. The facet joints at L5/S1 are primarily responsible for resisting this tendency, aided by ligamentous and muscular elements. The facets are oriented very close to the coronal plane, a configuration that offers the most resistance to spondylolisthesis.

From the lumbosacral junction, the weight of the body is passed through the sacroiliac joints and on to the hips and lower limbs. The sacroiliac articulation is mostly a fibrocartilaginous amphiarthrodial joint (i.e., no synovial capsule). A small diarthrodial (i.e., synovial capsule present) portion is located along the ventral aspect of the joint. The mechanical stability of this joint is conferred primarily by three characteristics: (1) its wedge-like configuration, which locks the sacrum into the dorsal pelvic ring; (2) the complementary irregularities in the articular surfaces of the sacrum and ilium; and (3) most importantly, the incredibly strong supporting ligaments.

The forward tilt of the sacrum causes the body load to be transmitted to the ventral surface of the sacrum as a potential rotatory force, with the axis centered at S2. The dorsal ligamentous complex, including the interosseous and dorsal sacroiliac ligaments, are the strongest ligaments binding the sacrum to the

From: *Current Clinical Oncology: Cancer in the Spine: Comprehensive Care.*
Edited by: R. F. McLain, K-U. Lewandrowski, M. Markman, R. M. Bukowski,
R. Macklis, and E. C. Benzel © Humana Press, Inc., Totowa, NJ

ilium. These ligaments resist forward rotation at the upper end of the sacrum. The sacrospinous and sacrotuberous ligaments are primarily responsible for resisting the tendency of the lower end of the sacrum and coccyx to rotate dorsally.

3. FUNCTIONAL CONSIDERATIONS

In sacral resections for tumors, sacral nerve roots may have to be sacrificed. Intuitively, the resulting deficits (sensory and motor deficits, urinary and fecal incontinence, and sexual dysfunction) depend primarily on the level and number of nerve roots that are taken. However, factors that may account for variations in the functional results after sacral resection include (1) anatomical variability between subjects, (2) the patient's preoperative neurological status, (3) the surgical technique and approach used, (4) the nature of postoperative complications, (5) the amount of follow-up time, and (6) the varied criteria used to evaluate the neurological deficits. Nevertheless, in a review of the literature, Biagini et al. (1) found some consistent correlations between the level of sacral resection and the extent of postoperative deficits.

Patients with amputations distal to S3 (with removal of the last sacral roots and the coccygeal plexus) generally have very limited deficits, with preservation of sphincter function in the majority and some reduced perineal sensation. Sexual function may be decreased, however. The highest variability in functional results is seen for transverse resections of S2–S3 (including removal of one to all four roots of S2–S3). There is seldom any relevant motor deficit, however, many patients have saddle anesthesia and a significant reduction in sphincter control. Nevertheless, clinical observations by Stener et al. (2) indicate that functional urinary and fecal continence is generally achievable if at least one S2 nerve root is preserved. Section of the S1 roots or levels proximal to this result in clinically relevant motor deficits (walking with external support) associated with loss of sphincter control and sexual ability. Removal of sacral roots (S1–S5) on only one side, which was studied extensively by Stener and Gunterburg (3), results in unilateral deficits in strength and sensitivity, however, sphincter control may be either preserved or only partially compromised.

No matter the level of resection, damage to the lumbosacral trunks or sciatic nerves may cause serious postoperative motor and sensory deficits. Likewise, damage to the parasympathetic and sympathetic plexus can compromise sexual ability and sphincter function.

4. INDICATIONS FOR SURGERY

A detailed discussion of the evaluation of patients with lumbosacral lesions, the clinicopathological characteristics of specific tumor types, and the various treatment options for different tumors is beyond the scope of this chapter. However, a discussion of some of the general indications for surgery is warranted.

Most primary lumbosacral tumors are resistant to radiation therapy and chemotherapy. *En-bloc* resection, even if only marginal, therefore remains the most effective treatment for long-term disease control and potential cure in these patients. Primary tumors can be classified on the basis of their biological behavior as benign tumors, low-grade tumors that are locally invasive, and high-grade malignancies. Benign encapsulated tumors may be treated with simple lesional resection. *En-bloc* resection that includes a margin of uninvolved tissue is necessary to effect cure for patients with low-grade malignancies, such as giant cell tumor or chordoma (4,5), and is also indicated for some patients with localized high-grade malignancies such as osteogenic sarcoma. However, some very high-grade primary malignancies may be best managed with radiation therapy and chemotherapy. Simple intralesional curettage or cryosurgery for benign and low-grade tumors is generally discouraged because of unacceptably high rates of local recurrence (6).

In cases of metastatic tumors, the primary goal is palliation—namely, to restore or preserve neurological function and help alleviate pain. The treatment of these patients is highly individualized and depends on several factors, including the clinical presentation, tumor type, anticipated radio-sensitivity, anatomic location of the tumor and extent of any local invasion, presence of any extraspinal disease, integrity of the spinal column, and the medical fitness and life expectancy of the patient. Because the surgical treatment of metastatic lesions is generally not curative, it is important to consider the effect of treatment on the quality of further survival. General indications for surgical intervention (including tumor resection and spinal reconstruction) in patients with metastatic lumbosacral tumors include (1) radio-resistant tumor, (2) evidence of instability or bony compression, (3) progressive neurological deterioration, (4) previous radiation exposure, (5) recurrent tumor, and (6) uncertain diagnosis. With regard to the latter, the diagnosis of malignancy can frequently be established on the basis of needle biopsy findings.

In addition to hematogenous metastases from distal sites, the sacrum may be invaded locally by tumors arising from the pelvic viscera. Some patients with adenocarcinoma of the rectum that is adherent to or invading the distal sacrum may benefit from extended abdominoperineal resection, including sacral amputation. Total pelvic exenteration, including a portion of the sacrum, has been reported for patients with recurrent anorectal cancer (7). Careful patient selection is paramount in ensuring a favorable outcome from these aggressive procedures (8).

Patients referred for the resection of primary or metastatic lumbosacral tumors should be assessed completely for evidence of local and systemic spread. This may require computed tomography of the chest and abdomen as well as a bone scan. Cystoscopy may be necessary in the assessment of some pelvic tumors. Cancers of the rectum and pelvic organs must be thoroughly staged. Repeated radiographic and clinical staging studies may be indicated for patients with primary lumbosacral tumors initially considered inoperable as a result of advanced local spread of disease, because these patients may become candidates for surgery following neoadjuvant chemotherapy or other therapy.

The need for careful patient selection can never be understated. It is important to discuss the operation at length with the patient before surgery. Wide lumbosacral resections are associated with significant morbidity and involve inherent functional consequences with regard to bladder, bowel, and sexual functions.

5. PRE-OPERATIVE MANAGEMENT

Appropriate pre-operative planning requires a keen appreciation of the anatomic, biomechanical, and functional aspects of the lumbosacral region. familiarity with the advantages and limitations of the different exposures, and a clear sense of the surgical objective.

Wide sacral resections may be complicated by significant blood loss. Pre-operative angiographic embolization is a worthwhile consideration, especially for highly vascularized lesions such as giant cell tumor (9). Good vascular access, including the placement of large-bore intravenous catheters, is necessary in order to administer large volumes of fluids and blood. Central venous pressure monitoring is almost always needed, a Swan-Ganz catheter may be warranted in selected patients. We have generally avoided use of the cell saver because of the potential for tumor dissemination.

Special attention must be given to preparation of the bowel before any sacral procedures. The lower extent of posterior sacral incisions is very near the anus, and, thus, wound contamination is of great concern. With anterior approaches, there is the risk of inadvertently entering the bowel during the procedure. A low-residue diet is advisable for several days before hospitalization. Pre-operatively, mechanical cleaning of the bowel is carried out using GoLYTELY®. In addition, we generally administer prophylactic antibiotics, such as second-generation cephalosporins, both pre-operatively and in the immediate postoperative period.

6. LUMBOSACRAL POSTEROLATERAL TRANSPEDICULAR RESECTION

Many medically fit patients with symptomatic L5 or S1 vertebral body tumors are not candidates for radical lumbosacral resections. This group includes patients with metastatic disease and patients with primary lumbosacral disease that is locally advanced or associated with extraspinal disease considered unresponsive to systemic therapy. Although basic oncological principles do not justify wide resection in these patients, the decompression of tumor ventral to the thecal sac at L5 or S1 may yield symptomatic benefits for some patients. The posterolateral transpedicular approach is useful for ventral tumor decompression at L5/S1 (10,11). This approach affords satisfactory tumor decompression, posterior segmental fixation, and reconstruction of the vertebrectomy defect with polymethylmethacrylate (PMMA) all in one procedure. In addition, the potential for morbidity is less than that associated with anterior approaches at this level of the spine.

Although Steinman pins may be used to help secure the PMMA to the vertebral bodies, the senior author has had excellent results with the chest tube technique (10). This technique involves the placement of a chest tube into the corpectomy defect, followed by injection of PMMA cement into the tube through a hole. This provides a well-contained and well-placed interbody strut. At the L5 level, this method of reconstruction is essentially no different from that used at other lumbar levels. However, an S1 reconstruction is somewhat problematic because the S2 vertebral body has only a small surface area on which to fix the cement. Even if the polymer is successfully secured to

the rostral and caudal vertebral bodies with the chest tube, the reliability of the lateral fixation to the alae may be questionable. These constructs should, therefore, always be supplemented with posterior segmental fixation (11).

7. SACRAL RESECTION

The exposure of the sacrum is complicated by many factors, including its location deep within the pelvis, its intimate relationships with neurovascular structures and pelvic organs, its lateral iliac articulations, and the dorsal overhang of the iliac crests (12). In addition, owing to the capacity of the sacral canal and pelvis to accommodate regional expansion, tumors of the sacral region may attain enormous dimensions before they are detected clinically. Because of tumor size and the constraints posed by regional anatomy, the standard unidirectional approaches (anterior, posterior, perineal, lateral) are frequently combined in order to achieve an adequate exposure. Combined approaches may be performed simultaneously (14,15), performed consecutively under the same anesthetic, or staged. Although a simultaneous dorsal and ventral approach to the sacrum can be performed, in our hands the lateral position makes neither exposure optimal for midline tumors requiring a high sacral amputation, we, therefore, favor a staged approach to these lesions. We reserve the combined simultaneous anterior and posterior approaches for patients requiring hemisacrectomy and for exposure of tumors in the region of the sacroiliac joint (see Subheading 7.1.).

7.1. LATERAL APPROACH FOR RESECTION AT THE SACROILIAC JOINT

A combined anteroposterior approach to the sacroiliac joint is useful for the *en-bloc* resection of malignant tumors that involve not only the sacroiliac joint but also the lateral sacral ala and medial iliac wing (16). Chondrosarcoma, for example, is notorious for its often eccentric location within the sacrum and typically involves the sacroiliac joint (17).

The patient is placed in the lateral decubitus position for the procedure. A curved incision is made just above the margin of the iliac crest, beginning a few centimeters behind the anterior superior iliac spine. The incision extends to the lumbosacral junction where it is joined by a posterior midline lumbosacral incision. The fascia of the abdominal muscles is incised near the iliac crest, leaving a 1-cm-wide cuff attached to the crest to later facilitate closure. The iliacus muscle is stripped from the inner aspect of the iliac wing using a Cobb elevator. Blunt dissection using a sponge-covered elevator is recommended as the sacroiliac joint and greater sciatic notch is approached. Damage to the femoral nerve and major vessels is prevented by remaining deep to the iliacus muscle. The nearby lumbosacral trunk, which passes over the pelvic inlet medial to the ventral surface of the sacroiliac joint, is also at risk during these maneuvers. Medial retraction of the iliacus and psoas muscles as well as the overlying viscera completes the ventral exposure of the sacroiliac joint.

Posteriorly, the attachments of the lumbodorsal fascia and gluteus maximus are detached from the iliac crest. The gluteus maximus is raised with a Cobb elevator in a subperiosteal fashion. It is important to proceed with care in the region of the greater sciatic notch to avoid damage to the sciatic nerve and the superior gluteal vessels. The ipsilateral erector spinae muscles are divided transversely below the level of the sacroiliac joint and raised subperiosteally as a lumbosacral flap, which is retracted laterally and rostrally. Depending on the extent of tumor, additional posterior exposure may be gained by transecting the sacrospinous and sacrotuberous ligaments and the piriformis muscle.

With the superior gluteal vessels mobilized and the neural structures protected, a Gigli saw is passed through the greater sciatic notch and the iliac osteotomy is performed. The anterior structures are retracted medially, and the sacrum is osteotomized in a posteroanterior direction, beginning just lateral to the upper three dorsal foramina. Although others have recommend using a curved osteotome, we prefer to use a high-speed drill to create sacral osteotomies because it offers better hemostasis and finer control. A diamond burr does not tend to entrain the adjacent soft tissues. After completing the osteotomy, the entire specimen can be removed *en bloc*.

Osseous bleeding is controlled with bone wax, and soft tissue hemostasis is obtained. Suction drains are placed within the resection cavity. The gluteus maximus can sometimes be reapproximated to the midline fascia. Anteriorly, the closure is performed in layers. The aponeurosis of the abdominal muscles is reattached to the soft tissue cuff left on the iliac crest during the exposure.

7.2. LOW SACRAL AMPUTATION

The techniques of sacral amputation were popularized by Stener and Gunterberg *(2)*. It must be emphasized that the goal of these procedures is to achieve an *en-bloc* resection with a margin of healthy, uninvolved tissue. In general, sacral amputation should be carried out one complete segment above the rostral level of tumor involvement, as determined from preoperative imaging studies. Low sacrectomy (S3 or below) is relatively straightforward because the osteotomy is performed below the level of the sacroiliac joint and therefore is not inherently destabilizing. Low sacral amputation can be performed as a single-stage procedure through a combined posterior and transperineal route, as described by McCarty et al. in 1952 *(18)*. A staged abdominosacral procedure is required for more complicated cases, such as in patients with recurrent tumor or rectal involvement.

The patient is placed in a Kraske (flexed prone) position over padded bolsters to allow the abdomen to hang free and minimize compression of the inferior vena cava. After careful skin preparation, draping, and temporary closure of the anal orifice with a purse-string suture, a midline incision is made from the region of the lumbosacral junction to the coccyx. The dorsal exposure should be tailored to incorporate any biopsy incision as well as the underlying tract. The erector spinae muscles are usually dissected subperiosteally and retracted laterally. However, if pre-operative imaging studies show that the tumor extends dorsally out of the sacrum, a layer of sacrospinalis musculature and fat should be left to cover the involved regions. Depending on the extent of soft tissue involvement, it may also be advantageous to transect the gluteus maximus several centimeters from its origin, leaving a cuff of gluteal musculature attached to the sacrum laterally. The lateral sacrococcygeal

attachments including the sacrotuberous and sacrospinous ligaments and the coccygeal and piriform muscles are then identified and transected close to their insertions. The pudendal and sciatic nerves as well as the gluteal arteries are carefully identified and preserved. The inferior edge of the sacroiliac joint is cleared of soft tissue using a Cobb elevator.

Division of the anococcygeal ligament allows entry into the presacral space. The rectum is gently mobilized away from the tumor surface by blunt-finger dissection. A limited sacral laminectomy, immediately rostral to the level of intended amputation, allows direct visualization of the nerve roots. For example, if the intent is to amputate the sacrum at the S2–S3 level with preservation of the third sacral nerve roots, a laminectomy from S1 to S3 is performed. The filum terminale externa is transected and the nerve roots below S3 are doubly ligated and transected within the sacral canal. The roots are also divided just distal to their exit from the ventral sacral foramina. An osteotomy of the sacral body is then performed using a high-speed drill with a diamond burr. The pelvic structures are protected during the osteotomy by keeping a finger in the presacral space. This maneuver also provides tactile sensation to help guide the osteotomy. The coccyx is included with the specimen.

Excellent hemostasis is essential because wide sacral resection results in a large cavity with the potential for postoperative hematoma or seroma formation. Suction drains are placed, and the wound is reapproximated in a layered fashion. Local soft-tissue flaps may be necessary to fill the defect and to facilitate a tensionless closure. Finally, the rectal purse-string suture is released.

7.3. HIGH SACRAL AMPUTATION

High (above S3) sacral amputation utilizing a staged ventral and dorsal approach was initially reported by Bowers in 1948 *(19)*. The authors favor staged rather than combined exposure, as discussed previously. This technique is very similar to that described by Stener and Gunterberg *(2)* (Fig. 1). The use of a transpelvic vertical rectus abdominis myocutaneous (VRAM) flap for the reconstruction of large sacral defects has significantly reduced problems with wound breakdown in our patients *(20)*.

The first stage is the transabdominal exposure, for which the patient is positioned supine. A midline celiotomy is performed. The abdomen contents are initially inspected to confirm the resectability of the tumor and to ensure that there are no other intra-abdominal masses that would preclude curative resection. The bowel is packed off, and the ureters and internal iliac vessels are identified and dissected free. Moistened umbilical tapes are loosely applied to secure the common iliac arteries and veins. The common iliac vessels must be completely mobilized. The internal iliac vessels as well as the anterior and lateral sacral vessels are all identified, ligated, and transected. Although the sacrum is somewhat devascularized by transection of the vessels, hemostasis of the robust presacral venous plexus is often difficult. If the rectum is to be spared, the retrorectal peritoneal reflection is incised, and the rectosigmoid colon is dissected away from the tumor capsule. The tumor is exposed carefully so that as much normal fatty presacral tissue as possible is included with the specimen.

The ventral sacral foramina serve as the best landmarks to guide the ventral sacral osteotomy, although the level may also

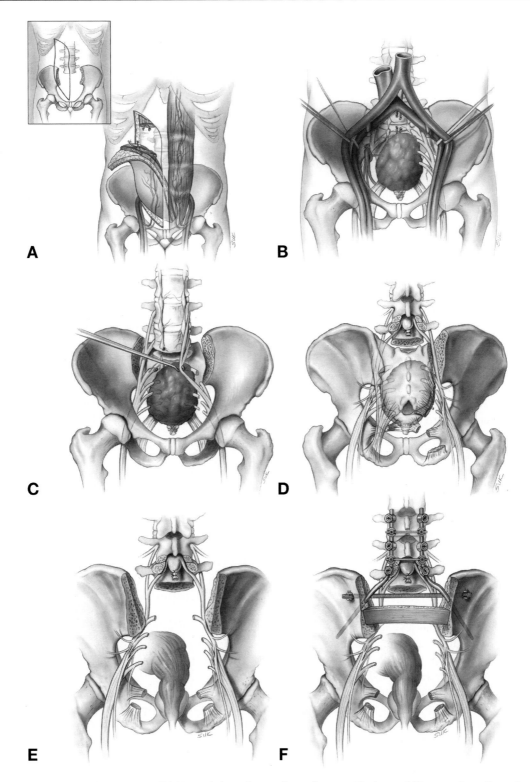

Fig. 1. Operative fields during total sacrectomy. **(A)** Ventral view after median celiotomy. The internal iliac vessels are ligated and the common iliac vessels are mobilized to provide a clear view of the L5–S1 disc space and the lumbosacral trunks. **(B)** Ventral view with the vessels removed. The nerve roots at S1–S3 are transected laterally and sacroiliac osteotomies are performed. **(C)** Ventral view of the abdominal wall. The vertical rectus abdominis myocutaneous flap is harvested based on the inferior epigastric vessels. **(D)** Dorsal view with the patient placed in the flexed-prone position (second stage). An L5 laminectomy, bilateral L5–S1 foraminotomies, an L5–S1 discectomy, and bilateral dorsal sacroiliac osteotomies are performed. The thecal sac is ligated distal to the takeoff of the L5 nerve roots bilaterally. **(E)** Dorsal view following total sacrectomy. The lumbar trunks and sciatic nerves are preserved. The cut ends of the sacrotuberous and sacrospinous ligaments are depicted. The dorsal rectal wall is visualized. **(F)** Dorsal view after reconstruction and stabilization. Pedicle screws at L3–L5 are attached to rods embedded between the cortices of the remaining ilia as per the Galveston technique. A threaded transiliac rod is placed ventral to the Galveston rods but dorsal to the lumbar trunk. A tibial allograft bridges the defect between the remaining ilia. (Reproduced with permission from ref. *23*.)

be confirmed using intra-operative radiography or fluoroscopy. At approximately one sacral level above the region of the planned osteotomy, the periosteum is incised transversely and reflected downward. The sympathetic trunks are unavoidably transected with this maneuver, along with the hypogastric plexus in the case of very high sacral amputations. If the planned osteotomy incorporates any of the ventral sacral foramina, the sacral nerves exiting at that level are first dissected out and preserved. It is not possible to spare any sacral nerves if the osteotomy must cross the body of S1 above the foramina. The sacral alae are dissected laterally, and the lumbosacral nerve trunks are exposed and freed. The nerve trunks are mobilized laterally during the osteotomy.

The anterior osteotomy only incises the anterior cortical bone and should not go deep enough to damage the dural contents. We prefer to use a high-speed drill with a diamond burr rather than an osteotome. The osteotomy proceeds inferolaterally to incorporate a small portion of the sacroiliac joints and anterior ilium. It is important to be able to feel the lateral extent of the anterior osteotomy through the sciatic notch as a guide during the posterior osteotomy.

If the rectum is to be included with the specimen, the superior rectal vessels are identified and ligated and the rectosigmoid junction is mobilized in preparation for division with a mechanical stapler. The bowel is transected, and the middle rectal vessels are ligated. The stapled stumps of bowel may be oversewn to decrease the risk of wound soilage. When the tumor involves other pelvic organs or the endopelvic fascia, pelvic excenteration is required if the surgery is to be curative.

A Silastic sheet may be placed into the plane of dissection between the sacral specimen with its associated presacral mass, and the ventral structures, including the iliac vessels, ureters, and sacral plexi. The VRAM flap, which is based on the inferior epigastric vessels, is harvested and secured within the pelvis until it is needed for the posterior closure. The anterior abdominal wall is closed in the standard fashion.

We previously preferred to stage these complex procedures on separate days. However, performing the two stages sequentially under the same anesthetic has several advantages. During the anterior procedure, the distal gastrointestinal tract is denervated, resulting in a consistent postoperative ileus. As a result, the second stage was previously delayed for 10 to 14 d. Because of concerns about maintaining flap viability during this prolonged interval, the VRAM flap was not harvested until the beginning of the second stage. Thus, the celiotomy incision had to be reopened with the patient in the supine position before we could proceed with the posterior approach. With more experience, we can now complete the entire operation (both the anterior and posterior stages) in 12 to 14 h.

The second stage begins with the patient in the Kraske (flexed prone) position on padded bolsters. The abdomen should be allowed to hang free. The anal orifice is temporarily closed with a purse-string suture. A midline incision is created from the tip of the coccyx to the lower lumbar level. If the rectum is to be included with the resection, the caudal end of the incision also involves a circumferential incision about the anus. Any skin and underlying soft tissue that are involved by tumor

or may be seeded with tumor cells as a consequence of a percutaneous biopsy should be incorporated with the specimen *en bloc*. Mobilizing the lumbosacral fascia and muscles rostrally rather than laterally permits a wide lateral and caudal exposure without causing ischemic damage and retractor-related muscular injury (Fig. 2).

Lateral flaps are elevated to expose the iliac crest. The gluteus maximus is transected while leaving a cuff of tissue attached to the sacrum. The underlying piriform muscles are also divided bilaterally. The superior and inferior gluteal vessels and the sciatic, pudendal, and posterior cutaneous femoral nerves should be identified and protected. If the resection is to spare the rectum, the anococcygeal ligament is divided and the sacrotuberous and sacrospinous ligaments as well as the coccygeal muscles are divided. If the rectum is to be included, the levator musculature is divided and the anus is freed circumferentially.

A wide L5 and upper sacral laminectomy is completed to expose the dural sac. The dural sac is doubly ligated and transected just below the exit of the last nerve root to be preserved. The floor of the sacral canal can thus be exposed for the dorsoventral osteotomy.

The ventral osteotomy cuts are palpated by introducing a finger presacrally via the perineal exposure, allowing the dorsal osteotomy to be guided tactilely. The osteotomy is performed in two stages, each beginning in the midline and extending through the lateral sacroiliac joint to exit at the greater sacroiliac notch. Once the specimen is freed, the sacral roots, which have already been sacrificed within the spinal canal, are divided just proximal to their connections with the sciatic nerve. Hemostasis is achieved with bone wax and electrocautery. The gluteal muscles may be re-approximated to each other or to bone. Suction drains are placed deep in the wound and tunneled to remote exit sites. The large sacral defect is closed using the VRAM flap, which is retrieved from the pelvis and sutured into place in a layered fashion. As an alternative, a microvascular free flap reconstruction may be performed. Free flap reconstruction is challenging in the sacral area because it is difficult to access adequate recipient vessels *(21)*. Gluteal rotation flaps are not a reliable option *(20)*.

If the rectum has been spared, the anal purse-string suture is removed. Patients with rectal resections are again turned to the supine position, and the celiotomy is reopened. Omental grafting of peritoneal defects may be required and a colostomy is completed. Lumbosacral reconstruction and stabilization is performed in the majority of cases (*see* Subheading 7.6.).

7.4. HEMISACRECTOMY

Hemisacrectomy generally involves unilateral removal of the sacroiliac joint and a portion of the ilium along with the hemisacrum. It may be performed as part of a more extensive internal or external hemipelvectomy *(22)*. The approach involves combined simultaneous retroperitoneal and posterior exposures with the patient in the lateral decubitus position. Dorsal and ventral osteotomies can thus be performed under direct vision. Resection of all the sacral nerves on one side results in expected deficits in sensitivity and strength, however, sphincter function may be normal or only partially compromised *(2)*.

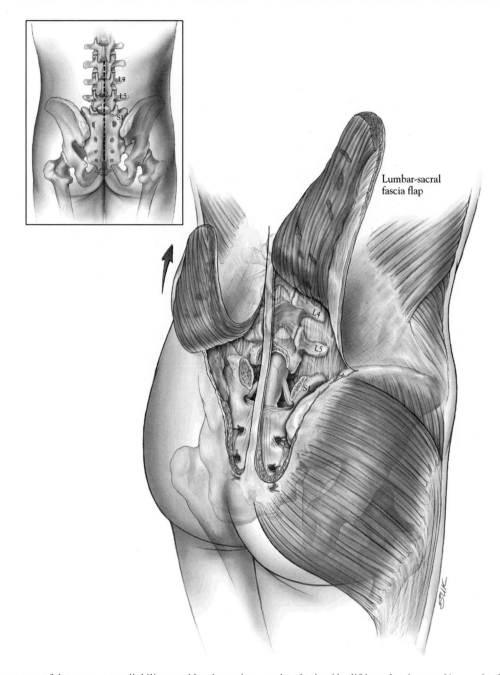

Fig. 2. Posterior exposure of the sacrum, medial ilium and lumbar spine may be obtained by lifting a lumbosacral/muscular flap off the sacrum and retracting it cephalad and laterally. Inset: The dashed line represents the posterior incision (Reproduced with permission from ref. *11*.)

7.5. TOTAL SACRECTOMY

Few cases of total sacrectomy have been reported in the literature *(23,24)*. Although it is not possible to spare any of the sacral roots during this procedure, careful preservation of the L4 and L5 nerve roots allows patients to ambulate postoperatively. Urinary bladder, rectosigmoid colon, and sexual functions are markedly altered, although manageable with rehabilitation.

The technique is essentially the same as that described for high sacral amputation, with some exceptions (Figs. 1 and 3). In the anterior approach, bilateral ventral osteotomies are performed along the entire length of the sacroiliac joints with the

lumbar nerve roots and lumbosacral trunks protected medially. Instead of a transverse osteotomy through the upper sacrum, a complete L5–S1 discectomy is performed. Finally, the S1–S3 ventral nerve roots are transected at their foramina, if they can be visualized. During the second stage of the procedure, an L5 laminectomy and bilateral L5–S1 foraminotomies are done to expose the L5 nerve roots, which are preserved. The posterior aspect of the iliac crests are removed with Leksell rongeurs, and a high-speed drill is used to complete the sacroiliac osteotomies from the posterior approach. The thecal sac is then ligated below the level of the L5 nerve roots, and the L5–S1 discectomy is completed. The sciatic notches are exposed bilat-

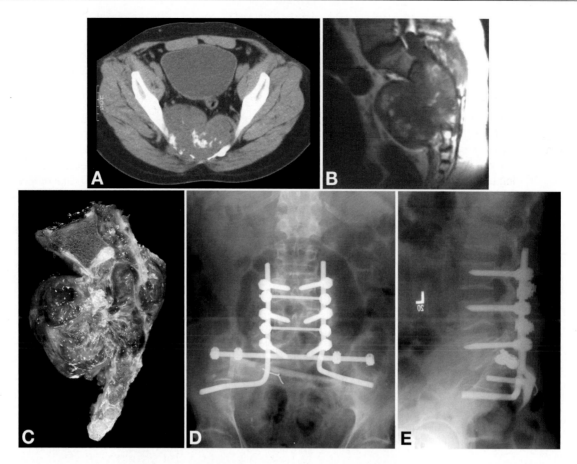

Fig. 3. Pre-operative computed tomography (CT) scan (**A**) and sagittal magnetic resonance imaging (**B**) reveal a sacral chordoma. (*Lower Left*) Hemisection of the gross pathological specimen (**C**) demonstrates complete *en-bloc* resection of the sacrum. Postoperative anteroposterior (**D**) and lateral (**E**) radiographs show the modified Galveston rod construct with lumbar pedicle screws, cross-links, the tibial allograft, and the transiliac threaded rod. (Reproduced with permission from ref. *11*.)

erally, and the S1–S5 roots are transected. Following division of the posterior ligamentous attachments, the sacrum can be removed *en bloc*. Lumboilial fixation is performed using a modification of the Galveston rod technique (*see* Subheading 7.7.2.). As described for high sacral amputation, resection of the rectum may be incorporated into the procedure, and the VRAM flap is routinely used to close the sacral defect.

7.6. LUMBOSACRAL RECONSTRUCTION AND STABILIZATION

In the resection of sacral tumors, spinopelvic stability is not greatly affected if the sacroiliac joints are left intact *(2,25)*. Although the sacrospinous and sacrotuberous ligaments are often transected in lower sacral amputations, the strong dorsal ligamentous complex confers stability. Gunterberg et al. *(25)* evaluated pelvic strength after major amputations of the sacrum. Fifteen cadaver pelvises were loaded to failure: five unresected, five after resection of the sacrum between S1 and S2, and five after resection about 1 cm below the promontory. In these dissections, the second group (resections between S1 and S2) had approximately one-third of the sacroiliac joint and the associated ligamentous structures resected. The third group (resection below the promontory) had approximately one-half of the sacroiliac joint and ligamentous structures removed. Weakening of the pelvic ring amounted to approx 30% in the second

group and 50% in the third group. In all of these experiments, the load to failure far exceeded physiological loads. The authors therefore concluded that weight-bearing was safe for patients after sacral resection, as long as 50% or more of the sacroiliac joint (corresponding to at least the upper half of the S1 segment) remained intact. Clinical reports have supported these conclusions *(26–28)*. Some partial sacrectomies may involve resection of a sacroiliac joint on only one side. Although such resections can be performed successfully without reconstruction, the patient may experience pain from proximal migration of the pelvis. We believe that some form of fixation is required in most of these cases, unless the contralateral joint is completely intact and there is no anterior pelvic deficiency *(29)*. Total sacrectomy results in complete dissociation of the spine from the pelvis and requires complex iliolumbar reconstruction for adequate mechanical support to preserve satisfactory walking ability *(11,23)*.

7.7. LUMBOSACRAL AND SPINOPELVIC FIXATION SYSTEMS

7.7.1.Sublaminar Devices, Hooks, Screws, Screw Plates, Intrasacral Rods, and Iliac Screw Fixation

Some of the earliest instrumentation methods for achieving fixation to the pelvis involved sublaminar wires or cables. However, the sacral laminae are often thin and inadequate to accommodate sublaminar devices. Luque *(30)* described a rod-sublaminar wire construct that involved driving the distal rods through the pelvic wings with a bicortical purchase. However, this method of fixation does not provide substantial resistance to extension or torsional loads. Fusion rates similar to those achieved without internal fixation have been reported. Sublaminar fixation in the lumbosacropelvic region has therefore been largely abandoned *(31)*.

Distraction instrumentation across the lumbosacral junction using hooks, such as with Harrington and Knodt rods, often results in poor fixation on weak sacral laminae. Although the sacral laminae are usually not strong enough to accommodate a compression hook, devices involving compression hooks distal to S1 screws have strength similar to that of intrasacral rods *(32)*.

Screws provide rigid stabilization and can be used for short-segment fixation across the lumbosacral junction. In a recent review of 100 consecutive procedures involving pedicle screw fixation for the management of malignant spinal tumors, the rate of screw-related late instrumentation failure was only 2% *(33)*. The S1 pedicle is larger than the lumbar pedicles and often can be fitted with 7- to 8-mm screws. Additional bony purchase can be obtained if the screw penetrates the anterior S1 cortex or the superior end plate of S1. Medially directed S1 pedicle screws that are cross-linked and attached to rods create a triangulation effect, which greatly increases torsional stability and resists pullout *(34–37)*. Triangulation with an oblique orientation also interferes less with the superjacent facet joint and allows more purchase with a longer screw *(38)*.

A method to enhance sacral fixation with screws is to place an additional pair of laterally directed bone screws into the sacral alae below the S1 level. This has a biomechanical advantage over a single pair of S1 pedicle screws *(35)*, however, the bone of the ala is usually of low density, and purchase may be tenuous *(32)*. Moreover, the risk of neurovascular injury from laterally directed screws in this region must be kept in mind.

Screw-plate devices such as the Tacoma plate (Sofamor-Danek, Memphis, TN) permit the insertion of multiple sacral screws and may be easily attached to the proximal lumbar component of the instrumentation. These plates provide a template for the insertion of laterally directed alar screws after placement of the S1 pedicle screws.

S2 (or lower level) pedicle screws are often of little use because the pedicles are very short. Biomechanical testing has shown that pedicle screws placed below the S1 level do not significantly enhance stability *(35)*. In addition, the thin sagittal dimension of the sacrum at lower levels increases the risk of penetration of its ventral surface, with a potential for injury to the adjacent vascular and visceral structures. Screws at lower sacral levels are often prominent dorsally and may even tent the overlying skin.

Sacral screw fixation may be sufficient for cases in which the fixation length is short (one or two levels) and there is minimal instability. If a long construct is placed, the sacral attachment is subjected to large cantilevered forces that may lead to screw pullout. Finally, the use of sacral screws may be precluded in certain cases, such as when the pedicles, body, or ala of the sacrum is involved with tumor.

A method to supplement sacral fixation has been devised that involves inserting rods into the lateral sacral bony masses distal to their connections with S1 pedicle screws *(39)*. These intrasacral rods provide fixation at a significant distance from the axis of rotation of the lumbosacral junction, thereby increasing the ability of the construct to resist flexion moments. The use of intrasacral rods also permits longer lever arms without having to cross the sacroiliac joint and involve the iliac crest. Obviously, this method cannot be used if the lateral sacral bony masses have been resected or are weakened by neoplastic disease.

A simple method of sacropelvic fixation involves the placement of long, variable-angle bone screws obliquely across the sacroiliac joint into the iliac bones. A tripod effect may be gained by combining the sacroiliac fixation with additional sacral fixation points *(40)*. Although this technique is relatively simple to perform, its disadvantages include those related to the placement of pedicle screws caudal to the S1 segment, as previously described.

7.7.2. Galveston Fixation

Allen and Ferguson *(41)* from Galveston, TX, were the first to describe a technique involving the insertion of an angled distal limb of a spinal fixation rod into the posterior iliac bones, just above the sciatic notch. Although the Galveston technique originally involved segmental spinal fixation using sublaminar techniques, we have employed lumbar pedicle screw fixation *(23)*. In addition, we place cross-links between the rods (Fig. 4).

The Galveston technique has become the benchmark for other spinopelvic fixation systems, however, the custom bending and insertion of the rod requires some technical skill to achieve the correct position with the rod remaining intracortical. Tube benders are used to create an initial sacro-iliac bend of approx 60°, and then a table vice is used to stabilize the distal ilial segment of the rod while an approx 110° lumbosacral bend is created (Fig. 5). Preformed rods are also available. Another option are iliac screws (ISOLA iliac screws, Depuy, Raynham, MA), which can be placed independently of the spinal rod, with the two subsequently linked together.

In the biomechanical testing of 10 different lumbosacral instrumentation techniques in a bovine model, McCord et al. *(35)*. found that the most effective construct entailed medially directed S1 pedicle screws and an iliac purchase in the Galveston-type fashion. The key structural element of this construct is mostly related to the resistance to flexion conferred by the anterior purchase obtained with iliac rods wedged between the hard cortical bone above the sciatic notch.

McCord et al. *(35)* explained the key to the strength of the Galveston construct by introducing the concept of the lumbosacral "pivot point." This point is located at the intersection of the osteoligamentous column in the sagittal plane and the lumbosacral intervertebral disc in the transverse plane. It represents the axis of rotation at the lumbosacral junction. The iliac rod in the Galveston technique extends anterior to the lumbosacral pivot point, providing a long lever arm within the ilium to counteract flexion moments exerted by the lumbar spine.

A concern about the Galveston technique is the theoretical problem of the instrumentation crossing the unfused sacroiliac joint. Cadaveric studies have revealed that autofusion of this

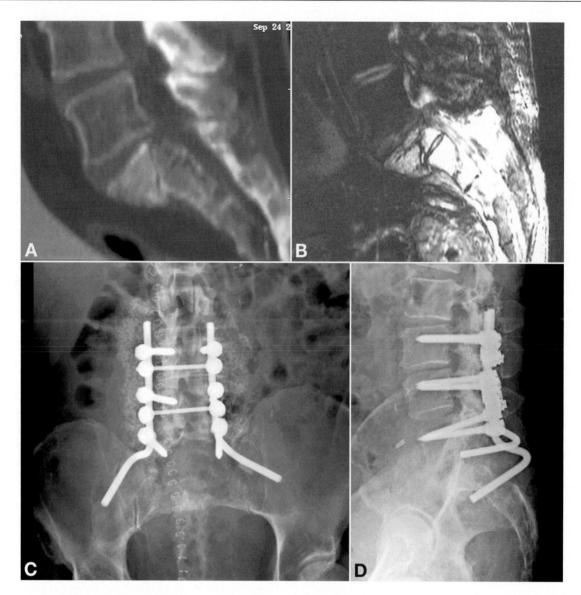

Fig. 4. Reconstructed sagittal computed tomography image (**A**) and sagittal magnetic resonance imaging (**B**) reveals metastatic renal cell carcinoma of S1 and an associated pathological fracture in a patient who presented with pain due to instability. Galveston stabilization was performed, as seen in the postoperative anteroposterior (**C**) and lateral (**D**) radiographs.

joint occurs in 75% of adults aged 50 yr or older *(42)*. In addition, we have not found fixation across the sacroiliac joint to be a problem in our series *(11)* or in other series *(43,44)*. Another reported disadvantage is that the rods lie within cancellous bone, any change in the orientation of the rods after the iliac limb has been implanted creates a small void in the bone with the potential for loosening. A 2- to 3-mm lucency around the iliac portion of the rod is often visible on X-ray studies, however, in our experience, this finding alone does not indicate construct failure or pseudoarthrosis.

7.8. RECONSTRUCTION FOLLOWING TOTAL SACRECTOMY

Total sacrectomy results in complete spinopelvic dissociation and requires technically challenging reconstructive techniques. A number of different constructs for reconstruction following total sacrectomy have been described in the litera-

ture. Some of the more frequently used methods involve the placement of transverse sacral bars *(45,46)* or Steinmann pins *(47,48)* to connect the posterior iliac wings. Sometimes, these bars are placed through the L5 vertebral body *(45)*. These devices may then be connected to the spinal instrumentation, such as Harrington rods *(45)* or Cotrel-Dubousset rods *(46–48)*. Massive bone grafting from the posterolateral aspects of the distal lumbar segments to the iliac wings bilaterally is performed. The major disadvantage of these constructs relates to the soft bone of the posterior ilium, which does not provide firm fixation. Additionally, these methods provide poor rotational stability *(47)*. The hook-and-rod systems used may accidentally disengage from the transverse sacral bars or Steinmann pins.

An alternative form of reconstruction for large sacral defects is the implantation of a prosthesis *(49)*. A custom-made device is required to fit the individual shape of the pelvis and accom-

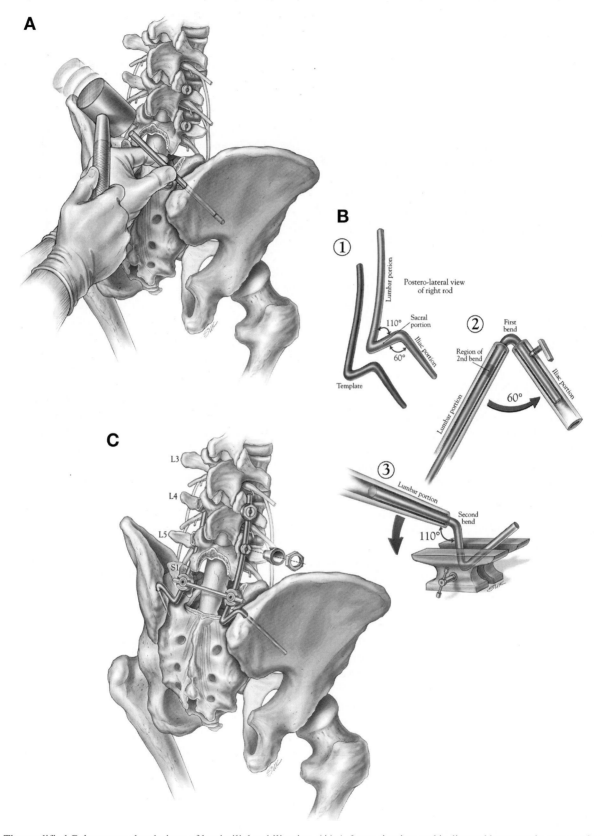

Fig. 5. The modified Galveston rod technique of lumboilial stabilization. (**A**) A 6-mm titanium rod is directed between the two cortices of the ilium to a depth of 6 to 9 cm to reach a point 1.5 cm above the sciatic notch. This temporary rod is used to create a path for the contoured rod. A 6-mm titanium rod is then contoured to match the template rod (wire) (**B1**). Tube benders are used to create the 60° sacroiliac bend (**B2**). A table vice is used to stabilize the sacral and iliac segments of the rod while a 110° bend is created between the lumbar and sacral segment (**B3**). Finally, the Galveston rod is tapped into the ilium and attached to the lumbar pedicle screws (**C**). Cross-links are placed between the rods. (Reproduced with permission from ref. *11*.)

modate for the amount of resection performed. The major disadvantage of a custom-made prosthesis is that it is impossible to make adjustments during surgery.

In cases requiring total sacrectomy, we supplement the Galveston technique by placing a threaded transiliac rod to resist axial rotation of the lumboiliac union (Fig. 1). This threaded rod helps reconstruct the pelvic ring, thereby preventing the open-book phenomenon. The rod is placed more anteriorly on the ilium, which avoids the slippage associated with anchorage into the softer posterior ilium. Locking collars are placed to prevent lateral migration of the rod. An alternative to the threaded rod (although the authors have not used this) is to place a large pelvic reconstruction plate, with pedicle screws at the fifth lumbar vertebra going through the plate and bicortical screws securing the plate to each iliac wing *(24)*.

Extensive bone grafting is essential to obtain a fusion. In addition to placing autogenous and allogenic corticocancellous bone extending from the transverse processes to the ilium bilaterally, the authors place a tibial allogenic strut graft to close the space between the two ilia and help facilitate fusion of the entire defect (Fig. 1).

After surgery, the patient remains in bed for 6 to 8 wk in order to allow at least a fibrous union of the reconstruction before the patient is mobilized. Although bone fusion takes a minimum of 6 mo, this fibrous union may be quite effective at providing enough structural support for ambulation. A thoracolumbosacral orthosis may be used for the first 6 mo after total sacrectomy, but may not be necessary in all cases.

In the authors' series of 13 patients who underwent Galveston fixation following the resection of metastatic or locally aggressive neoplasms of the lumbosacral region *(11)*, including 5 patients who required total sacrectomy, solid bone fusion was achieved in 4 (31%) and partial or unilateral fusion in 3 (23%). Five patients (38%) had no convincing evidence of fusion on radiographic studies. Because three of these five patients improved clinically, a satisfactory fibrous union may have occurred. Radiation therapy, chemotherapy, and neoplastic disease processes may have contributed to the lack of bony fusion in some patients. Only one hardware-related complication occurred: the rods fractured bilaterally at the transition point between the lumbar and sacral segments in one patient. This was corrected with double iliolumbar rod fixation. Ambulatory status improved in 62% (eight patients), and spine-related pain, as reflected by visual analog pain scores and medication consumption, was significantly reduced in 85% of our patients.

7.9. POSTOPERATIVE CARE

Patients undergoing major lumbosacral resections are managed in an intensive care unit postoperatively. Because a significant amount of blood is often lost during these procedures, ongoing assessment of fluid and blood product requirements is essential. Nursing the patient on an air bed helps prevent wound breakdown and decubitus ulcers. The wound should be observed closely for the development of infection, hematoma, or seroma. Antibiotics are continued until all suction drains have been removed from the wound. Pneumatic compression devices applied to the lower extremities and/or small intermittent doses

of subcutaneous heparin are important for the prevention of deep vein thrombosis. Denervation of the distal gastrointestinal tract during high sacral resections almost uniformly results in a significant postoperative ileus, with some patients requiring intravenous nutrition for a prolonged period.

Patients are mobilized as soon as possible, depending on functional reserve and the perceived stability of the dorsal pelvic ring. The input of rehabilitation physicians is essential for patients who undergo aggressive sacral resections. Progressive independence with walking, competence with intermittent catheterization, and management of fecal incontinence are some of the goals of rehabilitative therapy. The input of psychosexual counselors and reproductive health specialists may be valuable with regard to sexual function issues.

7.10. PITFALLS AND COMPLICATIONS

The highest incidence of wound infection in patients who undergo complex spinopelvic fixation is seen those who receive pre-operative radiation therapy. The authors routinely use soft tissue reconstructive techniques such as the transpelvic VRAM flap or a microvascular free flap to help reduce the risk of wound complications for patients who require high sacral resection or total sacrectomy.

Early failure of the lumbosacral instrumentation (i.e., within 6–12 wk) is usually owing to screw pullout. This is most commonly caused by repetitive stress at the bone-metal interface. If hook-and-rod systems are used, early failure may result from laminar fracture. Early failure of the construct may be prevented by the use of multiple sites of fixation in order to best distribute the forces at the bone-implant junction. In some cases, early loosening of the instrumentation may not prevent solid bony fusion, however, close radiological follow-up is required. Delaying revision surgery is reasonable until it is certain that it is required to achieve an acceptable result.

Reoperation is recommended if evidence of progressive deformity or painful pseudoarthrosis is observed. Revision surgery should address the cause for failure. For example, metal fatigue fracture suggests poor load sharing in the original construct, and new fixation points may need to be added. Screw pullout suggests the need for larger-diameter or longer bone screws to obtain a solid bony purchase on additional cortices. PMMA may enhance screw fixation in the setting of poor-quality bone. Finally, a more complex construct, such as the Galveston technique, may be required.

Surgery for failed spinal fixation should always involve additional bone grafting, preferably with autologous bone. Interbody fusion may be done to augment the dorsolateral fusion in some cases. No rigid ventral stabilizing device can be easily applied to the sacrum, although interbody grafts (allogenic or autogenic), cages, and techniques using PMMA *(11)* may be applied at the lumbosacral junction.

REFERENCES

1. Biagini R, Ruggieri P, Mercuri M, et al. Neurologic deficit after resection of the sacrum. Chir Organi Mov 1997; 82:357–372.
2. Stener B, Gunterberg B. High amputation of the sacrum for extirpation of tumors. Principles and technique. Spine 1978; 3:351–366.
3. Gunterberg B, Norlen L, Stener B, Sundin T. Neurological evaluation after resection of the sacrum. Invest Urol 1975; 13:183–188.

4. Turcotte RE, Sim FH, Unni KK. Giant cell tumor of the sacrum. Clin Orthop Relat Res 1993; 291:215–221.

5. York J, Kaczaraj A, Abi-Said D, et al. Sacral chordoma: 40-year experience at a major cancer center. Neurosurgery 1999; 44:74–80.

6. Camins M, Oppenheim J, Perrin R. Tumors of the vertebral axis: Benign, primary malignant, and metastatic tumors. In: Youmans J, ed. Neurological Surgery. Vol. 2. Philadelphia, PA: W. B. Saunders; 1996:3134–3167.

7. Weber KL, Nelson H, Gunderson LL, Sim FH. Sacropelvic resection for recurrent anorectal cancer. A multidisciplinary approach. Clin Orthop Relat Res 2000; 372:231–240.

8. Moffat F, Falk R. Radical surgery for extensive rectal cancer: is it worthwhile? Recent Results Cancer Res 1998; 146:71–83.

9. Broaddus WC, Grady MS, Delashaw JB, Ferguson RD, Jane JA. Pre-operative superselective arteriolar embolization: a new approach to enhance resectability of spinal tumors. Neurosurgery 1990; 27:755–759.

10. Akeyson E, McCutcheon I. Single-stage posterior vertebrectomy and replacement combined with posterior instrumentation for spinal metastasis. J Neurosurg 1996; 85:211–220.

11. Jackson R, Gokaslan Z. Spinal-pelvic fixation in patients with lumbosacral neoplasms. J Neurosurg (Spine 1) 2000; 92:61–70.

12. McCormick P, Post K. Surgical approaches to the sacrum. In: Doty J, Rengachary S, eds. Surgical Disorders of the Sacrum. New York, NY: Thieme, 1994:257–265.

13. Esses S, Botsford D. Surgical anatomy and operative approaches to the sacrum. In: Frymoyer J, ed. The Adult Spine: Principles and Practice. Vol. 2. Philadelphia, PA: Lippincott-Raven; 1997:2329–2341.

14. Localio S, Eng K, Ranson J. Abdominosacral approach for retrorectal tumors. Ann Surg 1980; 191:555–560.

15. Huth JF, Dawson EG, Eilber FR. Abdominosacral resection for malignant tumors of the sacrum. Am J Surg 1984; 148:157–161.

16. McDonald J, Lane J. Surgical approaches to the sacroiliac joint. In: Sundaresan N, Schidek H, Schiller A, Rosenthal D, eds. Tumors of the Spine: Diagnosis and Clinical Management. Philadelphia, PA: W. B. Saunders; 1996:426–431.

17. Camins M, Duncan A, Smith J, Marcove R. Chondrosarcoma of the spine. Spine 1978; 3:202–209.

18. McCarty C, Waugh J, Mayo C, Coventry M. The surgical treatment of presacral tumors: a combined problem. Proc Staff Meet Mayo Clin 1952; 27:73–84.

19. Bowers R. Giant cell tumor of the sacrum. A case report. Ann Surg 1948; 1:1164–1172.

20. Miles WK, Chang DW, Kroll SS, et al. Reconstruction of large sacral defects following total sacrectomy. Plas Reconstr Surg 2000; 105:2387–2394.

21. Hung S, Chen H, Wei F. Free flaps for reconstruction of the lower back and sacral area. Microsurgery 2000; 20:72–76.

22. Karakousis C, Emrich L, Driscoll D. Variants of hemipelvectomy and their complications. Am J Surg 1989; 158:404–408.

23. Gokaslan Z, Romsdahl M, Kroll S, et al. Total sacrectomy and Galveston L-rod reconstruction for malignant neoplasms. J Neurosurg 1997; 87:781–787.

24. Spiegel DA, Richardson WJ, Scully SP, Harrelson JM. Long-term survival following total sacrectomy with reconstruction for the treatment of primary osteosarcoma of the sacrum. A case report. J Bone Joint Surg Am 1999; 81:848–855.

25. Gunterberg B, Romanus B, Stener B. Pelvic strength after major amputation of the sacrum. Acta Orthop Scand 1976; 47:635–642.

26. Hayes R. Resection of the sacrum for benign giant cell tumor: a case report. Ann Surg 1953; 138:115–120.

27. Localio S, Francis K, Rossano P. Abdominosacral resection of sacrococcygeal chordoma. Ann Surg 1967; 166:394–402.

28. Gennari L, Azzarelli A, Guagliuolo V. A posterior approach for the excision of sacral chordoma. J Bone Joint Surg Br 1987; 69:565–568.

29. Bridwell K. Management of tumors at the lumbosacral junction. In: Margulies J, Floman Y, Farcy J-P, Neuwirth M, eds. Lumbosacral and Spinopelvic Fixation. Philadelphia, PA: Lippincott-Raven; 1996:109–122.

30. Luque E. Segmental spinal instrumentation for correction of scoliosis. Clin Orthop 1982; 163:192–198.

31. Ogilvie J, Bradford D. Sublaminar fixation in lumbosacral fusions. Clin Orthop 1991; 269:157–161.

32. Ogilvie J, Transfedt E, Wood K. Overview of fixation to the sacrum and pelvis in spinal surgery. In: Margulies J, Floman Y, Farcy J-P, Neuwirth M, eds. Lumbosacral and Spinopelvic Fixation. Philadelphia, PA: Lippincott-Raven, 1996:191-198.

33. Fourney D, Abi-Said D, Lang F, McCutcheon I, Gokaslan Z. The use of pedicle screw fixation in the management of malignant spinal disease: experience in 100 consecutive procedures. J Neurosurg (Spine 1) 2001; 94:25–37.

34. Carson W, Duffield R, Arendt M, Ridgely B, Gaines JR. Internal forces and moments in transpedicular spine instrumentation. The effect of pedicle screw angle and transfixation–the 4R-4bar linage concept. Spine 1990; 15:893–901.

35. McCord D, Cunningham B, Shono Y, Myers J, McAfee P. Biomechanical analysis of lumbosacral fixation. Spine 1992; 17:235–243.

36. Carlson G, Abitbol J, Anderson D, et al. Screw fixation in the human sacrum. An in vitro study of the biomechanics of fixation. Spine 1992; 17:196–203.

37. Smith S, Abitbol J, Carlson G, Anderson D, Taggart K, Garfin S. The effects of depth of penetration, screw orientation, and bone density on sacral screw fixation. Spine 1993; 18:1006–1010.

38. Krag M, Beynnon B, Pope M, DeCoster T. Depth of insertion of transpedicular vertebral screws into human vertebrae: effect on screw-vertebra interface strength. J Spinal Disord 1988; 1:287–294.

39. Jackson R. Jackson sacral fixation and contoured spinal correction techniques. In: Margulies J, Floman Y, Farcy J-P, Neuwirth M, eds. Lumbosacral and Spinopelvic Fixation. Philadelphia, PA: Lippincott-Raven; 1996:357–379.

40. Baldwin N, Benzel E. Sacral fixation using iliac instrumentation and a variable angle screw device. J Neurosurg 1994; 81:313–316.

41. Allen BJ, Ferguson R. The Galveston technique for L rod instrumentation of the scoliotic spine. Spine 1982; 7:276–284.

42. Brooke R. The sacroiliac joint. J Anat 1924; 58:297–301.

43. Allen BJ, Ferguson RL. The Galveston technique of pelvic fixation with L-rod instrumentation of the spine. Spine 1984; 9:388–394.

44. Allen BJ, Ferguson R. A 1988 perspective on the Galveston technique of pelivc fixation. Orthop Clin North Am 1988; 19:409–418.

45. Shikata J, Yamamuro T, Kotoura Y, Mikawa Y, Iida H, Maetani S. Total sacrectomy and reconstruction for primary tumors. J Bone Joint Surg 1988; 70–A:122-125.

46. Tomita K, Tsuchiya H. Total sacrectomy and reconstruction for huge sacral tumors. Spine 1990; 15:1223–1227.

47. Thompson J, Doty J. Sacral biomechanics and reconstruction. In: Doty J, Rengachary S, eds. Surgical Disorders of the Sacrum. New York, NY: Thieme Medical; 1994:253–256.

48. Santi MD, Mitsunaga MM, Lockett JL. Total sacrectomy for a giant sacral schwannoma. A case report. Clin Orthop 1993:285–259.

49. Wuisman P, Lieshout O, Sugihara S, Dijk Mv. Total sacrectomy and reconstruction: oncologic and functional outcome. Clin Orthop 2000; 381:192–203.

33 Neoplastic Disease of the Spinal Cord and the Spinal Canal

DANIEL SHEDID, MD, AND EDWARD C. BENZEL, MD

CONTENTS

1. INTRODUCTION

Spine tumors can be classified by their relation to the spinal canal and its coverings. Tumors can arise from the different tissue types around the spinal column, such as neural tissue, meningeal tissue, bone, and cartilage. Furthermore, distant primary tumors can metastasize to the spine by hematogenous or lymphatic routes. Both benign and malignant tumors may occur in either location and at any level of the spine.

Spine tumors can occur inside the spinal cord. These are termed intramedullary tumors (e.g., astrocytoma, ependymoma, hemangioblastoma). They may occur within the meninges and are termed intradural extramedullary tumors (e.g., schwannoma, meningioma). They can also arise between the meninges and the bony confines of the spine and are termed extradural (e.g., primary and secondary tumors). The most common tumors that metastasize to the spine are tumors of the lung, breast, prostate, kidney, lymphoma, melanoma, and gastrointestinal tract (1,2).

The clinical presentation of spinal canal tumors depends on their location, type, growth pattern, and the biological behavior. They may considerably affect the activities of daily living of the patient, and appropriate treatment should be offered. The treatment varies from conservative to aggressive depending on the characteristic of the tumor, the location of the tumor, and on the clinical presentation. In this chapter, the surgical treatment of spine tumors, especially on the indications, surgical approaches, and complications, are specifically addressed.

2. METASTATIC EPIDURAL TUMORS

The spine constitutes the most common site of skeletal metastases (3). Sixty percent of all spinal metastasis are sec-

From: *Current Clinical Oncology: Cancer in the Spine: Comprehensive Care.*
Edited by: R. F. McLain, K-U. Lewandrowski, M. Markman, R. M. Bukowski,
R. Macklis, and E. C. Benzel © Humana Press, Inc., Totowa, NJ

ondary to breast, lung, prostate carcinomas, myeloma, and lymphoma (4). A spinal metastasis is found in as many as 70 to 90% of patients dying of cancer (5,6). Ten percent of the patients presenting with symptomatic spinal metastasis have an unknown primary (7). Tumors are multiple in 10 to 40 % of cases (8). The most common site of the disease is the thoracic spine (70%), followed by the lumbar spine (20%), and the cervical spine (10%) (8).

2.1. SURGICAL CONSIDERATIONS

The primary goal of the treatment in patients with metastatic disease is to improve their quality of life by providing pain relief, maintaining or ameliorating neurological function, and by restoring structural integrity of the spinal column (3,9). Stabilization of the spine is often necessary for extensive lesions, because they may cause spinal instability as they erode through the normal bony structures.

By taking into consideration the general medical condition, histology of the primary tumor, and the extent of the metastatic disease, the indications for surgical intervention can be determined. They include: the presence of spinal instability, neurological compression owing to tumor or compression fracture failure to respond to radiation therapy, radio-resistant tumor, unknown primary tumor, and recurrence after surgical decompression or maximal radiation therapy. Relative contraindications include: poor medical condition, complete paralysis greater than 24 h, a life expectancy less than 4 mo, radiosensitive tumor (e.g., multiple myeloma, plasmocytoma, lymphoma), and the presence of extensive lesions throughout the entire spine (9–12).

2.2. SURGICAL TECHNIQUES

In choosing the optimal surgical approach, the surgeon must take into account multiple factors, including the location of the tumor, the extent of the disease, the presence of instability, the vascularity of the tumor, and the patient general condition. In

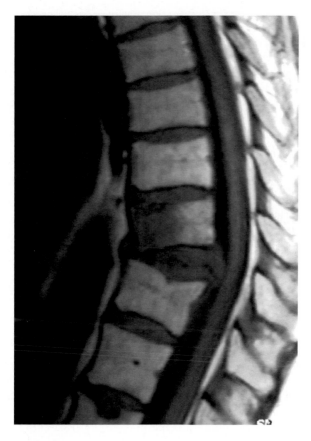

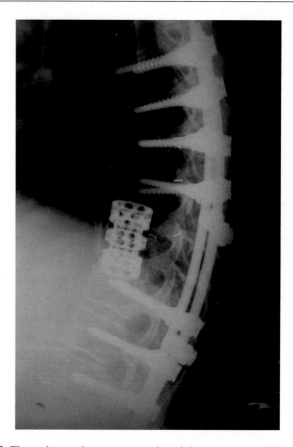

Fig. 1. Magnetic resonance imaging (T1 sagittal T1-weighted images) of a 43-yr-old female with a hypointense lesion at T9 and T10 owing to a metastasis of a breast carcinoma. Note spinal cord compression, the collapse of the vertebral body of T10, as well as the kyphotic deformity.

Fig. 2. The patient underwent a retropleural thoracotomy and T9 and T10 corpectomy. An expandable cage was put to restore the anterior column support followed by a fusion instrumentation from T5 down to L1.

general, the location of epidural compression should dictate the approach for decompression *(3)*.

In the rare cases, in which the compression is only located dorsal to the spinal cord, a decompressive laminectomy can be done for resection of the epidural tumor. Laminectomy alone can increase the instability and result in neurological injury when the pathology is ventral to the spinal cord or when the vertebral body collapse is present *(10,13)*. If the pathology is ventral or ventrolateral to the spinal cord (Figs. 1 and 2) and ventral (e.g., ventral cervical, transthoracic, retroperitoneal, transabdominal) or a dorsolateral approach and spinal reconstruction (e.g., costotransversectomy, transpedicular) can be done for tumor resection and instrumentation *(9, 14–17)*. In general, a ventral and dorsal stabilization may be necessary when both ventral and dorsal elements are disrupted *(18,19)*. Pre-operative embolization should be considered if the metastasis originates from a renal cell or thyroid carcinoma, because these lesions are notoriously vascular *(20)*.

2.3. SURGICAL COMPLICATIONS

The most important factor affecting prognosis of patients with epidural metastasis is the ability to ambulate at the time of initiation of treatment. Among the ambulatory patients, 60 to 80% retain the ability to walk after treatment, whereas among the paraparetic patients, 35% become ambulatory, and among

the paraplegics, 0 to 25% recover ambulation *(1,12,21,22)*. The presence of sphincter disturbances is a poor prognostic factor and is usually irreversible *(12)*. Rapid onset of neurological deficit also results in a suboptimal postoperative outcome *(9)*.

3. INTRADURAL EXTRAMEDULLARY TUMORS

Intradural extramedullary masses arise from inside the dura mater, but outside the spinal cord. The most common intradural extramedullary tumors are meningiomas and nerve sheath tumors (schwannomas and neurofibromas) (Fig. 3). Tumors that arise from within the dura mater are rarely metastatic and usually slow growing. Meningiomas, which arise from arachnoid cluster cells located at exit zones of nerve roots, are usually benign, but may be malignant. These tumors are more common in middle-aged and elderly women. Nerve sheath tumors arise from the nerve roots. This type of tumor is usually benign and slow-growing, and well circumscribed. In fact, it may be years before any neurological signs present *(2)*.

3.1. SURGICAL CONSIDERATIONS

The treatment for most intradural extramedullary tumors is complete surgical excision. The goal is total removal of the tumor with preservation of neurological function. Most nerve sheath tumors, which arise from the dorsal nerve roots, are dorsal or dorsolateral to the spinal cord, whereas meningiomas

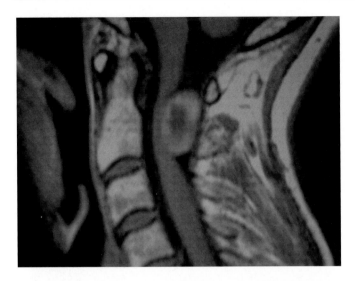

Fig. 3. Magnetic resonance imaging of the cervical spine sagittal view with gadolinium shows an enhancing intradural extramedullary lesion. The lesion, located at C2, compresses the spinal cord and was causing myelopathy. It was excised via a dorsal approach. The final diagnosis was a neurofibroma.

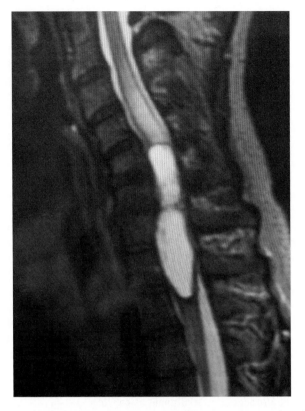

Fig. 4. A 40-yr-old female presented with a progressive myelopathy over a period of 6 mo. Note on the T2 saggital magnetic resonance imaging, the presence of an intramedullary lesion extending from C5 to T1 associated with a syrinx in the rostrally. The tumor was excised and the final diagnosis was of an intramedullary ependymoma.

are predominantly located ventrally or ventrolaterally. The latter pose more of a surgical challenge. In most cases, complete surgical resection is feasible with good functional outcome *(23)*.

3.2. SURGICAL TECHNIQUES

Surgical exposure should encompass the tumor with some rostral and caudal margins to allow for adequate visualization. When the lesion is located dorsally (schwannoma), a laminectomy and midline durotomy is necessary and the removal of the tumor can be accomplished with the use of an ultrasonic aspirator after opening the arachnoid. It is important to remain within the arachnoid plane to prevent violating the spinal cord. A foraminotomy may be performed if transforamminal extension is present. It is necessary to identify and divide the proximal and distal nerve root (the origins of the tumor). To remove the tumor, it is often necessary to sacrifice the nerve root of origin (thoracic spine) *(23,24)*.

Dumbell tumors with significant extension into the paraspinal region may require a combined approach. A dorsal approach may precede a thoracotomy (thoracic lesions) or a retroperitoneal approach (lumbar lesions) *(25)*.

When the lesion is situated ventrally or ventrolaterally (meningioma), it is frequently necessary to perform a unilateral medial facetectomy, in addition to a laminectomy. A costo-transversectomy or a lateral extracavitary approach can be performed to maximize the exposure and to attain a complete resection *(24–26))*. The dura mater is opened and tacked laterally to maximize the exposure. The arachnoid is opened and dissected off the tumor and adjacent spinal cord. The resection involves gradual debulking along the lateral aspect of the spinal canal. An ultrasonic aspirator may be useful here. It is usually possible to delineate an arachnoid plain and separate the tumor from the spinal cord. The ultimate surgical goal is to excise the tumor with minimal spinal cord manipulation. Thus, it is often

necessary to sacrifice one or more nerve roots. It is advisable to perform a complete removal of the dural origin in the case of a meningioma in order to complete the resection. A measure of safety may be added by utilizing a microscope and intra-operative neurophysiological monitoring *(23)*.

3.3. COMPLICATIONS

Recurrences are rare after complete surgical resection. The rate of clinical recurrences after subtotal removal is 50%. Therefore, patients should be followed with a serial magnetic resonance imaging (MRI) *(27)*. Surgical results are usually excellent and the outcome is related to the patient's pre-operative neurological status, age, and duration of symptoms *(23)*. The potential postoperative complications include wound infection, meningitis, arachnoiditis, cerebrospinal fluid fistula, spinal destabilization, and other medical complications *(28,29)*.

4. INTRAMEDULLARY TUMORS

Intramedullary tumors arise within the substance of the spinal cord. They represent aprrox 4% of central nervous system neoplasms *(30)*. Primary glial tumors (e.g., astrocytomas, ependymomas, gangiogliomas, oligodendrogliomas, and subependymomas) account for 80 to 90% of intramedullary tumors *(31)*. Astrocytomas are the most common pediatric intramedullay tumors, whereas ependymomas are the most common intramedullary tumors in adults *(32)* (Fig. 4). Hemangioblastomas account for 3 to 8% of intramedullary tumors

(33) and the remaining intramedullary pathology may be owing to metastases, inclusion tumors, cysts, nerve sheath tumors, and vascular pathology (e.g., cavernous malformations and arteriovenous malformations). Lung and breast are the most common primary neoplastic sites to metastasize to the spinal cord. The latter accounts for fewer than 5% of intramedullary spinal cord tumors *(32)*.

4.1. SURGICAL CONSIDERATIONS

Advances in imaging and microsurgical techniques have established microsurgical resection as the most effective treatment for most intramedullary tumors. Surgery can provide long-term control or cure for almost all ependymomas and many astrocytomas.

The primary surgical objective is a complete total resection. This can be achieved in the majority of ependymomas because of the presence of a well-defined tumor plane around the tumor and in many astrocytomas. Most astrocytomas infiltrate into the spinal cord and thus complete removal is difficult and hazardous. Apart from complete total resection, another important treatment objective is the preservation of the neurological function. This can be achieved by limiting the tumor resection to the plane between the tumor and the spinal cord and by simply debulking in the event of an infiltrative or adhesive lesion. Performing a biopsy in the case of a suspected malignant tumor may be prudent (e.g., malignant astrocytomas).

4.2. SURGICAL TECHNIQUE

Appropriate positioning is accomplished in accordance with the location of the tumor. Sensory and motor evoked potentials may be monitored during the surgery. The resection of an intramedullary tumor is accomplished through a midline incision. Pre-operative localization can be enhanced by fluoroscopy. A subperiosteal dissection is carried out, followed by a laminectomy (or a laminoplasty in the pediatric population). After opening the dura mater and suturing it laterally to the muscles, the microscope is brought into the field. The arachnoid is opened and the spinal cord is inspected for spinal cord enlargement. The use of ultrasonography is helpful in localizing the lesion, its extent, and the presence and type of associated cysts *(34)*. A midline myelotomy, extending over the entire rostrocaudal extent of the tumor, is performed through the dorsal midline septum. This septum is located between the dorsal nerve entry zones bilaterally and usually small veins can be seen exiting from the septum. The myelotomy is performed using microinstruments and bipolar forceps at low settings. After adequate exposure of the entire tumor, and after placing traction sutures in the pia matter, the tumor can be debulked using ultrasonic aspirator in the area where the spinal cord is maximally enlarged. In the event of a small ependymoma, the tumor may be removed in one piece, whereas bulky lesions must be excised in a piecemeal fashion in order to prevent excessive manipulation of adjacent neural tissue. Debulking should be avoided in the case of a hemangioblastoma, because these tumors are vascular (Figs. 5 and 6A) (bleeding may be difficult to control) and, therefore, the dissection should proceed around the tumor surface with cauterization of the feeding vessels and tumor capsule. Cysts in the poles are drained and can help in identifying the extent of the lesion (Fig. 6B). A well-

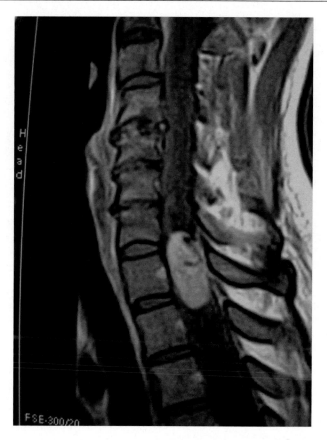

Fig. 5. A 45-yr-old female presented with myelopathy. The magnetic resonance imaging shows a C7–T1 intramedullary lesion that significantly enhances post gadolinium. The patient underwent a dorsal approach and complete resection. The diagnosis was compatible with a hemangioblastoma.

defined tumor plane should be sought and followed as in the case of ependymomas and some astrocytomas. In the case of an infiltrative tumor where a plane is absent, a biopsy should be performed. If the lesion is malignant, the procedure is terminated, and if it is benign, the removal or debulking can be continued by relying on the color (e.g., astrocytomas are gray, ependymomas are red or very dark gray), the texture of the lesion, and judgement of the surgeon. After satisfactory resection and adequate hemostasis, the dura is closed without closing the myelotomy. The dura mater should be closed in a watertight fashion, to minimize the occurrence of a cerebrospinal fluid fistula *(26,31,32)*.

4.3. COMPLICATIONS

Preservation of neurological function is a reasonable goal for the surgeon. Surgical morbidity is related to the pre-operative neurological condition, the location of the tumor, its histology, the duration of symptoms before diagnosis, the presence of spinal cord atrophy, and arachnoid scarring *(32,35)*. Most patients have a sensory loss (e.g., position-sense disturbances causing gait abnormalities) after the surgery. This sensory loss is a result of the midline myelotomy and may resolve within 3 mo *(35)*. Worsening of motor function is common but tends to be transitory. Among the serious complications, we note a more permanent picture of sensory and motor dysfunctions as well as sphincter disturbances. This picture may be related to an

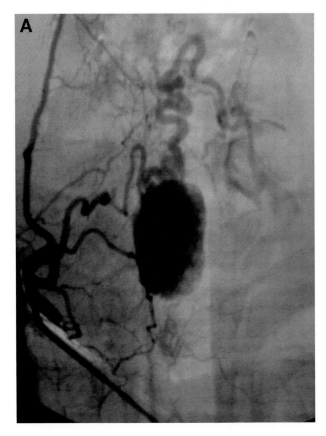
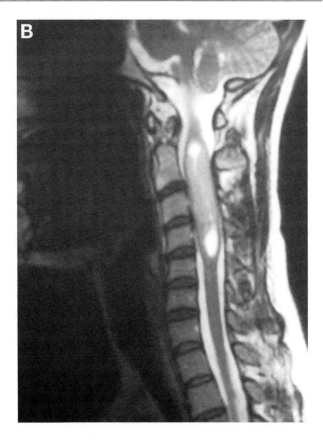

Fig. 6. **(A)** A pre-operative angiogram demonstrates a vascularized lesion. **(B)** A 27-yr-old female presenting with a history of myelopathy. The magnetic resonance imaging shows an intramedullary lesion extending from C2 down to C4. Note the presence of two cysts at the rostral and caudal extent of the lesion. A laminectomy, midline myelotomy, and tumor resection was accomplished. The diagnosis was intramedullary ependymoma.

aggressive removal of an infiltrative tumor. Postoperative deep venous thrombosis, pneumonia, cerebrospinal fluid fistula, and other complications should be treated aggressively in order to halt early ambulation and to maximize recovery (26,31,32).

These lesions tend to recur and patients warrant serial clinical and radiological (e.g., MRI) follow-up. As mentioned earlier, aggressive resection reduces the risk of local tumor recurrence, but involves a danger of major postoperative neurological dysfunction (2,31,32).

5. SUMMARY

The treatment of patients with spinal tumor continues to be a challenging problem. Spinal tumors range from those that are easily treatable to those that are incurable. The goals of treatment of spinal tumors are to obtain final diagnosis through biopsy or resection, institute the appropriate treatment, preserve the neurological function, relieve the patient's symptoms, and maintain the spinal column stability. The addition of a wide range of instrumentation capabilities has improved the ability to treat extradural tumors more radically allowing subsequent stabilization and patient mobilization.

REFERENCES

1. Gilbert RW, Kim JH, Posner JB. Epidural spinal cord compression from metastatic tumor: diagnosis and treatment. Ann Neurol 1978; 3:40–51.

2. Fehlings MG, Pao SC. Spinal cord and spinal column column tumors. In: Bernstein M, Berger MS, ed. Neuro-Oncology–The Essentials. New York, NY: Thieme; 2000:445–464.

3. Walker MP, Yaszemski MJ, Kim CW, Talac R, Currier BL. Metastatic disease of the spine: evaluation and treatment. Clin Orthop 2003; 415:S165–S175.

4. McLain RF, Weinstein JN. Tumors of the spine. Semin Spine Surg 1990; 2:157–180.

5. Black P. Spinal metastasis: current status and recommended guidelines for management. Neurosurgery 1979; 5:726–746.

6. Fornasier VL, Horne JG. Metastases to the vertebral column. Cancer. 1975; 36:590–594.

7. Camins MB, Jenkins AL, Singhal A, Perrin RG. Tumors of the vertebral axis: benign, primary malignant, and metastatic tumors. In: Winn RH, ed. Youmans Neurologic Surgery. 5th ed. Philadelphia, PA: Saunders; 2004:4835–4868.

8. Klimo P Jr, Kestle JRW, Schmidt MH. Treatment of metastatic spinal epidural disease: a review of the literature. Neurosurg Focus 2003; 15:1–8.

9. Riley LH 3rd, Frassica DA, Kostuik JP, Frassica FJ. Metastatic disease to the spine: diagnosis and treatment. Instr Course Lect 2000; 49:471–477.

10. Cooper PR, Errico TJ, Martin R, Crawford B, DiBartolo T. A systematic approach to spinal reconstruction after anterior decompression for neoplastic disease of the thoracic and lumbar spine. Neurosurgery 1993; 32:1–8.

11. Greenberg SH, Mark S, Greenberg MS. Handbook of Neurosurgery. Lakeland, FL: Greenberg Graphics; 2001.

12. Daw HA, Markman M. Epidural spinal cord compression in cancer patients: diagnosis and management. Cleve Clin J Med 2000; 67:497,501–504.

13. Onimus M, Schraub S, Bertin D, Bosset JF, Guidet M. Surgical treatment of vertebral metastasis. Spine 1986; 11:883–891.

14. Sundaresan N, Galicich JH, Lane JM, Bains MS, McCormack P. Treatment of neoplastic epidural cord compression by vertebral body resection and stabilization. J Neurosurg 1985 ;63:676–684.

15. Overby MC, Rothman AS. Anterolateral decompression for metastatic epidural spinal cord tumors. Results of a modified costotransversectomy approach. J Neurosurg 1985; 62:344–348.

16. Shaw B, Mansfield FL, Borges L. One-stage posterolateral decompression and stabilization for primary and metastatic vertebral tumors in the thoracic and lumbar spine. J Neurosurg 1989; 70:405–410.

17. Wetzel FT, Phillips FM. Management of metastatic disease of the spine. Orthop Clin North Am 2000; 31:611–621.

18. Johnston FG, Uttley D, Marsh HT. Synchronous vertebral decompression and posterior stabilization in the treatment of spinal malignancy. Neurosurgery 1989; 25:872–876.

19. Bell GR. Surgical treatment of spinal tumors. Clin Orthop 1997; 335:54–63.

20. Bhojraj SY, Dandawate AV, Ramakantan R. Pre-operative embolisation, transpedicular decompression and posterior stabilisation for metastatic disease of the thoracic spine causing paraplegia. Paraplegia 1992; 30:292–299.

21. Bruckman JE, Bloomer WD. Management of spinal cord compression. Semin Oncol 1978; 5:135–140.

22. Hall AJ, Mackay NN. The results of laminectomy for compression of the cord or cauda equina by extradural malignant tumour. J Bone Joint Surg Br 1973; 55:497–505.

23. McCormick PC, Post KD, Stein BM. Intradural extramedullary tumors in adults. Neurosurg Clin N Am 1990; 1:591–608.

24. Steck JC, Dietze DD, Fessler RG. Posterolateral approach to intradural extramedullary thoracic tumors. J Neurosurg 1994; 81: 202–205.

25. McCormick PC. Surgical management of dumbbell and paraspinal tumors of the thoracic and lumbar spine. Neurosurgery 1996; 38: 67–74.

26. McCormick PC, Torres R, Post KD, Stein BM. Intramedullary ependymoma of the spinal cord. J Neurosurg 1990; 72:523–532.

27. Seppala MT, Haltia MJ, Sankila RJ, Jaaskelainen JE, Heiskanen O. Long-term outcome after removal of spinal schwannoma: a clinicopathological study of 187 cases. J Neurosurg 1995; 83:621–626.

28. Levy WJ Jr, Bay J, Dohn D. Spinal cord meningioma. J Neurosurg 1982; 57:804–812.

29. Solero CL, Fornari M, Giombini S, et al. Spinal meningiomas: review of 174 operated cases. Neurosurgery 1989; 25:153–160.

30. Sloof JL, Kernohan JW, MacCarthy CS. Primary Intramedullary Tumors of the Spinal Cord and Filum Terminale. Philadelphia, PA: Saunders; 1964.

31. McCormick PC, Stein BM. Intramedullary tumors in adults. Neurosurg Clin N Am 1990; 1:609–630

32. Schwartz TH, McCormick PC. Spinal cord tumors in adults. In: Youmans Neurologic Surgery by Richard H Winn, fifth edition. Philadelphia, PA: Saunders;2004:4817–4834.

33. Neumann HP, Eggert HR, Weigel K, Friedburg H, Wiestler OD, Schollmeyer P. Hemangioblastomas of the central nervous system. A 10-year study with special reference to von Hippel-Lindau syndrome. J Neurosurg 1989; 70:24–30.

34. Epstein FJ, Farmer JP, Schneider SJ. Intra-operative ultrasonography: an important surgical adjunct for intramedullary tumors. J Neurosurg 1991 May; 5:729–733.

35. Hoshimaru M, Koyama T, Hashimoto N, Kikuchi H. Results of microsurgical treatment for intramedullary spinal cord ependymomas: analysis of 36 cases. Neurosurgery 1999; 44:264–269.

36. Benzel EC. Biomechanics of spine stabilization. Philadelphia, PA:American Association of Neurological Surgeons Publications, 2001.

34 Minimally Invasive Approaches to Spinal Metastases

Endoscopic Surgery and Vertebral Augmentation

JEAN-VALÉRY C. E. COUMANS, MD, A. JAY KHANNA, MD,
AND ISADOR H. LIEBERMAN, MD

CONTENTS

INTRODUCTION
APPROACHES
PERCUTANEOUS VERTEBRAL AUGMENTATION PROCEDURES
CONCLUSIONS
REFERENCES

1. INTRODUCTION

Approximately 50 to 70% of all cancer patients ultimately develop skeletal metastases, and the spine is the most common site of metastatic deposition. Most patients with spinal metastases are treated nonsurgically, commonly with radiation therapy, chemotherapy, radiopharmaceutical therapy, hormonal therapy, and antiresorptive therapy with bisphosphonates and analgesics *(1,2)*. Usually, surgery is considered only for patients with intractable pain, neurological compromise, and overt or impending instability. The goals of spinal tumor surgery are to decompress the spinal cord and nerve roots, stabilize the spine, alleviate pain, and, in some cases, establish a diagnosis. Occasionally, the goal of surgery for a patient with a primary neoplasm of the spine is to effect a cure.

However, some patients with spinal metastases are not good surgical candidates. For example, such patients are frequently too ill to undergo open surgical intervention, and the concurrent or recent administration of chemotherapy or radiation therapy increases the likelihood of surgical complications such as infection and wound dehiscence. In patients with poor life expectancy, minimizing pain and improving quality of life is of paramount importance. Because it is desirable to achieve the surgical goals of decompression, stabilization, and pain relief with the least possible amount of collateral tissue disruption and physiological disturbance, selecting a minimally invasive procedure, whenever feasible, may be the means of achieving this goal.

These minimally invasive procedures, which use endoscopic and percutaneous techniques, have had a profound effect on the

practice of general and oncological surgery by decreasing morbidity, recovery time, and postoperative pain. Many surgical procedures that were once involved open techniques are now performed primarily via endoscopic and percutaneous techniques *(3,4)*. As with any intervention, the risks and effectiveness of minimally invasive surgery must be balanced against the patient's life expectancy, quality of life, and willingness to undergo a procedure.

This chapter addresses different approaches (i.e., endoscopic approaches to the lumbar spine, thoracoscopic approaches, and the concurrent open and thoracoscopic approach to the thoracic spine), discusses the technique of endoscopic-assisted costotransversectomy, and reviews percutaneous vertebral augmentation procedures (vertebroplasty and kyphoplasty).

2. APPROACHES

2.1. ENDOSCOPIC LUMBAR APPROACHES

In spinal surgery, the term *minimally invasive surgery* has become synonymous with any surgical procedure involving endoscopic access to a body cavity or joint. This terminology emphasizes the philosophy of targeting the pathology and applying the therapeutic intervention with little or no damage to surrounding nonpathologic tissues. Thus, the term minimally invasive has truly come to mean much more than just endoscopy, which essentially refers to the use of a scope and light source for visualization and magnification through small percutaneous portals.

With the advances in endoscopy, anterior lumbar spine exposure has evolved from the traditional open transperitoneal, to open retroperitoneal, to muscle-sparing retroperitoneal, to endoscopic retroperitoneal, and to laparoscopic transperitoneal approaches. To date, there have been only anecdotal references

From: *Current Clinical Oncology: Cancer in the Spine: Comprehensive Care.*
Edited by: R. F. McLain, K-U. Lewandrowski, M. Markman, R. M. Bukowski,
R. Macklis, and E. C. Benzel © Humana Press, Inc., Totowa, NJ

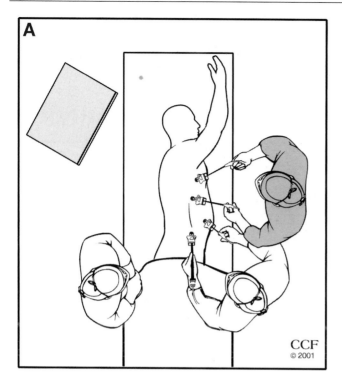

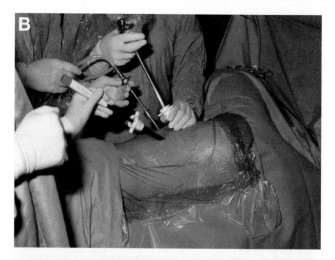

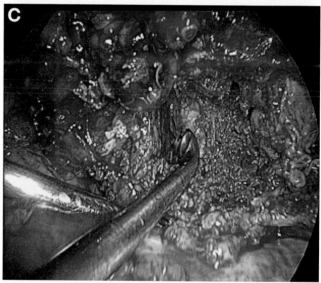

Fig. 1. The thoracoscopic approach. (**A**) Lateral decubitus positioning with surgeon (shaded) and assistants. (**B**) Portal placement (cranial right, caudal left). (**C**) Thoracoscopic view of curette during corpectomy.

to the use of true laparoscopic or retroperitoneal endoscopic techniques to facilitate spine exposure in the treatment of spinal metastases; most reports describe the use of these techniques as they relate to lumbar decompression and arthrodesis *(4–6)*. The benefits of these exposures are intuitive, but the complexity of the spinal reconstruction and the intimidating local anatomy may have limited the widespread use of these techniques to a few very experienced surgeons.

2.2. THORACOSCOPIC APPROACH

In 1970, the use of thoracoscopy was first described *(7)*. Advances in instrumentation and anesthetic techniques have allowed a multitude of operations, from biopsies to the resection of lung and mediastinal tumors, to be performed without a sternotomy or a thoracotomy *(8–10)*. In the thoracic surgery literature, clinical studies have unequivocally shown the benefits of thoracoscopic surgery compared with open approaches *(11,12)*. Thoracoscopic surgery is associated with less pain within the first year after surgery *(12)* and with better shoulder and pulmonary function in the early postoperative period *(11)*. Furthermore, the long-term survival of patients treated with resection of pulmonary metastases is comparable to that obtained with open thoracotomy *(8)*, suggesting that the goals of surgery can be accomplished equally well with thoracoscopic means. Spinal procedures are a recent development in thoracoscopic surgery *(3,13–17)* and have not been formally compared with open thoracic spinal approaches in a large trial. However, based on existing thoracic surgery studies, it is reasonable to assume that similar benefits in pulmonary dysfunction and pain could be obtained with thoracoscopic spinal surgery because much of the reported morbidity is related to the thoracotomy itself.

Thoracoscopic spinal surgery can be performed from either side (Fig. 1). The choice of side is dictated by the location of the pathology. For centrally located tumors, a right-side approach may be preferable in the upper and mid-thoracic spine because more space is available dorsal to the azygous vein than dorsal to the aorta *(3)*. In the lower thoracic spine, a left-side approach avoids the diaphragm, which is higher on the right.

The patient is intubated with a dual-lumen endotracheal tube and placed in the lateral decubitus position, as for a thoracotomy. The position, draping, and available instrumentation are planned so a thoracotomy could be performed rapidly in the event of a complication. Before making the incisions, the proper functioning of the dual-lumen tube is verified. The lung is deflated, and a portal is made in the anterior axillary line by dissecting over the appropriate rib or with the use of a trochar. To avoid injury to the diaphragm and abdominal viscera, it is advisable to remain above the eighth intercostal space with the initial trochar insertion *(17)*. The thoracoscope is inserted into the first portal and the pathology is localized. Under direct visualization, two to three additional portals are created in the mid or anterior axillary lines for the insertion of surgical instruments. If necessary, the lung can be depressed with a "fan" retractor or the table can be rotated to allow gravity to pull the

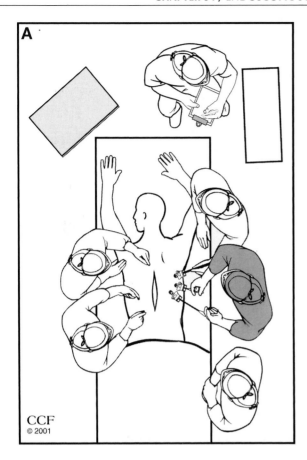

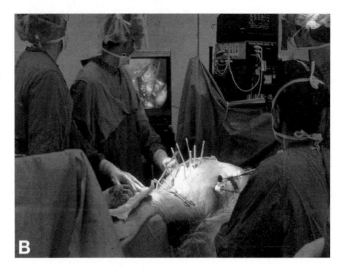

Fig. 2. The simultaneous posterior and thoracoscopic approach. (A) Prone positioning with the thoracoscopic surgeon (shaded) on right side and cosurgeons on the left side. (B) Intra-operative photograph showing posterior instrumentation in place and thoracoscopic portals on right side.

lung down. After the appropriate level has been identified, the pleura is dissected off the ribs and vertebrae, and the segmental vessels are ligated. With the diseased vertebral body exposed, the resection proceeds similarly to that of an open procedure. With a combination of rongeurs, curettes, osteotomes, and the high-speed drill, the tumor is excised. The vertebral body subsequently can be reconstructed with autologous bone graft, strut allograft, methylmethacrylate, or a metal/carbon corpectomy cage *(3)*. A plate can also be affixed, although this procedure can be technically difficult, and the portals must be planned accordingly *(13)*. At the completion of the procedure, chest tubes are placed through two of the portals.

The results of 17 thoracoscopic corpectomies (seven of which were performed for tumors) have been compared with a cohort of seven patients (two with tumors) who underwent the same operation through a thoracotomy *(3,13)*. The patients with thoracoscopic procedures had shorter surgeries with less blood loss, less chest tube drainage, half the number of days on intravenous or intramuscular narcotic medications, and approximately half the number of days in the intensive care unit and in the hospital. Although a prospective multicenter study of the complications associated with endoscopic spinal surgery made no comparison with patients undergoing thoracotomy, the results appear comparable to those typically obtained with open surgical intervention *(18)*. The authors prospectively analyzed 78 thoracoscopic spinal procedures, 13 of which were partial or complete corpectomies. There were no infections or permanent neurological or vascular injuries, in one case a conversion to an open thoracotomy was needed because of adhesions *(18)*. In

another series of 15 patients who underwent thoracic corpectomy (eight of the procedures were performed for tumors *[15]*), no substantial complications occurred, and the authors claimed results that were equal to or superior than those obtained by thoracotomy. Specifically, the authors described easier access to the T3–T4 and T12 regions endoscopically than with open techniques, which require mobilization of the scapula in the former region and of the diaphragm in the latter region.

As with any minimally invasive procedure, potential complications must be weighed against the benefits of surgery. Although it avoids a thoracotomy or sternotomy, thoracoscopic spine surgery still requires single-lung ventilation, which may be problematic in patients with lung cancer or pulmonary metastases. It is necessary to evaluate all patients who are being considered for this procedure with pulmonary function tests pre-operatively. The potential for vascular injury means that the procedure may have to be converted to an open procedure emergently in the event of a complication. Hence, a patient is not considered a candidate for thoracoscopic spinal surgery if deemed unable to tolerate an emergent conversion to an open procedure. This procedure is also contraindicated in patients who have pulmonary adhesions, such as patients with previous thoracotomies or those having undergone a pleurodesis, because of the inability to collapse the lung *(13)*.

2.3. CONCURRENT POSTERIOR AND THORACOSCOPIC APPROACHES

This technique represents a concurrent combination of the conventional posterior approach to the thoracic spine for instrumentation and stabilization and of the thoracoscopic approach for decompression and reconstruction *(19)*. It allows anterior access to the thoracic spine and concurrent exposure to the posterior thoracic spine without requiring an open thoracotomy and without the need to stage the procedure or reposition the patient (Fig. 2).

As with the thoracoscopic approach, the patient is intubated with a dual-lumen endotracheal tube. The patient is then placed in the prone position and draped widely to allow access to the anterior axillary line bilaterally. Unlike the lateral decubitus position used in thoracotomy or thoracoscopy, this position allows concurrent access to the ventral and dorsal thoracic spine. The dual endotracheal tube is checked before the start of the procedure. The dorsal exposure is then obtained by way of a midline incision, and the spine is decompressed and stabilized. Before accessing the anterior spine, the appropriate endotracheal tube lumen is clamped, and the lung is allowed to deflate. The first portal is created in the mid-axillary line by bluntly dissecting over the appropriate rib and entering the thoracic cavity as is done for the placement of a chest tube. After inserting a 30° endoscope, two other portals (one, two levels rostral, and the other, two levels caudal) are created under direct visualization to allow the passage of instruments. This approach allows concurrent dorsal decompression and stabilization of the spine, facilitates minimally invasive anterior tumor resection and stabilization, and avoids a more physiologically injurious procedure, such as a thoracotomy or a lateral extracavitary approach. Judicious positioning also precludes having to redrape and reposition the patient between the dorsal and ventral parts of the procedure.

2.4. ENDOSCOPICALLY ASSISTED THORACIC SURGERY

Recently, endoscopically assisted surgery has emerged as an alternative to open surgery. Strictly speaking, it is not a minimally invasive approach, but it can be considered less invasive than conventional approaches because it requires less dissection for a given surgery *(16,20,21)*. Endoscopically assisted thoracic surgery initially entails a posterolateral approach to the diseased vertebral body and the completion of a corpectomy with the aid of 30 and 70° endoscopes to visualize the dura, followed by strut graft reconstruction (Fig. 3). Its advantage lies in the novel use of readily available instruments to improve visualization and minimize tissue disruption.

The patient is placed prone on bolsters or a Wilson frame, maintaining thoracic kyphosis. A midline incision is made, and the lamina, transverse process, and proximal rib are exposed. The vertebral body is entered by the transpedicular route, and the visible part of the tumor is resected using a high-speed drill. A 4-mm 30° endoscope is then introduced, and the resection is continued with a combination of Epstein curettes and pituitary rongeurs. The dissection continues to the contralateral pedicle, and a 70° endoscope is then introduced to inspect the dura and to resect the remainder of the tumor. A curved bipolar is used to cauterize bleeding epidural veins. Involvement of the contralateral pedicle necessitates a bilateral approach. The intervertebral discs and endplates are cleared of tissue and prepared for graft placement. The corpectomy defect is reconstructed with a corpectomy strut filled with graft or suitable graft substitute. Posterior instrumentation is then placed in compression to lock the strut in place.

Although this technique does not change the prognosis of patients with spinal metastases, it can alleviate or prevent neurological deficits, with less morbidity than does transthoracic surgery. In a series of nine patients *(21)*, all patients with a

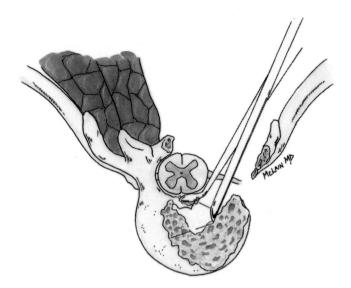

Fig. 3. Endoscopically assisted thoracic surgery performed via a lateral extracavitary approach with endoscope and curette in the operative field.

neurological deficit improved. The patients averaged 1.4 d in the intensive care unit, 6.4 d in the hospital, and an average blood loss of 1677 mL. Although no study directly compares endoscopically assisted surgery with other approaches, the preliminary experience suggests that this technique enables the resection of anterior lesions without the morbidity of anterior approaches.

3. PERCUTANEOUS VERTEBRAL AUGMENTATION PROCEDURES

3.1. VERTEBROPLASTY

Pain is the cardinal manifestation of metastatic spinal disease *(22)*. Several causes have been postulated, including stretching or irritation of the periosteum, instability, microarchitectural fractures, the release of nerve-stimulating factors (such as prostaglandins, bradykinins, substance P, and histamine) by the cancer cells, and the associated pathological fractures *(23)*. Because most metastases are osteolytic, vertebral compression fractures are a common complication of spinal metastases.

Vertebroplasty, first reported by Galibert et al. *(24)* in France in the 1980s, entails the injection of polymethylmethacrylate (PMMA) into a vertebra with the goal of relieving pain and stabilizing the collapsed vertebral body. Initially, vertebroplasty was used in the treatment of hemangiomas and osteolytic neoplasms *(25)*. With experience, its indications have been broadened to include the treatment of osteoporotic compression fractures *(26)*. This technique can be used for most patients with pathological compression fractures associated with spinal metastases, but it is contraindicated for patients who have nerve root or cord compression, who are coagulopathic or severely ill, or who have a disrupted posterior wall of the vertebral body.

Typically, vertebroplasty involves the percutaneous insertion of a 10- or 11-gage needle under fluoroscopic guidance into a diseased vertebral body. The transpedicular or extrapedicular routes can be used. A biopsy can be obtained if desired. Once in proper position, 5 mL of contrast material are injected to ensure that the needle tip is not located within a major venous outflow tract. A mixture of low-viscosity cement (such as PMMA) and an opacification powder (such as barium) is prepared. The preparation is loaded into syringes and injected under pressure while the injection site is monitored fluoroscopically for the extravasation (leakage of cement through the walls of the vertebral body or into the venous outflow tracts) (27). Breaches in the posterior wall of the vertebral body are a contraindication, and extravasation of the cement results in termination of the procedure. Some authors have advocated the use of a combination of computed tomography (CT) and fluoroscopy for monitoring purposes. CT is used to ensure accurate needle placement, and the contrast and cement injections are performed under fluoroscopic guidance (28).

Several clinical studies have documented the benefits of vertebroplasty. Weill et al. (29) retrospectively studied 37 patients who underwent 52 vertebroplasties for metastatic disease. In 26 of 33 procedures for the relief of pain, an immediate and durable improvement was obtained. Pain recurrence was associated with the development of new lesions at other levels. In 11 procedures for stabilization, no injected vertebral body collapsed during the average follow-up period of 13 mo. In a prospective study of osteoporotic compression fractures (30), significant and durable decreases in pain were associated with improvements in the Nottingham Health Profile scores. Improvements were statistically significant in the dimensions of pain, physical mobility, emotional reaction, energy, and social isolation, but not sleep. In a recent study (31), marked to complete pain relief was achieved in 24 of 38 patients treated for osteoporosis, and in 4 of 8 patients treated for vertebral malignancies. The improvement in pain, if it occurred, was observed immediately, and its persistence was documented at the 18-mo follow-up.

The mechanism by which vertebroplasty relieves pain is not understood. Stabilization of the fractured vertebra (30,31), and heat-induced (32) or cytotoxic necrosis of nerve endings (30) have been postulated as mechanisms. An in vitro study of temperature changes induced by the polymerization of cement inside cadaveric vertebral bodies showed that a peak temperature at the center of the vertebral body of 40 to 74°C was sufficient for necrosis of intra-osseous neural tissue. However, studies conducted in femoral implants have shown areas of osteonecrosis adjacent to PMMA that cannot be explained solely on the basis of temperature elevation (33,34). In addition to relieving pain, it has been suggested that PMMA has an anti-tumoral effect on a chemical basis, perhaps related to its acrylic content, but this hypothesis has been based, in part, on the unproven observation that tumors rarely recur in PMMA-treated bones (22). One study found that postmortem histological evaluation of PMMA-treated vertebral bodies revealed tumoral necrosis in the region of the implant (35). The necrosis extended 11 mm beyond the margin of the PMMA, supporting the hypothesis of an anti-tumoral factor.

Vertebroplasty confers stability to the diseased vertebra. One biomechanical study showed statistically significant improvements in strength and stiffness after the injection of 8 mL of cement (36). Another study (37) showed statistically significant increases in strength and stiffness whether the vertebral bodies were injected unilaterally with 6 mL or bilaterally with 5 mL per side; there was no significant difference between the two treatment groups. Other authors have shown significant improvements in cadaveric vertebral bodies with the injection of apatite cement (38) or that as little as 1 mL confers stability in vertebral body stiffness, leading to the clinical trend of injecting less cement into the vertebral body.

Although it restores strength, vertebroplasty does not restore height. Collapsed and kyphotic vertebrae create stress on adjacent vertebrae and predispose them, in turn, to collapse. Although prophylactic treatment of adjacent segments has been advocated (31), currently there is insufficient data to support the routine use of this treatment.

The complications of vertebroplasty are usually related to the extravasation (29) or systemic toxicity of cement (39). Extravasation is a common occurrence. Cortet et al. (30) used CT scans to show cement extravasation in 65% of patients treated for osteoporotic compression fractures. However, in no instance was the leak clinically significant. Weill et al. (29) reported leaks in 20 of 37 patients treated for metastases: in five cases, the leak was symptomatic and in one case the patient required surgical evacuation of the cement. Thus, it may be stated that although cement extravasation often occurs in patients treated with vertebroplasty, it is clinically significant in only a minority.

The results of vertebroplasty studies conducted over nearly two decades suggest that it is a useful adjunct to the management of spinal metastasis (40–43). It enables the restoration of vertebral strength and stiffness, relieves pain, does not interfere with adjunctive treatment such as chemotherapy and radiation therapy, and (despite its high rate of cement extravasation) is well tolerated.

3.2. KYPHOPLASTY

Kyphoplasty is a new technique combining the vertebroplasty experience and the balloon catheter technology developed for angioplasty. It involves the extra- or transpedicular cannulation of the vertebral body, under fluoroscopic guidance, followed by insertion of an inflatable bone tamp (Figs. 4 and 5). Once inflated, the tamp partially restores the vertebral body to its original height, reduces the fracture, elevates the endplate, and creates a cavity to be filled with bone cement (Fig. 4B). To reduce the risk of extravasation, the cement is injected under relatively low pressure (Fig. 4C).

Compared with vertebroplasty, kyphoplasty has several advantages. In biomechanical models of compression fractures (44), kyphoplasty has been shown to increase strength and to restore height to a greater extent than does vertebroplasty. In a series of 70 kyphoplasty procedures in 30 patients by Lieberman et al. (45), kyphoplasty restored 47% of lost height in 70% of the patients with osteoporotic compression fractures. The same study (45) also showed that kyphoplasty was effective at reducing pain: after kyphoplasty, there were significant improvements in SF-36 scores for bodily pain, physical function, role physical, vitality, and mental health, although general health and role emotional scores remained unchanged (45). Most importantly, cement extravasation occurred in only 6 of 70 treated vertebrae, and in all cases the extravasations were asymptomatic (45). This finding compares favorably with the

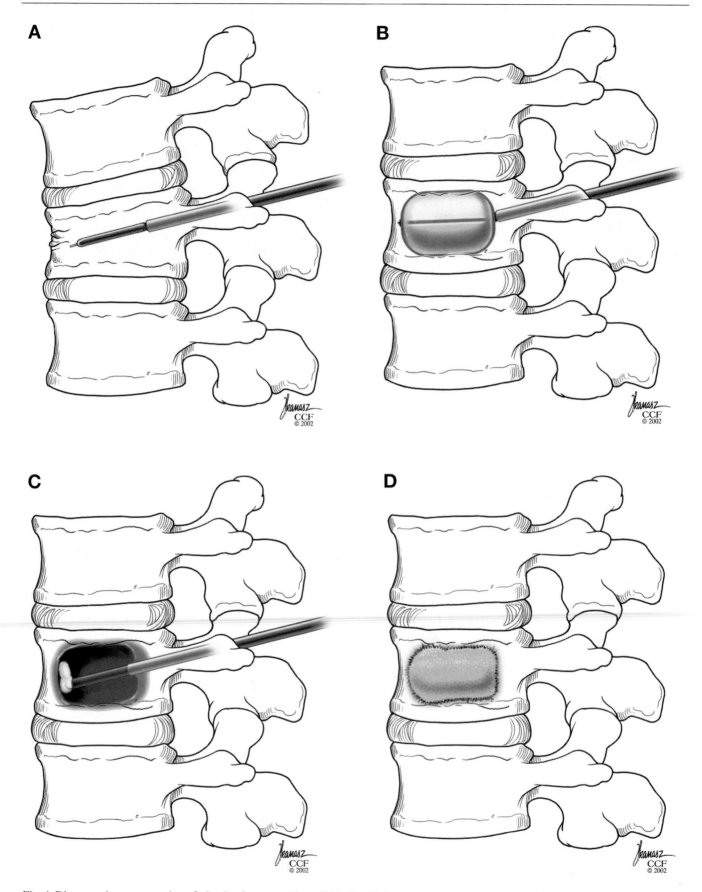

Fig. 4. Diagramatic representation of a kyphoplasty procedure. (**A**) Inflatable bone tamp inserted through working canula. (**B**) Cavity creation via inflatable bone tamp. (**C**) Cement injection. (**D**) Cement within cavity created by inflatable bone tamp.

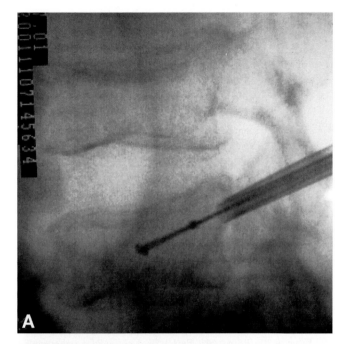

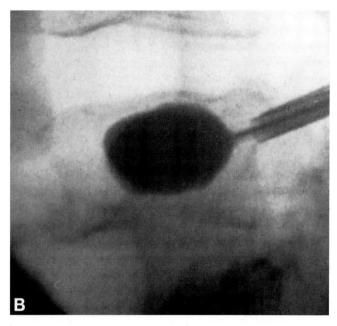

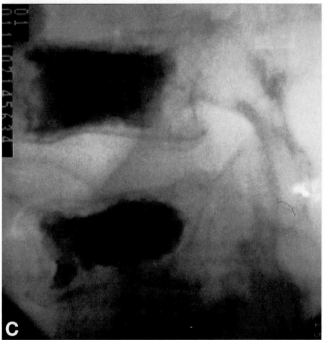

Fig. 5. Clinical images of a kyphoplasty procedure. (A) Inflatable bone tamp inserted through a working cannula. (B) Balloon inflation and cavity creation. (C) Cement within cavity created by inflatable balloon tamp.

high extravasation rate of vertebroplasty (41). The results of Lieberman et al. (45) have been updated by Coumans et al. (46) in a series of 188 kyphoplasty procedures in 78 patients with similar findings.

There are several reasons why fracture reduction, a step in kyphoplasty but not in vertebroplasty, is desirable. Biomechanically, a collapsed vertebra creates stresses on the adjacent levels, which predisposes them to collapse. In the case of osteoporosis, for example, it has been estimated that the risk of collapse is fivefold once a fracture has occurred, in large part owing to the altered biomechanics (47). In addition to causing pain and predisposing to additional fracture and deformity, compression fractures have a substantial impact on pulmonary

function (48). Therefore, the restoration of height and alignment whenever possible is potentially beneficial.

Because fracture reduction is part of this procedure, the best results are obtained with acute and subacute fractures. Magnetic resonance imaging scanning has proved useful in selecting the best candidates for fracture reduction (49). Frequently, it even allows the discrimination between benign and pathological fractures. Chronic osteoporotic fractures exhibit T1- and T2-weighted sequence signals that are isointense to normal vertebral bodies. Acute benign fractures show edema, often along one of the fractured endplates, manifested as a hypointense signal on T1-weighted images and hyperintensity on T2-weighted images. Malignant lesions frequently exhibit ill-defined borders and are usually hypointense on noncontrast T1-weighted images. Bone scanning can also be useful, showing increased radionuclide uptake in acute fractures compared with chronic fractures (49).

Myelomatous osteolytic destruction of the spinal column is common in patients with multiple myeloma and has become more of a clinical issue by virtue of their prolonged survival rates. Typically, the diffuse involvement that occurs results in painful progressive vertebral compression fractures at multiple levels over time. Treatment with bed rest, bracing, and analgesics is the standard of care for most of these patients, but it has proven to be of limited benefit, especially when considering the progressive spinal kyphosis and its subsequent consequences.

Kyphoplasty has been successfully used to treat the painful progressive osteolytic vertebral collapse associated with multiple myeloma (50). In a prospective series, 55 consecutive kyphoplasty procedures were performed over 27 sessions in 18 patients with osteolytic vertebral compression fractures resulting from multiple myeloma *(50)*. The mean age of patients was 63.5 yr (range of 48–79 yr), the mean duration of symptoms was 11 mo, and the mean follow up of 7.4 mo. The levels treated were T6 to L5. The authors reported no major complications related directly to use of this technique. On average, 34% of lost height was restored. Asymptomatic cement leakage occurred at only 2 of 55 levels (4%). The authors noted statistically significant improvement in SF-36 scores for bodily pain, physical function, vitality, and social functioning. They concluded that kyphoplasty was efficacious in the treatment of osteolytic vertebral compression fractures secondary to multiple myeloma and that it was associated with early clinical improvement of pain and function as well as some restoration of vertebral body height in these patients. Similar results have been reported by other authors, including Fourney et al. *(41)*, who reported on 32 cancer patients who underwent the kyphoplasty procedure and 65 who underwent the vertebroplasty procedure. Fourney et al. *(41)* found statistically significant improvements in visual analogue scale pain scores and analgesic consumption in both groups and no procedure-related complications in either group, except for a 9.2% (6/65) rate of asymptomatic cement leakage with vertebroplasty.

4. CONCLUSIONS

Minimally invasive approaches to the spine offer an important tool in the treatment of patients with metastatic disease: they provide a means of relieving symptoms with less physiological disturbance and trauma in patients with limited life expectancies. However, these techniques should not be used if doing so will preclude achieving the goals of surgery (i.e., to decompress the neural structures and stabilize the spine), nor should they be used in patients who are too ill to tolerate an emergent conversion to an open procedure in the event of a complication. Future developments likely will include a merging of endoscopic techniques and image guidance *(51,52)*. Such technological advances are likely to increase the spectrum of endoscopic and percutaneous approaches and permit increasingly complex procedures to be performed less traumatically.

The term "minimally invasive spinal therapy" means much more than the endoscopic techniques previously described, it now encompasses everything from traditional injection techniques (epidural injections, discography, facet, and nerve root blocks) to percutaneous therapeutic modalities (intradiscal electrothermal therapy, vertebroplasty, kyphoplasty) and true endoscopic procedures (endoscopic discectomies, endoscopic lumbar fusions, endoscopic transthoracic procedures). This definition will continue to evolve as new advances in technology (image-guided surgery), biology (bone substitutes and enhancers, nuclear regeneration), and diagnostic techniques are developed and impact on spinal treatment modalities. However, such evolution must be embraced with caution: although there is a clear trend showing that technological advances will improve spinal surgery, there is also a reciprocal trend showing that biological advances may decrease the need for surgical intervention in the spine.

REFERENCES

1. Body JJ, Bartl R, Burckhardt P, et al. Current use of bisphosphonates in oncology. International Bone and Cancer Study Group. J Clin Oncol 1998; 16:3890–3899.
2. Schachar NS. An update on the nonoperative treatment of patients with metastatic bone disease. Clin Orthop 2001; 382:75–81.
3. Dickman CA, Karahalios DG. Thoracoscopic spinal surgery. Clin Neurosurg 1996; 43:392–422.
4. Hanley E, Green NE, Spengler DM. An AOA critical issue. Less invasive procedures in spine surgery. J Bone Joint Surg 2003; 85:956–=961.
5. Staelin ST, Zdeblick TA, Mahvi DM. Laparoscopic lumbar spinal fusion: the role of the general surgeon. J Laparoendosc Adv Surg Tech 2000; 10:297–304.
6. Zdeblick TA. Laparoscopic spinal fusion. Orthop Clin North Am 1998; 29:635–645.
7. Jacobaeus HC. Possibility of th euse of the cystoscope for investigation of serious cavities. Munch Med Wochenschr 1910; 57:2090–2092.
8. Lin JC, Wiechmann RJ, Szwerc MF, et al. Diagnostic and therapeutic video-assisted thoracic surgery resection of pulmonary metastases. Surgery 1999; 126:636–641.
9. Lin JC, Hazelrigg SR, Landreneau RJ. Video-assisted thoracic surgery for diseases within the mediastinum. Surg Clin North Am 2000; 80:1511–1533.
10. Schwarz RE, Posner MC, Ferson PF, Keenan RJ, Landreneau RJ. Thoracoscopic techniques for the management of intrathoracic metastases. Results. Surg Endosc 1998; 12:842–845.
11. Landreneau RJ, Hazelrigg SR, Mack MJ, et al. Postoperative pain-related morbidity: video-assisted thoracic surgery versus thoracotomy. Ann Thorac Surg 1993; 56:1285–1289.
12. Landreneau RJ, Mack MJ, Hazelrigg SR, et al. Prevalence of chronic pain after pulmonary resection by thoracotomy or video-assisted thoracic surgery. J Thorac Cardiovasc Surg 1994; 107:1079–1085.
13. Dickman CA, Rosenthal D, Karahalios DG, et al. Thoracic vertebrectomy and reconstruction using a microsurgical thoracoscopic approach. Neurosurgery 1996; 38:279–293.
14. Han PP, Kenny K, Dickman CA. Thoracoscopic approaches to the thoracic spine: experience with 241 surgical procedures. Neurosurgery 2002; 51:S2-88–S2-95.
15. McAfee PC, Regan JR, Fedder IL, Mack MJ, Geis WP. Anterior thoracic corpectomy for spinal cord decompression performed endoscopically. Surg Laparosc Endosc 1995; 5:339–348.
16. McLain RF, Lieberman IH. Endoscopic approaches to metastatic thoracic disease. Spine 2000; 25:1855–1858.
17. Rosenthal D, Marquardt G, Lorenz R, Nichtweiss M. Anterior decompression and stabilization using a microsurgical endoscopic technique for metastatic tumors of the thoracic spine. J Neurosurg 1996; 84:565–572.
18. McAfee PC, Regan JR, Zdeblick T, et al. The incidence of complications in endoscopic anterior thoracolumbar spinal reconstructive surgery. A prospective multicenter study comprising the first 100 consecutive cases. Spine 1995; 20:1624–1632.
19. Lieberman IH, Salo PT, Orr RD, Kraetschmer B. Prone position endoscopic transthoracic release with simultaneous posterior instrumentation for spinal deformity: a description of the technique. Spine 2000; 25:2251–2257.
20. McLain RF. Endoscopically assisted decompression for metastatic thoracic neoplasms. Spine 1998; 23:1130–1135.
21. McLain RF. Spinal cord decompression: an endoscopically assisted approach for metastatic tumors. Spinal Cord 2001; 39:482–487.
22. Deramond H, Depriester C, Galibert P, Le Gars D. Percutaneous vertebroplasty with polymethylmethacrylate. Technique, indications, and results. Radiol Clin North Am 1998; 36:533–546.
23. Diener KM. Bisphosphonates for controlling pain from metastatic bone disease. Am J Health Syst Pharm 1996; 53:1917–1927.

24. Galibert P, Deramond H, Rosat P, Le Gars D. [Preliminary note on the treatment of vertebral angioma by percutaneous acrylic vertebroplasty]. Neurochirurgie 1987; 33:166–168.

25. Kaemmerlen P, Thiesse P, Jonas P, et al. Percutaneous injection of orthopedic cement in metastatic vertebral lesions [letter]. N Engl J Med 1989; 321:121.

26. Mathis JM, Petri M, Naff N. Percutaneous vertebroplasty treatment of steroid-induced osteoporotic compression fractures. Arthritis Rheum 1998; 41:171–175.

27. Jensen ME, Evans AJ, Mathis JM, Kallmes DF, Cloft HJ, Dion JE. Percutaneous polymethylmethacrylate vertebroplasty in the treatment of osteoporotic vertebral body compression fractures: technical aspects. AJNR Am J Neuroradiol 1997; 18:1897–1904.

28. Gangi A, Kastler BA, Dietemann JL. Percutaneous vertebroplasty guided by a combination of CT and fluoroscopy. AJNR Am J Neuroradiol 1994; 15:83–86.

29. Weill A, Chiras J, Simon JM, Rose M, Sola-Martinez T, Enkaoua E. Spinal metastases: indications for and results of percutaneous injection of acrylic surgical cement. Radiology 1996; 199:241–247.

30. Cortet B, Cotten A, Boutry N, et al. Percutaneous vertebroplasty in the treatment of osteoporotic vertebral compression fractures: an open prospective study. J Rheumatol 1999; 26:2222–2228.

31. Barr JD, Barr MS, Lemley TJ, McCann RM. Percutaneous vertebroplasty for pain relief and spinal stabilization. Spine 2000; 25:923–928.

32. Deramond H, Wright NT, Belkoff SM. Temperature elevation caused by bone cement polymerization during vertebroplasty. Bone 1999; 25:17S–21S.

33. Jefferiss CD, Lee AJC, Ling RSM. Thermal aspects of self-curing polymethylmethacrylate. J Bone Joint Surg 1975; 57:511–518.

34. Radin EL, Rubin CT, Thrasher EL, et al. Changes in the bone-cement interface after total hip replacement. An in vivo animal study. J Bone Joint Surg 1982; 64:1188–1200.

35. San Millan Ruiz D, Burkhardt K, Jean B, et al. Pathology findings with acrylic implants. Bone 1999; 25:85S–90S.

36. Belkoff SM, Maroney M, Fenton DC, Mathis JM. An in vitro biomechanical evaluation of bone cements used in percutaneous vertebroplasty. Bone 1999; 25:23S–26S.

37. Tohmeh AG, Mathis JM, Fenton DC, Levine AM, Belkoff SM. Biomechanical efficacy of unipedicular *versus* bipedicular vertebroplasty for the management of osteoporotic compression fractures. Spine 1999; 24:1772–1776.

38. Schildhauer TA, Bennett AP, Wright TM, Lane JM, O'Leary PF. Intravertebral body reconstruction with an injectable in situ-setting carbonated apatite: biomechanical evaluation of a minimally invasive technique. J Orthop Res 1999; 17:67–72.

39. Padovani B, Kasriel O, Brunner P, Peretti-Viton P. Pulmonary embolism caused by acrylic cement: a rare complication of percutaneous vertebroplasty. AJNR Am J Neuroradiol 1999; 20:375–377.

40. Alvarez L, Perez-Higueras A, Quinones D, Calvo E, Rossi RE. Vertebroplasty in the treatment of vertebral tumors: postprocedural outcome and quality of life. Eur Spine J 2003; 12:356–360.

41. Fourney DR, Schomer DF, Nader R, et al. Percutaneous vertebroplasty and kyphoplasty for painful vertebral body fractures in cancer patients. J Neurosurg 2003; 98:21–30.

42. Martin JB, Wetzel SG, Seium Y, et al. Percutaneous vertebroplasty in metastatic disease: transpedicular access and treatment of lysed pedicles—initial experience. Radiology 2003; 229:593–597.

43. Wenger M. Vertebroplasty for metastasis. Med Oncol 2003; 20:203–209.

44. Belkoff SM, Mathis JM, Fenton DC, Scribner RM, Reiley ME, Talmadge K. An ex vivo biomechanical evaluation of an inflatable bone tamp used in the treatment of compression fracture. Spine 2001; 26:151–156.

45. Lieberman IH, Dudeney S, Reinhardt MK, Bell G. Initial outcome and efficacy of "kyphoplasty" in the treatment of painful osteoporotic vertebral compression fractures. Spine 2001; 26:1631–1638.

46. Coumans JV, Reinhardt MK, Lieberman IH. Kyphoplasty for vertebral compression fractures: 1-year clinical outcomes from a prospective study. J Neurosurg 2003; 991 :44–50.

47. Heaney RP. The natural history of vertebral osteoporosis. Is low bone mass an epiphenomenon? Bone 1992; 13:S23–S26.

48. Leech JA, Dulberg C, Kellie S, Pattee L, Gay J. Relationship of lung function to severity of osteoporosis in women. Am Rev Respir Dis 1990; 141:68–71.

49. Do HM. Magnetic resonance imaging in the evaluation of patients for percutaneous vertebroplasty. Top Magn Reson Imaging 2000; 11:235–244.

50. Dudeney S, Lieberman IH, Reinhardt MK, Hussein M. Kyphoplasty in the treatment of osteolytic vertebral compression fractures as a result of multiple myeloma. J Clin Oncol 2002; 20:2382–2387.

51. Assaker R, Reyns N, Pertruzon B, Lejeune JP. Image-guided endoscopic spine surgery: Part II: clinical applications. Spine 2001; 26:1711–1718.

52. Assaker R, Cinquin P, Cotten A, Lejeune JP. Image-guided endoscopic spine surgery: Part I. A feasibility study. Spine 2001; 26:1705–1710.

35 Single-Stage Posterolateral Transpedicle Approach With Circumferential Decompression and Instrumentation for Spinal Metastases

MARK H. BILSKY, MD, TODD VITAZ, MD, AND PATRICK BOLAND, MD

CONTENTS

1. INTRODUCTION

Metastatic tumors to the spine account for significant morbidity in cancer patients. With treatment, one seeks to restore quality of life, reduce pain, and preserve or maintain neurological function. The roles for chemotherapy, radiation therapy (RT), and surgery continue to evolve, but clearly all play significant roles in treating metastatic spinal tumors. Initial attempts to treat tumors using a laminectomy approach proved no better than radiation alone. Inherently, laminectomy is ineffective for treating metastatic spine tumors because it does not effectively address anterior vertebral body or epidural tumor, and creates iatrogenic instability. The evolution of operative approaches for metastatic spine tumors, including anterior transcavitary and posterolateral, and the development of segmental fixation has markedly improved surgical outcomes (1–5,7–14,16–30). This chapter describes the authors' indications, operative techniques, and outcomes using a single-stage posterolateral transpedicle approach (PTA) (2), which provides exposure for epidural tumor and vertebral body resection, and anterior and posterior reconstruction.

2. INDICATIONS FOR OPERATION

Decision making for the treatment of metastatic spinal tumors is often difficult. RT remains the primary treatment modality,

From: *Current Clinical Oncology: Cancer in the Spine: Comprehensive Care.*
Edited by: R. F. McLain, K-U. Lewandrowski, M. Markman, R. M. Bukowski,
R. Macklis, and E. C. Benzel © Humana Press, Inc., Totowa, NJ

but a small subset of patients will benefit from early operation. Decisions can be made based either on a conceptual framework or a list of indications. A conceptual framework provides an algorithm to evaluate individual patients based on oncological, neurological, and biomechanical indications. Oncological issues reflect the radiation and/or chemo-sensitivity of a given tumor type, resection of residual tumor post neoadjuvant RT or chemotherapy, or biological pain (nocturnal or early morning) responsive to steroids. Neurological concerns include the presence and degree of radiculopathy, myelopathy, and degree of radiographic epidural spinal cord compression. Biomechanical issues include the presence of axial or incidental back pain, pattern of bone involvement, and the presence of coronal (scoliosis) and sagittal (kyphosis) plane deformities.

In general, RT is given to patients with moderate- to high-radiation-sensitive tumors who are biomechanically stable. With few exceptions, the degree of epidural compression is less likely to impact on the decision to radiate than the radiosensitivity of the tumor. Biomechanical stability is often defined by the quality of the back pain, specifically by the degree of incidental or movement-related back pain. This pain often does not resolve with RT. Conversely, patients with biological pain generally improve with RT or chemotherapy. Radiographic criteria are less helpful in defining instability and are dependent on the segmental level involved. For example, thoracic spine compression fractures rarely result in instability, but subaxial cervical spine compression fractures often present with intractable neck pain.

Surgery is reserved as first-line therapy for patients with radioresistant tumors (e.g., sarcoma, renal cell carcinoma), spinal instability, and/or a pathological fracture with bone in the spinal canal. In the authors' experience, bone in the spinal canal from a pathological fracture is rare. In addition, patients with high-grade spinal cord compression resulting from a circumferential epidural tumor that is moderately radiosensitive have a high probability of progression during RT when compared with other patterns of epidural tumor and are considered for surgery as initial treatment. A frequently reported indication for surgery is unknown diagnosis, but tumor histology can frequently be obtained using a computed tomography (CT)-guided needle or thoracoscopic biopsy.

Following prior RT that has reached spinal cord tolerance, patients are considered for surgery based on progression of neurological symptoms, radiographic progression of tumor, and spinal instability. Patients with residual radiographic tumor following radiation or chemotherapy may be considered for curative surgery (e.g., osteogenic sarcoma, Ewing's sarcoma, germ cell tumor). Contraindications to surgery include a limited life expectancy, significant medical co-morbidities and extensive disease. Additionally, paraplegic patients are rarely operated on because of the significantly low rate of recovery, particularly after 24 h.

3. GOALS OF OPERATION FOR METASTATIC SPINAL TUMORS

Once the decision to operate has been made, the operative approach is dictated by the location of the epidural, bone, and paraspinal tumor, as well as the overall medical and oncological status of the patient. The basic tenets of operations for metastatic spine tumors are fourfold: (1) relieve spinal cord compression (i.e., resect epidural tumor), (2) achieve mechanical stability, (3) maximize tumor resection (e.g., paraspinal mass, chest wall resection), and (4) tailor the operation to produce the least morbidity and best quality of life.

In many practices, the anterior, transcavitary approach is the primary operation used to treat metastatic spine tumors. This is an excellent approach for resection of the vertebral body and anterior paraspinal masses. Spinal cord compression can be relieved if the epidural tumor is primarily located anterolateral on the side of the approach by resection of the posterior longitudinal ligament and unilateral pedicle. Resection of the vertebral body without resection of the epidural tumor may result in early progression of neurological symptoms. Anterior reconstruction can be accomplished with Steinman pins and polymethylmethacrylate (PMMA), cage, or bone graft and an anterior plate, however, in some patients, augmentation with posterior instrumentation may be beneficial to prepare for disease progression at adjacent levels and to reinforce anterior instrumentation.

4. POSTEROLATERAL TRANSPEDICLE APPROACH INDICATIONS

In the authors' practice, a number of patients present with vertebral body tumor extending into the epidural space with 270° or circumferential compression resulting in high-grade spinal cord compression from radioresistant tumor (e.g., sar-

coma, renal cell carcinoma) or in patients who were previously radiated to spinal cord tolerance. To effectively treat these tumors, one would need an anterior transcavitary approach to resect the vertebral body combined with a posterolateral approach to resect the epidural tumor and decompress the spinal cord. For many patients, the morbidity from an anterior and posterior approach seems excessive in light of the patients' medical and oncological co-morbidities. Furthermore, anterior, transcavitary approaches may be difficult because of prior operations, previous radiation therapy, or unresectable ventral paraspinal masses. The solution is to extend the posterolateral approach to include resection of the vertebral body, which for simplicity sake is termed a "PTA" (posterolateral transpedicle approach with circumferential decompression and instrumentation). From a decompressive standpoint, other benefits became clear including the ability to resect three-column bone involvement and to correct sagittal plane deformities from a single approach. An advantage over anterior transcavitary approaches is the ability to initiate epidural tumor resection from a normal dural plane and to resect multilevel epidural tumor without the need to resect uninvolved vertebral bodies. The approach can be extended to include rib or chest wall resection and paraspinal tumors (e.g., psoas muscle) extending to the lumbosacral plexus.

In addition to decompressive benefits, circumferential fixation can also be accomplished from a PTA approach. The anterior column can be reconstructed using a standard Steinman pin and methylmethacrylate construct that has been used effectively in cancer patients for 30 yr. This, combined with posterior segmental fixation, makes a rigid, durable construct.

4.1. PTA TECHNIQUE

Patients are positioned prone on lateral chest supports. The head is placed in a Mayfield pin fixation device. A midline incision is made at least two segments above and below the level to be fused. The ligamentous attachments and muscle are taken off the spinous processes and laminae to the tips of the transverse processes. The rib heads are not exposed unless a chest wall resection is required. If the dorsal elements are involved with tumor, care must be taken to dissect the ligamentous attachments and muscle off the tumor without transmitting pressure to the spinal cord. This is often done with bipolar cautery and Metzenbaum scissors. Dorsal element and adjacent soft tissue tumor is then piecemeal resected to the level of the lamina.

4.2. TUMOR DECOMPRESSION

The dorsal bone work is initiated by removing the spinous processes with a rongeur. The authors have found that the M-8 burr on the Midas Rex drill (Fort Worth, TX) is used to thin the laminae to a cortical shell or to remove all of the bone exposing the ligamentum flavum, dura, or epidural tumor. Residual bone can be removed with a 2 mm Kerrison rongeur. The presence of a ventral mass compressing the spinal cord prohibits the use of large Kerrison rongeurs in the spinal canal. The laminectomy includes the bone overlying the disc spaces adjacent to the involved vertebral body segment and a normal dural plane adjacent to the epidural tumor. Bilateral facetectomies and complete pedicle resection to the base of the vertebral body are accomplished with the drill and curettes. In the lumbar spine, a unilateral facetectomy is often sufficient to gain exposure to the vertebral body tumor.

Following bone removal, the ligamentum flavum and epidural tumor are resected with tenotomy scissors starting at the interface between the tumor and dura. Bipolar cautery used on a low setting at this interface may help define the proper plane for dissection. Nerve roots are sacrificed only if they are enveloped by tumor in order to maximize the epidural tumor resection. The nerve roots are dissected free of tumor before ligation with vascular clips or suture ligatures. Nerve roots have not been sacrificed in the lumbar spine or when a major radicular feeding artery to the spine has been identified on preoperative angiogram.

Having dissected the epidural tumor from the dorsal and lateral dura, the disc spaces adjacent to the diseased vertebral body are exenterated to expose normal endplates (Fig. 1B). In the thoracic spine, it may be necessary to resect a portion of the pedicle caudal to the involved vertebral body to provide exposure of the caudal disc space. A cavity is created in the vertebral body by piecemeal resection of tumor using curettes and pituitary rongeurs.

The most common pattern of disease treated with PTA involves tumor extending from the vertebral body into the epidural space (Fig. 1A). With this pattern of disease, it is rare for tumor to insinuate between the posterior longitudinal ligament (PLL) and the dura. This pattern of tumor can often be predicted from the preoperative magnetic resonance imaging (MRI) scan. The ventral compressive tumor appears bilobed with a hypointense line, representing the PLL, between the vertebral body tumor and the spinal dura. On MRI, the authors have dubbed this the "v" sign (Figs. 2A and 3A). Resection of the intact PLL helps provide a gross resection of tumor at the ventral dura. In the thoracic spine, the plane between the dura and PLL may be difficult to identify, but can be sharply dissected with tenotomy scissors (Fig. 1D). Curettage or blunt dissection of the ligament may put excessive traction on the spinal dura and should be avoided. Once the anterolateral plane between the dura and PLL has been identified, the PLL can often be dissected along the ventral dura. The authors have not encountered significant epidural bleeding following this maneuver. Piecemeal resection of the vertebral body is then completed. The drill may be used to create a larger cavity or to resect infiltrated bone.

4.3. INSTRUMENTED STABILIZATION

Spinal reconstruction is initiated anteriorly. Right angle clamps are used to create starting holes in the vertebral body at the proper depth for placement of the Steinmann pins. The pin is generally bent at a 20° angle and driven into cranial vertebral body using a needle driver with a gentle rotational movement. The pin is then driven back into the caudal vertebral body. A pin is then placed on the contralateral side. Once radiographic confirmation shows good pin placement, PMMA mixed with 1 g of tobramycin is placed into the defect covering the Steinmann pins. The PMMA conforms well to the defect and endplates if allowed to harden slightly before administration and by drying the area of blood. The PMMA should cover the pins completely, so that the construct will remain secure and not rotate (Fig. 1C). The PMMA expands slightly just before it polymerizes, so it

should not directly abut the ventral dura, however, it should be compressed against the vertebral end plates with a Penfield 3 to prevent gaps from forming at the bone cement interface. For patients with primary tumors, bone graft or a cage (packed with bone) can be placed from a posterior approach.

Segmental fixation is then applied to the dorsal spine. In the thoracic spine, a claw construct is applied to one side of the spine and a compression construct on the contralateral side. Pedicle screw fixation is most often used in the lumbar spine and for selected thoracic fixation. Kyphosis correction may be achieved by under bending the rod and translating the spine into alignment. Cross-links are applied, unless they are too prominent (Fig. 1D). The wound is pulse irrigated with Bacitracin irrigant. Posterolateral bone graft may then be applied to decorticated bone for the patients with an expected survival of at least 1 yr.

5. POSTOPERATIVE CARE

Patients are placed in the intensive care unit for at least 24 h with neurological assessments performed every hour. Intravenous antibiotics are continued until the drains are discontinued. Patients are placed on flexicare bed (Hill-Rom, Batesville, IN) for 2 to 3 d, which seems to decrease the risk of wound dehiscence. Deep venous thrombosis prophylaxis consists of pneumatic compression boots. Patients who are predicted to ambulate early do not routinely receive subcutaneous heparin. Sitting in chairs is encouraged on d 1, ambulation on d 2, and walking stairs by d 4. An external orthosis is not used except for patients with instrumentation extending over the cervicothoracic junction who are placed in a soft cervical collar.

6. CASE STUDIES

6.1. CASE STUDY 1

In 1995, a 53-yr-old male presented with nonseminomatous germ-cell tumor and underwent a left orchiectomy, followed by radical lymph node dissection. He underwent three cycles of chemotherapy (cisplatin, vincristine, and bleomycin) and had no remaining evidence of tumor. He was asymptomatic until January 1998, when he developed lower back pain predominantly at night and in the early morning (biological), but no significant pain on ambulation or sitting (biomechanical). Chiropractic manipulation did not improve his pain. In July 1998, systemic evaluation revealed recurrent retroperitoneal tumor, lung nodules, and lytic destruction of the L2 vertebral body. Steroids resolved his back pain and he underwent salvage chemotherapy (cisplatin, etoposide, and ifosfamide) with a decrease in his α-fetoprotein (AFP) from 151,000 to 3000.

In January 1999, he developed intractable back and left L2 radicular pain on ambulation (mechanical radiculopathy) with an increase in AFP to 220,000. CT scan revealed a $15 \times 15 \times 12$ cm mass in the retroperitoneum causing lytic destruction of the L2 vertebral body and facet join and encasing the left L2 nerve root (Fig. 2A,B). The tumor was judged to be unresectable by the urologists because of the size of the mass and prior, extensive retroperitoneal surgery. The patient's expected survival was at least 6 mo. RT was a potential option, but had a low probability of resolving the mechanical instability pain or mechanical radiculopathy.

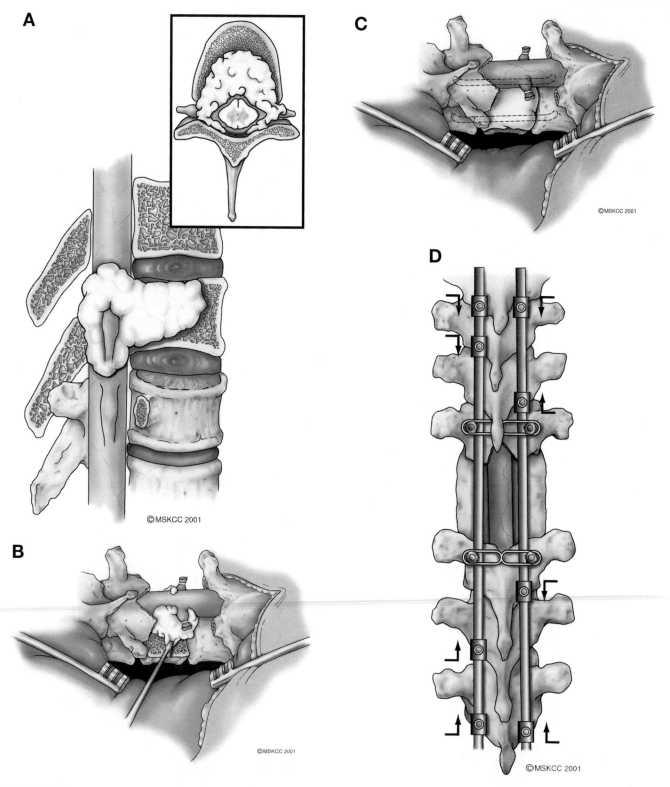

Fig. 1. **(A)** Diagram shows the typical pattern of tumor extending from the vertebral body, pushing the posterior longitudinal ligament posteriorly to compress the spinal cord bilaterally. **(B)** Following posterolateral decompression with a high-speed drill, the lateral dura is stripped of tumor and rhizotomy is performed with vascular clips. The vertebral body is then intralesional resected, followed by sharp dissection of the posterior longitudinal ligament to obtain an anterior dural margin. **(C)** Anterior reconstruction is accomplished with polymethylmethacrylate, impregnated with tobramycin, and Steinman pins. **(D)** Posterior segmental fixation is placed.

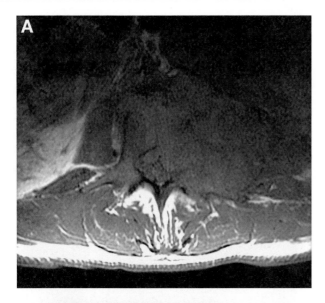

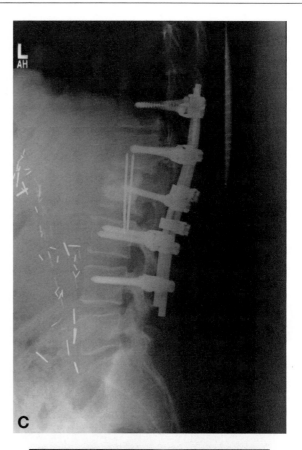

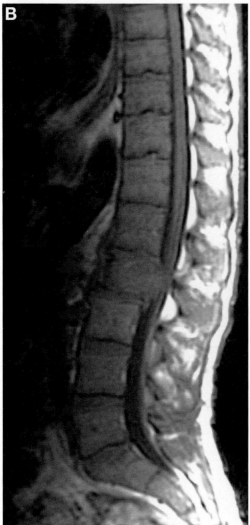

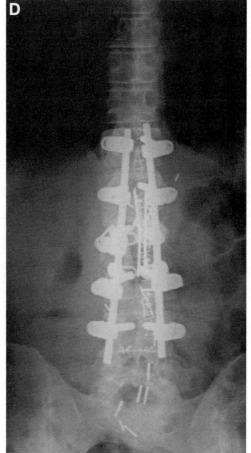

Fig. 2. Case 1. (**A,B**) Axial and sagittal magnetic resonance imaging images show L2 vertebral body replacement with high-grade epidural thecal sac compression and a massive left paraspinal tumor. (**C,D**) Anterior/posterior and lateral plain radiographs show anterior reconstruction with polymethylmethacrylate and pins and posterior segmental fixation with pedicle screws.

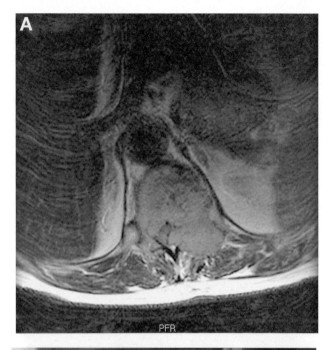

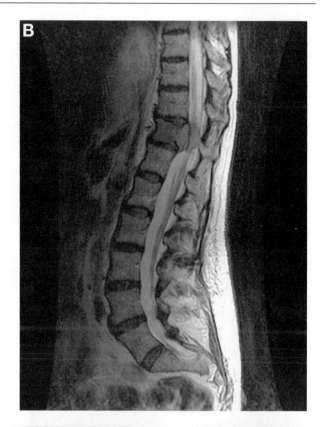

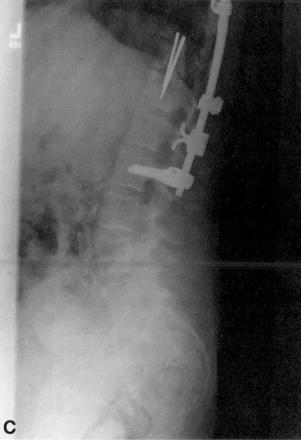

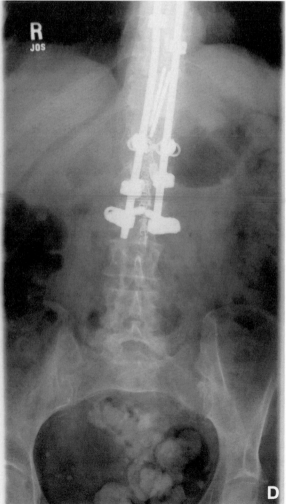

Fig. 3. Case 2. (A,B) Axial and sagittal magnetic resonance imaging
images show T11 vertebral body replacement extending into the left
T11–L2 facet joint resulting in high-grade spinal cord compression.
Anterior/posterior and lateral radiographs show anterior reconstruction with polymethylmethacrylate (PMMA) and pins and posterior
segmental fixation using a combination of hooks and screws. (C,D)
Anterior/posterior and lateral plain radiographs show anterior reconstruction with PMMA and pins and posterior segmental fixation with
pedicle screws and hooks.

A PTA was performed with unilateral left pedicle resection. The L2 nerve root was identified in the spinal canal and tumor was dissected from it to the level of the lumbosacral plexus. The L2 vertebral body was resected and anterior and posterior fixation were achieved (Fig. 2C,D). The patient's pain resolved and he was able to sit in a chair and ambulate without significant pain. He died of tumor progression at 5 mo following the operation.

6.2. CASE STUDY 2

A 67-yr-old female presented with a 4-mo history of nocturnal back pain. Two weeks before presentation, the back pain increased dramatically on ambulation. Chest CT scan showed a new right upper lobe mass. MRI showed a T11 vertebral body tumor extending to replace the left posterior elements and causing high-grade spinal cord compression (Fig. 3A,B) She was neurologically normal. Needle biopsy of the spinal lesion confirmed poorly differentiated non-small cell lung carcinoma.

The treatment decision to operate was based on the presence of mechanical instability resulting from vertebral body and facet involvement (biomechanical) and the relative radio-insensitivity of lung cancer (oncological) in the presence of high-grade spinal cord compression (neurological).

The patient underwent a PTA to treat circumferential bone involvement and epidural tumor involvement (Fig. 3C,D). She had resolution of her back pain and maintained normal neurological and functional status postoperatively. Six weeks after her operation, she underwent spinal irradiation to a total dose of 3000 cGy in 10 fractions and was subsequently started on chemotherapy. She maintained an excellent performance status until progression of tumor 14 mo following her diagnosis and ultimately died of disease 16 mo after her presentation.

7. RESULTS

The authors reported their initial experience with the PTA in 25 patients over a 15-mo period (2). The patients in this cohort had fairly advanced systemic tumor, generally could not tolerate an anterior and posterior approach to resect the vertebral body(ies), and had high-grade epidural spinal cord compression. All patients showed significant pain improvement of radicular, biological, and mechanical pain. Of the 21 patients presenting with severe or moderate pain, all had resolution to mild pain except 2, who had residual moderate pain. Pain improvement has been seen in 74 to 100% of patients in other series reporting this approach (1,3,13,16,19,24,26). Neurological assessments using the American Spinal Injury Association impairment scale (15), were stable or improved in 23/25 patients. Performance status assessment using Eastern Cooperative Oncology Group scores (6) showed 22/25 patients achieved a score of 2 or better, in essence able to ambulate and capable of self-care.

Complications in this group included Clostridium difficile colitis (1 patient), wound dehiscence (1 patient), gastrointestinal (GI) bleed (2 patients), and pulmonary embolism (1 patient). There was no evidence of fixation failures in the follow-up of these patients. Three patients (12%) died within 30 d. Of the perioperative deaths, two patients were fully ambulatory and had already been discharged from the hospital. One died from a massive GI bleed, presumably related to perioperative steroid administration. The second patient died from *Clostridium*

difficile colitis and the development of toxic megacolon. The third patient had progressive liver failure related to hepatocellular carcinoma.

The authors initially used the PTA approach for the sickest patient population, reserving anterior transcavitary or combined approaches for patients with less systemic disease and medical co-morbidities. Encouraged by the early results, the PTA has become the approach of choice at our institution for patients with high-grade epidural compression and vertebral body tumor. Including the initial 25 patients, the PTA has been used in 127/404 (31%) operated patients for metastatic spine tumors over the past 40 mo. The good pain, neurological, and functional outcomes make this a reliable approach to provide meaningful palliation in this patient population.

REFERENCES

1. Akeyson E, McCutcheon IE. Single-stage posterior vertebrectomy and replacement combined with posterior instrumentation for spinal metastasis. J Neurosurg 1996; 85:211–220.
2. Bilsky MH, Boland P, Lis E, Raizer JJ, Healey JH. Single-stage posterolateral transpedicle approach or spondylectomy, epidural decompression, and circumferential fusion of spinal metastases. Spine 2000; 25:2240–2250.
3. Bridwell K, Jenny A, Saul T, Rich KM, Grubb RL. Posterior segmental spinal instrumentation (PSSI) with posterolateral decompression and debulking for metastatic thoracic and lumbar spine disease: limitations and technique. Spine 1998; 13:1383–1394.
4. Cahill DW, Kumar R. Palliative subtotal vertebrectomy with anterior and posterior reconstruction via single posterior approach. J Neurosurg 1999; 90:42–47.
5. Cooper P, Errico T, Martin R, Crawford B, DiBartolo T. A systematic approach to spinal reconstruction after anterior decompression for neoplastic disease of the thoracic and lumbar spine. Neurosurgery 1993; 32:1–8.
6. Oken MM, Creech RH, Tomey DC, et al. Eastern Cooperative Group Performance Status Scale. Am J Clin Oncol 1982; 5:649–655.
7. Faccioli F, Lima J, Bricolo A. One-stage decompression and stabilization in the treatment of spinal tumors. J Neurosurg Sci 1985; 29:199–205.
8. Gokaslan ZL, York JE, Walsh GL, et al. Transthoracic vertebrectomy for metastatic spinal tumors. J Neurosurg 1998; 89:599–609.
9. Hall D, Webb J. Anterior plate fixation in spine tumor surgery. Indications, techniques, and results. Spine 1991; 3:S80–S83.
10. Harrington K. The use of methylmethacrylate for vertebral body replacement and anterior stabilization of pathological fracture-dislocations of the spine due to metastatic malignant disease. Journal of Bone Joint Surg Am 1981; 63:36–46.
11. Harrington K. Anterior cord decompression and spinal stabilization for patients with metastatic lesions of the spine. J Neurosurgery 1984; 61:107–117.
12. Harrington K. Anterior decompression and stabilization of the spine as a treatment for vertebral body collapse and spinal cord compression for metastatic malignancy. Clin Orthop 1988; 233:177–197.
13. Heller M, McBroom R, MacNab T, et al. Treatment for metastatic disease of the spine with posterolateral decompression and Luque instrumentation. Neuroorthopedics 1986; 2:70–74.
14. Hosono N, Yonenobu K, Fuji T, Ebara S, Yamashita K, Ono K. Vertebral body replacement with ceramic prosthesis for metastatic spinal tumors. Spine 1995; 20:2454–2462.
15. International Standards for Neurological and Functional Classifications of Spinal Cord Injury. American Spinal Injury Association. Chicago, IL: 1982;9 :78–98.
16. Johnston F, Uttley D, Marsh HT. Synchronous vertebral decompression and posterior stabilization in the treatment of spinal malignancy. Neurosurgery 1989; 25:872–876.
17. Lesoin F, Rousseaux M, Autricque A, et al. Posterolateral approach to tumors of the dorsolumbar spine. Acta Neurochir 1986; 81:40–44.

18. Lozes G, Fawaz A, Devos P, et al. Operative treatment of thoraco-lumbar metastases, using methylmethacrylate and Kempf's rods for vertebral replacement and stabilization. Report of 15 cases. Acta Neurochir 1987; 84:118–123.

19. Magerl F, Coscia M. Total posterior vertebrectomy of the thoracic and lumbar spine. Clin Orthop Rel Res. 1988; 232:62–69.

20. Moore A, Uttley D. Anterior decompression and stabilization of the spine in malignant disease. Neurosurgery 1989; 24:713–717.

21. Onimus M, Schraub S, Bertin D, Bosset JF, Guidet M. Surgical treatment of vertebral metastasis. Spine 1986; 11:883–891.

22. Perrin RG, McBroom RJ. Anterior versus posterior decompression for symptomatic spinal metastasis. Can J Neurol Sci 1987; 14:75–80.

23. Perrin RG, McBroom RJ. Spinal fixation after anterior decompression for symptomatic spinal metastasis. Neurosurgery 1998; 22:324–327.

24. Shaw B, Mansfield F, Borges L. One-stage posterolateral decompression and stabilization for primary and metastatic vertebral tumors in the thoracic and lumbar spine. J Neurosurg 1989; 70:405–410.

25. Siegal T, Siegal T. Surgical decompression of anterior and posterior malignant epidural tumors compressing the spinal cord: a prospective study. Neurosurgery 1985; 17:424–432.

26. Steffee AD, Sitkowski DJ, Topham LS. Total vertebral body and pedicle arthroplasty. Clin Orthop Rel Res 1986; 203:203–208.

27. Sundaresan N, Galicich JH, Lane JM, Bains MS, McCormack P. Treatment of neoplastic epidural cord compression by vertebral body resection and stabilization. J Neurosurg 1985; 63:676–684.

28. Sundaresan N, DiGiacinto G, Krol G, Hughes JE. Spondylectomy for malignant tumors of the spine. J Clin Oncol 1989; 7:1485–1491.

29. Sundaresan N, Steinberger AA, Moore F, et al. Indications and results of combined anterior-posterior approaches for spine tumor surgery. J Neurosurgery 1996; 85:438–446.

30. Walsh GL, Gokaslan ZL, McCutcheon IE, et al. Anterior approaches to the thoracic spine in patients with cancer: indications and results. Ann Thorac Surg 1997; 64:1611–1618.

36 Primary Benign Spinal Tumors

Gordon R. Bell, MD

Contents

1. INTRODUCTION

Primary bone tumors are rare, accounting for approx 0.4% of all tumors, and primary spine tumors represent only approx 10% of all bone tumors *(1,2)*. Overall, primary spine tumors are much less common than metastatic lesions to the spine. The nature of a primary bone tumor of the spine depends largely on the location of the lesion and the age of the patient. Lesions located within the vertebral body are far more likely to represent a malignancy, particularly a metastatic lesion, than lesions in the posterior elements. Up to 75% of tumors located within the vertebral body are malignant, compared with only 35% found in the posterior elements *(3)*. Metastatic lesions involve the vertebral body initially in approx 85% of cases, and are seven times more likely to involve the vertebral body than the posterior elements.

The age of the patient also plays a significant role in the likelihood of a bony spine lesion being malignant. Malignancies, in general, are far more common in older patients. Because the incidence of most carcinomas peaks in the fourth through sixth decades, lesions occurring at or beyond this age have a high likelihood of malignancy. It has been estimated that greater than 70% of primary tumors in patients older than 21 yr of age are malignant, compared to patients younger than 21 yr of age, where the majority of lesions are benign *(3)*. Therefore, the combination of a posterior element lesion in a young patient is very likely benign.

Tumors may be "malignant" either by their nature or by their location. Malignant lesions are aggressive by nature, and are characterized by their tendency to recur and to metastasize. Although many primary bone tumors of the spine are benign, they may have a high morbidity by virtue of their location and

their tendency to cause neural compression. Tumors causing spinal cord, conus medullaris, cauda equina, or nerve root compression may present difficult therapeutic and technical challenges and may require aggressive surgery, such as combined anterior and posterior approaches.

2. CLINICAL FEATURES

Primary benign bony tumors of the spine may either be asymptomatic or symptomatic. Although the most common presenting symptom is axial pain, that symptom is notoriously nonspecific, being present in up to 80% of the population at some time during their lives. Cancer is an uncommon cause of low back pain, being reported in less than 1% of patients presenting with back pain in a primary care practice *(4)*. The presence of pain with non-mechanical features, however, should raise clinical suspicion of another etiology. Persistent pain, pain at rest, and nocturnal pain warrants further investigation. Indeed, the combination of such pain with a neurological deficit should prompt suspicion of a primary or metastatic lesion. In a large retrospective study of 82 primary neoplasms of the spine, axial pain was present in 60.2% of patients and radicular pain in 24% *(3)*. The incidence was similar for both benign and malignant lesions. In that study, the duration of pain before diagnosis was nearly twice as long for benign lesions than for malignancies (19.3 vs 10.4 mo). Features suggesting a benign tumor rather than a malignancy included: younger patient age, absence of neurological deficit, and posterior location of the lesion.

The presence of a painful scoliosis, particularly in an adolescent, should raise the suspicion of a spinal tumor, because idiopathic scoliosis is not typically painful. Painful scoliosis associated with unilateral benign intra-osseous lesions such as osteoid osteoma and osteoblastoma has been reported *(5,6)*.

The etiology of pain in patients with spinal tumors is thought to result from growth of the tumor and its subsequent expan-

From: *Current Clinical Oncology: Cancer in the Spine: Comprehensive Care.*
Edited by: R. F. McLain, K-U. Lewandrowski, M. Markman, R. M. Bukowski,
R. Macklis, and E. C. Benzel © Humana Press, Inc., Totowa, NJ

sion. As a tumor expands within the confines of the vertebra, expansion of the vertebral cortical bony margin may occur with consequent stretching of the pain-sensitive periosteum. As this process progresses, pathological fracture may occur and instability may result. In addition, compression of adjacent structures may occur. These include neurological structures, such as spinal cord, conus medullaris, cauda equina, or nerve roots. Such compression may mimic the pain of lumbar disc disease *(7)*. Compression of non-neural structures, such as paravertebral soft tissues, may also produce pain.

Neurological deficit is more common with malignant tumors, either primary or metastatic, than with benign primary tumors *(3,8,9)*. However, approximately one-third of patients with benign lesions present with a neurological deficit, compared with slightly more than half of those with a primary malignant vertebral lesion *(3)*.

3. IMAGING

Initial imaging of suspected vertebral tumors should include standard radiographs. The choice of which subsequent radiographic investigations to order depends on many factors, including availability, cost, and patient conditions. In most cases this will include magnetic resonance imaging (MRI), but the patient may not be a candidate for this owing to factors such as claustrophobia, obesity, presence of a pacemaker, or metallic hardware from prior surgery in the location being imaged. When imaging for neural compression is required under such conditions, myelography, with computed tomography (CT), is performed. Other imaging, such as bone scanning, may be required as part of the overall work-up of an undiagnosed spinal lesion. Additional imaging studies are sometimes helpful in the diagnosis of some tumors, such as CT, which is useful for CT-guided biopsy of a suspected lesion.

3.1. PLAIN RADIOGRAPHY

Malignant bony lesions most commonly involve the vertebral body, where they are more than seven times more likely to be found, than in the posterior elements. In general, vertebral body lesions are more likely to be malignant, whereas posterior element tumors are more likely to be benign. The sensitivity of routine radiographs to detect bony spine tumors depends on the stage of the disease: lesions are more likely to be detected late, as the disease progresses, than early in its course. Nevertheless, the detection of primary bone tumors of the spine by routine radiography has been reported as high as 99% *(3)*.

Because there must be approx 30 to 50% loss of trabecular bone before a lesion is visible on a routine radiograph, lesions that involve cortical bone are detected earlier than those that involve cancellous bone. Because the posterior elements are composed largely of cortical bone, lesions there are typically detected earlier than lesions in the cancellous vertebral body (Fig. 1). Similarly, lesions involving the pedicle, because of its cortical bone content, are typically detected before they are recognized in the vertebral body. Therefore, scrutiny of the pedicles is mandatory for early detection of bone lesions, particularly metastatic lesions, which tend to involve the vertebral body. The absence of a pedicle ("winking owl sign") on the anteroposterior (AP) radiograph suggests involvement by a metastatic process. Benign spinal lesions, because of their pro-

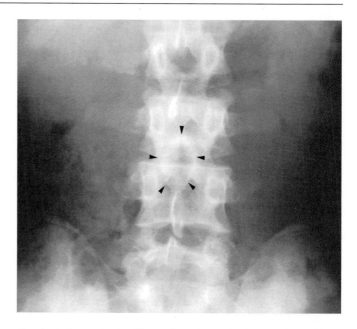

Fig. 1. Anteroposterior X-ray of lumbar spine in a patient with an osteoblastoma involving the spinous process of L3. Note the expansion of the enlarged margins *(arrows)* of the spinous process.

pensity to involve the posterior elements, are more likely to be detected early in the course of the disease than malignant lesions, many of which involve the vertebral body.

Rapidly growing lesions tend to produce a moth-eaten radiographic appearance, whereas slow-growing lesions produce a geographic pattern of bone destruction. The presence of a scalloped margin to a bony lesion suggests a slow growing tumor and therefore the likelihood of a benign lesion. Cortical destruction, on the other hand, indicates a more aggressive lesion and therefore the likelihood of malignancy.

For the lumbar spine standing AP and lateral X-rays, including a spot lateral of the lumbosacral junction, should be obtained. Oblique lumbar radiographs are rarely necessary and result in a significant additional X-ray exposure. Similarly, AP and lateral thoracic radiographs are indicated for a suspected thoracic lesion. For suspected cervical lesions, AP, lateral, and open-mouth odontoid X-rays are obtained. Oblique films are rarely indicated and dynamic flexion-extension views may be ordered later if instability is suspected.

Pathological compression fracture, in the absence of trauma, suggests either metabolic bone disease or tumor. The presence of an associated paravertebral soft tissue mass suggests either tumor or infection. Indeed, the association of vertebral body collapse with vertebral osteomyelitis has been reported, and infection should, therefore, be ruled out *(10)*. Disc space narrowing, particularly when associated with involvement of adjacent vertebral bodies, suggests pyogenic vertebral osteomyelitis rather than tumor because the disc is resistant to spread of tumor *(11)*.

3.2. RADIONUCLIDE IMAGING (BONE SCAN)

Bone scintigraphy (bone scanning) is a useful imaging modality that uses radiation emitted from radiopharmaceutical agents to detect variations in vascularity or osteogenesis *(12)*. Its primary use is in detecting infectious, traumatic, ischemic,

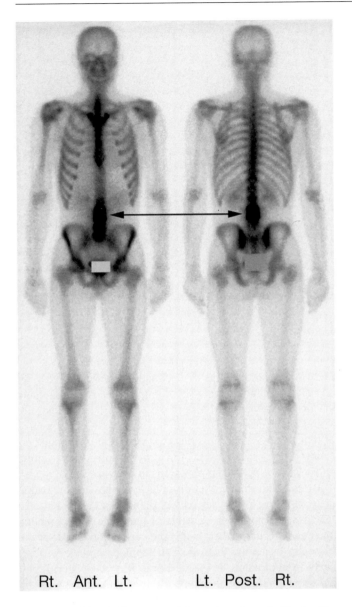

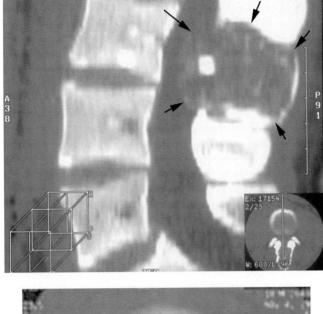

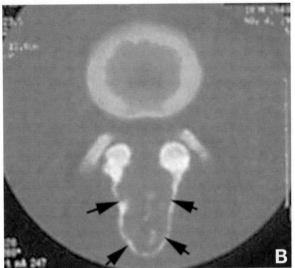

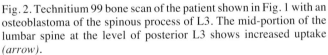

Fig. 2. Technitium 99 bone scan of the patient shown in Fig. 1 with an osteoblastoma of the spinous process of L3. The mid-portion of the lumbar spine at the level of posterior L3 shows increased uptake (*arrow*).

Fig. 3. Sagittal (**A**) and axial (**B**) computed tomography scan of the patient shown in Figs. 1 and 2, which clearly delineates the extent and margins (*arrows*) of the osteoblastoma of the L3 spinous process.

or neoplastic conditions. It is useful as a broad screening tool to image the entire skeleton, and is, therefore, particularly useful in detecting bony lesions, both primary and metastatic.

Technitium 99m, the most commonly used radiopharmaceutical agent for bone scanning, can detect any process that alters the normal balance between bone formation and bone resorption. Conditions that are characterized by an increase in osteoblastic activity result in increased uptake of technetium 99m (Fig. 2). Such conditions most commonly involve bone-forming conditions, such as fractures and bone tumors, but also include other diverse conditions such as osteomyelitis, pseudarthrosis, and avascular necrosis. This lack of specificity is a major drawback to the use of technetium 99m bone scanning. In addition, false-negative results may occur with some aggressive osteolytic conditions, such as multiple myeloma. It is important to correlate information from the bone scan with

both clinical information and ancillary imaging modalities, such as plain radiography, CT, and MRI.

3.3. CT AND CT MYELOGRAPHY

CT is a valuable diagnostic and surgical planning tool that visualizes the spine *directly*, and, therefore, provides precise knowledge of the nature of the compressing lesion. CT shows bony detail better than any other imaging modality, including MRI, and is, therefore, particularly useful in imaging for suspected bony lesions. CT provides more information when performed with sagittal reformation, thereby providing orthogonal (two-plane) imaging (Fig. 3). When ordered routinely, however, it images only the lower three lumbar levels and, thus, has the potential to miss proximal lumbar pathology. Therefore, when scanning for suspected tumors, careful attention must be paid to alerting the technician to the area of interest.

The accuracy of CT in identifying and delineating neural compression can be enhanced by its use following the introduction of water-soluble contrast agents (intrathecal contrast enhanced CT or myelo-CT). Myelography alone provides only *indirect* evidence of neural compression by demonstrating changes in the contour of normal contrast-filled structures. In this respect, it differs from both routine radiography, which gives no information about neural compression, and CT or MRI, both of which *directly* visualize and identify the source of neural compression. When combined with CT, myelography provides information about both the presence or absence of neural compression and its precise nature.

CT is also a useful adjunct for diagnosis when used for a CT-guided biopsy to confirm and identify a bony lesion.

3.4. MAGNETIC RESONANCE IMAGING

MRI images the spine by a matrix of numbers that have been assigned a shade of gray, based on the intensity of a radio wave signal emanating from the tissue. This is owing to the property of the hydrogen protons within the nuclei to be perturbed in the presence of a superimposed magnetic field and external radiofrequency pulse. Typically, osseous structures appear as areas of relative signal void, with cortical bone having a low intensity on MRI and cancellous bone, owing to its fat content, having high signal intensity. The distinction between a small contiguous cortical bone structure and an adjacent soft tissue structure on the T1-weighted sagittal image may be difficult, and precise differentiation between the two may require CT.

MRI, like myelography, images the entire spine and, therefore, can detect unsuspected pathology throughout the spine. MRI visualizes the spine *directly*, and therefore provides detail as to the nature and extent of lesions or neural compression (Fig. 4). Unlike routine CT, however, MRI routinely provides both sagittal and axial visualization of the spine and, therefore, provides orthogonal imaging. Furthermore, MRI provides parasagittal images that sequentially visualize the neural foramina and can detect lateral compressive pathology. MRI also distinguishes between soft tissue and neural tissue better than non-enhanced CT, but generally does not distinguish between bony and soft tissue compression as well as CT. When this distinction is deemed important, CT, particularly contrast-enhanced CT, is sometimes needed.

4. TYPES OF BENIGN PRIMARY BONY TUMORS

4.1. OSTEOCHONDROMA

Osteochondroma is a common, benign, osteocartilaginous exostosis characterized by a predominantly bony mass produced by progressive enchondral ossification of its growing cartilaginous cap *(13)*. It is thought to expand by growth of aberrant foci of cartilage on the surface of bone *(13)*. It is a growing lesion of childhood, ceasing its growth after puberty or when the epiphyses close. Osteochondromas are usually solitary lesions, but they may rarely have a familial tendency and affect many bones with multiple lesions. Such patients with multiple osteochondromas have a small, but definite, risk of developing secondary chondrosarcoma.

Approximately 60% of osteochondromas occur in males, and approximately the same percentage occurs in patients younger than 20 yr of age. Although this lesion may be found

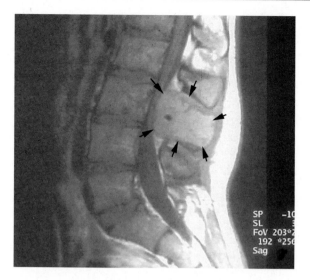

Fig. 4. T1-weighted sagittal magnetic resonance imaging of patient with an osteoblastoma of the L3 spinous process. Note the expansile lesion *(arrows)*, which is causing posterior neural compression of the cauda equina.

in any bone that develops by enchondral ossification, it typically occurs in the metaphysis of long bones. Approximately 50% of the osteochondromas in the Mayo Clinic series were located in the femur and humerus *(13)*. Only 3% were found in the spine. Osteochondromas account for a relatively high percentage of the benign lesions found in the spine, representing approx 23% of benign spine lesions in one series *(3)*.

Osteochondromas commonly arise at the site of tendon insertions, which may partially explain their tendency to be located in the posterior elements of the spine, where tendon attachment occurs, rather than in the vertebral body. They are frequently located at the tips of the spinous processes. They may be asymptomatic, or may present with pain or neural compression. Pain may be owing to local impingement on adjacent structures, or may occur from development of a painful bursitis overlying the osteocartilaginous growth. Osteochondromas may also occasionally cause neural compression, including spinal cord compression.

Malignant transformation in the cartilaginous cap of an osteochondroma is uncommon, but chondrosarcoma may occur in approx 1% of cases. In patients with the familial form of the disease exhibiting multiple lesions affecting many bones, the incidence of developing secondary chondrosarcoma is probably at least 10% *(13)*.

Treatment of osteochondromas is indicated if there is compression of adjacent neural structures, if there is a significant increase in size of the tumor, if there are other changes suggesting malignancy, if the diagnosis is uncertain or if there is localized pain. Fortunately, osteochondromas do not often cause neurological compression, because they do not tend to grow intraspinally. Treatment consists of surgical removal of both the bony lesion and the overlying cartilaginous cap. Recurrences following resection of the lesion are uncommon.

4.2. OSTEOID OSTEOMA AND OSTEOBLASTOMA

Osteoid osteoma and osteoblastoma are bone-forming lesions of young individuals, occurring nearly exclusively within the first three decades of life. Although thought to represent separate pathological entities, osteoid osteoma and osteoblastoma are histologically similar benign osteoblastic lesions that have similar clinical presentations. Pain is the predominant presenting symptom, particularly with osteoid osteoma. The pain from osteoid osteoma is typically more severe, is more commonly nocturnal and is characteristically better relieved by salicylates than that from osteoblastoma. More than 50% of patients with osteoid osteoma or osteoblastoma in the thoracolumbar spine present with painful scoliosis (6,14,15,19). When associated with scoliosis, the lesion is typically located on the concavity of the curve, and the apex is located within two vertebral levels of the tumor (6,15). Both lesions have a male preponderance, with the male:female ratio being approx 3:1 (16,17).

Osteoid osteoma is predominantly a lesion of the appendicular skeleton, whereas osteoblastoma is commonly located in the axial skeleton. In the Mayo Clinic series of bone tumors, 44% of osteoblastomas occurred in the spine and sacrum compared to only 6% of osteoid osteomas (16,17). In one review of 82 primary tumors of the spine, 7 of the 31 benign tumors were osteoblastomata and only 2 were osteoid osteomata. When occurring in the spine, osteoid osteoma and osteoblastoma are typically located in the posterior elements. The distinction between the two entities is based on the size of the lesion: a lesion less than 1 cm in diameter is arbitrarily designated osteoid osteoma, whereas a lesion larger than 2 cm in diameter is classified as osteoblastoma (18) (Figs. 1–4).

Osteoid osteoma is characterized by a well-delineated, radiolucent, central vascular nidus of woven trabecular bone with a surrounding region of reactive sclerosis. Although its radiographic appearance is usually typical, it may be poorly visualized when it occurs in juxta-articular cancellous bone or in the sacrum. Under such circumstances, diagnosis may be aided by technetium 99m bone scanning, CT, or MRI. A normal bone scan virtually rules out an osteoid osteoma or osteoblastoma. The appearance of the lesion by CT is characteristic, with a central radiolucent nidus and a surrounding halo of sclerotic bone (Fig. 5).

The natural history of untreated osteoid osteoma is unknown, but spontaneous regression of the lesion may apparently occur with resolution of symptoms. Treatment of osteoid osteoma and osteoblastoma is surgical excision. Intra-operative localization of these lesions, however, may be difficult. Use of intra-operative technetium 99m bone scanning or intra-operative CT may facilitate localization of the lesion, and intra-operative radiography of the resected specimen can confirm its removal. Treatment of osteoid osteoma is *en bloc* resection of the lesion. Because osteoblastoma is more aggressive than osteoid osteoma, excision is the preferred surgical option. Scoliosis associated with osteoid osteoma or osteoblastoma usually resolves following excision of the lesion, although delay in treatment can result in the development of a significant structural curve that may not fully resolve following surgery (6). Routine use of radiation therapy is controversial because of the risk of development of postradiation sarcoma.

4.3. ANEURYSMAL BONE CYST

Aneurysmal bone cyst (ABC) is a benign proliferative lesion of unknown etiology that is neither a true bone cyst, nor an

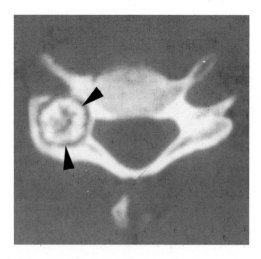

Fig. 5. Axial computed tomography scan of a young patient with an osteoid osteoma involving the right lateral mass of C5. Note the central radiolucency surrounded by sclerotic margin *(arrows)*.

aneurysm, nor neoplastic (19). It typically affects patients younger than 20 yr of age and has a slight female predominance. Presenting symptoms include axial pain, reduced range of spinal motion, and symptoms of neurological compression.

ABC affects the spine in approx 10 to 20% of cases, in which it has a predilection for the posterior elements 60% of the time (19,20). It is an expansile, osteolytic lesion of bone, often with sclerotic margins suggesting a slow growing process. As the lesion progresses, it may assume a soap bubble appearance with eggshell thin cortical margins, which may progressively expand and blow out (21) (Fig. 6). An unusual feature of ABC is its tendency to expand from one vertebra to another, a distinctly uncommon feature, which distinguishes it from other lesions (19).

Anatomically, ABCs have a tendency to involve both the anterior and posterior elements. In one large series of 22 patients with ABCs, all patients had involvement of the posterior elements (pedicle and/or lamina) and no patient had involvement of the vertebral body alone. Of the 22 patients, 14 (64%) had involvement of both the vertebral body and posterior elements (20). This suggests that the lesion most likely starts within the posterior elements and secondarily invades the vertebral body (20).

Treatment of ABC is surgical excision. Because of its highly vascular nature, preoperative embolization may be useful to reduce its vascularity. The addition of radiation therapy to partial surgical resection or curettage is controversial, but does not seem to provide an incremental benefit and may predispose to sarcoma formation (20). The use of radiation alone is associated with as much as a 50% recurrence rate and is, therefore, not recommended (20). Because the vertebral body is commonly involved, combined anterior and posterior surgical resection and reconstruction is frequently required. Where complete resection is not feasible, curettage may be performed, although it is associated with a higher rate of recurrence. Recurrence is nearly twice as common in long bone ABCs as in vertebral lesions and is nearly three times more common in patients younger than 15 yr of age than in patients older than 15 yr (19).

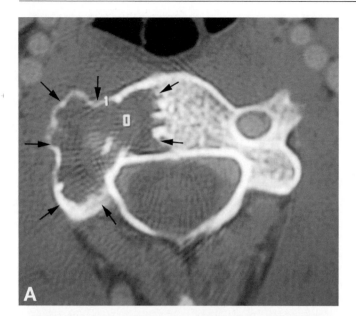

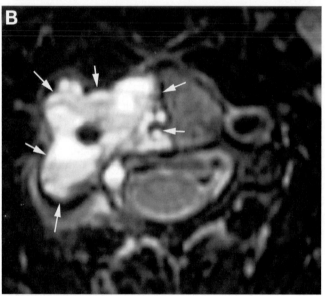

Fig. 6. Axial computed tomography scan (**A**) and axial magnetic resonance imaging (**B**) of an aneurysmal bone cyst. The lesion is expansile and well marginated *(arrows)* with a soap bubble appearance.

4.4. GIANT CELL TUMOR

Giant cell tumors are locally aggressive, slow-growing tumors that typically present between the second and fourth decades of life. In one study of 31 vertebral giant cell tumors above the sacrum, the female to male ratio was 3:1 *(1,22)*. Female predominance is also characteristic of giant cell tumors elsewhere in the body.

Giant cell tumors are uncommonly located in the spine. In a multicenter, multinational study of 1277 giant cell tumors, only 2.7% were localized to the spine *(7)*. They may be found in any region of the spine. Up to 70% of spinal giant cell tumors are located within the vertebral body, and are frequently associated with pedicle involvement. Only 15% are isolated to the posterior elements *(6)*. It typically appears as an area of rarefaction on routine X-ray. As the tumor expands, it may pro-

duce cortical expansion of the vertebra resulting in pathological fracture. CT is particularly helpful in characterizing the lesion, which may exhibit scalloped borders by CT. CT is also extremely helpful in the postoperative evaluation following surgical excision. Giant cell tumor may be confused with ABC and benign osteoblastoma. The presence of a lesion in the posterior elements, either exclusively or in conjunction with anterior vertebral body involvement, suggests the diagnosis of ABC rather than giant cell tumor.

Although considered a benign osseous lesion of the spine, giant cell tumor differs from other benign lesions by its more aggressive nature. It is considered by some to be a low-grade malignancy *(23)*. Accordingly, its prognosis is not as favorable as other primary bony lesions of the spine. Giant cell tumors are characterized by both their high local recurrence rate and by their more aggressive local extension. Overall recurrence rates as high as 40 to 50% have been reported for giant cell tumors of the spine *(22,24–26)*. In a study of 82 primary neoplasms of the spine, 31 of which were benign, local recurrence was seen in 21% of those undergoing surgery for their tumors, half of which occurred in patients having giant cell tumors *(3)*.

Because of its locally aggressive nature, surgical treatment of giant cell tumors must be radical *(22,27)*. Surgery for these tumors is challenging because of its anterior location, its frequent extension into the pedicle often necessitating combined anterior and posterior surgical approach, and its occasional profuse bleeding. Curettage of giant cell tumors should generally be avoided in favor of a more definitive and aggressive attempt at complete excision. *En-bloc* excision affords the best prognosis for cure and local control *(22,27,28)*. The use of postoperative radiation therapy is controversial and is generally not recommended if adequate resection is obtained. Sarcomatous change within the tumor has been reported in up to 10% of patients undergoing radiation therapy for giant cell tumor.

4.5. HEMANGIOMA

Hemangiomas are common spine lesions that are typically located within the vertebral body and are often noted as incidental findings by MRI (Fig. 7). Spinal occurrence is common, occurring in approx 10% of people *(29,30)*. In the Mayo Clinic series, 24% of all hemangiomas were located in the spine. It is likely that their current incidence in the spine might be even higher with incidental detection by MRI being common. They are generally thought not to cause symptoms, although they may occasionally be a source of pain if there is collapse of the vertebra.

Hemangiomas are easily identified by CT (Fig. 8) or MRI (Fig. 9), although they can be detected even on routine radiographs as a lytic area with characteristic vertical striations from abnormally thickened trabeculae and without cortical expansion (Fig. 10). In this respect they differ from Paget's disease, which is characterized by both vertical striations and bone expansion. For cases where the hemangioma is thought to be symptomatic, therapeutic options include radiation therapy, angiography with embolization of the tumor, or vertebral augmentation with polymethylmethacrylate.

Treatment of hemangiomas depend on the degree of symptomatology. In the spine these lesions are commonly asymp-

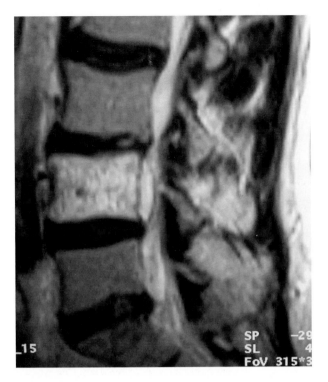

Fig. 7. Sagittal magnetic resonance imaging of patient with an asymptomatic hemangioma involving L4. Note the typical increased (white) signal intensity of the lesion.

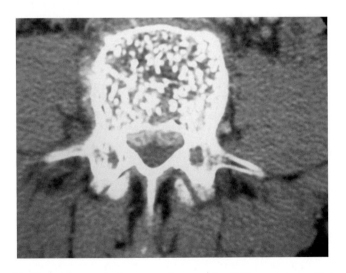

Fig. 8. Axial computed tomography scan of an L4 hemangioma. Note the stippled appearance of the lesion within the body of the vertebra.

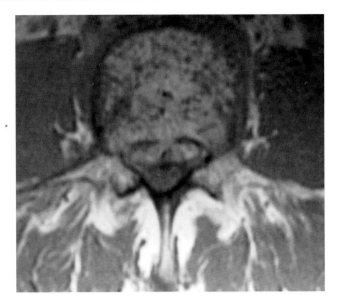

Fig. 9. Axial magnetic resonance imaging of the same patient shown in Fig. 8 with an L4 hemangioma.

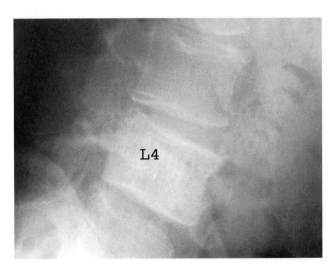

Fig. 10. Lateral lumbar X-ray of the patient with a hemangioma shown in Figs. 8 and 9. Note the vertical striations of the vertebral body without associated expansion of the margins of the bone.

tomatic and can be ignored. When symptoms such as pain are present in a patient with a hemangioma, it must first be determined whether or not the two conditions are causally related. If so, treatment with radiotherapy should be considered because these lesions are radiosensitive. If neurological symptoms from spinal cord, cauda equina, or nerve root are present, surgical excision is indicated. When spinal cord compression is present, angiography is indicated to determine the vascular supply to the cord and to determine the feasibility of preoperative embolization of the tumor.

4.6. EOSINOPHILIC GRANULOMA

Eosinophilic granuloma (EG) is a benign, self-limited condition of children and young adults. Initially described by Calvé *(31)*, it was originally thought to represent osteochondritis of the vertebral body. It is now considered one of the triad of entities (EG, Hand-Schuler-Christian disease, and Letterer-Siwe disease) comprising the histiocytosis X diseases (reticuloendotheliosese).

Skeletal lesions of EG most commonly involve the skull, but any bone is a potential target. Spinal lesions may occur in up to 10 to 15% of cases, most commonly in the lumbar spine *(29)*. In the spine, EG appears as a discreetly defined focal destructive lesion of bone that typically involves the vertebral body and pedicle. The spectrum of vertebral involvement ranges from a purely lytic lesion without collapse, to partial collapse and even complete collapse. The latter is termed *vertebra plana*.

Calvé *(31)* described the radiographic appearance as resembling the edge view of a silver dollar . Although EG is the most common cause of vertebra plana, this condition is also seen with other conditions such as tuberculosis, fungal infections, and malignancy.

Treatment of EG consists of observation and use of symptomatic bracing, as needed *(32)*. The condition is usually self-limited and the vertebral body may partially or completely reconstitute *(33,34)*. Vertebral body collapse may, however, be associated with neural compression and require decompressive surgery with stabilization *(35)*.

5. PROGNOSIS

Benign bony spinal tumors generally have a very good prognosis. With the exception of giant cell tumors, recurrences are uncommon. In one series of 31 patients with benign tumors, the overall 5-yr survival rate was 86% with local recurrences occurring in 21% of operated patients *(3)*. Half of the recurrences, however, occurred in patients with giant cell tumors, and two of the four patients with giant cell tumors eventually died from recurrence of their tumor associated with spinal cord compression. Overall, there was no association between the survival rate and the extent of the surgical excision.

6. CONCLUSION

Primary benign osseous lesions of the spine represent an uncommon neoplastic condition. Benign lesions are more commonly associated with younger patients, absence of a neurological deficit and localization in the posterior elements of the vertebrae. Radiographic features suggesting a benign, rather than malignant, lesion include well-defined borders with scalloped margins and absence of cortical breakthrough or paravertebral soft tissue mass. Features suggestive of malignancy include older patient age, progressive neurological deficit, nonmechanical pain (e.g., night pain), and location within the vertebral body. Because benign primary bone tumors of the spine are generally slow growing, are easily accessible from a posterior approach, and generally do not recur following excision, surgery is usually palliative and rewarding.

REFERENCES

1. Dahlin DC, Unni KK. Bone Tumors: General Aspects and Data on 8542 Cases. 4th ed. Springfield, IL: Charles C. Thomas; 1986.
2. Weinstein JN. Spinal tumors. In: Wiesel SW, Weinstein JN, Herkowitz HN, et al., eds. The Lumbar Spine. 2nd Ed. Philadelphia, PA: W.B. Saunders Company; 1996:917–944.
3. Weinstein JN, McLain RF. Primary tumors of the spine. Spine 1987; 12:843–851.
4. Deyo RA, Diehl AK. Cancer as a cause of back pain: frequency, clinical presentation and diagnostic strategies. J Gen Intern Med 1988; 3:230–238.
5. Kirwan EO, Hutton PAN, Pozo JL, Ransford AO. Osteiod osteoma and benign osteoblastoma of the spine. J Bone Joint Surg 1984; 66B:21–26.
6. Ransford AO, Pozo JL, Hutton PAN, Kirwan EO. The behavior pattern of the scoliosis associated with osteoid osteoma or osteoblastoma of the spine. J Bone Joint Surg Br 1984; 66:16–20.
7. Shankman S, Greenspan A, Klein MJ, Lewis MM. Giant cell tumor of the ischium: a report of two cases and review of the literature. Skeletal Radiol 1988; 17:46–51.
8. Sim FH, Dahlin DL, Stauffer RN, et al. Primary bone tumors stimulating lumbar disc syndrome. Spine 1989; 2:65–74.
9. Thommese P, Poulsen JO. Primary tumors in the spine and pelvis in adolescents: clinical and radiological features. Acta Orthop Scand 1976; 47:170–174.
10. Marsh BW, Bonfiglio M, Brady LP, Enneking W F. Benign osteoblastoma: range of manifestations. J Bone Joint Surg Am 1975; 57:1–9.
11. McHenry MC, Duchesneau PM, Keys TF, Rehm SJ, Boumphrey FR. Vertebral osteomyelitis presenting as spinal compression fracture. Arch Intern Med 1988; 148:417–423.
12. Bell GR, Modic MT. Radiology of the Lumbar Spine. The Spine. Vol. 1., 1999, 1992, 1982, 1975:109–134.
13. Dahlin DC. Osteochondroma (Osteocartilaginous Exostosis). Bone Tumors. 3rd ed. Springfield, IL: Charles C. Thomas Publisher; 1978:17–27.
14. Keim H, Reina E. Osteoid-osteoma as a cause of scoliosis. J Bone Joint Surg 1975; 57:159–163.
15. Pettine KA, Klassen RA. Osteoid-osteoma and osteoblastoma of the spine. J. Bone Joint Surg Am 1986; 68:354–361.
16. Dahlin DC. Benign Osteoblastoma (Giant Osteoid Osteoma) Bone Tumors. 3rd ed. Springfield, IL: Charles C. Thomas Publisher; 1978:86–98.
17. Dahlin DC. Osteoid Osteoma. Bone Tumors, 3rd ed. Springfield, IL: Charles C. Thomas Publisher;1978:75–85.
18. McLeod RA, Dahlin DC, Beabout JW. The spectrum of osteoblastoma. Am J Roentgenol 1976; 126:321–335.
19. Tillman BP, Dahlin DC, Lipscomb PR, Stewart JR. Aneurysmal bone cyst: an analysis of ninety-five cases. Mayo Clin Proc 1968; 93:478–495.
20. Campanna R, Albisinni U, Picci P, Calderoni P, Campanacci M, Springfield DS. Aneurismal bone cyst of the spine. J Bone Joint Surg 1985; 67:527–531.
21. Hay MC, Paterson D, Taylor TKF. Aneurysmal bone cysts of the spine. J. Bone Joint Surg Br 1978; 60:406–411.
22. Dahlin DC. Giant-cell tumor of vertebrae above the sacrum. Cancer 1977: 39:1350–1356.
23. Enneking WF, ed. Musculoskeletal Tumor Surgery. New York, NY: Churchill Livingstone; 1983:69–122.
24. Larsson SE, Lorentzon R, Boquist L. Giant cell tumor of bone. J Bone Joint Surg 1975; 57A:167–173.
25. Larsson SE, Lorentzon R, Boquist L. Giant cell tumors of the spine and sacrum causing neurologic symptoms. Clin Orthop 1975; 111:201–211.
26. Sanjay BKS, Sim F H, Unni KK, McLeod RA, Klassen RA. Giant-Cell tumors of the spine. J Bone Joint Surg Br 1993; 75:148–154.
27. Savini R, Gherlinzoni F, Morandi M, et al. Surgical treatment of giant-cell tumor of the spine. J Bone Joint Surg Am 1983; 65:1283–1289.
28. Stener B, Johnsen OE. Complete removal of three vertebrae for giant cell tumor. J Bone Joint Surg Br 1971; 53:278–287.
29. McLain RF, Weinstein JN. Tumors of the Spine. The Spine, Vol. II (38), pp. 1171-1206, 1999, 1992, 1982, 1975.
30. Weinstein JN. Differential diagnosis and surgical treatment of primary benign and malignant neoplasms. In: Frymoyer JW, ed. The Adult Spine: Principles and Practice. New York, NY: Raven Press; 1991:829–860.
31. Calve J. A localized affection of the spine suggesting osteochondritis of the vertebral body, with the clinical spect of Pott's disease. J Bone and Joint Surg 1925; 7:41–46.
32. Fowles JV, Bobechko WP. Solitary eosinophilic granuloma of bone. J Bone Joint Surg Br 1970; 52:238–243.
33. Ippolito E, Farsetti P, Tudisco C. Vertebral plana. J Bone Joint Surg 1984; A:1364–1368.
34. Nesbit M, Kieffer S, D'Angio G. Reconstitution of vertebral height in histiocytosis X: A long-term follow up. J Bone Join Surg 1969; 51A:1360–1368.
35. Green NE, Robertson WW, Kilroy AW. Eosinophilic granuloma of the spine associated with neutral deficit. J Bone Joint Surg Am 1980; 62:1198–1202.

37 Surgical Treatment of Primary Malignant Tumors

BRANCO PRPA, MD AND ROBERT F. MCLAIN, MD

CONTENTS

1. INTRODUCTION

The primary goal of treatment for patients with malignant primary spine tumors is to provide cure, or the best chance of cure, if possible. If cure is not possible, we seek to palliate pain and provide early return to function and activity, to maintain or improve neurological function, and to provide a stable spinal column. The "upside" to an aggressive resection of a primary spinal malignancy has never been higher, making the "downside" to a poorly planned or executed surgery all the more unacceptable. With improved medical and radiotherapies, the treating physician now has the opportunity—and the obligation—to carefully tailor treatment to the biology and stage of each specific spine tumor (Table 1). The role of surgery differs depending on tumor type, stage, and location.

2. INDICATIONS FOR SURGERY

Not all patients with spine tumors require surgery, but few primary malignancies will be treated entirely without surgery. Patients with clearly benign tumors may simply be observed, and those with diffuse metastases may be treated with local radiotherapy and systemic chemotherapy. Primary malignancies found in the spine, however, are better managed with more aggressive surgical methods, both in terms of local control and long-term survival. Surgical resection is indicated when the patient presents with an isolated primary lesion or a solitary site of recurrence amenable to *en-bloc* resection, when the primary lesion requires surgery for local control because of radio-resistance, whether widely respectable or not, or when the tumor causes severe pain, neural compression, or segmental instabil-

Table 1
General Treatment Approach for Spine Tumors

Therapeutic option	Appropriate applications
Observation	Indolent and clearly benign tumors (hemangioma, osteochondroma, bone island, bone infarct)
Radiotherapy	Metastatic lesions from a known radiosensitive primary (multiple myeloma, breast carcinoma)
Chemotherapy	Metastatic lesions from a known chemosensitive primary (thyroid)
Intralesional excision, curettage	Benign tumors with limited potential for recurrence (aneurysmal bone cyst, osteoblastoma), radiosensitive metastatic lesions with adjuvant radiation therapy
Marginal excision +/− adjuvant cryotherapy or radiotherapy	Locally aggressive benign lesions (giant cell tumor), radiosensitive primary and metastatic lesions (plasmacytoma, breast and prostate carcinoma), low-grade malignancies
Wide excision	All primary malignancies without known metastases (osteosarcoma, chondrosarcoma, chordoma), solitary metastases with likelihood of prolonged survival (breast, prostate, renal cell carcinoma), locally aggressive benign tumors (giant cell tumor)

ity, irrespective of metastatic status. The relative importance of surgical treatment to outcome depends on the tumor type. Radio-resistant chondrosarcomas or chordomas are rarely cured unless an adequate surgical margin is obtained. A radiosensitive plasmacytoma may benefit from surgical stabilization and

From: *Current Clinical Oncology: Cancer in the Spine: Comprehensive Care.*
Edited by: R. F. McLain, K-U. Lewandrowski, M. Markman, R. M. Bukowski,
R. Macklis, and E. C. Benzel © Humana Press, Inc., Totowa, NJ

311

reduction of tumor burden, but radiotherapy provides excellent local control in most cases.

3. STAGING BEFORE SURGERY

The anatomic extent of the primary lesion must be defined in three dimensions before a rational and successful surgery can be planned. Extension of the tumor beyond regional barriers and into vital tissues must be recognized and accounted for in the surgical plan. Although true anatomic compartments (as defined by Enneking [1]) do not exist in the spinal column, certain anatomic structures provide natural planes for dissection and wide excision (Chapter 4). The vertebral body, anterior and posterior longitudinal ligaments, the intervertebral disks, and the dura may all be resected to avoid leaving residual tumor behind. Neural, muscular, and some vascular structures may all be sacrificed to obtain a clear surgical margin in primary malignancies. Some vital structures (aorta, trachea/esophagus) can be resected and reconstructed when survival depends on the surgical margin, but only if proper planning is carried out in advance. Such an aggressive approach is as well justified in the spine as in extremity surgery: a complete resection provides the best chance for both local control and cure of the disease.

4. CLASSIFYING TUMORS

To select the best approach to tumor resection, the vertebral body may be divided into four zones, I–IV, and tumor extension can be defined as A–C for contained (intra-osseous), local extension (extra-osseous), or metastatic spread (Fig.1) (2). A zone IA lesion would be contained within portions of the spinous process and laminae, pars interarticularis, and/or inferior facets. Zone IIA includes the superior articular facets, transverse processes, and the pedicle from the level of the pars to its junction with the vertebral body. Zone IIIA includes the anterior three-fourths of the vertebral body, whereas zone IVA designates involvement of the posterior one-fourth of the body, that segment immediately anterior to the cord. Type B lesions begin in the involved zone, but extend beyond the boundaries of the cortical bone. Type C lesions have developed regional or distant metastatic spread.

The best surgical approach is determined by the zones involved and the extent of the local tumor spread. Although the patient's survival and outcome depend on the stage, type, and grade of tumor, an aggressive surgical approach to tumor control can provide a survival benefit even when true *en-bloc* excision is not achieved (3,4).

5. MALIGNANT PRIMARY TUMORS

The surgical approach varies depending on tumor type, as well as stage. The various aspects of tumor biology and clinical behavior that influence surgical planning are illustrated by the tumor types listed in Subheadings 5.1.–5.5.

5.1. OSTEOSARCOMA

Approximately 2% of all primary osteogenic sarcomas arise in the spine, almost always in the vertebral body. This high-grade sarcoma expands rapidly within the bone, and is quick to extend beyond the cortical margins into the adjacent soft tissues. Patients typically present with pain and often have neu-

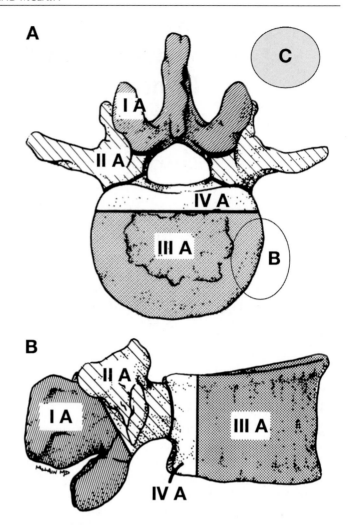

Fig. 1. Anatomic extent of spine tumors by zone. **(A)** Axial cut through L2 zones I–IV. A (intra-osseous lesions confined within the boundaries of the cortical spine), B (extra-osseous extension), and C (distant metastases) stages. **(B)** Lateral views of L2 zones I–IV.

rological compromise. Metastases occur early and often. Vertebral osteosarcoma arising from Paget's disease or previous radiation therapy has an even more grim prognosis (5–7). Radiographic studies demonstrate cortical destruction, soft tissue calcification, and vertebral collapse in advanced cases. Computed tomography (CT) and magnetic resonance imaging (MRI) demonstrate intraspinal and paraspinal soft tissue masses, permitting comprehensive pre-operative planning (Fig. 2, Telangiectatic OGS).

Treatment of high-grade sarcoma of the spinal column is most challenging, and the outcome in these tumors has traditionally been poor. Limited tumor excision and radiotherapy provided median survival ranging only from 6 to 10 mo (5,6). A more aggressive surgical approach, with a serious attempt at *en-bloc* resection, has resulted in longer survival times and a measurable rate of cure (3,4,7,8). In A- and B-stage lesions, complete excision with a cuff of normal tissue (muscle, pleura, nerve root) offers the best opportunity for local control and cure. When a clear margin cannot be obtained, the best attempt should be made to resect any contaminated margins, including sections of dura. Improvements in adjuvant radiotherapy and

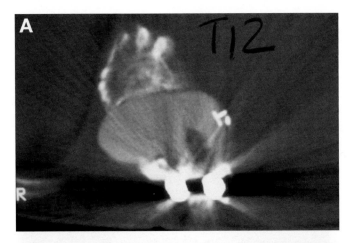

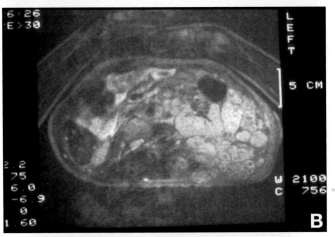

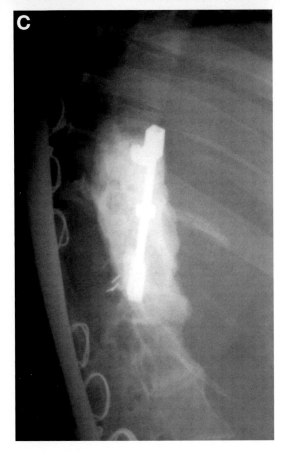

chemotherapy protocols have provided greatly improved survival and disease-free survival in these circumstances.

5.2. EWING'S SARCOMA

Approximately 3.5% of all Ewing's tumors arise in the spinal column, many originating in the sacrum (9,10). Patients usually present in the second or third decade of life, and neurological signs are present 58 to 64% of the time (9,10). These tumors usually emanate from the vertebral body, but extension into the posterior elements and canal can occur. Ewing's tumors present a permeative appearance on radiographs, making diagnosis difficult even in advanced disease. Collapse of the vertebral body creates a vertebra plana that may be indistinguishable from eosinophilic granuloma (11). Surgical treatment to decompress the neural elements and stabilize the vertebral column is beneficial, but effective treatment of Ewing's sarcoma involves multi-agent chemotherapy and high dose radiotherapy. Combining surgical extirpation with systemic chemo- and radiotherapy may further improve prognosis (12).

5.3. CHORDOMA

Chordoma is a relatively rare malignancy occurring predominantly in older patients. The tumor arises from remnants of the primitive notochord (13) found in the sacrococcygeal and suboccipital regions of the spine, and occasionally from notochordal rests within thoracic or lumbar vertebrae (14). Although this low-grade lesion is characterized by slow, relentless local spread, chordoma is a fully malignant lesion capable of distant metastases. Early symptoms are usually mild and unrecognized, and pain and neural dysfunction progress slowly as the tumor expands. Chordomas may reach a considerable size before symptoms of constipation, urinary frequency, or nerve root compression prompt the patient to see a physician. A firm, fixed presacral mass can usually be palpated on rectal exam.

CT is helpful to define the destruction of bony architecture and MRI is mandatory to define the extent of the tumor for presurgical planning. Patient survival depends on local control of the tumor, and surgical extirpation of the tumor, with a wide margin, is the only curative procedure, as these lesions are notoriously resistant to radio and chemotherapy (Fig. 3). *En-bloc* excision is associated with the least risk of local recurrence, but may be terrifically challenging (14,15). Sacropelvic reconstruction after extensive resection may require multiple stages to complete, and morbidity is universal among patients with large lesions.

Fig. 2. (**A–C**) Neurofibrosarcoma: degenerative sarcoma arising in a previously benign neurofibroma. (**A**) A 26-yr-old patient with previous fusion for scoliosis resulting from her neurofibromatosis, presented with acute paraplegia. Computed tomography scan demonstrates a large extramedullary tumor within the spinal canal. (**B**) At the time of presentation, this extremely aggressive tumor had filled the left hemithorax, making the routine thoracotomy impossible. (**C**) An emergent decompression was performed, with complete vertebrectomy. However, considering the patient's poor prognosis for survival, the reconstruction was performed using polymethymethacrylate, which provides immediate stability and strength, but may begin to loosen after 6–12 mo.

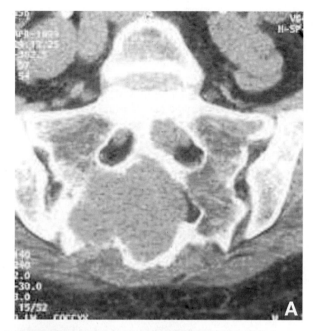

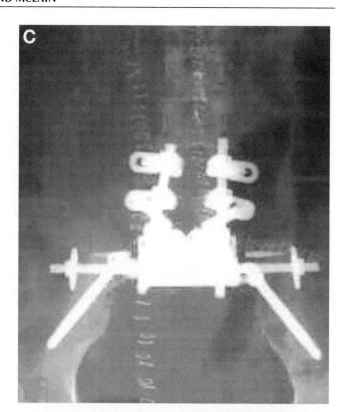

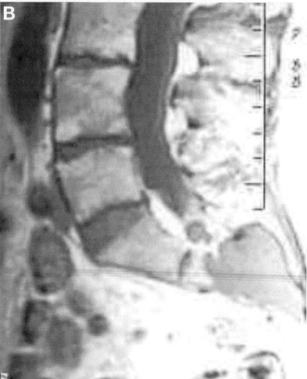

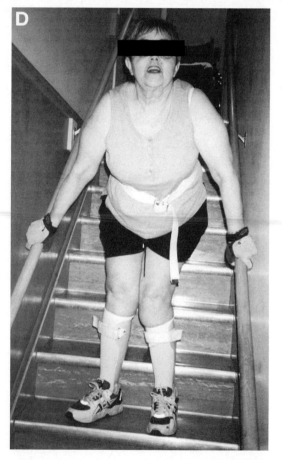

Fig. 3. (A,B) Illustration of reconstruction performed for L3 chordoma. (C,D) Lateral X-ray views taken postoperatively. No signs of recurrence to date. (A,B) Computed tomography and sagittal magnetic resonance imaging of sacral chordoma, demonstrating involvement of S1 vertebra. Tumor extended proximally into the spinal canal involving S1 vertebra and nerve roots. (C) Resection of tumor necessitated removal of S1 vertebra. Reconstruction with sacral prosthesis allowed early mobilization and protected weight bearing. (D) Six months postoperatively patient was ambulating in braces, with an L5 level of motor control. Three years after surgery the patient remains disease free.

5.4. CHONDROSARCOMA

Approximately 7 to 10% of chondrosarcomas arise in the spinal column (16,17). Most of these tumors are low grade, so they grow slowly and are relatively resistant to radiotherapy and chemotherapy. A high rate of recurrence leads to the poor prognosis of spinal chondrosarcoma.

Radiographically, chondrosarcoma has a fairly characteristic appearance. In advanced disease, there is a large area of bone destruction and an associated soft tissue mass with flocculent calcifications within it. If there is no soft tissue mass the vertebral lesion may be primarily lytic, with sclerotic margins, and with no mottled calcification (18).

Complete surgical excision is required to cure spinal chondrosarcoma. This may be impossible to obtain in some vertebral lesions. In 1971, Stener (19) pioneered en-bloc excision of chondrosarcoma of the spine. All of the larger series since then have demonstrated the importance of obtaining negative margins in an en-bloc fashion to disease-free survival (17,20–22). Excision of the overlying soft-tissue capsule, muscle, pleura or peritoneum, and as wide a margin of vertebral bone as possible, is crucial to success.

5.5. SOLITARY PLASMACYTOMA

Multiple myeloma and solitary plasmacytoma are two manifestations in a continuum of B-cell lymphoproliferative diseases. Because the natural history of these two lesions differs so significantly, the clinical distinction between solitary plasmacytoma and multiple myeloma is important.

True solitary plasmacytoma is an uncommon entity, comprising 3% of all plasma cell tumors. Although the course of multiple myeloma is often rapidly progressive and lethal, solitary plasmacytoma may allow prolonged survival if local control can be obtained. Prior to recent advances in bone marrow transplantation, the 1-yr mortality rate for patients with multiple myeloma involving the spine was 76%, and the 4-yr mortality nearly 100% (23). At that same time the 5-yr disease-free survival for solitary plasmacytoma was roughly 60% (24).

The treatment of choice in spinal lesions of either solitary plasmacytoma or multiple myeloma is radiation. Because of the radiosensitivity of this tumor, surgical treatment has less influence in determining outcome than it does in other tumor types. Surgical intervention is usually reserved for cases with cord compromise or spinal instability, though resection of large solitary lesions may also reduce the body's tumor burden before radiotherapy. Palliative stabilization of fractured vertebrae through either kyphoplasty or vertebraplasty may offer immediate pain relief for patients undergoing systemic therapy or radiation.

6. SURGICAL TREATMENT

6.1. SURGICAL APPROACH

Choosing the correct approach is, perhaps, the most important step in treating primary spinal malignancies. The approach selected must provide adequate access for tumor excision and for stabilization of the spine thereafter. If both operations cannot be performed through the same incision, the surgeon must plan for a combined approach. An ill-planned approach may leave the surgeon unable to complete the excision of the tumor, compromising the outcome and complicating every treatment step thereafter.

Zone I lesions are best approached posteriorly, and the extent of excision must be based on any soft-tissue extension seen on pre-operative studies (Fig. 4). Zone II lesions are also more easily excised through a posterior or posterolateral approach and should be similarly stabilized. The need for stabilization following zone I and II resections depends to a great extent on the spinal segment involved. Extensive laminectomies in the cervical or thoracic spine routinely lead to progressive kyphosis, and posterior instrumentation prevents this by restoring a posterior column tension band to combat the normal tensile loads seen in these segments. In the lumbar segments kyphosis is less of a concern than translational deformities and back pain.

Zone III lesions should be approached anteriorly. Adequate resection of zone IIIA lesions can usually be obtained, but zone IIIB lesions should be carefully evaluated for invasion or adherence of tumor to the great vessels of the thoracic cavity, retroperitoneal structures of the abdomen, or critical neurovascular elements, esophagus, or trachea in the cervical region. Reconstruction may be performed with or without internal fixation depending on the extent of the resection and the inherent stability of the residual elements.

Zone IV lesions indicated for en-bloc excision must be managed through a combined anterior and posterior surgical approach. These lesions provide major technical challenges to the surgeon before, during, and after the actual tumor resection. Zones I, II, and/or III must be crossed at some point to provide access to zone IV, and frequently more than one zone is involved with tumor. Complete excision of IVA lesions can be accomplished, but tumor margins must often be violated. En-bloc excision requires vertebrectomy, essentially separating zone II from zones III and IV through combined approaches, and in such cases both anterior and posterior columns must be stabilized. Failure to provide sure fixation and an adequate bone graft may result in loss of fixation, with catastrophic neurological complications if hardware migrates into the canal or if excessive kyphosis develops (17).

After the appropriate work-up has been completed, the surgeon must incorporate three crucial elements into a coherent surgical plan: (1) determine the proper margin of resection, (2) assess the need for neurological decompression, and (3) plan the reconstruction.

6.2. RESECTION MARGINS

The ideal resection margin is determined by the biology of the tumor and its stage (Table 1). Obtaining a wide or marginal margin rather than an intra-lesional margin improves survival and protects against local recurrence in both primary malignancies (25) and isolated metastases (26–29). Obtaining the widest margin possible is essential in many locally aggressive or malignant primary tumors, particularly those that do not respond well to irradiation. A wide margin can be obtained in most isolated lesions in zones IA through IIIA because the tumor can usually be completely resected. Type IVA lesions can often be resected cleanly, but only by removing the surrounding compartments as well.

An adequate margin can be difficult to obtain in type B lesions. Type B lesions may not be completely resectable without resecting nerve roots, producing serious neurological defi-

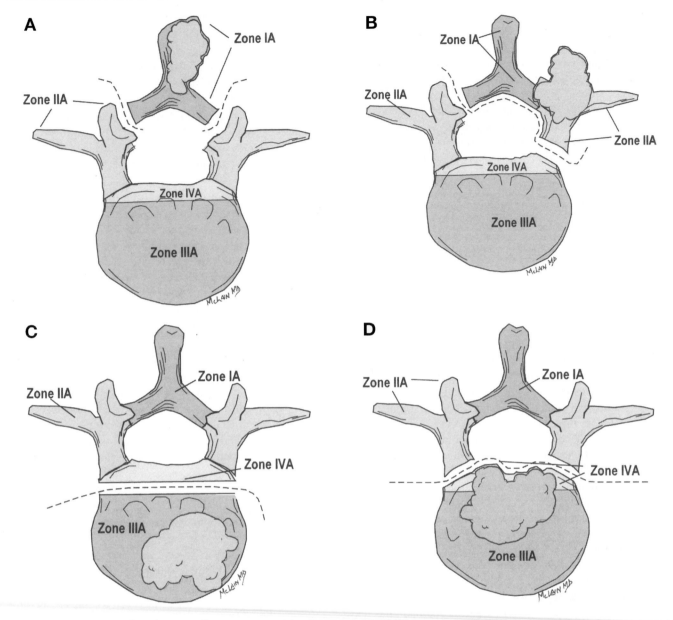

Fig. 4. Resection planes for primary malignant tumors arising in zones I–IV. (**A**) Approach to zone IA tumor involving spinous process or lamina. A wide laminectomy separating the spinous process from the bordering facets and pars interarticularis allows the dorsal lesion to be removed with an ample cuff of surrounding tissue. (**B**) Approach to zone IIA lesion involving facet, transverse process, or pedicle. A contralateral laminectomy combined with an osteotomy of the ipsilateral pedicle allows the lesion to be removed with a wide margin of bone and a cuff of overlying tissue. (**C**) Approach to zone IIIA primary tumor involving anterior vertebral body. A direct anterior approach permits the surgeon to develop a circumferential plane over the vertebral body, leaving the anterior cuff of soft tissues undisturbed. After discectomy to further free the involved body, an osteotome is used to cut out the segment containing the lesion. In high-grade lesions the pedicles may be osteotomized and the body removed *en bloc*. (**D**) Approach to zone IVA tumor involving vertebral body and posterior cortex. Zone IV lesions also involve zone III, by definition. This two-stage approach begins with a posterior decompression and removal of the lamina, facets, and both pedicles down to the vertebral body. The annulus of the disc is divided at this point and the pedicles packed with bone wax or polymethylmethacrylate cement to prevent hemorrhage from the vertebral body to contaminate the field with tumor cells. An anterior approach permits formal corpectomy, removing the tumor and any soft tissue mass *en bloc* with the overlying capsule. If tumor is adherent to the dura, the decision to excise the dura is made based on the tumor's sensitivity to adjuvant radio- or chemotherapy.

cits. The decision to attempt a wide or radical resection in these cases must be weighed against the risk of neurological deficit.

Special mention should be made of sacral tumors. Partial or total sacrectomy with a combined anterior and posterior approach is essentially an internal amputation, with the poten-

tial for a wide margin in selected cases. The complication rate is high, mostly because of wound problems and infectious complications. If nerve roots can be spared, bladder and anorectal function can be retained *(30,31)*.

6.3. NEURAL COMPRESSION

Spinal cord or cauda equina compression may result from one of four processes: (1) direct compression by an enlarging soft tissue mass, (2) pressure owing to fracture and retropulsion of bony fragments into the canal, (3) severe kyphosis following vertebral collapse, or (4) pressure owing to intradural metastases *(32)*. The most common cause of cord compression is mechanical pressure from tumor tissue or bone extruded from the collapsing vertebral body *(33)*.

The most reliable way to optimize neurological function in these patients is to maintain it in the first place. The behavior of each neoplasm is determined by its intrinsic biology *(27,34–36)*, and understanding the tumor biology allows the surgeon to predict which lesions will endanger neurological structures and how rapidly. Severe neurological deficits are difficult to recover from: 60 and 95% of the patients who can walk at the time of diagnosis will retain that ability following treatment, but only 3 to 65% of paraplegic patients will regain the ability to walk, and fewer than 30% of quadraplegic patients will walk again *(34,35,37–39)*. The *rate* at which the neurological deficit progresses also influences the likelihood of recovery. A patient who progresses from intact status to a major deficit in less than 24 h has a poor prognosis for recovery irrespective of treatment. Conversely, compression that has evolved over a period of months has a far more favorable prognosis for recovery following treatment *(33)*.

Primary malignancies commonly arise in the vertebral body, and when they encroach on the spinal cord the anterior columns are compressed first. The patient typically loses motor function first, with progressive loss of sensory function as the cord is pressed back against the lamina. Laminectomy is usually a poor choice for these patients as it does not directly decompress the cord, rarely allows a satisfactory resection margin, and it may add to the instability of the spinal column *(33)*. Anterior resection has far better track record for neural improvement and tumor control.

6.4. RECONSTRUCTION

After resection of a tumor, some form of reconstruction will be needed to restore the mechanical stability of the spine and compensate for the loss of bony elements. The stabilizing construct must restore the anterior weight-bearing column whenever a significant amount of the vertebral body has been resected at one or more levels. Without reconstruction, collapse and kyphosis will result. Likewise, segmental instrumentation must be applied after extensive laminectomy to restore the posterior tension band, especially in cases where facet joints have been removed. This will help to prevent kyphosis and can compensate for resected musculature. Finally, combined anterior and posterior reconstructions should be performed following extensive resection for larger tumors. Problems of construct failure can be avoided by extending the fixation construct several levels above and below the tumor, combining anterior and posterior instrumentation, and by maximizing the number of fixation points. Although radiation therapy will impair the process, strive for biological fusion in patients who are likely to survive more than 3 to 6 mo.

6.5. PLANNING SURGICAL TREATMENT

The cumulative experience of many authors has led to the following recommendations:

1. Use a posterior approach for tumors of the upper cervical spine.
2. Anterior approaches are optimal for the majority of lower cervical, thoracic, and lumbar lesions because most tumors are located in the body in these regions *(37,39–41)*.
3. A posterior approach in the lower cervical, thoracic, and lumbar spine is desirable only for tumors of the posterior elements.
4. Use costotransversectomy and intra-lesional approaches only for tumors that are clearly sensitive to radio- or chemo-therapy or when cure by surgical route is not possible *(42–44)*.
5. Use a combined anterior and posterior approach for *en-bloc* spondylectomy *(19,29,45–49)*.

6.5.1. Instrumentation

Although Harrington distraction rods and Luque rods with sublaminar wires were used successfully in the past, they have been supplanted by newer segmental instrumentation systems. These systems are versatile, with hook and screw fixation possible at multiple levels. The superior strength and resiliency of these constructs allows them to be used even in cases where the posterior elements have been completely resected or destroyed by tumor. The surgeon can contour rods or plates to restore sagittal alignment and can either compress or distract separately at each intercalary level. Pedicle screws offer more secure anchorage than hooks, and can be used in both the thoracic and lumbar spine with good results (Fig. 5) *(50)*.

Because most implant systems are now available in titanium, these systems also allow better postoperative imaging and follow-up than was possible in the past. Despite their greater versatility, however, these new systems cannot overcome biomechanically unsound circumstances without additional support or compensation. In areas of excessive bending stress, such as the transitional zones between the occiput and upper cervical spine, and the cervicothoracic and thoracolumbar junctions, fixation may have to be extended over more levels to avoid loosening or failure. Also, in cases where a significant portion of the anterior and middle spinal columns is missing or collapsed, posterior instrumentation can fatigue and fail, either through hook or screw failure, or breakage of the longitudinal rod *(51)*. An anterior strut graft or cage, added to the posterior construct, compensates for the excessive axial loads and insures a successful reconstruction. Finally, pedicle screws can be augmented with polymethylmethacrylate (PMMA) to provide reliable, lasting fixation in poor quality bone *(52)*.

6.5.2. Anterior Reconstruction

Anterior spinal reconstruction using PMMA remains somewhat controversial. Although use in traumatic spinal instability has led to significant complications and failure, most authors agree there is a role for cement in stabilizing metastatic spinal lesions. This role has become more limited, however, as better alternatives have become available, and particularly in primary spinal lesions where the expectation after a successful excision

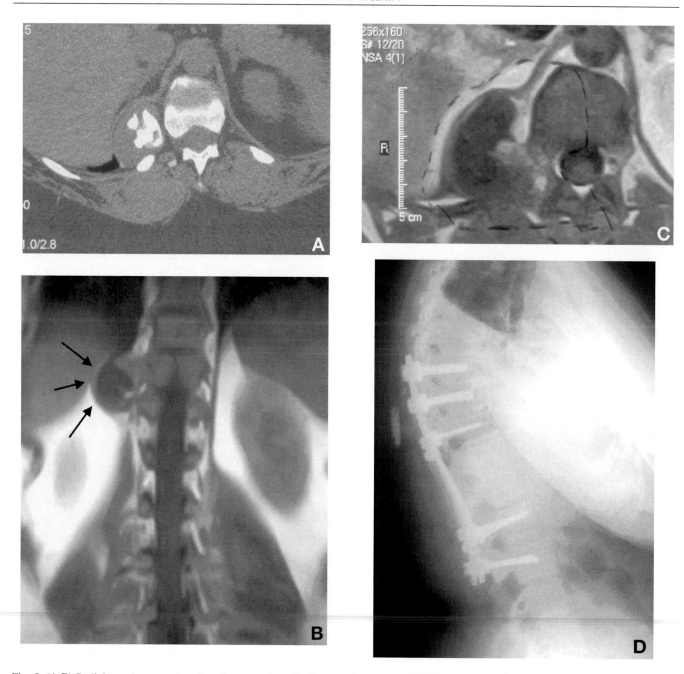

Fig. 5. (**A,B**) Pedicle screw reconstruction after resection of primary spine tumor. (**C,D**) Zombar. (**A**) Axial computed tomography scan of chondrosarcoma originating from T11 osteochondroma in a 45-yr-old woman. Lesion involved structures from zones II, III, and IVB, without metastasis or invasion through the parietal pleura. (**B**) Coronal magnetic resonance imaging demonstrates cartilage mass of T11 chondrosarcoma. Lesion involved structures from zones II, III, and IVB, without metastasis or invasion through the parietal pleura. Soft tissue pseudocapsule can be seen *(arrows)*. (**C**) Resection plan for chondrosarcoma using a midline posterior approach. (**D**) Pedicle screw and rod reconstruction after successful resection. Disease free at 2-yr follow-up.

is for continued local control and a significant disease-free survival. PMMA is resilient in compression, but has no potential for biological integration. It should be used only as a spacer, providing a temporary internal splint in anticipation of eventual bony arthrodesis or inevitable demise. If arthrodesis is not obtained, it is only a matter of time before the methacrylate construct fails; only patients with a very limited life expectancy should be indicated for methacrylate fixation without bone grafting. Longitudinal Steinmann pins may be incorporated

into the PMMA mass to enhance both the bending resistance of the construct and its fixation to the adjacent vertebral bodies. Anterior plates can also be used to increase the rigidity of this construct *(53)*. Care must be taken to avoid contact of the PMMA with the dura, to maintain enough space for the sac, and to prevent thermal injury. This is especially important when the patient is supine, in which case a sheet of Gelfoam may be used to shield the thecal sac while the cement polymerizes under a constant flow of saline irrigation *(54)*.

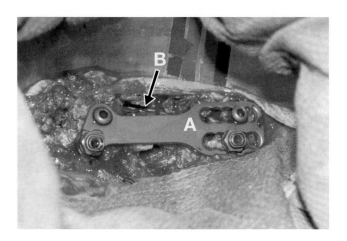

Fig. 6. Anterior reconstruction after L1 vertebral resection. Longitudinal plate (**A**) controls motion in all planes and prevents strut graft and cage from migrating or collapsing. The cage (**B**) shares the axial loads of the spine and prevents the screws placed in T12 and L2 from loosening or breaking. The patient is mobilized to a chair the evening of surgery, and begins transfers the next day.

Prosthetic cages with morselized autograft, tricortical strut grafts, and allograft bone struts are used for patients with a longer anticipated survival. Grafts should be keyed into the vertebral endplates, whereas the endplates should not be violated when using titanium cages. These devices and struts need to be combined with anterior or posterior instrumentation to provide stable fixation suitable to allow the patient out of bed in a brace (Fig. 5). The goal is complete bony arthrodesis and results in attaining this have been good *(55,56)*.

Anterior plate fixation may be combined with anterior column reconstruction to restore sagittal, coronal, and torsional rigidity following vertebrectomy, eliminating the need for posterior instrumentation in some patients (Fig. 6) *(57)*. Plate fixation also minimizes the likelihood that the strut graft or cage will displace. There is less need to key the graft into the adjacent vertebral bodies, and the graft can be impacted directly into the hard vertebral endplates. Because the graft or cage rests on the endplates, there is less chance of subsidence over time. Expandable cages make fitting into the vertebral defect easier and also allow the surgeon to correct kyphosis at the time of placement (Fig. 7).

Several carbon fiber vertebral replacement prostheses have become available recently, which can provide both the mechanical support necessary for axial stability and the potential for bone ingrowth or arthrodesis without the morbidity of harvesting large tricortical autografts. These can be connected to the posterior instrumentation providing a stable construct for large defects. Modularity and radiolucency are other advantages *(58)*.

7. SUMMARY

The prognosis for survival has improved dramatically for patients with primary spinal neoplasms over the past 30 yr. New approaches to systemic disease have improved survival and quality of life even in those patients who cannot be cured. As adjuvant therapies have improved, the importance of managing spinal column disease and protecting cord function has increased.

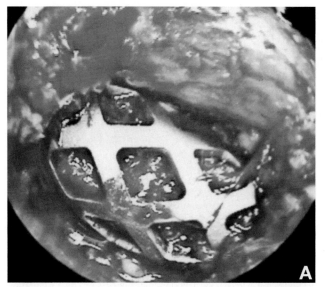

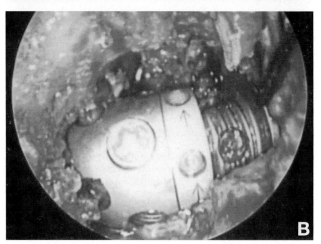

Fig. 7. (**A,B**) Anterior reconstruction with titanium cages. (**A**) Mesh titanium cages can be cut to fit the vertebrectomy defect. Packed with autograft bone, they provide a weight-bearing strut until fusion occurs. In cases where life expectancy is limited, the cages may be filled with methylmethacrylate cement. (**B**) Expandable cages provide the same mechanical benefits, but can be adjusted in place to correct residual deformity and provide optimal fit.

Advances in surgical technique and biomaterials have reduced many of the postoperative complications that plagued earlier treatment techniques. Newer fixation techniques have eliminated many of the instrumentation failures previously seen, and now allow rapid mobilization with limited or no bracing. Patient recovery is quicker, and return to normal function and independence more rapid and assured.

Improved medical management, antibiosis, and preoperative planning, along with techniques of pre-operative embolization and early postoperative mobilization have made surgical management less risky. Treatment of primary spinal malignancies can now focus aggressively on cure and rapid return to normal activity and function.

REFERENCES

1. Enneking WF, Spanier SS, Goodmann MA. A system for the surgical staging of musculoskeletal sarcoma. Clin Orthop 1980; 153:106–120.

2. Weinstein JN. Surgical approach to spine tumors. Orthopaedics 1989; 12:897–905.

3. Sundaresan N, Rosen G, Huvos AG, Krol G. Combined treatment of osteosarcoma of the spine. Neurosurgery 1988; 23:714–719.

4. Weinstein JN, McLain RF. Primary tumors of the spine. Spine 1987; 12:843–851.

5. Barwick KW, Huvos AG, Smith J. Primary osteogenic sarcoma of the vertebral column. Cancer 1980; 46:595–604.

6. Shives TC, Dahlin DC, Sim FH, Pritchard DJ, Earle JD. Osteosarcoma of the spine. J Bone Joint Surg 1986; 68A:660–668.

7. Spiegel DA, Richardson WJ, Scully SP, Harrelson JM. Long-term survival following total sacrectomy with reconstruction for the treatment of primary osteosarcoma of the sacrum. A case report. J Bone Joint Surg 1999; 81:848–855.

8. Ozaki T, Flege S, Liljenqvist U, et al. Osteosarcoma of the spine: experience of the Cooperative Osteosarcoma Study Group. Cancer 2002; 94:1069–1077.

9. Grubb MR, Currier BL, Pritchard DJ, Ebersold MJ. Primary Ewing's sarcoma of the spine. Spine 1994; 19:309–313.

10. Pilepich MV, Vietti TJ, Nesbit ME, et al. Ewing's sarcoma of the vertebral column. Int J Radiat Oncol Biol Phys 1981; 7:27–31.

11. Poulsen JO, Jensen JT, Tommesen P. Ewing's sarcoma simulating vertebra plana. Acta Orthop Scand 1975; 46:211–215.

12. Hadfield MG, Quezado MM, Williams RL, Williams RL, Luo VY. Ewing's family of tumors involving structures related to the central nervous system: a review. Pediatr Dev Pathol 2000; 3:203–210.

13. Yamaguchi T, Yamato M, Saotome K. First histologically confirmed case of a classic chordoma arising in a precursor benign notochordal lesion: differential diagnosis of benign and malignant notochordal lesions. Skeletal Radiol 2002; 31:413–418.

14. Boriani S, Chevalley F, Weinstein JN, et al. Chordoma of the spine above the sacrum: treatment and outcome in 21 cases. Spine 1996; 21:1569–1577.

15. Bergh P, Kindblom LG, Gunterberg B, Remotti F, Ryd W, Meis-Kindblom JM. Prognostic factors in chordoma of the sacrum and mobile spine: a study of 39 patients. Cancer 2000; 88:2122–2134.

16. Dahlin DC. Bone Tumors: General Aspects and Data on 6,221 Cases. 3rd ed. Springfield, IL: Charles C. Thomas; 1978.

17. Shives TC, McLeod RA, Unni KK, Schray MF. Chondrosarcoma of the spine. J Bone Joint Surg 1989; 71:1158–1165.

18. Hermann G, Sacher M, Lanzieri CF, Anderson PJ, Rabinowitz JG. Chondrosarcoma of the spine: an unusual radiographic presentation. Skeletal Radiol 1985; 14:178–183.

19. Stener B. Total spondylectomy in chondrosarcoma arising from the seventh thoracic vertebra. J Bone Joint Surg 1971; 53B:288–295.

20. Bergh P, Gunterberg B, Meis-Kindblom JM, Kindblom LG. Prognostic factors and outcome of pelvic, sacral, and spinal chondrosarcomas: a center-based study of 69 cases. Cancer 2001; 91:1201–1212.

21. Boriani S, De Iure F, Bandiera S, et al. Chondrosarcoma of the mobile spine: report on 22 cases. Spine 2000; 25:804–812.

22. York JE, Berk RH, Fuller GN, et al. Chondrosarcoma of the spine: 1954 to 1997. J Neurosurg 1999; 90:73–78.

23. Valderrama JAF, Bullough PG. Solitary myeloma of the spine. J Bone Joint Surg 1998; 50B:82–90.

24. McLain RF, Weinstein JN. Solitary plasmacytomas of the spine: a review of 84 cases. J Spinal Disord 1989; 2:69–74.

25. Talac R, Yaszemski MJ, Currier BL, et al. Relationship between surgical margins and local recurrence in sarcomas of the spine. Clin Orthop 2002; 397:127–132.

26. Abdel-Wanis MS, Kawahara N, Murata A, et al. Thyroid cancer spinal metastases: report on 25 operations in 14 patients. Anticancer Res 2002; 22:2509–2516.

27. Bohm P, Huber J. The surgical treatment of bony metastases of the spine and limbs. J Bone Joint Surg 2002; 84:521–529.

28. Jackson RJ, Gokaslan ZL, Loh SC. Metastatic renal cell carcinoma of the spine: surgical treatment and results. J Neurosurg 2001; 94:18–24.

29. Murakami H, Kawahara N, Abdel-Wanis ME, Tomita K. Total *en bloc* spondylectomy. Semin Musculoskel Radiol 2001; 5:189–194.

30. Nakai S, Yoshizawa H, Kobayashi S, Maeda K, Okumura Y. Anorectal and bladder function after sacrifice of the sacral nerves. Spine 2000; 25:2234–2239.

31. Raque GH Jr, Vitaz TW, Shields CB. Treatment of neoplastic diseases of the sacrum. J Surg Oncol 2001; 76:301–307.

32. Boland PJ, Lane JM, Sundaresan N. Metastatic disease of the spine. Clin Ortho 1982; 169:95–102.

33. Harrington KD. Metastatic disease of the spine. J Bone Joint Surg 1986; 68:1110–1115.

34. Constans JP, Divitiis E, Donzelli R, Spaziante R, Meder JF, Haye C. Spinal metastases with neurological manifestations: review of 600 Cases. J Neurosurg 1983; 59:111–118.

35. Helweg-Larsen S, Sorensen PS, Kreiner S. Prognostic factors in metastatic spinal cord compression: a prospective study using multivariate analysis of variables influencing survival and gait function in 153 patients. Int J Radiat Oncol Biol Phys 2000; 46:1163–1169.

36. Tatsui H, Onomura T, Morishita S, Oketa M, Inoue T. Survival rates of patients with metastatic spinal cancer after scintigraphic detection of abnormal radioactive accumulation. Spine 1996; 21:2143–2148.

37. Harrington KD. Anterior decompression and stabilization of the spine as a treatment for vertebral collapse and spinal cord compression from metastatic malignancy. Clin Ortho 1988; 233:177–197.

38. Klekamp J, Samii H. Surgical results for spinal metastases. Acta Neurochir 1998; 140:957–967.

39. Kostuik JP. Anterior spinal cord decompression for lesions of the thoracic and lumbar spine, techniques, new methods of internal fixation, results. Spine 1983; 8:512–531.

40. Gokaslan ZL, York JE, Walsh GL, et al. Transthoracic vertebrectomy for metastatic spinal tumors. J Neurosurg 1998; 89:599–609.

41. Kanayama M, Ng JTW, Cunningham BW, Abumi K, Kaneda K, McAfee PC. Biomechanical analysis of anterior versus circumferential spinal reconstruction for various anatomic stages of tumor lesions. Spine 1999; 24:445–450.

42. Akeyson EW, McCutcheon IE. Single-stage posterior vertebrectomy and replacement combined with posterior instrumentation for spinal metastasis. J Neurosurg 1996; 85:211–220.

43. Bilsky MH, Boland P, Lis E, Raizer JJ, Healey JH. Single-stage posterolateral transpedicle approach for spondylectomy, epidural decompression, and circumferential fusion of spinal metastases. Spine 2000; 25:2240–2250.

44. McLain RF. Endoscopically assisted decompression for metastatic thoracic neoplasms. Spine 1998; 23:1130–1135.

45. Boriani S, Biagini R, De Iure F, et al. *En bloc* resections of bone tumors of the thoracolumbar spine: a preliminary report on 29 patients. Spine 1996; 21:1927–1931.

46. Fourney DR, Abi-Said D, Rhines LD, et al. Simultaneous anterior-posterior approach to the thoracic and lumbar spine for the radical resection of tumors followed by reconstruction and stabilization. J Neurosurg 2001; 94:232–244.

47. Heary RF, Vaccaro AR, Benevenia J, Cotler JM. *En bloc* vertebrectomy in the mobile lumbar spine. Surg Neurol 1998; 50:548–556.

48. Krepler P, Windhager R, Bretschneider W, Toma CD, Kotz R. Total vertebrectomy for primary malignant tumours of the spine. J Bone Joint Surg 2002; 84:712–715.

49. Tomita K, Kawahara N, Baba H, Tsuchiya H, Fujita T, Toribatake Y. Total *en bloc* spondylectomy: a new surgical technique for primary malignant vertebral tumors. Spine 1997; 22:324–333.

50. Fourney DR, Abi-Said D, Lang FF, McCutcheon IE, Gokaslan ZL. Use of pedicle screw fixation in the management of malignant spinal disease: experience in 100 consecutive procedures. J Neurosurg 2001; 94:25–37.

51. McLain RF, Sparling E, Benson DR. Failure of short segment pedicle instrumentation in thoracolumbar fractures: complications of Cotrel-Dubousset instrumentation. J Bone Joint Surg 1993; 75:162.

52. Jang JS, Lee SH, Rhee CH, Lee SH. Polymethylmethacrylate-augmented screw fixation for stabilization in metastatic spinal tumors. Technical note. J Neurosurg 2002; 96:131–134.

53. Caspar W, Pitzen T, Papavero L, Geisler FH, Johnson TA. Anterior cervical plating for the treatment of neoplasms in the cervical vertebrae. J Neurosurg 1999; 90:27–34.

54. Miller DJ, Lang FF, Walsh GL, Abi-Said D, Wildrick DM, Gokaslan ZL. Coaxial double-lumen methylmethacrylate reconstruction in the anterior cervical and upper thoracic spine after tumor resection. J Neurosurg 2000; 93:181–190.

55. Akamaru T, Kawahara N, Tsuchiya H, Kobayashi T, Murakami H, Tomita K. Healing of autologous bone in a titanium mesh cage used in anterior column reconstruction after total spondylectomy. Spine 2002; 27:E329–E333.

56. Munting E, Faundez A, Manche E. Vertebral reconstruction with cortical allograft: long-term evaluation. Eur Spine J 2001; 10:S153–S157.

57. Hall DJ, Webb JK. Anterior plate fixation in spine tumor surgery. Indications, technique, and results. Spine 1991; 16:580–583.

58. Boriani S, Biagini R, Bandiera S, Gasbarrini A, De LF. Reconstruction of the anterior column of the thoracic and lumbar spine with a carbon fiber stackable cage system. Orthopedics 2002; 25:37–42.

38 Complications of Surgical and Medical Care

Anticipation and Management

REX A. W. MARCO, MD AND HOWARD S. AN, MD

CONTENTS

1. INTRODUCTION

Complications related to the treatment of spinal neoplasms are often associated with inaccurate pre-operative assessment and diagnosis, as well as the definitive surgical procedure. A careful history and physical examination can lead to the appropriate diagnosis *(1)* and identify co-existing premorbid conditions, which may require further evaluation before operative intervention. Appropriate radiological and laboratory studies are important because they may lead to the correct diagnosis and direct proper treatment *(2)*. In general, once a lesion is identified, a biopsy should be obtained to make a definitive diagnosis. Exact techniques of the biopsy and the definitive treatment should be tailored to the nature and location of the lesion and the patient's general condition and life expectancy. A multidisciplinary team approach consisting of surgical, medical, and radiation oncologists, combined with experienced radiologists and pathologists, helps optimize patient care. The goals of operative intervention of spinal tumors are pain control, maintenance, or improvement of neurological function, eradication of the tumor, and maintenance of spinal stability, and the attainment of normal coronal and sagittal alignment. Attention to details and appropriate goal-oriented intervention should help decrease the incidence of complications related to spinal surgery. The anticipation and management of complications of the treatment of spinal tumors are discussed in this chapter.

From: *Current Clinical Oncology: Cancer in the Spine: Comprehensive Care.*
Edited by: R. F. McLain, K-U. Lewandrowski, M. Markman, R. M. Bukowski,
R. Macklis, and E. C. Benzel © Humana Press, Inc., Totowa, NJ

2. PRE-OPERATIVE PLANNING

Many complications could be obviated by a careful initial evaluation. The history is often helpful in separating neoplastic processes from other causes of back pain. Pain associated with tumors is characteristically persistent, progressive, worse at night, and present at rest. The age of the patient helps narrow the differential diagnosis. Metastatic disease, multiple myeloma, and chordoma are more common in patients older than 40 yr. Eosinophilic granuloma, osteoid osteoma, osteoblastoma, and Ewing's sarcoma are more common in children and young adults. Leukemia and neuroblastoma are malignancies found in the younger child. A previous history of cancer increases the likelihood that the lesion is a metastatic deposit.

Intradural, extramedullary tumors are mostly benign and frequently grow in relation to a nerve root. Radicular pain that is worse at night is common. Intramedullary tumors are often painless. Centrally located tumors can affect pain and temperature sensation in a segmental fashion without affecting light touch or position sense because the fibers controlling pain and temperature are located centrally in the spinal cord. This "segmental differential sensory deficit" or "dissociated sensory loss" is characteristic of an intramedullary tumor *(3)*. The most common location of intramedullary tumors is the cervical spinal cord and, therefore, the hands are frequently affected early. Subsequently, long tract signs, weakness, and incontinence may develop. The evolution of these symptoms is almost invariably slow, and this fact, associated with the absence of pain, is responsible for misdiagnoses such as multiple sclerosis and cervical spondylosis.

The physical examination should include a general survey, because primary tumors from breast, prostate, lung, rectum, or thyroid may be detected. Sacral chordoma are often palpable on rectal examination. A careful neurological examination is mandatory to detect early signs of spinal cord compression. An elderly patient with a new onset of persistent back pain should have an evaluation to rule out tumors or infections. Signs and symptoms of spinal cord compression include persistent back pain, difficulty maintaining balance, wide-based gait, fatigue after a short walk, bowel or bladder incontinence, paresthesias, and weakness of the extremities. Early diagnosis of spinal cord compression, and the commencement of appropriate treatment may prevent irreversible neurological deficits and deformity.

Complete blood cell count with differential, erythrocyte sedimentation rate, and C-reactive protein may help differentiate neoplastic from inflammatory disorders. Prostate specific antigen, serum protein electrophoresis, and thyroid function tests should be ordered if the diagnosis is unclear. Calcium, phosphate, and alkaline phosphatase levels are altered in metabolic diseases such as osteomalacia, Paget's disease, and hyperparathyroidism. Roentgenographically, severe osteoporosis is often difficult to distinguish from multiple myeloma. Paget's disease also mimics osteoblastic tumors such as prostate carcinoma. Further metastatic studies, such as mammography and chest or abdominal computed tomography (CT), should be obtained in accordance with the suspected primary carcinoma. Although metastatic lesions are the most common tumors of the spine, primary tumors including benign and malignant bone tumors, intraspinal tumors, and cysts should be considered in the differential diagnosis. Metabolic disorders such as osteoporosis (Fig. 1) and Paget's disease should also be considered in the differential diagnosis (4). Spinal infections should be ruled out, particularly in immunocompromised patients. Occasionally, an infection and tumor may exist in the same individual (5).

Conventional high-quality roentgenographs are non-invasive, low-cost studies utilized to evaluate the level of the lesion, the local anatomy, and the overall alignment. CT helps define bony architecture and integrity, whereas magnetic resonance imaging (MRI) provides additional information on soft tissue and neural involvement (6). MRI is useful to differentiate malignant spinal tumors from infections (7) and benign compression fractures (8). Vertebral osteomyelitis usually involves the disk space and adjacent vertebral body end plates with decreased signal intensity on the T1-weighted images and increased signal intensity on the T2-weighted images (Fig. 2). Spinal tumors do not usually involve the disc space. Malignant compression fractures of the spine, as compared to benign compression fractures, are more likely to demonstrate bony destruction, involvement of the pedicle, and a soft tissue epidural component (Fig.3).

Pre-operative angiography is invaluable for tumors with significant vascularity. Metastatic renal cell carcinoma and myeloma are particularly vascular. Pre-operative embolization may be effective in reducing blood loss (9–12). Angiography also identifies the feeding artery to the spinal cord, which may be involved by tumor. Additionally, if the tumor is close to a major artery, angiography will help define this relationship and its clinical significance.

3. BIOPSY

A biopsy of the lesion is often essential before rendering definitive treatment (13). The clinician must provide adequate and representative tissue for interpretation without compromising further intervention. The careful planning and execution of the biopsy decreases the likelihood of adverse effects on the prognosis and on treatment options. Confirmation of the tissue diagnosis is preferred. Many definitive procedures are performed, based on frozen section analysis. If the diagnosis is equivocal on frozen section analysis, the definitive procedure should be postponed, if possible. Image-guided large-bore core needle biopsies are usually diagnostic when evaluated by an experienced pathologist (14). Needle biopsies minimize soft tissue contamination and hematoma formation compared to an open biopsy. Open biopsies are performed if the needle biopsy is nondiagnostic or if the patient has spinal cord compression that requires emergent decompression. The definitive procedure can be performed if the frozen section analysis is diagnostic and the surgeon is prepared to perform the appropriate procedure. Proceeding with a definitive procedure is not prudent if equivocal frozen section analysis results are rendered or if the diagnosis is consistent with a primary bone tumor. Cultures and sensitivities for bacteria, fungus, and mycobacterium should be sent if the frozen section analysis is nondiagnostic.

Needle biopsies for the thoracic, lumbar, and sacral spine is usually performed in the prone position under fluoroscopic or CT guidance (15). Local anesthesia minimizes injury to neural structures because the patient can communicate abnormal sensations, which may indicate proximity of the needle to important structures. An estimate of the point of needle insertion is obtained by placing the needle over the lesion in the midline. The distance from the tip of the localization needle to the lesion should equal the distance from the insertion point of the biopsy needle to the midline if a 45° angle is used for the needle trajectory (16). This distance is usually 8 to 10 cm in the lumbar spine, 6 to 7 cm in the thoracolumbar junction, and 4 to 5 cm in the thoracic spine (17–19). A local anesthetic is infiltrated using a long 22-gage needle. The needle should point at a 45° angle, while image guidance monitors the progress of the needle. Constant aspiration on the needle will help identify vessels if encountered. The periosteum and the needle tract are anesthetized. The large-bore core needle biopsy is advanced in the same tract under image guidance. A piece of gel foam is inserted into the biopsy site through the needle if excessive bleeding is encountered. An experienced pathologist should confirm that an adequate amount of representative tissue was obtained. Following biopsy, the patient should be closely monitored for bleeding complications. Percutaneous needle biopsy is also utilized to access anterior cervical spine lesions (20). C2 lesions can be biopsied through an oblique, submucosal transoral approach through the buccal space under general anesthesia under CT guidance. Complications associated with needle biopsies include neural injury, paraspinal hematoma, infection, pneumothorax, meningitis, and death (21–25).

An open biopsy can be incisional or excisional. Dorsal lesions are occasionally amenable to an excisional biopsy by performing a laminectomy. Ventral cervical exposure is utilized for

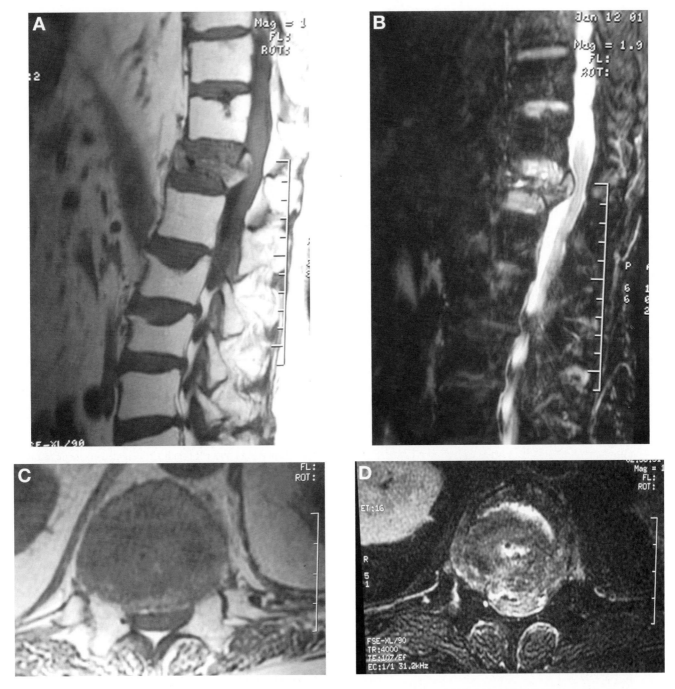

Fig. 1. Osteoporotic burst fracture initially treated as metastatic cervical carcinoma. A 69-yr-old female with a L1 osteoporotic burst fracture, severe back pain, and paraparesis. The patient had a remote history of cervical cancer. T1- and T2-weighted sagittal, (**A,B**) and axial, (**C,D**) magnetic resonance imaging (MRI). A pathological fracture associated with metastatic cervical carcinoma was presumed, and radiation therapy was initiated. Radiation therapy was stopped after consultation with the spinal surgery team. No evidence of malignancy was identified on histological examination of the vertebral body. Careful evaluation of the MRI shows that there is no soft tissue mass, no epidural extension, and no pedicle or posterior element involvement.

incisional biopsies of ventral cervical spine lesions. Open biopsies for ventral lesions located in the thoracic and lumbar spine frequently employ the transpedicular approach (30). The precise localization of the thoracic and lumbar pedicles is important. Intra-operative imaging is helpful. Costotransversectomy and dorsolateral approaches are occasionally utilized for thoracic and lumbar lesions. Recently, use of endoscopy has become popu-lar for thoracic lesions for biopsy or excision of lesions (26). An experienced pathologist should confirm that an adequate amount of viable and representative tissue was obtained. If not, more tissue should be obtained. If the definitive procedure is not performed at the time of the biopsy, meticulous hemostasis should be obtained before skin closure to minimize risk of hematoma formation.

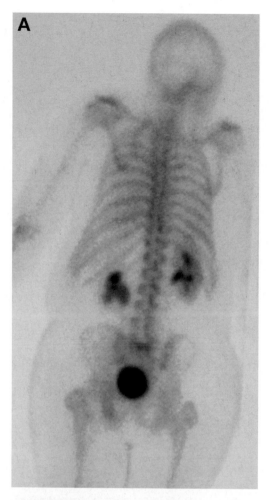

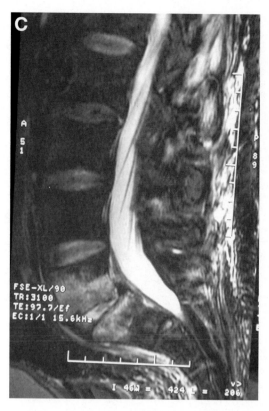

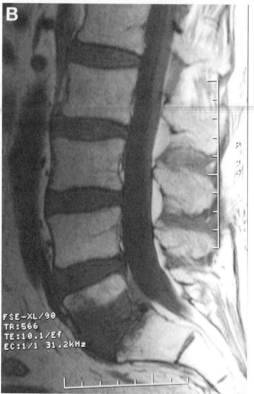

Fig. 2. Discitis initially diagnosed as an osteoporotic compression fracture. A 67-yr-old male with metastatic colon cancer to the liver presented with a 5-mo history of low back pain. A bone scan showed increased uptake at L5 (**A**). T1- and T2-weighted magnetic resonance imaging of the lumbar spine showed abnormal signal at L5, S1, and the L5–S1 disc (**B,C**). The radiologist felt that these findings were consistent with an osteoporotic compression fracture. However, osteoporotic compression fractures do not usually result in increased signal in two adjacent vertebral bodies and the disc on T2-weighted images. A computed tomography-guided biopsy demonstrated acute inflammatory cells and gram positive diplococci. Pan-sensitive coagulase negative staphylococcus was identified. His back pain improved with intravenous antibiotics.

Prolonged survival and decreased incidence of local recurrence has been reported with complete excision of malignant primary bone tumors of the spine as compared to incomplete resection *(27–29)*. Suboptimal performance of the biopsy may decrease the ability to perform complete excision of the tumor *(30,31)*.

4. SURGICAL APPROACH

Before performing a specific procedure, indications for surgery should be strictly defined. Most primary tumors of the spine that are malignant or locally aggressive should be surgically removed, provided that radiation therapy and chemotherapy, or in combination, are not sufficiently effective alone. The surgical indications and considerations for metastatic tumors include the presence of significant neurological deficits, deformity, failure of non-operative treatment, medical status, and oncological prognosis of the patient. The surgical approach obviously depends on the type and location of the tumor. As in any other primary tumors in the extremities, surgical margins should be respected when possible. Even for

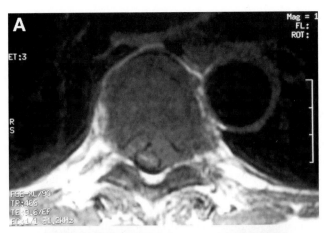

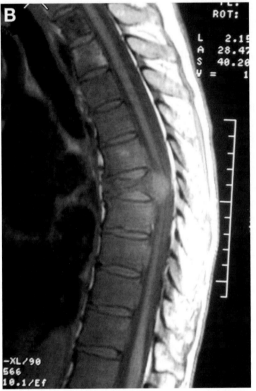

Fig. 3. Spinal cord compression from metastatic rhabdomyosarcoma. A 61-yr-old female with a history of nasopharyngeal rhabdomyosarcoma presented with a 2 wk history of severe mid-thoracic back pain. The axial and sagittal magnetic resonance imaging (MRI) (A,B) showed a compression fracture of the T7 vertebral body with epidural extension. The radiologist did not feel that these findings were consistent with metastatic tumor. However, the bilobed appearance of the epidural extension is commonly seen on the axial MRI in patients with spinal cord compression secondary to metastatic tumor. A computed tomography-guided biopsy at T7 confirmed the presence of metastatic rhabdomyosarcoma. She was treated with corticosteroids and radiation therapy.

certain metastatic tumors such as hypernephroma and thyroid carcinoma, *en-bloc* excision should be attempted if feasible. Most metastatic tumors in the spinal column are present in the vertebral body, and therefore, a ventral approach is most frequently used to perform corpectomy or vertebrectomy. Spinal reconstruction includes fusion and stabilization, which should

be rigid and stable whenever possible. Postoperative fixation failure and pseudarthrosis frequently occur owing to inadequate spinal fusion and instrumentation techniques. Dorsal augmentation of fusion and instrumentation should be considered to maximize the rigidity of the surgical construct and fusion success. Thorough familiarity of surgical anatomy and surgical approaches to the cervical, thoracic, and lumbar spine is important to prevent intra-operative complications.

5. POSITIONING

Avoidance of abnormal pressure on the eyes can prevent corneal abrasions and blindness. Constant attention by the surgeon and the anesthesiologist helps minimize ocular pressure. Foam headrests with open areas over the eyes and Mayfield tongs or headrests are devices that minimize direct pressure on the eyes.

Avoiding shoulder abduction beyond 80° minimizes the likelihood of brachial plexus traction injuries. Avoiding direct pressure on the ulnar nerves decreases the likelihood of ulnar nerve neuropraxia. Padding the knees helps prevent pressure ulcers. Minimizing external pressure on the abdomen increases blood flow through the inferior vena cava, which probably decreases blood flow through the epidural venous system resulting in decreased blood loss and increased visibility during excision of the tumor. An axillary roll is utilized in the lateral decubitus position to prevent brachial plexopathy of the down arm. Padding over the greater trochanter prevents pressure ulcers and protection of the peroneal nerve of the down leg prevents peroneal nerve injuries.

The axillary roll and flexion of the table at the waist invariably creates a scoliotic deformity. Minimizing the size of the axillary roll and the flexion in the table will help decrease the deformity. Reversing the flexion of the table, combined with appropriate manipulation of the spinal instrumentation, also helps minimize the deformity.

6. APPROPRIATE LEVEL AND SIDE

Identifying the appropriate spinal level is facilitated by intra-operative examination and radiographs. The level of the clavicle and mandible relative to the cervical level are readily visible on a lateral radiograph. The hyoid bone is usually at C3, the thyroid cartilage overlies C4 and C5, and the cricoid cartilage usually overlies C6. Following a ventral approach, a spinal needle placed within the disc helps confirm the appropriate level. A bayonet bend at the end of the needle helps prevent posterior over penetration of the needle into the spinal canal.

Palpation of the last rib and counting the ribs from within the thoracic cavity help identify the appropriate thoracic level during ventral thoracic approaches. Lateral radiographs and palpation of the L1 transverse process and the last rib help identify the thoracolumbar junction during dorsal approaches. Palpation of the iliac crest in comparison to the corresponding lumbar level combined with an intra-operative radiograph and palpation of the sacrum, help identify the target site in the lumbar spine (32). Ultimately, a soft tissue mass, tumor, and local bone destruction or collapse, usually assist in confirming the appropriate level.

7. COMPLICATIONS

7.1. NEUROLOGICAL COMPLICATIONS

Although neurological improvements are often observed after tumor resection, patients who have advanced neurological deficits pre-operatively may have worsening of their deficit postoperatively. Awake intubation with the aid of a fiberoptic light is helpful to prevent excessive cervical manipulation during intubation of patients with cervical spine tumors. Ventrally, the tumor is removed with a combination of rongeurs and curettes. Careful removal of tumor, bone, or disc material in the lateral corner near the uncovertebral joint may help avoid nerve root injury. Careful utilization of a diamond burr along the posterior longitudinal ligament may be of assistance. Removal of the posterior longitudinal ligament removes microscopic deposits of tumor and may decrease the rate of local recurrence. Dorsolateral decompressions utilize a laminectomy at the involved level and the bone overlying the rostral and caudal disc spaces adjacent to the involved level. The use of a burr, curettes, and small caliber Kerrison rongeurs minimizes forces on the previously compromised thecal sac and underlying cord or cauda equina.

Inadvertent penetration of the spinal canal should be avoided. Evaluation of the radiological studies helps identify areas of weak bone and relatively wide interlaminar spaces. The utilization of broad elevators over large interlaminar spaces or posterior arch deficiencies is preferred over utilization of sharp-pointed instruments, which can pass through the defects. Gentle subperiosteal dissection of the soft tissue at levels of the spinal cord compression is recommended to minimize motion and pressure during exposure of the dorsal elements. A diamond burr or very small Kerrison rongeur may be utilized to perform the laminectomy at this level.

The depth of ventral grafts, cages, or cement may be assessed intraoperatively by examination and lateral radiographs. The stability of the graft should be maintained by compressive forces placed on the graft. If neurological complications are discovered postoperatively, a lateral radiograph may be obtained to determine the position of a ventral interbody strut and the administration of steroids may be considered. CT or MRI can be helpful. If a hematoma or bone graft malalignment is suspected, exploration usually is recommended.

Injury to the sympathetic chain can result in a Horner's syndrome. The cervical sympathetic chain lies on the ventral surface of the longus colli muscles just dorsal to the carotid sheath. Subperiosteal dissection helps prevent damage to these nerves. Horner's syndrome is usually temporary but can be permanent in approx 1% of patients (33). The lumbar sympathetic chain lies medial to the psoas muscle. Transection of this structure usually results in vasodilation of the vessels to the ipsilateral extremity.

7.2. DURAL TEARS

Perforations of the dura mater may lead to cerebrospinal fluid leakage, neurological impairment, pseudomeningocele formation, cerebrospinal fluid fistula, meningitis, or wound healing problems. Dural tears may occur during excision of the ligamentum flavum, but more commonly during manipulation of the dural sac to free adhesions. Burrs, curettes, and rongeurs should be used in a cautious manner. Dural tears should be closed primarily using a 4:0 or 5:0 nonabsorbable suture while avoiding constriction of the spinal cord or cauda equina. Fibrin adhesive sealant helps reinforce the repair (34). Local fascial graft, free fat graft, collagen-based dural graft matrix, and gel foam are often utilized to augment the repair (35). Large tears may require repair with fascial grafts, allograft dura, or synthetic dural material. The anesthesiologist should increase intrathoracic pressure by Valsalva maneuver to distend the dura and ensure proper sealing of the repair. The paraspinous muscle, overlying fascia, subcutaneous tissue, and skin should be closed in multiple layers in a water-tight manner. Drains are usually avoided, although some authors advocate utilization of a drain if an adequate repair was performed (36). Postoperative spinal fluid leaks and pseudomeningoceles, paradoxically, are more likely to occur with small perforations in the dura mater compared to large openings. Pre-operative radiation therapy increases the incidence of wound dehiscence and spinal fluid leakage. If skin dehiscence is present, skin closure with a running nonabsorbable suture may stop further leakage. Insertion of a lumbar subarachnoid or subcutaneous drain may allow healing of the wound and ultimate closure of the fistulous tract. These bedside procedures are not predictable, and are associated with bed confinement for several days and the potential for infection. Empiric broad-spectrum intravenous antibiotics are instituted until wound drainage ceases and the drain is removed. If prompt improvement is not observed, the surgeon is encouraged to explore the wound and repair the dural leak. If the exact site of leakage is difficult to discover, a lumbar injection of 10 mL of indigo-carmine may help to identify the dural opening. Intrathecal methylene-blue is avoided because of its neurotoxicity. Subarachnoid-pleural fistulas are difficult to treat because the negative intrathoracic pressure encourages flow from the intrathecal space into the intrathoracic cavity. Pedicled flaps may be required to augment these repairs (37).

7.3. COMPLICATIONS ASSOCIATED WITH SPINAL INSTRUMENTATION

Complications related to posterior spinal instrumentation include hook dislodgement, neural element encroachment, pedicle screw failure, hardware prominence, and junctional kyphosis. Erosion of visceral or vascular structures, penetration of the spinal canal, and interbody instrumentation dislodgement can occur with ventral spinal instrumentation. The goal of instrumentation is to provide sufficient spinal stability to allow early mobilization and to maintain spinal alignment. Instrumentation also improves the likelihood of spinal fusion in patients with prolonged life expectancies.

Patients with metastatic disease often present with multilevel spinal column involvement. A screening cervical, thoracic, and lumbar spine sagittal MRI will help define the extent of tumor involvement. Posterior spinal instrumentation should have a normal vertebra cephalad and caudal to the construct to help prevent junctional failures. Transverse process hooks are reserved for levels with uninvolved dorsal elements and are used sparingly in patients with myeloma or osteoporosis because the transverse process is more susceptible to fracture in these situations. Pedicle screws and supralaminar or infralaminar hooks may provide better fixation in these patients. Polymethylmeth-acrylate (PMMA) injected into the vertebral body before pedicle screw fixation may improve screw purchase. Patients with osteoporosis or diffuse spinal involvement should be instrumented *in situ*. Excessive correction forces on the instrumentation may lead to dislodgement of the instrumentation. Precise contouring of the rod in the sagittal plane may help minimize junctional failures. Lower profile instrumentation should be utilized in thin patients to prevent prominent hardware. Supplemental fixation with offset laminar hooks at the end of the construct decreases pedicle screw bending moments and migration, which may provide a more durable construct *(38)*.

Single-level vertebral body involvement can often be treated with a vertebral body reconstruction and ventral instrumentation. PMMA has a similar modulus of elasticity to cancellous bone and provides a broad surface with structural support. Securing the cement to the adjacent vertebral bodies helps prevent dislodgement *(39–41)*. Careful contouring of the cement, as well as saline irrigation during the exothermic reaction, helps prevent impingement of the dura and thermal damage. PMMA usually provides durable structural support when utilized in compression as an interbody strut *(39–41)*. However, loosening and failure of fixation have been reported with PMMA supplementation of dorsal fixation *(42)*. Structural bone graft and carbon fiber and titanium cages also provide durable structural support. Utilizing a cage with a broad surface area should help prevent failure of the cage secondary to cage instability or penetration into the endplate. Ideally, slight distraction of the spinal column is performed to help place the cage followed by gentle compressive forces to enhance stability of the cage. Ventral spinal instrumentation improves the stability of the construct and may prevent dislodgement of the interbody instrumentation. Vertebral body screws should be directed away from the spinal canal to avoid canal penetration. The instrumentation should be placed away from visceral structures and vessels to avoid erosion of these structures. Low profile, locking cervical plates with unicortical screws can help prevent esophageal erosion, screw loosening and canal penetration.

7.4. VISCERAL INJURY

Esophageal perforation can occur during ventral cervical spine procedures. Sharp retractors should be avoided. Use of a nasogastric tube helps identify the esophagus during surgery. If an esophageal perforation is suspected, then methylene blue injected in the nasogastric tube can identify occult esophageal injuries. An intra-operative consultation with a head and neck or general surgeon is recommended and primary repair is usually performed. Unrecognized esophageal perforations can present later as an abscess, a tracheosophagcal fistula, or mediastinitis. The usual treatment consists of intravenous antibiotics, nasogastric feeding, drainage, debridement, and repair by a surgeon with expertise in treatment of esophageal disorders *(43)*.

Injury to the lung can occur during exposures of the rib or costovertebral junction during anterior or posterolateral spinal procedures. Careful subperiosteal dissection of the ribs usually provides exposure of the rib without violating the parietal pleura. Holding ventilation and utilization of a double lumen endotracheal tube (T1–T6) during transthoracic approaches

before entering the pleura helps minimize risk of injury to the lung during anterior procedures. A tube thoracostomy is usually placed if the pleura is entered during the dorsolateral approach and almost always after anterior approaches.

Transection of the anococcygeal ligaments allows careful separation of the rectum from the sacrum during the posterior portion of distal sacrectomy and coccygectomy procedures. Placement of a rectal tube can facilitate identification of the rectum.

7.5. PULMONARY COMPLICATIONS

Pulmonary complications commonly occur after reconstructive spinal procedures in patients with cancer. Atelectasis, pneumonia, pneumothorax, and aspiration are the most frequently encountered complications. Expansion of the lung before extubation, deep breathing, coughing, and early mobilization are techniques utilized to prevent atelectasis and pneumonia. Aggressive pulmonary toilet, early mobilization, bronchoscopy, and antibiotics are utilized to treat pneumonia. A small apical pneumothorax following chest tube removal usually resolves with observation, but a persistant, symptomatic, or large pneumothorax may require replacement of a tube thoracostomy. A pneumothorax refractory to non-operative treatment may require further investigation and treatment. Aspiration is prevented by elevation of the head of the bed, control of nausea and vomiting, judicial utilization of nasogastric suction, and minimizing oversedation.

7.6. GENITOURINARY COMPLICATIONS

Ureteral injuries usually occur during retroperitoneal dissections around the bifurcation of the common iliac vessels (Fig. 4) *(44–47)*. Ureteral stents enhance identification of the ureter, and are recommended for reoperations in the retroperitoneal space and for sacral lesions with a large soft tissue component. Retrograde ejaculation can occur if the superior hypogastric sympathetic plexus is injured during dissection on the ventral portion of the upper sacrum. Bowel, bladder, and sexual dysfunction are common after a total sacrectomy. Near normal bowel, bladder, and sexual function are expected with bilateral S2 nerve root or unilateral S2, S3, and S4 preservation. Patients with neurogenic bladders are treated with intermittent clean catheterization, which has a lower incidence of urinary tract infections compared to prolonged indwelling bladder catheters *(47)*.

7.7. DYSPHAGIA AND HOARSENESS

Dysphagia after ventral cervical surgery may be caused by hemorrhage, edema, denervation, or infection *(49)*. A hematoma can cause airway obstruction or spinal cord compression *(50)*. Meticulous hemostasis, placement of a drain, and elevation of the head in the immediate postoperative period can help prevent these complications. Careful identification and ligation of the superior or the inferior thyroid artery can prevent arterial bleeding. Airway obstruction after extubation may occur in the postoperative period. Airway exchange is confirmed before extubation. Prolonged retraction of the soft tissues can result in retropharyngeal edema. Postoperative intubation *(51)* and corticosteroids are considered until the edema decreases.

If persistent dysphagia is present, a barium swallow or an endoscopy should be considered. Minor hoarseness or sore

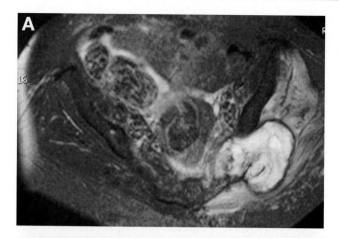

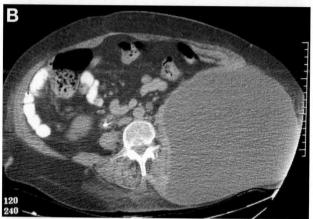

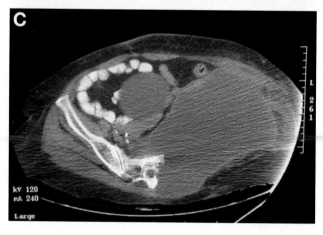

Fig. 4. Left retroperitoneal urinoma secondary to left distal ureteral perforation. A 55-yr-old female with a left sciatic notch pleomorhphic liposarcoma. T2-weighted axial magnetic resonance imaging (**A**). A hemipelvectomy and partial sacral excision was performed. The patient developed a large, retroperitoneal fluid collection that was in continuity with the sacrum (**B,C**). She denied headaches. The fluid collection spontaneously drained and the wound sealed. The patient declined a radionucleotide cysternogram to evaluate for cerebrospinal fluid leakage. The fluid recollected, and a percutaneous aspiration revealed a creatinine level of 19 mg/d. The urinoma was treated with percutaneous drainage and a left nephrostomy tube. A subsequent left nephrostogram demonstrated left distal ureteral extravasation of contrast. The distal ureteral injury was treated with a ureteral stent. The ureter crosses the bifurcation of the common iliac artery or the beginning of the external iliac artery, and can be injured during anterior approaches to the lumbar or sacral spine.

throat after a ventral cervical approach is usually caused by edema or endotracheal intubation. Occasionally, laryngeal nerve palsy causes hoarseness (52,53). The external branch of the superior laryngeal nerve travels along with the superior thyroid artery to innervate the cricothyroid muscle. Damage to this nerve may result in hoarseness, but often produces symptoms such as easy fatiguing of the voice. The inferior laryngeal nerve is a recurrent branch of the vagus nerve, which pierces the cricothyroid membrane and innervates all of the laryngeal muscles except for the cricothyroid muscle. On the left side, the recurrent laryngeal nerve travels under the arch of the aorta and is protected in the left tracheoesophageal groove. On the right side, the recurrent laryngeal nerve passes around the subclavian artery, and then dorsomedially to the side of the trachea and esophagus. It is vulnerable as it passes from the subclavian artery to the right tracheoesophageal groove. The right inferior laryngeal nerve is occasionally nonrecurrent, and travels directly from the vagus nerve and carotid sheath to the larynx. This anomaly occurs when the right subclavian artery arises directly from the aortic arch, rather than from the innominate artery (8,80). The subclavian artery then passes dorsal to the esophagus and recurrence of the inferior laryngeal nerve does not develop. If hoarseness persists for more than 6 wk following anterior cervical surgery, laryngoscopy should be done to evaluate the vocal cord and laryngeal muscles. Treatment of inferior laryngeal nerve palsy includes observation to allow for spontaneous recovery of function. Further treatment or surgery by an otolaryngologist may be necessary in persistent cases.

7.8. ILEUS/GASTROINTESTINAL

Postoperative ileus can occur after spinal procedures, particularly following ventral procedures at the thoracolumbar, lumbar, or sacral levels. Ileus is often treated with nasogastric tube suction, iv fluids, and delayed oral intake until intestinal function returns.

7.9. VASCULAR COMPLICATIONS

Vascular injuries can occur during ventral and dorsal approaches to the spine. The common carotid artery, branches of the external carotid artery, the vertebral artery, and the internal jugular vein can be injured during anterior cervical approaches. Palpation of the common carotid artery, followed by careful dissection ventrally between the trachea and the carotid sheath, helps prevent injuries to the common carotid and internal jugular. Gentle retraction followed by palpation of the temporal artery helps assure adequate blood flow through the common carotid. Exposure of the upper cervical spine may require dissection and ligation of branches of the external carotid artery. The vertebral arteries and veins are usually located within the transverse foramen of C2–C6. Examination of the pre-operative axial images helps define the interforaminal distance between the transverse foramina, thus facilitating orientation during anterior decompressive procedures (54). The vertebral veins are usually located medial to the arteries, and will, thus, be injured more frequently than the vertebral arteries. Hemostasis is usually managed with gentle packing with thrombotic agents. Persistent hemorrhage may require further decompression and exposure of the vessels followed by bipolar electrocautery, repair, or ligation of the vessel. Ligation of the vertebral artery is associated with an increased risk of neuro-logical deficit, thus repair is often preferred, if possible *(55)*. The dominance of the artery should enter this decision-making process. The smaller of the two ventral arteries, if sacrificed, poses less of a neurological risk than the sacrifice of the larger artery.

Dorsally, the lateral aspect of the vertebral foramen is located 9 to 12 mm from the midpoint of the lateral mass at a 5 to 6° medially directed angle in the C3 and C5 vertebrae. The angle is laterally directed 5 to 6° at C6 *(56)*. Laterally directed place-ment of lateral mass screws should help avoid injury to the vertebral arteries and nerve roots *(57)*. The vertebral artery emerges from the foramen of C2, and then courses medially on the superior portion of C1 within the vertebral artery groove. The distance from the midline of C1 to the medial aspect of the groove ranges from 12 to 23 mm on the dorsal aspect of the ring and from 8 to 13 mm on the rostral aspect of the ring in adult vertebrae *(58)*. Dorsal dissection on the C1 ring should, there-fore, remain within 12 mm lateral of midline, and deep dissec-tion on the rostral aspect of the ring should remain within 8 mm of midline to minimize risk of injury to the vertebral artery.

The arch of the aorta with its innominate, left common carotid, and left subclavian artery branches, as well as the right and left brachiocephalic veins, are at risk of injury during exposures of tumors involving C7–T3 through low cervical or median sternotomy approaches *(59,60)*. The subclavian ves-sels and the origin of the vertebral artery are at risk for injury during procedures for superior sulcus tumors. Knowledge of the anatomy and careful retraction and protection can prevent injuries to these vessels. The azygos vein is located on the right ventrolateral aspect of the thoracic vertebral bodies from T4 through T12 and hemiazygos and accessory hemiazyous veins lie on the left side of the thoracic vertebral bodies and usually cross over at T8 or T9 to join the azygos vein. The descending aorta is at risk for injury during left-sided ventral approaches from T4 to L4 and the inferior vena cava is at risk for injury during procedures involving L1–L4 *(61)*. Protection of the aorta, inferior vena cava, azygous, and hemiazygous veins with a malleable retractor helps prevent injuries to these structures. Ligation of the segmental vessels, followed by gentle dissec-tion off the vertebral body, helps identify the plane between the anterior longitudinal ligament and the larger vessels. Careful utilization of curettes and pituitary ronguers combined with protection of the vessels with a laparotomy pad or malleable retractors helps prevent injuries to the large vessels. Identifica-tion and ligation of the iliolumbar vein aids visualization of the lower lumbar spine and increases the mobility of the common iliac vein. Ligation or mobilization of the internal iliac vessels and its branches helps decrease blood loss during total and partial sacrectomies.

The radicular artery of Adamkiewicz contributes to the an-terior spinal artery and provides the main blood supply to the lower spinal cord. It usually originates from the left side and accompanies the ventral root of T9, T10, or T11, but can origi-nate anywhere from T5 to L5. The artery of Adamkiewicz usu-ally originates from a segmental artery at the level of the costotransverse joint, and then enters the intervertebral fora-men *(62)*. Ligation of segmental vessels over the midportion of the vertebral body may help minimize risk of injury to the artery of Adamkiewicz. Dissection or electrocautery near the foramen and disarticulation of the costotransverse and costo-vertebral joints can injure the artery or important collateral vessels. Paraplegia resulting from segmental vessel ligation is rare if vessel ligation is unilateral and normotensive anaesthe-sia is utilized *(63)*.

Injury to the aorta, azygos, inferior vena cava, and iliac vessels can also occur during dorsal approaches to the spine. Most injuries occur during the discectomy. Knowledge of the width of the vertebral body and attention to the depth of pen-etration of pituitary rongeurs and curettes within the interver-tebral space should prevent over penetration of instruments *(64)*. Similar precautions help prevent vessel injuries during dorsolateral vertebrectomy procedures. Subperiosteal dissec-tion of the segmental vessels away from the vertebral body followed by gentle dissection and protection of the great ves-sels helps prevent injuries to the aorta, azygous, and inferior vena cava during dorsal *en-bloc* spondylectomy procedures *(29,65,66)*.

Late hemorrhage owing to erosion, leakage, or false aneu-rysm formation of the vessel has been reported. This complica-tion is usually associated with prominent metal implants *(67)*.

7.10. THORACIC DUCT INJURY

The thoracic duct is at risk for injury during ventral approaches to the spine *(68–70)*. The cisterna chyli is the beginning of the thoracic duct and usually lies on the surface of the second lum-bar vertebra between the right crus and the aorta. The thoracic duct remains between the aorta and the azygos vein in the lower thoracic spine and then crosses over to the left side at about T5. The thoracic duct ascends into the neck as high as C6 before it descends to empty near the internal jugular and subclavian vein junction. If damaged, the thoracic duct should be doubly ligated both proximally and distally to prevent chylothorax. A fat-free, high-carbohydrate, high-protein diet combined with aspiration is often effective treatment of chylothorax. Tube thoracostomy drainage, intravenous hyperalimentation, and no oral intake are instituted for persistent leaks. Exploration and thoracic duct ligation may be required if non-operative mea-sures fail.

7.11. THROMBOEMBOLIC DISEASE

The incidence of thromboembolic complications following major spine surgery is probably between 1 and 10 % *(70,72,73)*. Postoperative compression boots and early mobilization prob-ably lowers the incidence of thrombosis and pulmonary embo-lism. The efficacy and safety of prophylactic anticoagulation with aspirin, heparin, low molecular weight heparin, or war-farin is unclear. Therapeutic heparinization for the treatment of non-fatal pulmonary emboli following major spine surgery is associated with a high incidence of complications, including wound hematoma, deep wound infection, upper gastrointesti-nal bleeding, cauda equina syndrome secondary to epidural hematoma, and paraplegia secondary to epidural formation *(74)*. Placement of a vena cava filter is probably associated with lower complication rates than heparinization and should be considered for patients that develop pulmonary emboli after major spinal surgery. The treatment of clinically significant deep venous thrombosis should be individualized from patient to patient.

7.12. INFECTION

Spinal procedures for metastatic disease are associated with higher wound infection rates as compared to procedures for other disease processes *(75)*. Weinstein et al. *(75)* reported the incidence of spinal wound infection in 2391 consecutive index procedures. They noted 20% (4/20) incidence of wound infection in patients with cancer metastatic to the spine compared with 0.86% after discectomy, 1.5% after decompressive laminectomy, 0.4% after fusion without instrumentation, and 3.2% after fusion with instrumentation. Utilization of instrumentation, prolonged operative times, previous operations, neutropenia, history of chronic infections, alcohol abuse, recent hospitalization, and prolonged postoperative wound drainage are associated with an increased incidence of wound infection *(75–77)*. The incidence of wound infection is approx 2.5 times greater with dorsal procedures compared to ventral procedures. The utilization of peri-operative and intra-operative antibiotics decreases the incidence of wound infection *(76)*. Temperature, white blood cell count, C-reactive protein, and erythrocyte sedimentation rate are often elevated in patients with wound infection. Wound erythema, warmth, and tenderness are suggestive of a wound infection. Early cellulitis may be treated with antibiotics, but exploration is indicated for persistent signs of infection. Purulent drainage warrants exploration, irrigation, and debridement. Wound exploration is also considered in patients with persistent wound drainage. The fascia should be opened unless the infection is clearly localized to the superficial layer. A thorough debridement and irrigation is recommended for deep wound infections. Loose bone graft should be removed. Instrumentation should remain unless the infection persists despite proper irrigation and debridement. Wound closure over drains is preferred, but occasionally the wound is left open and delayed primary closure is performed. Broad spectrum antibiotics are initially utilized until final culture and sensitivity results allow narrowing of the antibiotic spectrum. Intravenous antibiotics are usually administered for 6 to 8 wk.

7.13. WOUND COMPLICATIONS

Radiation therapy, chemotherapy, pre-operative embolization, poor nutrition, and immobility contribute to increased wound complications in patients with cancer. Ventral decompressive procedures through a thoracotomy, thoracolumbar, or retroperitoneal approach may decrease the incidence of wound complications *(78,79)* compared to dorsal procedures utilizing a midline dorsal incision.

Patients that received myelosuppressive doses of chemotherapy or pre-operative radiation therapy are predisposed to wound complications *(78,80)*. An absolute neutrophil count less than 1500 cells/mm^3 is associated with higher wound complication rates *(81,82)*. G-CSF effectively increases the absolute neutrophil count in most patients with neutropenia. The incidence of wound complications is higher in patients who received pre-operative radiation therapy within a week of the operation compared to patients that had surgery several weeks after radiation therapy *(78)*.

Minimizing pressure on the wound helps prevent wound complications, especially in patients undergoing simultaneous ventral and dorsal approaches through a T-shaped incision. Maintaining a 90° angle at the intersection of the two arms of the T-shaped incision helps decrease the likelihood of epidermolysis and wound dehiscence. Early mobilization, log rolling, and specialized mattresses diminish pressure and length of time lying on the wound. Local flaps utilizing the latissimus or trapezius muscle may prevent or treat wound complications associated with prominent or exposed hardware *(9,83)*.

7.14. RADIATION-ASSOCIATED COMPLICATIONS

Radiation therapy is an effective adjuvant and treatment modality utilized to treat symptomatic metastatic carcinoma to the spine and to decrease the rate of local recurrence. Radiation therapy before surgical intervention for spinal cord compression is associated with a higher wound complication rate compared to patients that receive radiation therapy after surgical decompression *(78)*. Ventral approaches may have fewer wound complication rates compared to dorsal approaches. However, Bilsky et al. *(9)* reported low wound complication rates (1 out of 20 patients) after dorsolateral decompression and stabilization in patients that received radiation therapy prior to decompression. Judicious use of local flaps and the utilization of low-profile instrumentation may decrease wound complications. If postoperative radiation therapy is planned, a delay of at least 2 wk may decrease the incidence of wound complications.

7.15. COMPLICATIONS ASSOCIATED WITH CORTICOSTEROID UTILIZATION

Corticosteroids are frequently administered to patients with spinal cord compression. High doses of dexamethasone (100 mg iv bolus followed by 24 mg orally or intravenously every 6 h) and moderate doses of dexamethasone (10 mg iv bolus followed by 4 mg orally or intravenously every 6 h) have similar neurological outcomes *(84,84)*. Fewer corticosteroid related complications occur utilizing moderate doses of dexamethasone compared to high doses *(86,87)*. A steroid taper is usually begun after initiation of radiotherapy or after surgery if the patient is neurologically stable. H$_2$-receptor antagonists are administered to prevent steroid-associated stress ulcers *(88,89)*. Neuroleptics are utilized to treat or prevent steroid-associated psychiatric disturbances such as mania, psychosis, and depression *(90)*. Patients receiving prolonged corticosteroid therapy are more susceptible to *Pneumocystis carinii* pneumonia, and are therefore given prophylactic sulfamethoxazole and trimethoprim *(91)*.

7.16. DEFORMITY

Patients with tumors involving the vertebral body have an increased risk of developing a kyphotic deformity (Fig. 5). If non-operative treatment is indicated, the use of a molded thoracolumbar spinal orthosis may prevent collapse of the vertebral body during radiation therapy. A laminectomy alone is reserved for patients with lesions that only involve the dorsal elements. A laminectomy performed in a patient with ventral column involvement increases the likelihood of the development of a pathological fracture of the vertebral body, and a subsequent kyphotic deformity. Stabilization of the ventral

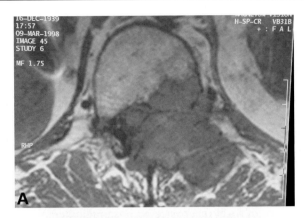

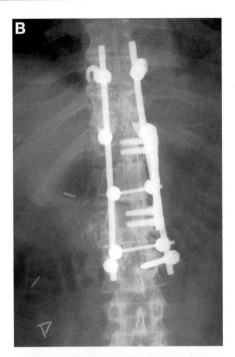

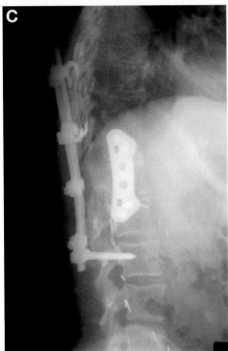

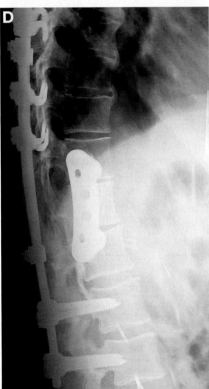

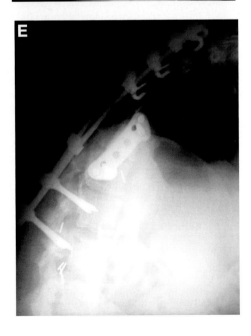

Fig. 5. A 58-yr-old male with a solitary T12 metastatic renal cell carcinoma. T1-weighted axial magnetic resonance imaging (A). Marginal excision via simultaneous anterior thoracolumbar and posterior midline approaches with anterior and posterior instrumentation and posterior spinal fusion from T9–L2 was performed (B,C). He developed a deep wound infection and a left pleural effusion 2 mo later. An irrigation and debridement of the thoracolumbar and posterior midline incision was performed followed by extension of the posterior instrumentation from T8–L3 (D). The infection resolved, but he developed a progressive kyphotic deformity with loss of fixation cephalad and caudal to the T12 laminectomy 23 mo after the previous procedure (E).

column should help prevent the development of a kyphotic deformity. Corpectomy, combined with a vertebral body reconstruction and stabilization, helps maintain sagittal alignment for most patients with a single level metastatic lesion of the spinal column (39–41,48). A single-stage dorsolateral transpedicle corpectomy with vertebral body reconstruction and dorsal spinal stabilization can help prevent postlaminectomy kyphosis in patients with ventral and dorsal element involvement or in patients with multi-level spinal column involvement (9,92,93). Laminectomy with dorsal stabilization is occasionally indicated for patients requiring short-term palliation (27,94,95).

Postlaminectomy and post irradiation kyphosis also occur after treatment of spinal cord tumors and radio-sensitive tumors located near the spinal column. Children with tumors in the cervical spine and cervicothoracic junction are more likely to develop deformity than older patients (96–98). Yasuoka et al. (98) noted that 12 of 26 patients (46%) younger than age 15 developed a postlaminectomy deformity. Eight of these patients required surgical intervention. Patients between 15 and 25 yr of age did not develop postoperative deformities with the exception of two patients (6%). These two patients developed mild deformities that did not progress after maturity and did not require further treatment. Spinal deformity is more likely after unilateral or bilateral facet excision has been performed along with the laminectomy. An acute angular kyphosis is more likely to occur after facetectomies compared to a more gradual rounded kyphosis after laminectomies alone. Irradiation affects the growing cartilage cells in the growth plate of the vertebral bodies and may contribute to the development of spinal deformities. Laminoplasty techniques may decrease the risk of developing a kyphotic deformity by allowing reconstitution of the posterior elements. Expansive open door laminoplasty may be appropriate in some cases. Fusion at the time of the initial decompressive laminectomy may be appropriate in those patients with a high risk for postoperative deformities. Close observation is essential for early recognition of spinal deformities. Regular follow-up visits with lateral radiographs are essential during the first year after the operation and the adolescent growth spurt.

Operative intervention of postlaminectomy and postradiation deformities is usually recommended because bracing is usually ineffective. A ventral or ventral combined with a dorsal spinal fusion are associated with higher fusion rates compared to dorsal fusion alone (64).

7.17. FLUID AND ELECTROLYTE IMBALANCE

Careful fluid and electrolyte balance is needed to prevent pulmonary congestion, dehydration, and cardiac arrhythmia. Patients with diffuse skeletal metastases may develop hypercalcemia with associated complications such as nausea, vomiting, abdominal pain, or cardiac symptoms. Early mobilization, hydration, and utilization of bisphosphonates may prevent or treat hypercalcemia.

7.18. RECURRENCE OF TUMOR

Recurrence of tumor is related to the biology of the primary tumor and the surgical margin achieved during the initial operation. Prevention of local recurrence decreases the likelihood of recurrent spinal cord compression and subsequent revision surgical intervention. Wide excision (27,28) is associated with a lower incidence of local recurrence (<5%) compared to intralesional excision (10–20%) (9,100). A wide excision may be indicated in patients with primary bone tumors of the spinal column, superior sulcus tumors, non-metastatic lung carcinoma with spinal column invasion, and solitary spinal column metastases. Intralesional excisions are indicated for patients with aggressive tumors with multiple bone or visceral organ involvement. These procedures usually provide adequate intermediate or short-term local tumor control (27). Removal of all visible tumor and the posterior longitudinal ligament provides an immediate partial response, and probably decreases the incidence of local recurrence because radiotherapy is more effective against microscopic disease.

8. CONCLUSION

Attention to the details of obtaining the correct diagnosis, pre-operative planning, meticulous surgery, and postoperative care can minimize the incidence of complications. Prompt and judicious treatment of complications should decrease the long-term morbidity.

REFERENCES

1. Rougraff BT, Kneisl JS, Simon MA. Skeletal metastases of unknown origin. A prospective study of a diagnostic strategy. J Bone Joint Surg Am 1993; 75:1276–1281.
2. Simon MA, Finn HA. Diagnostic strategy for bone and soft-tissue tumors. J Bone Joint Surg Am 1993; 75:622–631.
3. Simeon FA, Lawner PM. Intraspinal neoplasms. In: Rothman RH, Simeon FA, eds. The Spine. Philadelphia, PA: W.B. Saunders; 1982:1041–1054.
4. Gruszkiewicz J, Doron Y, Borovich B, Zaaroor M. Spinal cord compression in Paget's disease of bone with reference to sarcomatous degeneration and calcitonin treatment. Surg Neurol 1987; 27:117–125.
5. Eismont FJ, Green BA, Brown MD, Ghandur-Mnaymneh L. Coexistent infection and tumor of the spine. A report of three cases. J Bone Joint Surg Am 1987; 69:452–458.
6. Benassi MS, Ragazzini P, Gamberi G, et al. Adhesion molecules in high-grade soft tissue sarcomas: correlation to clinical outcome. Eur J Cancer 1998; 34:496–502.
7. An HS, Vaccaro AR, Dolinskas CA, Cotler JM, Balderston RA, Bauerle WB. Differentiation between spinal tumors and infections with magnetic resonance imaging. Spine 1991; 16:S334–S338.
8. An HS, Andreshak TG, Nguyen C, Williams A, Daniels D. Can we distinguish between benign versus malignant compression fractures of the spine by magnetic resonance imaging? Spine 1995; 20:1776–1782.
9. Bilsky MH, Boland P, Lis E, Raizer JJ, Healey JH. Single-stage posterolateral transpedicle approach for spondylectomy, epidural decompression, and circumferential fusion of spinal metastases. Spine 2000; 25:2240–2249.
10. Graham JJ, Yang WC. Vertebral hemangioma with compression fracture and paraparesis treated with preoperative embolization and vertebral resection. Spine 1984; 9:97–101.
11. Hekster RE, Luyendijk W, Tan TI. Spinal-cord compression caused by vertebral haemangioma relieved by percutaneous catheter embolisation. Neuroradiology 1972; 3:160–164.
12. Roscoe MW, McBroom RJ, St Louis E, Grossman H, Perrin R. Preoperative embolization in the treatment of osseous metastases from renal cell carcinoma. Clin Orthop Relat Res 1989; 238:302–307.
13. Simon MA, Biermann JS. Biopsy of bone and soft-tissue lesions. J Bone Joint Surg Am 1993; 75:616–621.
14. Ayala AG, Raymond AK, Ro JY, Carrasco CH, Fanning CV, Murray JA. Needle biopsy of primary bone lesions. M.D. Anderson experience. Pathol Annu 1989; 24:219–251.

15. Mick CA, Zinreich J. Percutaneous trephine bone biopsy of the thoracic spine. Spine 1985; 10:737–740.

16. Alexander AH. Chymopapain chemonucleolysis, discography, and needle biopsy technique. In: Chapman MW, ed. Operative Orthopaedics. Philadelphia, PA: J.B. Lippincott; 1988:2125–2135.

17. Bender CE, Berquist TH, Wold LE. Imaging-assisted percutaneous biopsy of the thoracic spine. Mayo Clin Proc 1986; 61:942–950.

18. Fyfe IS, Henry AP, Mulholland RC. Closed vertebral biopsy. J Bone Joint Surg Br 1983; 65:140–143.

19. Laredo JD, Bard M. Thoracic spine: percutaneous trephine biopsy. Radiology 1986; 160:485–489.

20. Ottolenghi CE, Shajowicz F, DeSchant FA. Aspiration biopsy of the cervical spine. Techniques and results in twenty-four cases. J Bone Joint Surg Am 1964; 46A:715–733.

21. Ambrose GB, Alpert M, Neer CS. Vertebral osteomyelitis. A diagnostic problem. JAMA 1966; 197:619–622.

22. Armstrong P, Chalmers AH, Green G, Irving JD. Needle aspiration/biopsy of the spine in suspected disc infection. Br J Radiol 1978; 51:333–337.

23. Debnam JW, Staple TW. Needle biopsy of bone. Radiol Clin North Am 1975; 13:157–164.

24. Gladstein MO, Grantham SA. Closed skeletal biopsy. Clin Orthop Relat Res 1974; 0:75–79.

25. McLaughlin RE, Miller WR, Miller CW. Quadriparesis after needle aspiration of the cervical spine. Report of a case. J Bone Joint Surg Am 1976; 58:1167–1168.

26. McLain RF. Spinal cord decompression: an endoscopically assisted approach metastatic tumors. Spinal Cord 2001; 39:482–487.

27. Tomita K, Kawahara N, Kobayashi T, Yoshida A, Murakami H, Akamaru T. Surgical strategy for spinal metastases. Spine 2001; 26:298–306.

28. Boriani S, Biagini R, De Iure F, et al. En bloc resections of bone tumors of the thoracolumbar spine. A preliminary report on 29 patients. Spine 1996; 21:1927–1931.

29. Tomita K, Kawahara N, Baba H, Tsuchiya H, Fujita T, Toribatake Y. Total en bloc spondylectomy. A new surgical technique for primary malignant vertebral tumors. Spine 1997; 22:324–333.

30. Mankin HJ, Lange TA, Spanier SS. The hazards of biopsy in patients with malignant primary bone and soft-tissue tumors. J Bone Joint Surg Am 1982; 64:1121–1127.

31. Mankin HJ, Mankin CJ, Simon MA. The hazards of the biopsy, revisited. Members of the Musculoskeletal Tumor Society. J Bone Joint Surg Am 1996; 78:656–663.

32. Ebraheim NA, Inzerillo C, Xu R. Are anatomic landmarks reliable in determination of fusion level in posterolateral lumbar fusion? Spine 1999; 24:973–974.

33. Flynn TB. Neurologic complications of anterior cervical interbody fusion. Spine 1982; 7:536–539.

34. Cain JE Jr, Dryer RF, Barton BR. Evaluation of dural closure techniques. Suture methods, fibrin adhesive sealant, and cyanoacrylate polymer. Spine 1988; 13:720–725.

35. Eismont FJ, Wiesel SW, Rothman RH. Treatment of dural tears associated with spinal surgery. J Bone Joint Surg Am 1981; 63:1132–1136.

36. Wang JC, Bohlman HH, Riew KD. Dural tears secondary to operations on the lumbar spine. Management and results after a two-year-minimum follow-up of eighty-eight patients. J Bone Joint Surg Am 1998; 80:1728–1732.

37. Heller JG, Kim HS, Carlson GW. Subarachnoid—pleural fistulae—management with a transdiaphragmatic pedicled greater omental flap: report of two cases. Spine 2001; 26:1809–1813.

38. Yerby SA, Ehteshami J. R.; and McLain, R. F.: Offset laminar hooks decrease bending moments of pedicle screws during in situ contouring. Spine, 22(4): 376-81, 1997.

39. Boland PJ, Lane JM, Sundaresan N. Metastatic disease of the spine. Clin Orthop Relat Res 1982; 169:95–102.

40. Gokaslan ZL, York JE, Walsh GL, et al. Transthoracic vertebrectomy for metastatic spinal tumors. J Neurosurg 1998; 89:599–609.

41. Harrington KD. The use of methylmethacrylate for vertebral-body replacement and anterior stabilization of pathological fracture-dis-

locations of the spine due to metastatic malignant disease. J Bone Joint Surg Am 1981; 63:36–46.

42. McAfee PC, Bohlman HH, Ducker T, Eismont FJ. Failure of stabilization of the spine with methylmethacrylate. A retrospective analysis of twenty-four cases. J Bone Joint Surg Am 1986; 68:1145–1157.

43. Talmi YP, Knoller N, Dolev M, et al. Postsurgical prevertebral abscess of the cervical spine. Laryngoscope 2000; 110:1137–1141.

44. Cleveland RH, Gilsanz V, Lebowitz RL, Wilkinson RH. Hydronephrosis from retroperitoneal fibrosis after anterior spine fusion. A case report. J Bone Joint Surg Am 1978; 60:996–997.

45. Isiklar ZU, Lindsey RW, Coburn M. Ureteral injury after anterior lumbar interbody fusion. A case report. Spine 1996; 21:2379–2382.

46. Johnson RM, McGuire EJ. Urogenital complications of anterior approaches to the lumbar spine. Clin Orthop 1981; 81:114–8.

47. Nygaard IE, Kreder KJ. Spine update. Urological management in patients with spinal cord injuries. Spine 1996; 21:128–132.

48. Silber I, McMaster W. Retroperitoneal fibrosis with hydronephrosis as a complication of the Dwyer procedure. J Pediatr Surg 1977; 12:255–257.

49. Shen YS, Cheung CY, Nilsen PT. Chylous leakage after arthrodesis using the anterior approach to the spine. Report of two cases. J Bone Joint Surg Am 1989; 71:1250–1251.

50. U, HS, Wilson CB. Postoperative epidural hematoma as a complication of anterior cervical discectomy. Report of three cases. J Neurosurg 1978; 49:288–291.

51. Epstein NE, Hollingsworth R, Nardi D, Singer J. Can airway complications following multilevel anterior cervical surgery be avoided? J Neurosurg 2001; 94:185–188.

52. Bulger RF, Rejowski JE, Beatty RA. Vocal cord paralysis associated with anterior cervical fusion: considerations for prevention and treatment. J Neurosurg 1986; 62:657–661.

53. Heeneman H. Vocal cord paralysis following approaches to the anterior cervical spine. Laryngoscope 1973; 83:17–21.

54. Heary RF, Albert TJ, Ludwig SC, et al. Surgical anatomy of the vertebral arteries. Spine 1996; 21:2074–2080.

55. Smith MD, Emery SE, Dudley A, Murray KJ, Leventhal M. Vertebral artery injury during anterior decompression of the cervical spine. A retrospective review of ten patients. J Bone Joint Surg Br 1993; 75:410–415.

56. Ebraheim NA, An HS, Xu R, Ahmad M, Yeasting RA. The quantitative anatomy of the cervical nerve root groove and the intervertebral foramen. Spine 1996; 21:1619–1623.

57. An HS, Gordin R, Renner K. Anatomic considerations for plate-screw fixation of the cervical spine. Spine 1991; 16:S548–S551.

58. Ebraheim NA, Xu R, Ahmad M, Heck B. The quantitative anatomy of the vertebral artery groove of the atlas and its relation to the posterior atlantoaxial approach. Spine 1998; 23:320–333.

59. An HS, Vaccaro A, Cotler JM, Lin S. Spinal disorders at the cervicothoracic junction. Spine 1994; 19:2557–2564.

60. Sundaresan N, Shah J, Foley KM, Rosen G. An anterior surgical approach to the upper thoracic vertebrae. J Neurosurg 1984; 61:686–690.

61. Baker JK, Reardon PR, Reardon MJ, Heggeness MH. Vascular injury in anterior lumbar surgery. Spine 1993; 18:2227–2230.

62. Lu J, Ebraheim NA, Biyani A, Brown JA, Yeasting RA. Vulnerability of great medullary artery. Spine 1996; 21:1852–1855.

63. Wise JJ, Fischgrund JS, Herkowitz HN, Montgomery D, Kurz LT. Complication, survival rates, and risk factors of surgery for metastatic disease of the spine. Spine 1999; 24:1943–1951.

64. Harbison SP. Major vascular complications of intervertebral disc surgery. Ann Surg 1954; 140:342–348.

65. Kawahara N, Tomita K, Baba H, et al. Cadaveric vascular anatomy for total en bloc spondylectomy in malignant vertebral tumors. Spine 1996; 21:1401–1407.

66. Stener B. Complete removal of vertebrae for extirpation of tumors. A 20-year experience. Clin Orthop Relat Res 1989; 245:72–82.

67. Dwyer AP. A fatal complication of paravertebral infection and traumatic aneurysm following Dwyer instrumentation. J Bone Joint Surg 1979; 61B:239.

68. Colletta AJ, Mayer PJ. Chylothorax: an unusual complication of anterior thoracic interbody spinal fusion. Spine 1982; 7:46–49.

69. Eisenstein S, O'Brien JP. Chylothorax: a complication of Dwyer's anterior instrumentation. Br J Surg 1977; 64:339–341.

70. Shen YS, Cheung CY, Nilsen PT. Chylous leakage after arthrodesis using the anterior approach to the spine. Report of two cases. J Bone Joint Surg Am 1989; 71:1250–1251.

71. Catre MG. Anticoagulation in spinal surgery. A critical review of the literature. Can J Surg 1997; 40:413–419.

72. Dearborn JT, Hu SS, Tribus CB, Bradford DS. Thromboembolic complications after major thoracolumbar spine surgery. Spine 1999; 24:1471–1476.

73. Lee HM, Suk KS, Moon SH, Kim DJ, Wang JM, Kim NH. Deep vein thrombosis after major spinal surgery: incidence in an East Asian population. Spine 2000; 25:1827–1830.

74. Cain JE, Major MR, Lauerman WC, West JL, Wood KB, Fueredi GA. The morbidity of heparin therapy after development of pulmonary embolus in patients undergoing thoracolumbar or lumbar spinal fusion. Spine 1995; 20:1600–1603.

75. Weinstein MA, McCabe JP, Cammisa FP Jr. Postoperative spinal wound infection: a review of 2,391 consecutive index procedures. J Spinal Disord 2000; 13:422–426.

76. Klekamp J, Spengler DM, McNamara MJ, Haas DW. Risk factors associated with methicillin-resistant staphylococcal wound infection after spinal surgery. J Spinal Disord 1999; 12:187–191.

77. Lonstein J, Winter R, Moe J, Gaines D. Wound infection with Harrington instrumentation and spine fusion for scoliosis. Clin Orthop Relat Res 1973; 96:222–233.

78. Ghogawala Z, Mansfield FL, Borges LF. Spinal radiation before surgical decompression adversely affects outcomes of surgery for symptomatic metastatic spinal cord compression. Spine 2001; 26:818–824.

79. McPhee IB, Williams RP, Swanson CE. Factors influencing wound healing after surgery for metastatic disease of the spine. Spine 1998: 23:726–732.

80. Pascal-Moussellard H, Broc G, Pointillart V, Simeon F, Vital JM, Senegas J. Complications of vertebral metastasis surgery. Eur Spine J 1998; 7:438–444.

81. Dick J, Boachie-Adjei O, Wilson M. One-stage versus two-stage anterior and posterior spinal reconstruction in adults. Comparison of outcomes including nutritional status, complications rates, hospital costs, and other factors. Spine 1992; 17:S310–S316.

82. Seltzer MH, Bastidas JA, Cooper DM, Engler P, Slocum B, Fletcher HS. Instant nutritional assessment. JPEN J Parenter Enteral Nutr 1979; 3:157–159.

83. Hochberg J, Ardenghy M, Yuen J, et al. Muscle and musculocutaneous flap coverage of exposed spinal fusion devices. Plast Reconstr Surg 1998; 102:385–389.

84. Sorensen S, Helweg-Larsen S, Mouridsen H, Hansen HH. Effect of high-dose dexamethasone in carcinomatous metastatic spinal cord compression treated with radiotherapy: a randomised trial. Eur J Cancer 1994; 30A: 22–27.

85. Vecht CJ, Haaxma-Reiche H, van Putten WL, de Visser M, Vries EP, Twijnstra A. Initial bolus of conventional versus high-dose dexamethasone in metastatic spinal cord compression. Neurology 1989; 39:1255–1257.

86. Delattre JY, Arbit E, Rosenblum MK, et al. High dose versus low dose dexamethasone in experimental epidural spinal cord compression. Neurosurgery 1988;22:1005–1007.

87. Heimdal K, Hirschberg H, Slettebo H, Watne K, Nome O. High incidence of serious side effects of high-dose dexamethasone treatment in patients with epidural spinal cord compression. J Neurooncol 1992; 12:141–144.

88. DePriest JL. Stress ulcer prophylaxis. Do critically ill patients need it?. Postgrad Med 1995; 98:159–161.

89. Ellershaw JE, Kelly MJ. Corticosteroids and peptic ulceration. Palliat Med 1994; 8:313–319.

90. Goggans FC, Weisberg LJ, Koran LM. Lithium prophylaxis of prednisone psychosis: a case report. J Clin Psychol 1983; 44:111–112.

91. Slivka A, Wen PY, Shea WM, Loeffler JS. Pneumocystis carinii pneumonia during steroid taper in patients with primary brain tumors. Am J Med 1993; 94:216–219.

92. Akeyson EW, McCutcheon IE. Single-stage posterior vertebrectomy and replacement combined with posterior instrumentation for spinal metastasis. J Neurosurg 1996; 85:211–220.

93. Magerl F, Coscia MF. Total posterior vertebrectomy of the thoracic or lumbar spine. Clin Orthop Relat Res 1988; 232:62–69.

94. Bauer HC. Posterior decompression and stabilization for spinal metastases. Analysis of sixty-seven consecutive patients. J Bone Joint Surg Am 1997; 79:514–522.

95. Siegal T, Tiqva P. Vertebral body resection for epidural compression by malignant tumors. Results of forty-seven consecutive operative procedures. J Bone Joint Surg Am 1985; 67:375–3825.

96. Fraser RD, Paterson DC, Simpson DA.:Orthopaedic aspects of spinal tumors in children. J Bone Joint Surg Br 1977; 59:143–151.

97. Otsuka NY, Hey L, Hall JE. Postlaminectomy and postirradiation kyphosis in children and adolescents. Clin Orthop Relat Res 1998; 354:189–194.

98. Yasuoka S, Peterson HA, MacCarty CS. Incidence of spinal column deformity after multilevel laminectomy in children and adults. J Neurosurg 1982; 57:441–445.

39 Bracing for Patients With Spinal Tumors

Kai-Uwe Lewandrowski, md, Robert F. McLain, md, and Edward C. Benzel, md

Contents

1. ROLE OF BRACING

The literature regarding the use of braces in patients with spinal tumors is sparse. In fact, most references on spinal bracing relate to (1) idiopathic adolescent scoliosis *(1–6)*, (2) osteoporotic compression fractures *(7–10)*, and (3) thoracolumbar spine fractures *(11–14)*. The role of bracing is much less well defined for the operative and non-operative treatment of spinal tumors. However, they are commonly used in the immediate postoperative period after tumor resection and surgical stabilization to protect both the patient and the integrity of the spinal construct. Although long-term bracing may be successfully used as the sole way of treating spinal instability resulting from tumor, the role of long-term bracing for patients with spinal tumors appears limited. In this setting, with or without the additional use of neoadjuvant chemo- and radiation therapy, biological capacity to achieve spinal fusion may be limited or absent. High pseudoarthrosis rates should, therefore, be expected. If life expectancy is limited to less than 6 mo, braces are frequently applied in one form or another for the purpose of palliation, particularly if surgical treatment is not contemplated or feasible, but spinal instability is of concern. In the latter scenario, braces are used as an adjunct to other forms of palliative care, including chemo- and radiation therapy.

Braces provide an additional form of external support to a segment of the spine that is compromised by tumor. The goals of spinal bracing include (1) restriction of motion, (2) realignment of the spine, and (3) trunk support *(15)*. However, the use of braces is not without controversy. There remain concerns, for instance, regarding the efficacy of bracing *(16–20)*. These concerns are primarily based on the fact that the efficacy of spinal braces is susceptible to the thickness of the soft tissue overlying the spine. In fact, there is an inverse relationship to the thickness of the soft tissues covering the spine (under the inner surface of the brace) and its effectiveness *(15)*. The aforementioned is related to the length-to-width ratio of the brace. Longer braces provide more efficient spinal stabilization than shorter ones.

When using external splinting techniques, such as spinal braces, it is important to understand the mechanisms by which they function. It is, therefore, prudent for the spine surgeon to realistically understand the principles of bracing.

2. BIOMECHANICAL PRINCIPLES OF BRACING

Braces can be divided into cylindrical body shell braces (Fig. 1), and open braces, such as the Jewett brace (Fig. 2). Open braces apply three-point bending forces to the torso. Both concepts have advantages and disadvantages. Although cylindrical body shell braces are capable of providing significant trunk support by increasing the stability of the ventral and dorsal spinal elements *(15,21)*, three-point bending braces are possibly better at providing correction and control of sagittal plane spinal deformity (Fig. 3). On the other hand, the latter type of brace lends very little control of lateral bending and rotation. In comparison, the cylindrical shell body brace, such as a thoracolumbosacral orthosis (TLSO), is susceptible to poor fit. The latter factor is very important because its ultimate efficacy depends on conformation to the torso. A poor fit between the halves of a brace allows parallelogram deformation of the brace (Fig. 4) *(15)*. This sliding of one-half past the other can be minimized by the rigid attachment of the torso halves to each other.

2.1. BRACING OF THE CERVICAL SPINE

The cervical spine is perhaps the single region of the spine that is most suitable for bracing. This is because of the relatively thin soft tissue mass that separates the spine from the

From: *Current Clinical Oncology: Cancer in the Spine: Comprehensive Care.*
Edited by: R. F. McLain, K-U. Lewandrowski, M. Markman, R. M. Bukowski,
R. Macklis, and E. C. Benzel © Humana Press, Inc., Totowa, NJ

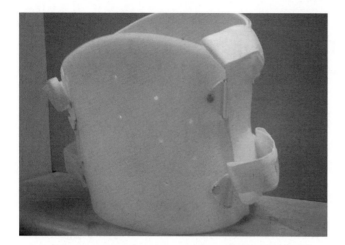

Fig. 1. Shell whole body thoracolumbar orthosis.

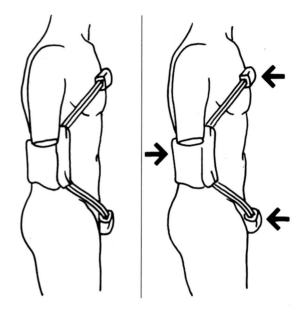

Fig. 3. Three-point bending forces applied by the Jewett brace (arrows) with minimized body contact. (Reproduced with permission from ref *15*.)

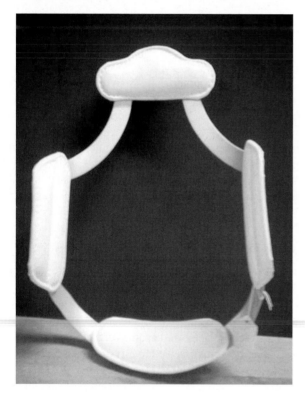

Fig. 2. Jewett three-point bending brace.

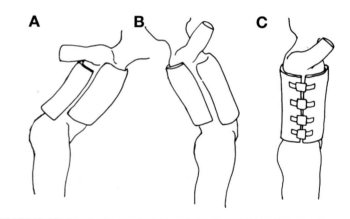

Fig. 4. The disadvantage of a poorly fitted brace, in which the ventral and dorsal halves are allowed to slide past each other, is depicted. In this case, flexion (**A**) and extension (**B**) are not significantly restricted because of this phenomenon. The elimination of this sliding motion, and accompanying tight security between the halves (causing the brace to function as a single solid unit), minimize this problem (**C**). (Reproduced with permission from ref *15*.)

brace. In addition, effective points of "fixation" such as the cranium rostrally and the thoracic cage caudally, are available. However, problems with control of lateral bending and rotation have been identified (*17,22–24*). The parallelogram effect is particularly relevant in the cervical spine because of its significant mobility, particularly at the occipitocervical junction. Attempts have been made to minimize this affect by using additional fixation points, such as the mandible. However, subsequent investigations have shown that these types of devices actually worsen the parallelogram effect by applying exaggerated forces to the brace with the mandible acting as an extended moment arm (*25*). If true immobilization of the upper cervical

spine is required, motion in the mid to lower cervical spine can be limited by utilizing thoracic fixation points (Fig. 5) (*15*).

This addresses the fact that all other forms of limited cervical bracing, such as most forms of soft collars, do not substantially restrict cervical movement. Therefore, they should essentially be regarded as comfort measures. Cervical braces with mandible and/or shoulder extensions (Philadelphia collar) provide a slight improvement over limited motion collars regarding their stabilization effect. Nevertheless, the parallelogram effect remains a significant concern (*15*). This is illustrated by the fact that true cervical flexion-extension move-

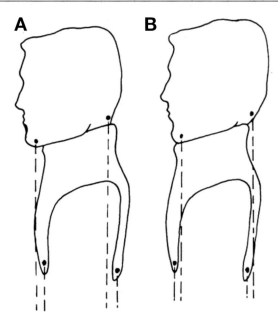

Fig. 5. The parallelogram-like bracing effect depicted here can be significantly diminished by the minimization of movement in the low cervical and cervicothoracic regions, via a three-point bending mechanism. This significantly restricts true neck flexion-extension (**A,B**). (Reproduced with permission from ref. *15*.)

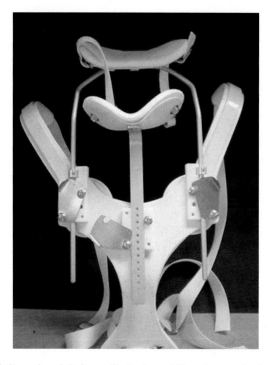

Fig. 6. Sternal occipital mandibular immobilizer three-point bending brace for immobilization across the cervicothoracic junction.

ments are essentially unimpeded by most forms of shoulder mounted cervical braces *(25,26)*.

2.2. CRANIAL-CERVICO-THORACIC IMMOBILIZATION TECHNIQUES

Traditionally, the halo has been regarded as the "gold standard" for the bracing of cervical lesions *(15)*. It has been gradually replaced with Minerva type devices because the use of the halo is associated with a number of problems. These are not limited to pin site infections and lack of efficacy *(16,27,28)*. There exists an increased morbidity and mortality related to prolonged halo use, particularly in the elderly *(29–31)*. Newer Minerva type devices minimize the parallelogram effect, resulting in an overall reduction of extension-flexion between the head and thorax. However, there still exists significant motion at each individual motion segment. This has been referred to as snaking *(15)*. The sum of these segmental motions can be quite substantial *(22)*. In fact, this effect can be exaggerated by the rigid fixation of the head by the halo. Because segmental instability, rather than global instability, is of concern in most spine tumor patients, snaking should be kept in mind when treating cervical lesions with a halo-type device. When comparing the halo and Minerva devices, it becomes apparent that Minerva type devices are better at controlling subaxial cervical spine motion and sagittal balance. In comparison, the halo is much better at controlling capital extension and flexion.

2.3. CERVICOTHORACIC BRACING

Lesions of the lower cervical and upper thoracic spine require inclusion of the thoracic spine by the brace to provide stability across the cervicothoracic junction. A commonly utilized device for this purpose is the sternal occipital mandibular immobilizer (SOMI) (Fig. 6) or four-poster brace. The halo

may be applicable to the lower subaxial and upper thoracic spine as well, because increased efficacy has been shown to become manifest as one descends into the more caudal regions of the spinal column *(32)*.

2.4. THORACIC AND LUMBAR SPINE BRACING

Although bracing in the thoracic spine is relatively straightforward, it is much less so in the lumbar and lumbosacral spine. Fixation for bracing in the thoracic spine can be achieved via the axial segments above and below the pathology. Although actual restriction of motion data are lacking, bracing in this area is generally successful. This can be inferred from the clinical data regarding the successful non-operative management of thoracolumbar fractures *(7–9)* and adolescent idiopathic scoliosis *(1–3)*.

In the lumbar spine, fixation to at least four to five vertebral levels above and below the segment of instability are required to achieve stability *(15)*. Stabilization of more caudal lumbopelvic levels is more difficult because of the short distance between the unstable segment and the pelvis. Hip flexion aggravates this problem further and makes adequate immobilization, even with application thigh-extensions (Fig. 7), nearly impossible *(19)*. In addition, lumbosacral orthoses with thigh extension are poorly tolerated. This raises concerns of the overall efficacy of these types of braces, which have been suggested to be effective by "irritating and reminding the patient to restrict motion" at the lumbosacral junction *(33)*. Although motion restriction data on bracing in the lumbosacral spine is scarce, the efficacy of the bracing is suggested by the fact that uninstrumented lumbar fusions have been shown to be associated with higher fusion rates when braced for 5 mo, as opposed to 3 mo postoperatively *(34)*.

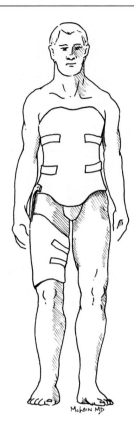

Fig. 7. Thoracolumbosacral orthosis with thigh extension.

3. THE CHOICES

Bracing is often used as an adjunct to rehabilitation in post-surgical patients following tumor resection. The ultimate goal of spinal bracing after the surgical stabilization of metastatic lesions is to protect the spinal elements during radio- and chemotherapy and after decompression surgery and to reduce pain for the patients in the immediate postsurgical convalescence period. In general, recommendations for spinal bracing depend on the location of the lesion *(35)*. However, it is well known that most spinal metastases are located in the anterior column. Hence, this has to be taken into consideration when choosing the size, type, and rigidity of the brace. Naturally, more rigid braces should be chosen in cases of significant bony destruction.

For lesions in the cervical spine, cervical collars, such as the Philadelphia collar, the four-poster brace, the Yale orthosis, the SOMI brace, the thermoplastic Minerva body jacket, and the halo can be used for immobilization of the spine (Table 1) *(35)*. As described above, the Philadelphia collar limits flexion/extension somewhat, but does little to restrict lateral bending and rotation. Instead, it is frequently a source of pain *(35)*. As a modification of the Philadelphia collar, the Yale collar is more rigid and is capable of limiting flexion/extension more efficiently than the Philadelphia collar. The SOMI brace should be used for stable fractures and after fusion. It is particularly useful when weaning a patient from the halo.

In the thoracic and lumbar spine, a TLSO, such as the Knight-Taylor, a molded TLSO, or a Jewett brace may be used *(35)*. Although most TLSO braces are three-point bending devices,

the Williams brace is somewhat different, because it holds the lumbar spine in flexion, thereby providing some lateral bending control *(36)*. If more significant limitation of motion is desired, the molded TLSO is the brace of choice as it provides near total contact. If lesions are present in the upper thoracic spine (T1–T6), a cervical extension should be added to the TLSO brace *(35)*. In the case of stable compression fractures owing to metastatic lesions, a Jewett extension type brace can be used. However, such a brace is unsuitable for unstable factures, which should not be maintained in extension *(35)*.

4. COMPLICATIONS

The use of spinal braces may be associated with a number of problems. These include "…(1) pain, (2) pressure, (3) psychological dependence, (4) poor hygiene, (5) axial muscle weakness and disuse atrophy, (6) restriction of activity, (7) aggravation of spinal symptoms, (8) vascular (venous) compromise, and (9) ineffective stabilization" *(15)*. Halo bracing may present with additional complications, such as pin site infections, cosmetic problems, osteomyelitis, brain abscess, and other soft tissue and wound-healing problems *(15)*. Another severe, but fortunately very rare complication, can be observed as a result of exceptionally tight spinal bracing, the body cast syndrome. This syndrome may be caused by duodenal obstruction. If unrecognized, acute gastric dilatation with vomiting may ensue, thus, setting the stage for aspiration, airway compromise, cardiac arrest, or gastric perforation and peritonitis *(15)*. Removal of the brace and other symptomatic therapy may be urgently required *(37)*. The rarity of this syndrome is owing to the rarity of extremely tight applications of lumbar braces, and to the infrequent use of casts that are not removed or loosened.

5. SUMMARY

Spinal orthoses should be used as an adjunct to surgical, and other non-operative treatments of palliation. Their role in patients with spinal tumors is to protect the spinal elements during the immediate postoperative period, or during periods of palliative chemo- and radiation therapy. They stabilize the spine and prevent deformity by providing trunk support.

Clear goals of spinal bracing should be established regardless of whether operative, or non-operative treatment is chosen. Long-term bracing may neither be efficacious, nor advantageous for the patient, particularly if live expectancy is longer than 6 mo. It should be noted that the different types of spinal orthoses are not equally efficacious in immobilizing the spine. In fact, segmental instability may be worsened by phenomena, such as the snaking and the parallelogram effects. Therefore, spinal braces should be used judiciously to avoid complications. More importantly, they "should be employed only as long as they offer a therapeutic advantage" *(15)*.

REFERENCES

1. Castro FP, Jr. Adolescent idiopathic scoliosis, bracing, and the Hueter-Volkmann principle. Spine J 2003; 3:180–185.
2. Climent JM, Sanchez J. Impact of the type of brace on the quality of life of Adolescents with Spine Deformities. Spine 1999; 24:1903–1908.
3. Korovessis P, Kyrkos C, Piperos G, Soucacos PN. Effects of thoracolumbosacral orthosis on spinal deformities, trunk asymme-

TABLE 1
Choice of Bracing for Stable and Unstable Spinal Lesions

Location of lesion	Stable lesion	Unstable lesion
Occipital–cervical junction		Four-poster brace TMBJ
		Halo
Cervical spine	Philadelphia Collar	TMBJ
	Aspen Collar	Yale orthosis
	SOMI brace	Halo
Cervicothoracic junction	Cervical braces with thoracic extensions	
Thoracic spine	Jewett brace	TLSO
Thoracolumbar spine	Jewett brace	Custom-molded TLSO
	TLSO	
Lumbar spine	LSO	
Lumbosacral junction	LSO with thigh extensions	

TMBJ, thermoplastic Minerva body jacket; SOMI, sternal occipital mandibular immobilizer; TLSO, thoracolumbosacral orthosis; LSO, lumbosacral orthosis.

try, and frontal lower rib cage in adolescent idiopathic scoliosis. Spine 2000; 25:2064–2071.

4. Noonan KJ, Weinstein SL, Jacobson WC, Dolan LA. Use of the Milwaukee brace for progressive idiopathic scoliosis. J Bone Joint Surg.Am 1996; 78:557–567.

5. Rigo M, Reiter C, Weiss HR. Effect of conservative management on the prevalence of surgery in patients with adolescent idiopathic scoliosis. PediatrRehabil 2003; 6:209–214.

6. Skaggs DL, Bassett GS. Adolescent idiopathic scoliosis: an update. AmFamPhysician 1996; 53:2327–2335.

7. Benzel EC, Larson SJ. Postoperative stabilization of the posttraumatic thoracic and lumbar spine: a review of concepts and orthotic techniques. JSpinal Disord 1989; 2:47–51.

8. Cantor JB, Lebwohl NH, Garvey T, Eismont FJ. Nonoperative management of stable thoracolumbar burst fractures with early ambulation and bracing. Spine 1993; 18:971–976.

9. Chow GH, Nelson BJ, Gebhard JS, Brugman JL, Brown CW, Donaldson DH. Functional outcome of thoracolumbar burst fractures managed with hyperextension casting or bracing and early mobilization. Spine 1996; 21:2170–2175.

10. Melchiorre PJ. Acute hospitalization and discharge outcome of neurologically intact trauma patients sustaining thoracolumbar vertebral fractures managed conservatively with thoracolumbosacral orthoses and physical therapy. Arch Phys Med Rehabil 1999; 80:221–224.

11. Bajaj S, Saag KG. Osteoporosis: evaluation and treatment. CurrWomens Health Rep 2003; 3:418–424.

12. Lin JT, Lane JM. Nonmedical management of osteoporosis. Curr Opin Rheumatol 2002; 14:441–446.

13. Lukert BP. Vertebral compression fractures: how to manage pain, avoid disability. Geriatrics 1994; 49:22–26.

14. Schroeder S, Rossler H, Ziehe P, Higuchi F. Bracing and supporting of the lumbar spine. Prosthet Orthot Int 1982; 6:139–146.

15. Benzel EC. Spinal bracing. In: Benzel EC, ed. Biomechanics of the Spine. 2nd ed. Stuttgart: Thieme; 2001:331–341.

16. Anderson PA, Budorick TE, Easton KB, Henley MB, Salciccioli GG. Failure of halo vest to prevent in vivo motion in patients with injured cervical spines. Spine 1991; 16:S501–S505.

17. Askins V, Eismont FJ. Efficacy of five cervical orthoses in restricting cervical motion. A comparison study. Spine 1997; 22:1193–1198.

18. Axelsson P, Johnsson R, Stromqvist B. Effect of lumbar orthosis on intervertebral mobility. A roentgen stereophotogrammetric analysis. Spine 1992; 17:678–681.

19. Axelsson P, Johnsson R, Stromqvist B. Lumbar orthosis with unilateral hip immobilization. Effect on intervertebral mobility determined by roentgen stereophotogrammetric analysis. Spine 1993; 18:876–879.

20. Benzel EC, Larson SJ, Kerk JJ, et al. The thermoplastic Minerva body jacket: a clinical comparison with other cervical spine splinting techniques. JSpinal Disord 1992; 5:311–319.

21. Morris JM, Lucas DB. Biomechanics of Spinal Bracing. ArizMed 1964; 21:170–176.

22. Benzel EC, Hadden TA, Saulsbery CM. A comparison of the Minerva and halo jackets for stabilization of the cervical spine. J Neurosurg 1989; 70:411–414.

23. Hart DL, Johnson RM, Simmons EF, Owen J. Review of cervical orthoses. Phys Ther 1978; 58:857–860.

24. Hartman JT, Palumbo F, Hill BJ. Cineradiography of the braced normal cervical spine. A comparative study of five commonly used cervical orthoses. Clin Orthop 1975; 97–102.

25. Johnson RM, Owen JR, Hart DL, Callahan RA. Cervical orthoses: a guide to their selection and use. Clin Orthop 1981; 34–45.

26. Kauppi M, Neva MH, Kautiainen H. Headmaster collar restricts rheumatoid atlantoaxial subluxation. Spine 1999; 24:526–528.

27. Tomonaga T, Krag MH, Novotny JE. Clinical, radiographic, and kinematic results from an adjustable four-pad halovest. Spine 1997; 22:1199–1208.

28. Whitehill R, Richman JA, Glaser JA. Failure of immobilization of the cervical spine by the halo vest. A report of five cases. J Bone Joint Surg Am 1986; 68:326–332.

29. Bucholz RD, Cheung KC. Halo vest versus spinal fusion for cervical injury: evidence from an outcome study. J Neurosurg 1989; 70:884–892.

30. Muller EJ, Wick M, Russe O, Muhr G. Management of odontoid fractures in the elderly. Eur Spine J 1999; 8:360–365.

31. Schroder J, Liljenqvist U, Greiner C, Wassmann H. Complications of halo treatment for cervical spine injuries in patients with ankylosing spondylitis–report of three cases. Arch Orthop Trauma Surg 2003; 123:112–114.

32. Koch RA, Nickel VL. The halo vest: an evaluation of motion and forces across the neck. Spine 1978; 3:103–107.

33. Sypert GW. External spinal orthotics. Neurosurgery 1987; 20: 642–649.

34. Johnsson R, Stromqvist B, Axelsson P, Selvik G. Influence of spinal immobilization on consolidation of posterolateral lumbosacral fusion. A roentgen stereophotogrammetric and radiographic analysis. Spine 1992; 17:16–21.

35. Lin JT. Bony pathology in the cancer patient. J Womens Health (Larchmt.) 2002; 11:691–702.

36. Millington PJ, Ellingsen JM, Hauswirth BE, Fabian PJ. Thermoplastic Minerva body jacket–a practical alternative to current methods of cervical spine stabilization. A clinical report. Phys Ther 1987; 67:223–225.

37. Berk RN, Coulson DB. The body cast syndrome. Radiology 1970; 94:303–305.

40 Rehabilitation in Patients With Tumors of the Spinal Column

LEAH MOINZADEH, PT AND SANDEE PATTI, OT

CONTENTS

1. INTRODUCTION

Rehabilitation is a critical part of the interdisciplinary approach to treating cancer patients suffering from tumors of the spinal column. Early mobilization and physical therapy (PT) intervention play and important role in preventing complications (*see* Fig. 1) *(1)* and improving quality of life. Rehabilitation is an integral part of the spine oncology team. It includes physical therapy, occupational therapy (OT), nursing, social work, case management, and physicians. This chapter discusses the role of PT and OT in patients with spinal tumors.

The focus of this section is to highlight the interventions and goals of PT for patients across an episode of care. PT and/or OT should be consulted in the immediate postoperative phase as well as during any other hospital admissions for medical treatment of spinal tumors and metastases. Rehabilitation should occur across all settings ranging from the acute hospital, to acute and long-term rehabilitation facilities, home care, outpatient, and hospice care facilities. Therapists and physicians work closely with case management to establish realistic rehabilitation goals while in house, and identify the most appropriate discharge setting and follow-up services. Discussions regarding anticipated discharge plans should begin immediately after the initial PT and OT evaluations.

2. REHABILITATION PLANNING

Regardless of the setting, patients should undergo a thorough examination and evaluation by the physical and occupational therapist to determine the appropriate care plan, addressing all impairments and functional limitations. Although PT and OT employ different interventions and methods, they share similar goals for maximizing quality of life and independent living. Impairments and functional limitations are assessed at the time of initial examination (*see* Fig. 1). The evaluation incorporates strategies used during the operative and non-operative treatment of the spine, as well as the results of the examination, social and environmental factors, patient goals, and status before admission. Patients may present with primary or metastatic spinal column tumors, spinal cord compression, and/or vertebral fractures. Regardless of diagnosis, patient goals, prior level of function, occupation, family support, home environment, and prognosis are all considered when establishing a plan of care.

3. EXAMINATION

The PT examination includes data collection for a history, systems review, and tests and measures *(2)*. The history is gathered from the patient/family/caregiver interview, medical record, and through team communication. Areas covered include medical/surgical history, social/work history, home environment, medications, mobility status before admission, and level of independence or assist required before admission. Objective data is gathered through tests and measures, selected by the physical therapist. PT examination of the patient with a spinal tumor may include the tests and measures included in Table 1.

4. CARE PLAN

The care plan is established after the initial PT examination, and includes the evaluation, diagnosis, and prognosis *(2)*. The *evaluation* is a clinical judgment based on the data gathered from the history, systems review, and test and measures *(2)*.

From: *Current Clinical Oncology: Cancer in the Spine: Comprehensive Care.*
Edited by: R. F. McLain, K-U. Lewandrowski, M. Markman, R. M. Bukowski,
R. Macklis, and E. C. Benzel © Humana Press, Inc., Totowa, NJ

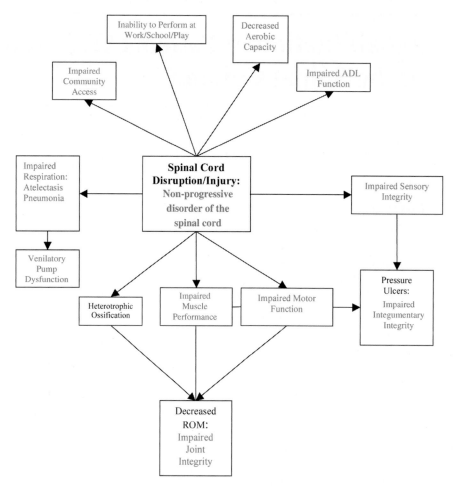

Fig 1. Impairments and functional limitations.

Factors that influence the complexity of the evaluation include the clinical findings, extent of loss of function, chronicity or severity of the problem, possibility of multi-site or multi-system involvement, preexisting conditions, potential discharge destination, social considerations, physical function, and overall health status.

To better assign appropriate rehabilitation strategies to the complexity of patients with spine tumors, diagnostic labels proposed by the American Physical Therapy Association (APTA) may be used. The *diagnosis* is a label encompassing a cluster of signs and symptoms, syndromes or categories. The diagnostic label indicates the primary dysfunction(s) toward which the therapist will direct interventions *(2)*.

The APTA has established the *Guide to Physical Therapist Practice (2)*. This guide was created to describe physical therapist practice, content, and processes, both for members of the physical therapy profession and for health care policy makers and third-party payers. The guide uses Preferred Practice Patterns[SM] that improve interdisciplinary communication, promote appropriate utilization of health care services, increase efficiency, and reduce unwarranted variation in the provision of services. Patients with tumors of the spinal column are included in practice pattern (5H) Impaired Motor Function, Peripheral

Nerve Integrity, and Sensory Integrity Associated with Non-progressive Disorders of the Spinal Cord *(2)*.

Another goal of rehabilitation planning is to establish the *prognosis* as the determination of the predicted optimal level of improvement in function and the amount of time needed to reach that level. The care plan identifies specific interventions, proposed frequency and duration of the interventions, anticipated goals, expected outcomes, and discharge plans. The anticipated goals and expected outcomes should be measurable and time limited. Frequency and duration may vary greatly among patients based on a variety of factors that the PT considers throughout the evaluation process *(2)*.

5. INTERVENTION

Intervention includes the interaction between the therapist and the patient, family, surgical and medical teams, and other individuals involved with patient care across multiple settings.

5.1. INPATIENT SETTING

Members of the rehabilitation team should be consulted as soon as the patient is admitted. Mobilization should begin as soon as spine stability has been assessed or restored, and when the patient is medically stable for intervention. The effects of bed rest far outweigh the risks of early mobilization *(3)*.

Table 1
Tests and Measures

- Aerobic capacity and endurance
- Anthropometric characteristics
- Arousal, attention, and cognition
- Assistive and adaptive devices
- Circulation (arterial, venous, and lymphatic)
- Cranial and peripheral nerve integrity
- Environmental, home, and work (job/school/play) barriers
- Ergonomics and body mechanics
- Gait, locomotion, and balance
- Integumentary integrity
- Joint integrity and mobility
- Motor function (motor control and motor learning)
- Muscle performance (including strength, power, and endurance)
- Neuromotor development and sensory integration
- Orthotic, protective, and supportive devices
- Pain
- Posture
- ROM, including muscle length
- Reflex integrity
- Self-care and home management (including ADL and IADL)
- Sensory integrity
- Ventilation and respiration/gas exchange
- Work (job/school/play), community, and leisure integration or reintegration (including IADL)

ROM, range of motion; ADL, activities of daily living; IADL, instrumental activities of daily living (2).

In addition to mobilization, the inpatient hospital setting provides an opportunity for education on prevention, functional adaptation, support, and the role of therapy regardless of the phase or extent of the disease process. Patients who have undergone spine surgery, radiation, or chemotherapy for spinal tumors will require education about brace application (see Chapter 39) and potential limitations on lifting, bending, or twisting. Transfers and early gait training is emphasized in the immediate postoperative phase. The log roll technique and positioning are emphasized to aide with bed mobility and comfort. Ambulation is the primary form of exercise in the first 4 to 8 wk following surgery. For patients with advanced weakness and impaired proximal strength, future stabilization exercise with a focus on abdominal and extensor strengthening is recommended as follow up in an outpatient setting (see Fig. 2).

5.2. INPATIENT REHABILITATION

Inpatient rehabilitation serves as a bridge between the acute hospital setting and home or a long-term care facility. Acute facilities are designed for the complex patient who can tolerate up to 3 h of PT and OT per day. The sub-acute setting is a less intense environment with a slower pace therapy program for elderly patients, or patients with decreased activity tolerance. The PT goals remain focused on maximizing independence and safety with functional mobility, aerobic conditioning, self-pacing, and precautions. Functional mobility and support at home are important factors when deciding between an inpatient facility and home following and acute hospital stay (see Fig. 2)

5.3. HOME CARE

Patients who are safe for discharge home are usually independent, or have supervision from family or home health care providers. Home therapy usually includes a home evaluation with attention to environmental safety as well as adaptive equipment. The frequency and duration of treatment is determined by the therapist based on patient prognosis, functional mobility, and support services (see Fig. 2).

5.4. OUTPATIENT THERAPY

Outpatient therapy plays an important role in educating patients with spinal tumors regarding spinal stabilization and body mechanics, regardless of whether the patient is a surgical or non-surgical candidate. Treatment for patients with spinal tumors may include bracing, ultrasound, hot packs, or transcutaneous electrical nerve stimulation to alleviate pain (4). Patient teaching and education may focus on extensor strengthening exercises to help maintain good posture if deemed appropriate by the treating spinal surgeon (5). Spinal stabilization exercises begin with low-level isometric abdominal and lumbar strengthening exercises, and may progress to resistive strength training with elastic bands or weights. Such educational programs may assist the patient in adjusting his routine to decrease pain and muscle fatigue. Overall lifestyle adaptation is important to allow for a healthy existence and decreased overall pain for patients with spinal column tumors (see Fig. 2).

6. OCCUPATIONAL THERAPY

OT centers on task adaptation and activities of daily living (ADL) including self-care, adaptive equipment, bathroom transfers, and kitchen and household tasks with the goal of maximizing independence. In the acute care setting, patients who are medically stable to mobilize should undergo an OT evaluation. The focus at this time is on patient education regarding postoperative precautions, particularly while performing ADL. This includes proper transfer techniques while moving onto and off of a toilet, in and out of a shower stall or tub/shower combination, and safe kitchen mobility during simple homemaking tasks.

6.1. ADAPTIVE EQUIPMENT

If the patient is interested in maximizing independence or working with a caregiver at home, instruction will be provided regarding appropriate dressing and bathing techniques utilizing adaptive equipment (AE). OT interventions are focused on impairments, which vary with spinal tumor location.

For most patients, lower extremity dressing and bathing is very difficult to perform because of pain and/or following spine surgery owing to postoperative precautions. Some commonly used devices can address these issues including reachers, sockaides, long-handled shoehorns, and elastic shoe laces (Fig. 3).

Cervical and upper thoracic spinal tumors can lead to impaired upper extremity strength, sensation, and fine motor control. The functional limitations that follow may impact feeding, upper extremity dressing, and toileting. AE is used to increase independence and decrease pain. Commonly used devices include wide-handled utensils, buttonhooks, and perineal tongs. Therapeutic exercise for the upper extremity is used to increase strength, coordination, and fine motor skills required for ADL.

6.2. OT ACROSS MULTIPLE SETTINGS

Spinal rehabilitation begins in the acute setting and continues in the inpatient rehabilitation setting. The focus remains on education regarding safe functional transfers and ADL perfor-

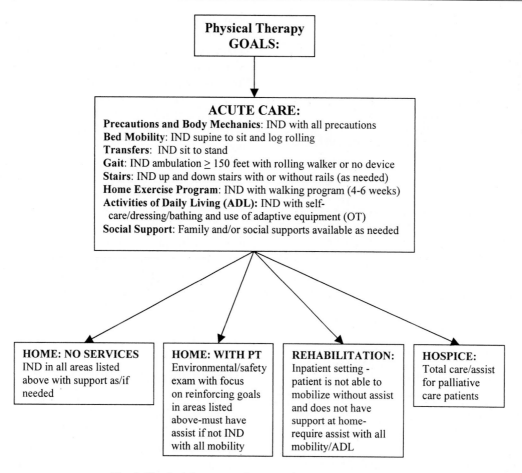

Fig. 2. Physical therapy goals across the continuum of care.

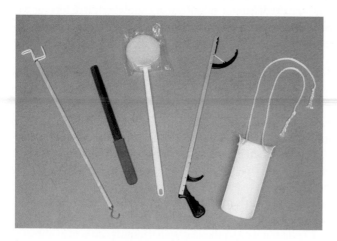

Fig. 3. Adaptive equipment.

mance. This is also the time when AE and durable medical equipment (DME) such as raised toilet seats and commodes are issued (Fig. 4).

Most patients benefit from home OT to address home safety and ensure proper carryover of all tasks and use of devices in the home setting. Attention is paid to environmental barriers in the kitchen as well as other areas of the home where potential safety hazards may exist.

Instrumental activities of daily living (IADL) can also be addressed in either the home or outpatient setting following spinal surgery or diagnosis with a tumor. These include cooking, shopping, gardening, community reintegration, and any other task that brings meaning to the individual patient's life.

Occupational therapy can have a profound effect on the lives of patients suffering from spinal column tumors. Patients are provided with the opportunity to regain or maximize independence and successfully adapt to or modify their environment. Increased awareness of the role of OT in this population is essential to providing the highest quality of care to the patient, providing them with the best possible outcome.

7. COMMUNICATION

A team approach to patient care should include open communication between the spinal tumor team and PT and OT. Designating a member of the rehabilitation team to attend rounds assists with therapist to doctor interactions and can provide for a concise care plan and discharge disposition. Good communication is essential to maximizing outcomes and providing safe mobilization, particularly with the complex patient. The therapist should complete a thorough analysis of the operative report followed by a discussion with the surgical/medical

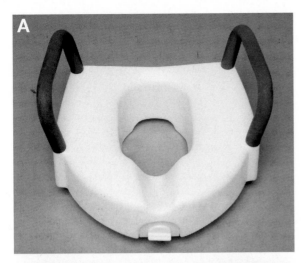

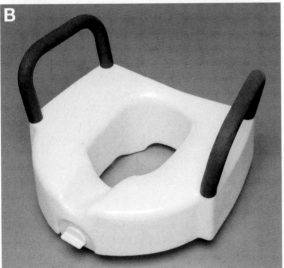

Fig. 4. Raised toilet seat with grab bars.

team regarding level of permitted mobility, precautions, and bracing needs. Once an appropriate plan for initial mobilization has been established, information should be passed to the team of caregivers interacting with the patient, allowing for improved patient safety and continuity of care.

REFERENCES

1. Somers MF. Spinal Cord Injury Functional Rehabilitation. East Norwalk, CT: Appleton and Lange; 1992.
2. APTA - American Physical Therapy Association. Guide to Physical Therapy Practice. 2nd ed. Phys Ther. 2001;81:9–744.
3. Bunting RW. Rehabilitation of cancer patients with skeletal metastases. Clin Orthop 1995; 312:197–200.
4. Spychalski J, Thomas B. Treatment and rehabilitation of pathologic fractures. Phys Med Rehabil 1995; 9:77.
5. Lukert BP. Vertebral compression fractures: how to manage pain, avoid disability. Geriatrics 1994; 49:22–26.

41 The Management of Pain in Spinal Malignancies

Susan B. LeGrand, md and Declan Walsh, md

Contents

1. INTRODUCTION

The management of pain caused by malignant involvement of the spine can be challenging. The pain is often multifactorial with somatic and neuropathic elements and may be complicated by pre-existing non-malignant pain from arthritis, spinal stenosis, or other chronic back syndromes. The mechanics of the back increase the likelihood of incident pain that may be particularly difficult to control. Excellent pain management requires a team approach that might include palliative medicine, anesthesia pain management, orthotics, and physical medicine and rehabilitation. This chapter focuses on medical management with opioid and adjuvant analgesic agents.

Despite evidence that 90% of cancer-related pain can be effectively controlled with oral medications or rarely needed invasive methods, too many patients continue to suffer from significant pain that negatively impacts their quality of life and interferes with function (1–3). Barriers to effective pain management are multifactorial and are physician- and patient-related (1,4). Physician related barriers include (1) confusion about the development of addiction, dependence, or tolerance, (2) unrealistic fear of side effects, particularly respiratory depression, and (3) fear of regulatory oversight. Because most physicians have minimal exposure to effective pain management during their medical school and residency training,

this educational lack contributes to ineffective treatment. This chapter begins with a discussion of the pertinent definitions, pathophysiology of pain, and pharmacology of opioid medications. The role of adjuvant analgesic medications, general principles of management, and suggestions for a multidisciplinary approach to the pain from spinal malignancies will follow.

2. DEFINITIONS

In discussing pain, specific terminology will be used throughout this chapter.

- *Constant or baseline pain*: Pain experienced the majority of the time.
- *Breakthrough pain*: Worsening of the baseline pain in an unpredictable fashion.
- *Incident pain*: Pain provoked by a particular movement or activity, voluntary or involuntary.
- *End-of-dose failure*: Pain that predictably occurs at the end of the effective half-life of a medication.

Three troublesome definitions interfere with appropriate pain management.

- *Addiction*: This is more appropriately termed *psychological dependence*. Addiction is a psychological illness in which the need for pain medication becomes paramount. It is characterized by compulsive drug-seeking behavior and illicit drug use despite negative consequences on health, work, and relationships. It is not a consequence of the appropriate use of pain medication for the management of cancer-related pain (5,6). Cancer patients whose pain has

From: *Current Clinical Oncology: Cancer in the Spine: Comprehensive Care.*
Edited by: R. F. McLain, K-U. Lewandrowski, M. Markman, R. M. Bukowski, R. Macklis, and E. C. Benzel © Humana Press, Inc., Totowa, NJ

been relieved by treatment are readily tapered from opioids. There is a syndrome called pseudoaddiction *(7)* seen in patients who have never had adequate pain control. They use their medication more rapidly than expected with frequent calls for additional medication prompting identification as drug abusers by health care professionals. These behaviors are not seen when adequate pain control is obtained.

- *Dependence*: More appropriately termed *physiological dependence*, this occurs with many medications including opioids. If a medication is stopped suddenly, there will be an expected withdrawal syndrome. It is not associated with psychological dependence or drug-seeking behaviors and does not imply addiction.

- *Tolerance*: Tolerance is the reduced efficacy of a medication after prior exposure to that medication. Although it is clear that tolerance develops at variable rates to both the side effects and the pain relieving effects of opioid medications, the dose increases required in cancer pain are predominantly related to progression of disease *(5,8,9)*. Allowing patients to suffer in the present in an unscientific fear that future medication will be ineffective is not justified.

3. PATHOPHYSIOLOGY

The pain seen in spinal malignancy is predominantly secondary to the involvement of the vertebral bodies with corresponding bone pain and the consequences of compression fracture, nerve compression or nerve root infiltration. The pathophysiology of bone pain is multifactorial. Contributing factors include (1) release of chemical mediators, (2) increased pressure within the bone, (3) microfractures, (4) stretch of the periosteum, and (5) reactive muscle spasm *(10,11)*. In the common classification used for pain pathophysiology, nociceptive vs neuropathic, it is clear that both will potentially be involved in the spine. The key differentiating feature is the transmission of pain sensation along normal nerves (nociceptive) vs abnormal nerves (neuropathic) *(12)*. Nociceptive pain may be subdivided into somatic and visceral with bone pain the prototypic somatic pain. Many cancer patients will have more than one type of pain. This may be secondary to the disease, treatment of the disease, or unrelated problems including preexisting pain from arthritis or chronic back pain. Careful assessment, characterization, and documentation, independently, of each pain is critical to appropriate management. The suspected pathophysiology can guide the choice of testing, therapeutic intervention, medication, and the use of adjuvant analgesics.

4. PHARMACOLOGY (FIG. 1)

The World Health Organization guidelines have been widely used to improve management of pain *(3,13,14)*. Revisions that include invasive techniques or eliminate the concept of "weak" and "strong" opioids have been suggested. For the purposes of this discussion these guidelines for medication will be used. The section on adjuvant analgesic agents will discuss the step 1 drugs. The preferred medications for management of moderate or severe pain are step 2 and 3 medications. Step 2 medications include tramadol and the μ-agonists (codeine, hydrocodone, and oxycodone) in combination with acetaminophen or aspirin. The

preferred step 3 medications are morphine, hydromorphone, oxycodone, fentanyl, and methadone.

4.1. MORPHINE

Morphine remains the medication of choice for moderate and severe cancer pain. There are individual studies that suggest different side effect profiles for other opioids, specifically less constipation with fentanyl *(15,16)* and fewer hallucinations with oxycodone *(17,18)*, but these are small studies with few patients. Relative costs of the different medications favor the use of morphine or methadone. Because most physicians have less experience with methadone, and the dosing may be more problematic, morphine remains the preferred medication for initial use.

Morphine may be given via multiple routes: oral, rectal, subcutaneous (sq), intravenous (iv), intramuscular (im), intraspinal, and sublingual. There is conflicting data on the value of sublingual or buccal administration *(19–21)*. Anecdotal studies suggested this was a means of obtaining a more rapid onset of pain relief. Other studies suggest that time to onset is actually delayed and occurs by gastrointestinal absorption of swallowed medication. There is no indication for intramuscular administration because sq is equally effective and less uncomfortable. The ratio of oral to parenteral (iv, sq, im) dosing in non-naïve individuals is 3:1. The oral to rectal ratio is 1:1 (Table 1).

Morphine is rapidly absorbed via the gastrointestinal tract, but undergoes extensive first pass metabolism in the liver via glucuronidation. Morphine 3-glucuronide (M3G) is the predominant metabolite and is pharmacologically inactive but thought to contribute to neurotoxicity. Morphine 6-glucoronide (M6G) is active and more potent than the parent compound but present in small quantities. In patients with renal insufficiency, the metabolites may accumulate and increase the potential for side effects. Morphine can be used safely in patients with stable renal insufficiency with careful titration. An alternative medication is preferred if renal function is rapidly declining *(22)*.

Peak plasma levels and therapeutic effects occur within 5 min of iv administration, 15 to 20 min after sq, and 30 to 90 min following oral dosing. The time to peak level for sustained release morphine products is 150 min *(22)*. The effective half-life of immediate release preparations is 3 to 4 h but may vary individually. The common practice of prescribing every 6-h dosing is, therefore, inappropriate.

4.2. HYDROMORPHONE

Hydromorphone is available for oral, rectal, iv, sq, and intraspinal use. The pharmacology is similar to morphine *(23)*. It has a significant but variable first pass effect with 62% ±33% bioavailablity. It is metabolized in the liver via glucuronidation that leads to an inactive metabolite (hydromorphone-3-glucuronide) and active metabolites in small quantities (dihydromorphine and dihydroisomorphine). The metabolites may accumulate in renal failure and lead to neurotoxicity as seen with morphine.

The onset of action is within 5 min for iv administration and 30 min for oral and rectal administration. There is no specific data available on buccal or sublingual absorption, but because hydromorphone is hydrophilic these routes are not likely to be useful. Hydromorphone has the advantage of increased potency

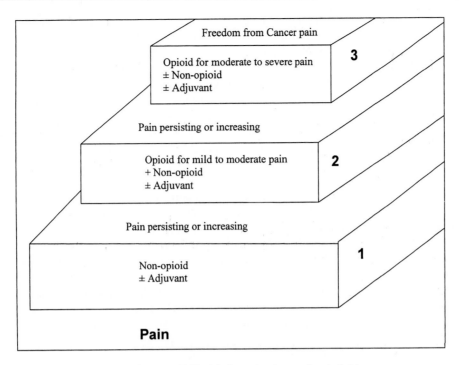

Fig. 1. The World Health Organization analgesic ladder.

Table 1
Equianalgesic Dosing of Preferred Opioids

Opioid	iv/sq	Oral
Morphine	10 mg	30 mg
Hydromorphone	2 mg	7.5 mg
Oxycodone	NA	30 mg
Methadone	1/2 Oral dose	Variable[a]
Fentanyl	0.1 mg[b]	NA

NA, not applicable.
[a]Ratio differs depending on prior opioid dose (40).
[b]Variable ratios (range 66 µg:1 mg–100 µg:1 mg) identified (109).

compared with morphine (1:5) that can be advantageous if large dosages are required (24,25). This can be particularly helpful in subcutaneous infusions where volume can be problematic (26). The oral to iv ratio is less well established but often quoted as 5:1. The lack of a sustained release preparation in the United States (available in United Kingdom and Canada) limits its use. Chronic use requires every 4-h dosing.

4.3. OXYCODONE

Oxycodone is available in the United States only in an oral preparation. It is commonly used in combination with acetaminophen that limits dose increases but is also available as a single agent allowing unrestricted dose adjustments. Oxycodone has a higher bioavailability from the gastrointestinal tract than morphine or hydromorphone. It is metabolized via demethylation to noroxycodone and oxymorphone. The parent compound is the predominant pharmacologically active agent. Clearance of all three compounds—oxycodone, noroxycodone, and oxymorphone—will be reduced in renal failure leading to a potential for accumulation. Half-life is prolonged in hepatic

failure and alternate medications should be used. Effective oral half-life is the same as morphine or hydromorphone, i.e., 3 to 4 h (27).

4.4. FENTANYL

Unlike morphine, hydromorphone, and oxycodone, fentanyl is highly lipophilic. Given the rapid redistribution into muscle and fat it has an initial short duration of action but accumulates with repeated dosing. It is metabolized in the liver with the metabolites felt to have little analgesic activity. Less than 10% is excreted by the kidney and, therefore, it was thought to be a reasonable choice in progressive renal impairment. There is evidence to suggest that clearance correlates with azotemia and the potential for accumulation exists with a corresponding potential for toxicity (28). Fentanyl is available for iv, intraspinal, transdermal, and transmucosal use (29).

The transdermal preparation requires an initial transfer of drug from the reservoir to the skin. This skin depot must be filled before vascular absorption and remains after the patch is removed. This results in a significant delay to initial effect (range 14–28 h) and a terminal half-life after patch removal of 16 to 25 h (29,30). Therefore, transdermal fentanyl should not be used in a patient in acute distress unless immediate release medications are also given. It is not recommended when rapid titration is needed. Use in narcotic-naïve patients is not recommended because deaths have occured and the FDA has increased required warnings. The transdermal preparation is particular useful for patients who cannot swallow. It may also be useful in patients who have difficulty maintaining regular schedules of medication. Cost can be of concern for hospice and individuals with limited insurance benefits.

Because fentanyl is lipophilic, it is the most appropriate choice for transmucosal administration. The oral transmucosal fentanyl citrate was created to manage breakthrough or incident pain when rapid onset of effect is desired. Dose titration is needed to identify the effective dose and this dose does not correlate with the doses used for sustained medications *(31,32)*. Utilization of this preparation may be limited by cost concerns. There is a report of the use of the injectable fentanyl and sufentanil via buccal route with rapid effect in incident pain *(33)*.

4.5. METHADONE

Methadone is a unique opioid that has particular utility in the management of pain related to malignancy in general and the spine in particular. (1) In addition to μ-agonist action it inhibits the *N*-methyl-D-asparate receptor and prevents monoamine uptake in the peri-aquiductal gray. (2) It does not have neuroactive metabolites, therefore, it is useful in renal failure. (3) It can function as sustained and immediate release. (4) It is relatively inexpensive. Methadone has been shown to be useful in pain, particularly neuropathic, that has not responded well to other opioids *(34–38)*. Unfortunately, physicians and patients may be reluctant to use it given the association with addiction management. The unique pharmacokinetics also contribute to physician discomfort with its use.

Methadone is well absorbed from the gastrointestinal tract with three times the bioavailability of morphine. It can be given by oral, rectal, iv, and intraspinal routes *(36–38)*. The sq route can be irritating but addition of corticosteroids to the infusion has allowed safe administration *(39)*. It is metabolized by the cytochrome P450 enzymes (CYP3A4) with, therefore, an increased potential for drug interactions compared with other opioids *(35)*. There is wide interpersonal variability in bioavailability with a half-life that can range from 10 to 75 h. Given this, as needed (PRN) dosing is recommended at initiation. Conversion ratios with other agents are also difficult to determine. Previously published conversion tables have proved to be inaccurate. The ratio varies substantially based on the morphine equivalent dose *(38,40,41)*. For example, at low doses of morphine, the ration of morphine to methadone may be 4:1. At higher doses the ratio may be 14:1. Use of published conversion protocols is recommended *(42)*.

4.6. TRAMADOL

Tramadol is a step 2 medication that is substantially different from other μ-agonists. It is neither an opium derivative nor a semi-synthetic derivative of morphine. It is a weak μ-agonist that also inhibits monoamine (noradrenaline and serotonin) uptake. Both mechanisms of action contribute to the analgesic effect *(43,44)*. It has been used successfully in cancer pain and is one of the more commonly used medications outside the United States *(45,46)*. Side effects are similar but less common than those seen with other opioid medications. Seizures have been seen at higher doses *(47,48)* that limit dose escalation (ceiling effect). It has the advantage of not being a controlled substance.

4.7. SUSTAINED RELEASE (SR) PREPARATIONS

Oxycodone and morphine are both available in sustained release forms *(49,50)*. These have facilitated improvement in pain control by eliminating the need for every 4-h dosing schedules. Sustained release hydromorphone is available in other countries *(51)*. The tablet forms of oxycodone and morphine

consist of an acrylic matrix that releases medication over a 12-h period. There are also morphine preparations with 24-h duration of action consisting of a gelatin capsule with polymer-coated micropellets *(52,53)*. The SR oxycodone has a biphasic pattern with an initial rapid release followed by a slower sustained phase *(54)*. The tablets (morphine or oxycodone) should not be crushed as this alters the sustained absorption.

Studies have shown that the sustained release tablets of morphine and oxycodone can be effectively dosed at 12-h intervals *(55,56)*. Despite this evidence, dosing intervals of every 8 h or even every 6 h are still seen. There is no evidence to support routine use of every 8-h dosing schedules. Rare individuals will develop end-of-dose failure *(55)*. These individuals give a consistent history of awakening in pain and requiring breakthrough medication routinely several hours before the next scheduled dose. End-of-dose failure may be managed either by increasing the 12-h dose or changing to an 8-h dosing schedule. This is the only circumstance in which every 8-h dosing should be needed. There is no justification for dosing intervals shorter than 8 h. A similar pattern can be seen with transdermal fentanyl. Some patients will notice poor pain control after 48 to 60 h. As with morphine the dose can either be increased or the patch may be changed earlier but not at intervals less than 48 h.

5. MEDICATIONS NOT RECOMMENDED FOR USE

Multiple commonly prescribed medications are not recommended for use in the management of cancer-related pain. These include codeine, hydrocodone, meperidine, and the agonist/antagonist combinations. The rationale for these recommendations are discussed in Subheadings 5.1.–5.4.

5.1. CODEINE

Clinical experience suggests codeine is more constipating, produces more nausea, and has more neuropsychological complications. It requires conversion to morphine for activity using an enzyme with ethnic polymorphism *(57)*. Some individuals are, therefore, unable to metabolize codeine and obtain no benefit.

5.2. HYDROCODONE

Hydrocodone in combination with acetaminophen is commonly prescribed for general pain complaints. There is no data available on use in cancer pain. It has the disadvantages of co-analgesic agents with a ceiling effect and only oral preparations. These products and codeine containing products are not schedule 2 medications and therefore, have the advantage of call-in prescriptions and refills.

5.3. MEPERIDINE

Although one of the more commonly prescribed parenteral analgesic agents, this medication is not recommended for regular use in pain management. Meperidine has a toxic metabolite, normeperidine, which accumulates in 2 to 3 d, even without renal impairment, and is associated with neuroexcitation, delirium, and seizures *(58–60)*. It also has very poor oral bioavailability with a 6:1 oral to iv ratio. Meperidine has no advantage over other opioid medications and should therefore be abandoned.

5.4. AGONIST/ANTAGONIST

These preparations are not recommended for several reasons: (1) there is a higher incidence of psychotomimetic events (pentazocine). (2) They are available only in parenteral forms (butorphanol, buprenorphine, and nalbuphine). Butorphanol also comes in a nasal spray and buprenorphine may be given sublingual but the doses are not practical for this patient population. (3) They may precipitate withdrawal symptoms in patients previously taking μ-agonists. (4) They have a ceiling effect *(61)*. A transdermal preparation of buprenorphine is in study and may make this a more useful product.

6. SIDE EFFECTS OF OPIOID MEDICATION

Successful management of pain requires prevention and treatment of opioid side effects *(62)*. Tolerance will develop to most side effects, with the exception of constipation. Education of patients to expect certain effects and the reassurance that these will resolve in several days with consistent use can prevent premature discontinuation of medication.

6.1. COMMON SIDE EFFECTS

6.1.1. Nausea

Opioid medications cause nausea by several mechanisms including stimulation of the chemoreceptor trigger zone, increased vestibular sensitivity and delayed gastric emptying. Of patients, 50–75% will experience transient nausea with morphine *(63)*. This can be readily treated with D_2 antagonist agents such as prochlorperazine or metaclopromide and generally resolves with continued use. Patients should be advised of the potential for nausea and given anti-emetics either routinely or PRN for the first several days. Occasionally, severe persistent symptoms develop that warrant drug rotation. A history of prior emesis with morphine should generate a more detailed exploration of the length of prior administration and concomitant problems (anesthesia, and others). Unless there is evidence of nausea with sustained use, it is reasonable to try morphine again.

6.1.2. Sedation

Mild sedation should be expected when starting opioid medications in a naïve patient. Although tolerance develops within several days, it may recur with subsequent dose increases. Patients should be advised of this whenever the doses are adjusted. There are reports of successful management of sedation with dextroamphetamine or methylphenidate *(64–66)*.

6.1.3. Pruritis

Pruritis is a non-allergic symptom the cause of which has not been clearly determined. Histamine release or effects of the opioid receptors are considered possibilities. It is seen more commonly with epidural or intrathecal administration. Antagonist agents such as nalbuphine and naloxone have been effective in relieving the symptom during postoperative intraspinal analgesia *(67,68)*. This would support a causative role for the opioid receptor. Reassurance that this is not allergy and provision of benadryl or hydroxyzine may be helpful. In occasional patients this may be bothersome enough to warrant drug rotation.

6.2. NEUROPSYCHIATRIC SIDE EFFECTS

In addition to sedation, other central nervous system complications may develop *(69)*. These include delirium and myoclonus. Delirium in the advanced cancer patient is usually multifactorial but there is little question that opioid medications contribute. The development of delirium can be addressed

by a decrease in dose, if possible, with or without specific medication for the delirium such as haloperidol. If the symptom does not resolve then drug rotation may be required *(70)*.

Myoclonus can develop with higher doses of all opioid medications although rarely reported with methadone *(71,72)*. Family members may be more aware of this symptom than the patient, particularly during sleep. If it is troublesome to the patient then dose reduction is the management strategy of choice. If pain control is inadequate, then the addition of adjuvant medication for an opioid sparing effect with dose reduction of the opioid or drug rotation may be needed. Symptomatic management has been predominantly with benzodiazepines *(73)*.

6.2.1. Constipation

This is the most common and troubling side effect of opioids *(74)*. Tolerance does not occur and the symptom may worsen with increasing doses. It can be so severe that patients will choose to remain in significant pain rather than risk worsening constipation. It is imperative that the prescribing physician initiates an aggressive bowel regimen whenever opioid medications are begun. Constant vigilance is required. The combination of a stool softener with a stimulant is usually effective *(70)*. Bulk agents are discouraged as they may exacerbate discomfort. New agents to manage constipation, methylnalhexone and alvimopan, are under study *(75,76)*.

6.3. RESPIRATORY DEPRESSION

The most feared side effect of opioids is respiratory depression. The unrealistic fear of this complication contributes to undertreatment of pain. There have been trials that clearly show the antagonizing effects of pain to the respiratory effects of opioids *(77,78)*. Tolerance also develops rapidly. In the non-naïve patient, sedation and delirium will develop before respiratory depression. Mild sedation (normal respiratory rate, easily aroused but returns to sleep) can be managed by decreasing the next scheduled dose, changing to a smaller patch or decreasing the rate of a continuous infusion. Other medications that may be contributing to sedation (i.e., anxiolytic, gabapentin, antiemetic agents) should be stopped. If the sedation is more severe (minimally arousable with adequate respiratory rate) then further medication should be withheld (patch removed) until improvement. Naloxone should be given only in the event of life-threatening hypoventilation. To avoid symptoms of withdrawal or an exacerbation of pain, naloxone (0.4 mg) should be diluted in 10 cc normal saline and then injected 1 cc every minute until hypoventilation resolves *(63)*. If the cause of sedation is the opioid then 1 to 2 cc is usually all that is needed. Because the half-life of naloxone is shorter than that of most opioids, repeated doses may be required or initiation of a continuous infusion.

6.4. ADJUVANT ANALGESIC MEDICATIONS

When comparing the side effect profiles of the adjuvant analgesic agents to the opioid medications it is important to note that irreversible toxicity and end organ damage are only seen with the non-opioid medications. Despite this fact and documented frequency of hospital admissions for complications of these medications, physicians are much more comfortable with their use. It is clear they have a role in the management of cancer-related pain particularly in combination with an opioid. They may have opioid sparing effects that can ameliorate delirium, sedation, opioid related constipation, etc. Choice of medication is predicated, to a degree, by the suspected pathophysiology of the pain.

6.4.1. Acetaminophen

Given in the appropriate dosage, this is the safest of the analgesic agents for mild pain. There are no renal, gastrointestinal, or cardiovascular side effects of concern. There is a recognized risk of hepatic necrosis with doses over 4 mg/d. There may be some increased risk at lower dose in individuals with pre-existing liver disease. It can be a useful adjuvant in bone or visceral pain. It has minimal activity as a single agent in the management of neuropathic pain.

6.4.2. Non-Steroidal Anti-Inflammatory Agents

Despite the common use of non-steroidal anti-inflammatory agents (NSAIDs) as single agents or in combination with opioid medications for malignant bone pain, there are no randomized controlled trials that confirm bone specific efficacy in cancer patients (79,80). The probability of response and the choice of medication are completely unpredictable. It is clear that some patients will respond to one agent from a class and not to others of the same class or may respond to a different class of agents. A sequential trial of different agents within a class or different classes of NSAIDs is reasonable.

6.4.3. Bisphosphonates

Bisphosphonates are routinely used in breast and myeloma patients with osteolytic bone involvement. They were developed for management of malignant hypercalcemia and their activity is primarily secondary to osteoclast inhibition. There have now been multiple trials (including placebo-controlled) that have demonstrated not only a decrease in skeletal events such as fracture or need for radiation therapy, but also a statistically significant increase in quality of life with decreased pain (81–83). Bisphosphonates are routinely used in breast and myeloma patients with osteolytic bone involvement. They were developed for management of malignant hypercalcemia and their activity is primarily secondary to osteoclast inhibition. There have now been placebo-controlled trials with both pamidronate and zoledronic acid demonstrating not only a decrease in skeletal events, such as fracture or need for radiation therapy, but also a statistically significant increase in quality of life with decreased pain (81–84). The medications are usually well-tolerated with the most common side effect being a flu-like syndrome with fever and chills that occurs within 24–48 h of administration. A Cochrane review concluded that their benefit was modest but real and should not be the first choice for pain control (85). Concerns with renal function and recently reported osteonecrosis of the jaw may also impact their use (86).

6.4.4. Muscle Relaxants

Although clinically it seems obvious that muscle spasms contribute to the pain of spinal malignancy, no trials documenting their significance could be found. Baclofen, diazepam, tizanidine, and dantrolene are approved for use in spasticity associated with neurological disease, i.e., amyotrophic lateral sclerosis, multiple sclerosis, and spinal cord injury. Cochrane reviews of agents for spasticity in spinal cord injury and multiple sclerosis found insufficient evidence to recommend a particular approach (87,88). There are no trials to evaluate the relative efficacy of these agents in patients with malignancy. Therapeutic trials of one of these agents would be reasonable when muscle spasms contribute to pain.

6.4.5. Corticosteroids

Corticosteroids, particularly dexamethasone, have multiple uses in the management of spinal malignancies. The value in symptomatic spinal cord compression is unquestioned (89). Although functional improvement is the ultimate goal, improvement in pain control also occurs. In addition, there is evidence to support the value of corticosteroids in nerve compression and bone pain (90). They can be particularly helpful in steroid responsive diseases, such as myeloma, that commonly involve the spine. While some studies have shown a rapid improvement in pain with high dose dexamethasone (96–100 mg) in spinal cord compression others have not confirmed this finding (91,92). Side effects, such as gastrointestinal hemorrhage, gastrointestinal perforation, myopathy, and neuropsychological toxicity, are greater with higher doses (93). In the acute setting, particularly cord compression, their value is clear although the specific dosage to use is still unsettled. For long-term management of bone or neuropathic pain risks and benefits must be carefully considered and the lowest effective dose should be used.

6.4.6. Antidepressants

There is significant experience in the use of tricyclic antidepressant medications in the management of neuropathic pain in diabetic neuropathy, post-herpetic neuralgia, and some headache syndromes (94,95). Typically these agents are used for burning, dysesthetic pain. The agent tested most often has been amitriptyline, but given the higher incidence of anticholinergic side effects, alternative agents have also been used with less available data. Starting doses should be low (10–25 mg of amitriptyline) and then increased gradually as required. Responses are seen at doses significantly lower than required for treatment of depression. Studies of the selective serotonin uptake inhibitors have been conflicting but generally have shown less efficacy (96). There are case reports that have shown efficacy for venlafaxine (97). Duloxetine is approved for diabetic neuropathy but has not been tested in cancer pain.

6.4.7. Anti-Convulsant Medications

Disease in the spine is often complicated by neuropathic pain and because this may be more difficult to manage with opioids alone, anticonvulsant medications are frequently used as adjuvant analgesics (95). As with the antidepressant medications, most data is from diabetic neuropathy, post-herpetic neuralgia, or trigeminal neuralgia. It is not clear that this data can be extrapolated to the pain from malignant nerve compression or invasion. A Cochrane review in 2001 found few well-constructed trials that confirmed the efficacy of anticonvulsants in pain management, no trials comparing different medications and only one study that included cancer pain (98). Their conclusion was to try other interventions before initiating these medications. The choice of agent must include consideration of cost, dosing frequency, side effect profile, and potential drug interactions. The most commonly used medications are carbamazepine, sodium valproate, and gabapentin. Gabapentin has the advantage of fewer drug interactions and fewer side effects but must be dosed more often. The Cochrane Palliative Care group found no evidence that gabapentin was superior to carbamazepine *(99)*. The somnolence seen with gabapentin may be of more concern in patients taking opioid medications. Newer agents, such as pregabalin and lamotrigine, have not been tested, but could have value.

6.4.8. Calcitonin

Numerous reports document the ability of calcitonin to contribute to pain control *(99–101)*. It has been found effective by sq *(102)*, nasal *(103)*, and subarachnoid *(104)* routes. Dosages used and length of therapy have varied substantially making specific recommendations difficult. Effects have typically been brief but on occasion long lasting relief has been obtained. Given the prolonged action of the bisphosphonates and their lack of tachyphylaxis, calcitonin is rarely used now for pain control in malignancy.

6.5. INVASIVE TECHNIQUES

Invasive techniques include intraspinal infusion of medication, neurolytic blockade, neuroablative procedures, and spinal stimulation techniques. Although there is extensive literature on various invasive techniques in the management of chronic non-malignant pain, their role in the management of cancer related pain is less clear. The various neurolytic blocks are more useful in visceral pain although an isolated nerve root compression from a spinal lesion could be managed this way. Multiple nerve levels are more commonly involved rendering these techniques less useful. As the oral/parenteral management of pain improves and with increasing experience using intraspinal infusions, neuroablative interventions are rarely needed. Spinal stimulators have been used for the management of non-malignant back pain but there is no literature on their use in cancer-related pain. Therefore, the only invasive technique discussed in this chapter will be the intraspinal administration of medications.

Even with optimal multidisciplinary pain management techniques a subset of patients will not have adequate pain control or will develop unacceptable side effects. These individuals may benefit from intraspinal (epidural or intrathecal) administration of medication. The percentage of patients in this group is less clear. There are no prospective trials in a multidisciplinary pain management setting that evaluate the need for intraspinal medications. Two retrospective reports referred 10% (included neurosurgical referrals) and less than 2% of patients for invasive techniques *(105,106)*. Indications for a trial of intraspinal analgesia are: (1) inadequate pain control despite appropriate attempts at management by other routes including the use of adjuvant medications and (2) unacceptable toxicity from oral/parenteral opioids after appropriate drug rotations and adjuvant analgesic agents.

The choice of epidural vs intrathecal and the choice of medication depend on the location of the pain symptoms. Relatively localized pain (particularly lower extremity or pelvis can usually be managed with an epidural catheter placed near the level of the nerves involved. For more generalized pain complaints, intrathecal administration may be a better option. The most commonly used medications are morphine, hydromorphone,

and fentanyl. If pain remains uncontrolled then bupivocaine and/or clonidine may be added. Patients with incident somatic pain were most often controlled with morphine alone, whereas those with neuropathic pain usually required the addition of bupivacaine for successful pain control *(106)*.

There are different techniques used to deliver intraspinal medications. It can be done using a tunneled external catheter, a tunneled catheter to an sq port, or an implantable infusion system. The external catheter and the port are then connected to an external pump. There are multiple issues to consider in the choice of technique.

1. Cost. Implantable pumps have a significant up front expense.
2. Life expectancy. Data suggest the pump becomes cost effective after 3 mo *(107)*.
3. Availability of personnel to fill/maintain the implantable pump. As patients become more ill, they may need more frequent changes in pain management and be less able to come to a clinic. Home care/hospice personnel would need to have the equipment and experience to adjust doses in the home.

Complications of intraspinal medications can be significant but vary by technique. Complications occurred in 30 to 50% of patients with external catheters. These included: (1) catheter dysfunction (dislodged or broken), (2) infection, (3) hematoma, or (4) hyperesthesia *(106)*. The implantable pump has the lowest risk of infection presuming frequent access for refills is not required. The subcutaneous injection port appears to have fewer complications than an external catheter and may be the best alternative in the patient with advanced disease and shorter life expectancy *(107,108)*.

7. PRINCIPLES OF PAIN MANAGEMENT

- Careful assessment. This should include an assessment of (1) time course. Is the pain constant or intermittent? Is there breakthrough pain? Incident pain? (2) Location and radiation pattern for each pain. (3) Pain quality (sharp, dull, burning, and so on). (4) Pain intensity. Intensity should be determined at baseline, before and after breakthrough dosing and for incident pain, if present. (5) The presence of modifying/exacerbating factors. (6) The functional and emotional impact. (7) The results of prior medication trials. What medications and dosages have been tried? Has there been intolerance to a particular pain medication? (8) Prior disease altering treatment, i.e., chemotherapy, hormonal therapy, radiation therapy, surgery, and others.
- Choose a medication appropriate to the severity. Moderate or severe pain (>4 on a scale of 0–10) should be managed with a step 2 or 3 medication *(3)*. Step 3 medications such as morphine do not have a dose ceiling and may be increased PRN until adequate pain control is obtained. It is not necessary to start at step 1 and progress to step 3. The choice of medication is determined by the severity of the pain (i.e., a patient presenting with level 7/10 pain on no current analgesic would be given morphine).
- Constant pain requires constant medication. This can be accomplished by scheduled dosing of immediate- or sustained-release products.

- Dosing should be based on the pharmacology of the medication and the patient report of efficacy and duration of effect. Immediate release opioid medications alone or in combination have an effective half-life of 3 to 4 h. Therefore every 4-h dosing is needed. Tramadol may be given every 6 h. Methadone, with its individual variability, should be dosed on PRN schedule initially, usually at 3-h intervals (34).
- Patients on sustained release medications or continuous parenteral infusions must also have immediate release medications available for breakthrough dosing.
- Use of adjuvant analgesic agents (NSAIDS, anti-convulsants, and tricyclic anti-depressants) should be tailored to the specific characteristics of the pain. For example, adding an NSAID for musculoskeletal pain, an anti-convulsant, or tricyclic for neuropathic pain.
- Frequent reassessment of the efficacy of the medication chosen, side effects, and need for breakthrough dosing is mandatory with adjustment in management as required. When initiating pain medication or adjusting doses, it is appropriate to have phone contact within several days and physician follow-up within 2 wk.
- Titrate to effect or development of an intolerable side effect using one opioid +/– adjuvant. There is no indication for more than one sustained-release opioid. Immediate-release medications should be the same opioid when possible (an exception is fentanyl).

8. INITIATION OF THERAPY

The method chosen to initiate treatment for constant pain depends on the severity. Patients with mild pain may be started on non-opioid medications. Those with moderate pain may manage well with the institution of an oral regimen. Parenteral treatment with subsequent conversion to oral medications is appropriate for someone in severe distress. In the opioid naïve the steps are as follows:

- Step 1. Initiate every 4-h as needed dosing. Begin with 5 to 10 mg of oral immediate release morphine or oxycodone. Have the person keep a diary of the doses used and the pain level before and after taking the medication. Verify the effectiveness of the PRN dose within 24 h.
- Step 2. After 48 h determine the efficacy of each dose and calculate the 24-h consumption. Initiate sustained release morphine by dividing the 24-h consumption by two. This is the 12-h sustained release dose. Immediate release preparations will still be needed to manage breakthrough and/or incident pain.
- Step 3. Frequent reassessment. Assess the level of constant pain, the number of breakthrough doses needed on average, and the efficacy of the breakthrough medication. If the constant pain is not well-controlled or frequent breakthrough dosing is required, calculate the 24-h breakthrough dosage, divide by two and add this to the sustained release dose.

Case Study 1:

Mr. J has metastatic disease to the spine. He comes to the office for his first visit and complains of aching pain of 4/10 severity. He has tried over-the-counter medications without success. He is given morphine elixir 5 to 10 mg every 4 h PRN and initiates a bowel regimen. He returns later that week for re-evaluation. He found the 5-mg dose ineffective and has consistently used 10 mg every 4 h. His 24-h consumption is 60 mg. You start him on 30 mg sustained-release morphine every 12 h and give him morphine 10 mg tablets for breakthrough. One month later, he complains of worsening pain. He is using his breakthrough dose more often but it continues to be effective. He is now using it five times a day for a 24-total of 50 mg. While evaluating the cause of worsening symptoms, you increase his SR morphine from 30 to 60 mg every 12 h (50/2 = 25. Next available dose size = 30 mg). No change is made in his breakthrough medication.

8.1. NON-NAÏVE PATIENTS

Management of the non-naïve patient is similar, except sustained release medications can be started after calculating the current dose and increasing proportional to the degree of relief obtained.

Case Study 2:

Mr. S comes to see you for pain management of prostate cancer metastatic to spine. He has had radiation therapy and hormonal therapy but continues to have pain. He is currently taking 100 mg of SR morphine every 12 h with 30 mg of immediate release as breakthrough. He is using his breakthrough medication four times a day and the dose relieves his pain 50%. You calculate his usage as 320 mg (200 mg SR plus additional 120 mg breakthrough) and increase his SR morphine to 160 mg every 12 h. You increase his breakthrough dose by 50% to 45 mg. (Other interventions would also be appropriate, but only the morphine is addressed for the purposes of discussion.)

8.2. MANAGEMENT OF INCIDENT PAIN

Incident pain can be particularly difficult to manage. It is relatively common in malignancies involving the spine. Typically this is seen with a positional change such as from sitting to standing or occasionally just rolling over in bed. If pain is adequately controlled at rest then increasing levels of the continuous medication may result in oversedation. Options for management include:

- Premedication with oral breakthrough medication before activity known to cause pain.
- Specific treatment directed to the etiology (i.e., radiation therapy, vertebral augmentation, and others).
- Bracing techniques.
- Patient-controlled parenteral medication.
- Oral transmucosal fentanyl citrate.

8.3. MANAGEMENT OF POSTOPERATIVE PAIN IN PATIENTS WITH CHRONIC PAIN

There is nothing written that specifically addresses the management of postoperative pain in patients on chronic opioids for cancer-related pain. In making recommendations, there are two issues to consider. (1) Will the surgery have an impact on the severity of the baseline pain for which the opioids were ordered? (2) How long before the patient will resume oral medication? It is unfortunate, but common, for a patient with chronic pain to go to surgery for unrelated problems and be placed on patient-controlled analgesia (PCA) at doses appropriate for the opioid naïve. Severe uncontrolled pain is the result.

If the surgery is unlikely to improve the baseline pain, and oral intake will resume immediately after surgery then maintaining the sustained release medication as scheduled is easiest. Postoperative pain can then be managed using normal or increased doses of breakthrough medication (oral, sq, iv). Alternatively parenteral (PCA) without a basal rate can be given for the postoperative pain. If the patient will be unable to take oral medication for some period of time, then a continuous infusion equivalent to the sustained release medication should be started with PCA dosing for the postoperative pain. Appropriate oral to iv conversions must be used.

If the surgery may have a significant impact on the level of baseline pain, then dose reduction may be necessary. At least 25% of the current medication level is needed to avoid withdrawal. A continuos infusion of at least this dose should be started. The breakthrough dose should be similar to the preoperative levels that were demonstrated to be safe and effective. The dose is subsequently adjusted based on response.

9. MULTIDISCIPLINARY TREATMENT

As noted at the beginning, the pain of spinal malignancy is often multifactorial and usually requires the integration of multiple modalities. The following scenario will address how these might be incorporated.

Case Study 3:

Mrs. S presents to the office with severe back pain that has been gradually progressive but with a sudden worsening. She has constant bone pain (7/10) and severe incident pain (10/10) when she tries to sit up. Additionally, she has weakness in her legs and some difficulty initiating urination. Physical exam demonstrates pain to palpation of several levels in her spine plus mild neurological weakness in her lower extremities. Laboratory evaluation is consistent with multiple myeloma. A magnetic resonance imaging (MRI) reveals involvement of multiple areas in spine with an early compression fracture at T7 and epidural disease with thecal sac impingement at T4. She is currently taking 10 mg of morphine immediate release every 4 h with minimal improvement.

You admit her to the hospital for management. She is given dexamethasone and radiation oncology is consulted to begin urgent treatment of the epidural disease. A continuous infusion of morphine is begun and a bowel regimen started. As an outpatient, her 24-h consumption was 60 mg. The iv equivalent would be 20 (oral:iv = 3:1). Given her severe pain, one could increase the dose 100%, but because the dexamethasone will also contribute to pain control, you begin an infusion at 1.5 mg/h sq. (36 mg/24 h). A PRN (or PCA) dose of 3 mg is available every 2 h. She is administered a dose of pamidronate.

At the completion of radiation therapy, her neurological function is normal and her pain is well-controlled at rest but with continued severe incident pain. At this time she is seen by a surgeon for vertebral augmentation. After the procedure, her incident pain is completely relieved and, she is converted to oral SR morphine 45 mg every 12 h (36 mg × 3 = 108 mg oral). She continues monthly pamidronate and chemotherapy for her myeloma.

In outpatient follow-up she is doing well except she feels she cannot stand up straight and finds her muscles tire as the day progresses. She is sent to orthotics for a corset for additional support. This effectively resolves her symptom.

10. SUMMARY

The management of pain related to spinal malignancy should proceed by the standards define by the World Health Organization and the American Pain Society. Given the numerous treatments available, there is no excuse for uncontrolled pain. Effective management requires a multidisciplinary team approach and integration of medical, surgical, rehabilitative, psychological, and spiritual modalities. Complimentary and alternative modalities may also be helpful for individual patients. Physicians managing these patients should be comfortable with the use of opioid medications and aware of the contribution of other modalities for appropriate consultation.

REFERENCES

1. Pargeon KL, Hailey BJ. Barriers to effective cancer management: a review of the literature. J Pain Symptom Manage 1999; 18:358–368.
2. Jacox A, Carr DB, Payne R, et al. Management of Cancer Pain: Adults. Clinical Practice Guideline No. 9 (no.95-0592). Rockville, MD: U.S. Department of Health and Human Services, Public Health Service; 1994.
3. World Health Organization. World Health Organization Technical Support Series. Cancer Pain Relief and Palliative Care (804). Geneva: WHO; 1990.
4. Hill CS Jr. The barriers to adequate pain management with opioid analgesics. Semin Oncol 1993; 20:1–5.
5. Kanner RM, Foley K. Patterns of narcotic drug use in a cancer pain clinic. Ann N Y Acad Sci 1981; 362:161–172.
6. Porter J, Jick H. Addiction rare in patients treated with narcotics. N Engl J Med 1980; 302:123.
7. Weissman DE, Haddox JD. Opioid pseudoaddiction –an iatrogenic syndrome. Pain 1989; 36:363–366.
8. Foley KM. Changing concepts of tolerance to opioids. What the cancer patient has taught us. In: Chapman CR, Foley KM, eds. Current and Emerging Issues in Cancer Pain: Research and Practice.. New York, NY: Raven Press; 1993:331–350.
9. Sawe J, Svensson JO, Rane A. Morphine metabolism in cancer patients on increasing oral doses–no evidence for autoinduction or dose dependence. Brit J of Clin Pharmacol 1983; 16:85–93.
10. Haegerstam GA. Pathophysiology of bone pain, a review. Acta Orthop Scand 2001; 72:308–317.
11. Ripamonti C, Fulfaro F. Malignant bone pain: pathophysiology and treatments. Current Review of Pain 2000; 4:187–196.
12. Payne R, Gonzalez, GR. Pathophysiology of pain in cancer and other terminal diseases. In: Doyle D, Hanks GW, MacDonald N, eds. Oxford Textbook of Palliative Medicine. . Oxford: Oxford Medical Publications; 1998:299-310.
13. World Health Organization. Cancer Pain Relief. Geneva. 1986.
14. Zech DFJ, Grond S, Lynch J, Hertel D, Lehmann KA. Validation of World Health Organization guidelines for cancer pain relief. A 10 year prospective study. Pain 1995; 634:65–76.
15. Allan L, Hays H, Jensen NH, et al. Randomized crossover trial of transdermal fentanyl and sustained release oral morphine for treating chronic non-cancer pain. Br Med J 2001; 322:1154–1158.
16. Radbruch L, Sabatowsku R, Loick G, Kulbe C, Kasper M, Grond S. Lehmann KA. Constipation and the use of laxatives: a comparison between transdermal fentayl and oral morphine. Palliat Med 2000; 14:111–119.
17. Kalso E, Vainio A. Morphine and oxycodone hydrochloride in the management of cancer pain. Clin Pharmacol Ther 1990; 47:639–646.
18. Poyhia R, Vainio A, Kalso EJ. A review of oxycodone's clinical pharmacokinetics and pharmacodynamics. J Pain Symptom Manage 1983; 8:63–67.

19. Weinberg DS, Inturrisi CE, Reidenberg B, et al. Sublingual absorption of selected opioid analgesics. Clin Pharmacol Ther 1998; 44:335–342.

20. Hoskins PJ, Hanks GW, Aherne GW, et al. The bioavailability and pharmacokinetics of morphine after intravenous, oral and buccal administration in healthy volunteers. Brit J Clin Pharmacology 1989; 27:499–505.

21. Ripamonti C, Bruera E. Rectal, buccal and sublingual narcotics for management of cancer pain. J Palliat Care 1991; 7:30–35

22. Glare PA, Walsh TD. Clinical pharmacokinetics of morphine. Ther Drug Monit 1990; 13:1–23.

23. Sarhill N, Walsh D, Nelson KA. Hydromorphone: pharmacology and clinical applications in cancer patients. Support Care Cancer 2001; 9:84–96.

24. Bruera E, Pereira J, Watanabe S, Hanson J. Opioid rotations in patients with cancer pain: a retrospective comparison of dose ratios between methadone, hydromorphone and morphine. Cancer 1996; 78:852–857.

25. Lawlor P, Turner K, Hanson J, Bruera E. Dose ratio between morphine and hydromorphone in patients with cancer pain: a retrospective study. Pain 1997; 72:79–85.

26. Miller MG, McCarthy N, O'Boyle CA, Kearney M. Continuous subcutaneous infusion of morphine vs. hydromorphone: a controlled trial. J Pain Symptom Manage 1999; 18:9–16.

27. Leow KP, Smith MT, Williams B, et al. Single-dose and steady-state pharmacokinetics and pharmacodynamics of oxycodone in patients with cancer. Clin Pharmacol Ther 1992; 52:487–495.

28. Davies G, Kingswood C, Street M. Pharmacokinetics of opioids in renal dysfunction. Clin Pharmacokinet 1996; 31:410–422.

29. Peng PW, Sandler AN. A review of the use of fentanyl analgesia in the management of acute pain in adults. Anesthesiology 1999; 90:576–579.

30. Southarn MA. Transdermal fentanyl therapy: system design, pharmacokinetics and efficacy. Anti-Cancer Drugs, 1995; 6(supplement 3):26-34.

31. Portenoy RK, Payne R Coluzzi P, et al. Oral Transmucosal fentanyl citrate (OTFC) for the treatment of breakthrough pain in cancers patients: a controlled dose titration study. Pain 1999; 79:303–312.

32. Chandler S. Oral transmucosal fentanyl citrate: a new treatment for breakthrough pain. Am J Hosp Palliat Care 1999; 16:489–491.

33. Gardner-Nix J. Oral transmucosal fentanyl and sufentanil for incident pain. Journal of pain and symptom management 2001; 22:627–631.

34. Inturrisi CE, Colburn WA, Kaiko RF, Houde RW, Foley KM. Pharmacokinetics and pharmacodynamics of methadone in patients with chronic pain. Clin Pharmacol Ther 1987; 41:392–401.

35. Davis MP, Walsh D. Methadone for relief of cancer pain: a review of pharmacokinetics, pharmacodynamics, drug interactions and protocols of administration. Support Care Cancer 2001; 9:73–83.

36. Ripamonti C, Zecca E, Bruera E. An update on the clinical use of methadone for cancer pain. Pain 1997; 70:109–115.

37. Mercadante S, Casuccio A, Fulfaro F, Groff L, Boffi R, Gebbia V, Ripamonti C. Switching from morphine to methadone to improve analgesia and tolerability in cancer patients: a prospective study. J Clin Oncol 2001; 19:2898–2904.

38. Morley JS, Makin MK. The use of methadone in cancer pain poorly responsive to other opioids. Pain Reviews 1998; 5:51–58.

39. Mathew P, Storey P. Subcutaneous methadone in terminally ill patients: manageable local toxicity. J Pain Symptom Manage 1999; 18:49–52.

40. Ripamonti C, Groff L, Brunelli C, Polastri D, Stavrakis A, De Conno F. Switching from morphine to oral methadone in treating cancer pain: what is the equianalgesic dose ratio? J Clin Oncol 1998; 16:3216–3221.

41. Ripamonti C, De Conno F, Groff L, et al. Equianalgesic dose/ratio between methadone and other opioid agonists in cancer pain: comparison of two clinical experiences. Ann Oncol 1998; 9:79–83.

42. Ripamonti C, Bianchi M. The use of methadone for cancer pain. Hematolo Oncol Clin North Am 2002; 16:543–555.

43. Dayer P, Collart L, Desmeules J. The pharmacology of tramadol. Drugs 1994; 47:3–7.

44. Raffa RB, Friderichs E, Reimann W, Shank RP, Codd EE, Vaught JL. Opioid and non-opioid components independently contribute to the mechanism of action of tramadol, an 'atypical' opioid analgesia. J Pharmacol Exp Ther 1992; 260:275–285.

45. Wilder-Smith CH, Schimke J, Osterwalder B, Senn HJ. Oral tramadol, a mu-opioid agonist and monoamine reuptake-blocker, and morphine for strong cancer-related pain. Ann Oncol 1994; 5:141–146.

46. Grond S, Zech D, Lynch J, Schug S, Lehmann KA. Tramadol-a weak opioid for relief of cancer pain. Pain Clinic 1992; 5:241–247.

47. Jick H, Derby LE, Vasilakis C, Fife D. The risk of seizures associated with tramadol. Pharmacotherapy 1998; 18:607–611.

48. Kahn LH, Alderfer RJ, Graham DJ. Seizures reported with tramadol. JAMA 1997; 278:1661.

49. Kaiko RF, Benziger DP, Fitzmartin RD, Burke BE, Reder RF, Goldenheim PD. Pharmacokinetic-pharmacodynamic relationships of controlled-release oxycodone. Clin Pharmacol Ther 1996; 59:52–61.

50. Savarese JJ, Goldenheim PD, Thomas GB, Kaiko RF. Steady-state pharmacokinetics of controlled release oral morphine sulphate in healthy subjects. Clin Pharmacokinet 1986; 11:505–510.

51. Davis M, Wilcock A. Modified release opioids. European Journal of Palliative Care 2001; 8:142–146.

52. Broomhead A, Kerr R, Tester W, et al. Comparison of a once-a-day sustained-release morphine formulation with standard oral morphine for treatment of cancer pain. J Pain Symptom Manage 1997; 14:63–73.

53. Portenoy RK, Sciberras A, Eliot L, Loewen G, Butler J, Devaine J. Steady-state pharmacokinetic comparison of a new, extended-release, once-daily morphine formulation, Avinza, and a twice-daily controlled-release morphine formulation in patients with chronic moderate-to-severe pain. J Pain Symptom Manage 2002;l 23:292–300.

54. Mandema JW, Kaiko RF, Oshlack B, Reder RF, Stanski DR. Characterization and validation of a pharmacokinetic model for controlled-release oxycodone. Br J Clin Pharmacol 1996; 46:747–756.

55. Warfield CA. Controlled-release morphine tablets in patients with chronic cancer pain. Cancer 1998; 82:2299–2306.

56. Hanks GW. Controlled release morphine tablets in chronic cancer pain: a review of controlled clinical trials. In: Benedetti C, Chapman CR, Giron G, eds. Advances in Pain Research and Therapy. Vol. 14. New York, NY: Raven Press; 1990:269–274.

57. Sindrup SH, Brosen K. The pharmacogenetics of codeine hypoalgesia. Pharmacogenetics 1995; 5:335–346.

58. Hagmeyer KO, Mauro LS, Mauro VE. Meperidine-related seizures associated with patient-controlled analgesia pumps. Ann Pharmacother 1993; 27:29–32.

59. Eisendrath SJ, Goldman B, Douglas J, Dimatteo L, Van Dyke C. Meperidine-induced delirium. Am J Psychiatry 1987; 144:1062–1065.

60. Kaiko RF, Foley KM, Grabinski PY, et al. Central nervous system excitatory effects of meperidine in cancer patients. Ann Neurol 1983; 13:180–185.

61. Hoskin PJ, Hanks GW. Opioid agonist-antagonist drugs in acute and chronic pain states. Drugs 1991; 41:326–344.

62. Portenoy RK. Management of common opioid side effects during long-term therapy of cancer pain. Ann Acad Med 1994; 23:160–170.

63. Hanks G, Cherny N. Opioid analgesic therapy. In: Doyle D, Hanks GWC, MacDonald N, eds. Oxford Textbook of Palliative Medicine. Oxford: Oxford Medical Publications; 1998:331–355.

64. Yee JD, Berde CB. Dextroamphetamine or methylphenidate as adjuvants to opioid analgesia for adolescents with cancer. J Pain Symptom Manage 1994; 9:122–125.

65. Kreeger L, Duncan A, Cowap J. Psychostimulants used for opioid-induced drowsiness. J Pain Symptom Manage 1996; 11:1–2.

66. Bruera E, Chadwick S, Brenneis C, Hanson J, Mac Donald N. Methylphenidate associated with narcotics in the treatment of cancer pain. Cancer Treat Rep 1987; 71:67–70.

67. Charuluxanan S, Kyokong O, Somboonviboon W, Lertmaharit S, Mgamprasertwong P. Nalbuphine versus propofol for treatment of

intrathecal morphine-induced pruritis after cesarean delivery. Anesth Analg 2001; 93:162–165.

68. Somrat C, Oranuch K, Ketchada U, Siriprapa S, Thipawan R. Optimal dose of nalbuphine for treatment of intrathecal morphine-induced pruritis after caesarian section. J Obstet Gynaecol Res 1999; 25:209–213.

69. Bruera E, MacMillan E, Hanson J, et al. The cognitive effects of the administration of narcotic analgesics in patients with cancer pain. Pain 1989; 39:13–16.

70. Walsh, D. Pharmacological management of cancer pain. Semin Oncol 2000; 27:45–63.

71. Mercandante S. Pathophysiology and treatment of opioid-related myoclonus in cancer patients. Pain 1998; 74:5–9.

72. Hagen N, Swanson R. Strychnine-like multifocal myoclonus and seizures in extremely high-dose opioid administration. J Pain Symptom Manage 1997; 14:81–88.

73. Ferris DJ. Controlling myoclonus after high-dosage morphine infusions. Am J Health Syst Pharm 1999; 56:1009–1010.

74. Bruera E, Suarea-Almazor M, Velason A, et al. The assessment of constipation in terminal cancer patients admitted to a palliative care unit: A retrospective review. J Pain Symptom Manage 1994; 9:515–519.

75. Schmidt WK. Alvimmopan (ADL 8-2698) is a novel peripheral opioid antagonist. Am J Surg 18:27s–38s.

76. Foss JF. A review of the potential role of methylnaltrexone in opioid bowel dysfunction. Am J Surg 2001; 172:19s–26s.

77. Borgbjerg FM, Neilsen K, Franks J. Experimental pain stimulates respiration and attenuates morphine-induced respiratory depression: a controlled study in human volunteers. Pain 1996; 64:123–128.

78. Moertel GG: Treatment of cancer pain with orally administered medications. JAMA 1980; 244:2448–2450.

79. Caraceni A, Gorni G, Zecca E, De Conno F. More on the use of nonsteroidal anti-inflammatories in the management of cancer pain. J Pain Symptom Manage 2001; 21:89–91.

80. Jenkins CA, Bruera E. Non-steroidal anti-inflammatory drugs as adjuvant analgesics in cancer patients. Palliat Med 1999; 13:183–196.

81. Mannix K, Ahmedzai SH, Anderson H, Bennett M, Lloyd-Williams M, Wilcock A. Using bisphosphonates to control the pain of bone metastases: evidence-based guidelines for palliative care. Palliat Med 2000; 14:455–461.

82. Koeberle D, Bacchus L, Thuerlimann B, Senn HJ. Pamidronate treatment in patients with malignant osteolytic bone disease and pain: a prospective randomized double-blind trial. Support Care Cancer 1999; 7:21–27.

83. Hutborn R, Gunderson S, Ryden S, et al. Efficacy of pamidronate in breast cancer with bone metastases: a randomized, double blind placebo controlled multicenter study. Anticancer Res 1999; 19:3383–3392.

84. Vogel CL, Yanagihara RH, Wood AL, et al. Safety and pain palliation of zoledronic acid in patients with breast cancer, prostate cancer, or multiple myeloma who previously received bisphosphonate therapy. Oncologist 2004; 9:687–695.

85. Wong R, Wiffen PJ. Bisphosphonates for the relief of pain secondary to bone metastases. Cochrane Database Syst Rev 2005; 3.

86. Durie BG, Katz M, Crowley J. Osteonecrosis of the jaw and bisphosphonates. N Engl J Med 2005; 353:99–102.

87. Shakespeare DT, Boggild M, Young C. Anti-spasticity agents for multiple sclerosis. Cochrane Database Syst Rev 2001; 4:CD001332.

88. Taricco M, Adone R, Pagliacci C, Telaro E. Pharmacological interventions for spasticity following spinal cord injury. Cochrane Database of Syst Rev 2000; 2:CD001131.

89. Loblaw DA, Laperriere NJ. Emergency treatment of malignant spinal cord compression: an evidence-based guideline. J Clin Oncol 1998; 16:1613–1624.

90. Portenoy, RK. Adjuvant analgesics in pain management. In: Doyle D, Hanks GWC, MacDonald, N, eds. Oxford Textbook of Palliative Medicine.. Oxford: Oxford Medical Publications; 1998.

91. Sorenson S, Helweg-Larsen S. Mouridsen H, Hansen HH. Effect of high-dose dexamethasone in carcinomatous metastatic spinal cord compression treated with radiotherapy: a randomized trial. Eur J Cancer 1994; 30:22–27.

92. Vecht CJ, Haaxma-Reiche H, van Putten WL, de Visser M, Vries EP, Twijnstra A. Initial bolus of conventional versus high-dose dexamethasone in metastatic spinal cord compression. Neurology 1989; 39:1255–1257.

93. Heimdal K, Hirschberg H, Slettebo H, Watne K, Nome O. High incidence of serious side effects of high-dose dexamethasone treatment in patients with spinal cord compression. J Neurooncol 1992; 12:141–144.

94. Lynch ME. Antidepressants as analgesic: a review of randomized controlled trials. J Psychiatry Neurosci 2001; 26:30–36.

95. Sindrup SH, Jensen TS. Efficacy of pharmacological treatments of neuropathic pain: an update and effect related to mechanism of action. Pain. 83:389–400.

96. Ansari A. The efficacy of newer antidepressants in the treatment of chronic pain: a review of the literature. Harv Rev of Psychiatry 2000; 7:257–277.

97. Sumpton JE, Moulin DE. Treatment of neuropathic pain with venlafaxine. Ann Pharmacother 2001; 35:557–559.

98. Wiffen P, Collins S, McQuay H, Carroll D, Jadad A, Moore A. Anticonvulsant drugs for acute and chronic pain. Cochrane Database Syst Rev. 2000; 3:CD001133.

99. Hindley AC, Hill EB, Leyland MJ, Wiles AE. A double blind controlled trial of salmon calcitonin in pain due to malignancy. Cancer Chemother Pharmacol 1982; 9:71–74.

100. Allan E. Calcitonin in the treatment of intractable pain for advanced malignancy. Pharmatherapeutica 1983; 3:482–486.

101. Pecile A. Calcitonin and relief of pain. Bone Miner 1992; 16:187–189.

102. Schiraldi GF, Soresi E, Locicero S, Harari S, Scoccia S. Salmon calcitonin in cancer pain: comparison between two different treatment schedules. Int J Clin Pharmacol Ther Toxicol 1987; 25:229–232.

103. Szanto J, Ady N, Jozsef S. Pain killing with calcitonin nasal spray in patients with malignant tumors. Oncology 1992; 49:180–182.

104. Blanchard J, Menk E, Ramamurthy S, Hoffman J. Subarachnoid and epidural calcitonin in patients with pain due to metastatic cancer. J Pain Symptom Manage 1990; 5:42–45.

105. Cherny NI, Arbit E, Jain S. Invasive techniques in the management of cancer pain. Hematol Oncol Clin North Am 1996; 10:121–137.

106. Hogan Q, Haddox JD, Abram S, Weissman D, Taylor ML, Janjan N. Epidural opiates and local anesthetics for the management of cancer pain. Pain 1991; 46:291–299.

107. Bedder MD, Burchiel K, Larson A. Cost analysis of two implantable narcotic delivery systems. J Pain Symptom Manage 1991; 6:368–373.

108. Meenan D, Lagares-Garcia JA, Kurek S. Craig D, Green J, Fritz W. Managing intractable pain with an intrathecal catheter and injection port: technique and guidelines. Am Surg 1999; 65:1054–1060.

109. Pereira J, Lawlor P, Vigano A, Dorgan M, Bruera E. Equianalgesic dose ratios for opioids: a critical review and proposals for long-term dosing. J Pain Symptom Manage 2001; 22:672–687.

42 Surveillance and Screening During Disease-Free Survival

RICHARD PLACIDE, MD, KAI-UWE LEWANDROWSKI, MD,
AND ROBERT F. MCLAIN, MD

CONTENTS

1. INTRODUCTION

After surgery for cancer of the spine, follow-up care to detect recurrence is an expected part of the overall postoperative care. Components of disease-free surveillance include periodic physical examinations, radiological studies, and blood work to follow or detect tumor markers. Establishing standards for routine follow-up may be difficult owing to the variability of cancers involving the spine (low-grade sarcomas, high-grade sarcomas, and metastatic disease) and the extent of involvement throughout the spine or body.

Cancer screening has been undertaken in certain populations to try to detect early stages of various cancers in hopes of providing earlier and more effective treatment (1–3). However, in the case of spinal surgery for cancer, the follow-up care changes from screening to detect early cancer to more frequent and, in some cases, aggressive surveillance to detect recurrence.

When following a patient after cancer surgery of the spine, whether the disease is a primary tumor or a metastatic process, periodic follow-up is necessary to assess patients' functional status and to evaluate for cancer recurrence. Unfortunately, there are no standards to guide the spine surgeon regarding the frequency of follow-up appointments or what sort of testing (blood work and radiographic imaging) should be performed. There are, however, certain factors outlined in this chapter that may help determine the aggressiveness of required follow-up care.

Most importantly, follow-up must not be neglected, either by the patient or their caregiver. Five years of disease-free survival does not suggest that the patient with a chondrosarcoma or chordoma of the spine is "out of the woods." Likewise, any patient with a history of spinal neoplasia presenting with the cardinal signs of systemic disease (weight loss, fatigue, malaise, pain, night pain, neurological impairment) should be re-evaluated with respect to both local (spinal) disease and systemic spread.

2. CLINICAL GUIDELINES FOR CANCER SURVEILLANCE

Clinical surveillance programs for spinal cancer following surgical resection largely dependent on (1) the type of the primary lesion, (2) its stage, (3) or in the case of sarcomas its grade (high- vs low-grade), and (4) the extent of spine involvement. These for factors directly impact the potential for a cure. Obviously, the smaller the tumor, the more feasible it becomes to perform a wide excision with clean margins. Typically, overall management should mimic the treatment of the primary lesion whether that is some type of adenocarcinoma metastatic to the spine, or a sarcoma or some other type of tumor arising from the spine. Clinical practice guidelines have been developed by expert panels of the American Society of Clinical Oncology for cancer surveillance for some types of tumors that may metastasize to the spine. Some of these clinic practice guidelines will be reviewed in the following sections (4,5).

From: *Current Clinical Oncology: Cancer in the Spine: Comprehensive Care.*
Edited by: R. F. McLain, K-U. Lewandrowski, M. Markman, R. M. Bukowski,
R. Macklis, and E. C. Benzel © Humana Press, Inc., Totowa, NJ

3. SURVEILLANCE AND FOLLOW-UP CARE FOR BREAST CANCER

Most recurrences of breast cancer occur within the first 5 yr after the primary therapy (6–9). Coordination of care is encouraged and should be performed at regular intervals by a health care provider, who is experienced in cancer surveillance programs and in breast examination, including the examination of irradiated breasts (10).

3.1. HISTORY AND PHYSICAL EXAMINATION

"All women should have a careful history every 3 to 6 mo for the first 3 yr after primary therapy, then every 6 to 12 mo for the next 2 yr, then annually. It is prudent to recommend that all women perform monthly breast self-examination" (11).

3.2. MAMMOGRAPHY

Annual mammography is recommend in all women previously diagnosed with breast cancer (11). In women who underwent breast-conserving therapy, a post-treatment mammogram should be performed 6 mo after completion of radiotherapy (6,11). Moreover, it should be performed for surveillance of abnormalities or annually. Once mammographic findings were found to be stable, yearly mammographic evaluations may be performed thereafter (6,11). However, women should be informed about symptoms of recurrence because most recurrences may occur between scheduled visits (8).

3.3. UNNECESSARY ROUTINE SURVEILLANCE FOR BREAST CANCER

There is no sufficient data to support the routine use of complete blood count, basic chemistry studies, chest X-rays, bone scans, ultrasounds of the liver, and computed tomography (CT) (6,11). In addition, a number of breast cancer tumor markers have been found to be unsuitable for routine surveillance. These include the cancer antigen CA 15-3, the CA 27.29 tumor marker, and the carcinoembryonic antigen (CEA) (6,11).

4. SURVEILLANCE AND FOLLOW-UP CARE FOR COLORECTAL CANCER

According to The American Society of Clinical Oncology, which publishes evidence-based clinical practice guidelines on colorectal cancer surveillance, the following clinical practice guidelines for surveillance of colorectal cancer have been recommended by an expert panel (12–15).

4.1. HISTORY AND PHYSICAL EXAMINATION

Although there is very little clinical data to support that history and physical examination influences outcomes of colorectal cancer surveillance, it is recommended that a clinical history and pertinent physical examination should be performed every 3 to 6 mo for the first 3 yr and annually thereafter (16,17).

4.2. CARCINOEMBRYONIC ANTIGEN

If resection of liver metastases was required, postoperative serum CEA testing should be performed every 2 to 3 mo in patients with stage II or III disease for 2 yr or more after diagnosis. If an elevated CEA level is found and confirmed by retesting further work-up for metastatic disease is recommended. However, this typically does not justify the institution of systemic therapy for presumed metastatic disease (13,18,19).

The utility of CEA testing was demonstrated in a study from the Eastern Cooperative Oncology Group, who followed 421 patients with recurrent disease after surgical resection for high-risk stage B2 and C colon carcinoma. "For the subgroup of resectable patients, the first test to detect recurrence was the CEA test (n = 30), chest X-ray (n = 12), colonoscopy (n = 14), and other tests (n = 40)." This study did not show that physical examination was able in finding resectable disease (19).

4.3. COLONOSCOPY AND FLEXIBLE PROCTOSIGMOIDOSCOPY

It is recommended that all patients should have a colonoscopy pre-operatively and postoperatively. Clinical evidence suggests that colonoscopy should be performed every 3 to 5 yr and not as routine annual colonoscopies. Guidelines differ somewhat for rectal cancer, particularly in individuals who did not have combined chemotherapy and pelvic radiation for stages II and III rectal cancer. In these patients, periodic inspection of the rectum via flexible proctosigmoidoscopy is recommended at periodic intervals. By contrast, patients who did receive pelvic radiation, "direct imaging of the rectum (except for colonoscopy at 3 to 5 years) is not suggested" (13,15,18,19).

4.4. UNNECESSARY ROUTINE SURVEILLANCE FOR COLORECTAL CANCER

In asymptomatic patients, who have received surgical resection and radiation for colorectal cancer, data are sufficient to suggest against routine pelvic imaging or CT. In addition, there is no sufficient data to support the routine use of liver function tests, or testing for fecal occult blood, and complete blood count. A chest X-ray should be ordered only to evaluate pulmonary abnormalities prompted by an elevated CEA test or for patients with symptomatic pulmonary disease suggestive of metastasis (15).

5. SURVEILLANCE AND FOLLOW-UP CARE FOR LUNG CANCER

5.1. HISTORY AND PHYSICAL EXAMINATION

"For patients treated with curative intent, in the absence of symptoms, a history and physical examination should be performed every 3 months during the first 2 years, every 6 months thereafter through year 5, and yearly thereafter" (4,5).

5.2. CHEST RADIOGRAPHS

"For patients treated with curative intent, there is no clear role for routine studies in asymptomatic patients and for those in whom no interventions are planned. A yearly chest X-ray to evaluate for potentially curable second primary cancers may be reasonable" (20).

5.3. UNNECESSARY ROUTINE SURVEILLANCE FOR LUNG CANCER

In asymptomatic patients and those patients not undergoing therapeutic interventions, there is no proven benefit of routine CT scan of the chest/abdomen; CT scan/magnetic resonance imaging (MRI) of the brain, fluorodeoxyglucose-positron emission tomography scan, bone scan, bronchoscopy; complete blood count, and routine chemistries and liver function tests. These tests should only be performed if recurrence is suspected (20–22).

5.4. LOW-DOSE HELICAL CHEST CT

This test has been found to be more sensitive than chest X-ray for the identification of second primary cancers. However, its merit has only been investigated for non-small cell lung cancer and has been deemed investigational for routine follow-up of patients with unresectable disease (20).

6. SURVEILLANCE AND FOLLOW-UP CARE FOR PLASMACYTOMA AND MYELOMA

6.1. HISTORY AND PHYSICAL EXAMINATION

Patients treated for solitary plasmacytoma may survive disease-free for decades before the malignant form of the disease emerges. Annual or biannual serum immunoglobulin profiles provide the most reasonable and sensitive form of surveillance. Radiographs are not sensitive to early lesions, and bone scans may appear negative even in patients with known bony disease. The patient presenting with fatigue, malaise, and anemia should spark concern in their physician.

6.2. CHEST RADIOGRAPHS

Recurrence of disease involves the bones, and skeletal manifestations are seen first. Chest X-ray may be remarkable only for osteoporosis and compression fractures, but these herald the emergence of myeloma in its malignant state.

6.3. ROUTINE SURVEILLANCE FOR MULTIPLE MYELOMA

In many patients the disease course of myeloma never gives enough respite to allow a surveillance period. Suppressive therapy and bone marrow transplantation are providing longer survivals, however, and even patients with persistent disease may enjoy long periods of symptom-free survival. Follow-up must include careful scrutiny of red cell counts, as well as surveys of marrow aspirates for plasma cell concentrations. Routine assay of serum immunoglobulins will signal an increase in the pathological cell line early on, allowing modification of suppressive therapy.

6.4. SPINE IMAGING

Spinal involvement is very common among myeloma patients. Spinal compression fractures are a major cause of pain and dysfunction. Identifying fractures when back pain first occurs can allow earlier intervention before deformity becomes profound. Screening studies (MRI) can demonstrate the extent of disease and guide prophylactic treatment of impending fractures through kyphoplasty or vertebraplasty techniques.

7. SURVEILLANCE AND FOLLOW-UP CARE FOR SARCOMA

Sarcomas of soft tissue and bone must be irradicated locally if long-term survival is expected. Local recurrence is often the first sign of treatment failure, and may be seen before systemic spread in some cases. Surveillance of the local tumor bed is crucial for early detection of recurrence.

Patient should undergo careful examination of the tumor site for any evidence of nodules or mass that may herald recurrence of tumor in the suture-line or margins of the resection. An MRI at 3 to 6 mo may still be confusing owing to edema and scar formation, but between 6 mo and 1 yr the tissues should be stable and new masses or nodules should be distinguishable from more benign conditions. Annual MRI is advisable from then on.

After 7 to 10 yr, it is reasonable in many cases to progress to every 2-yr MRI, but chordoma and chondrosarcoma patients should still be followed on an annual basis, as disease progression at the 7 to 10 yr point is still quite common.

On the anniversary of completing the treatment protocol indicated for the given sarcoma, a complete screening study is indicated. Sedimentation rate, bone scan and pulmonary CT are carried out, and abdominal CT or ultrasound to evaluate the liver.

Any recurrence of pain at the resection site, or any signs of systemic disease should trigger an aggressive screening study in any patient thought to have obtained a disease-free status.

REFERENCES

1. Grunfeld E, Gray A, Mant D, et al. Follow-up of breast cancer in primary care vs specialist care: results of an economic evaluation. Br J Cancer 1999; 79:1227–1233.
2. Grunfeld E, Mant D, Yudkin P, et al. Routine follow up of breast cancer in primary care: randomised trial. BMJ 1996; 313:665–669.
3. Winn RJ. The role of oncology clinical practice guidelines in the managed care era. Oncology (Huntingt) 1995; 9:177–183.
4. Smith RA, Cokkinides V, von Eschenbach AC, et al. American Cancer Society guidelines for the early detection of cancer. CA Cancer J Clin 2002; 52:8–22.
5. Smith TJ, Somerfield MR. The ASCO experience with evidence-based clinical practice guidelines. Oncology (Huntingt) 1997; 11:223–227.
6. American Society of Clinical Oncology. Recommended breast cancer surveillance guidelines. J Clin Oncol 1997;15:2149–2156.
7. Grunfeld E, Mant D, Vessey MP, Fitzpatrick R. Specialist and general practice views on routine follow-up of breast cancer patients in general practice. Fam Pract 1995; 12:60–65.
8. Lelli G, Indelli M, Modonesi C, Gulmini L, Durante E. [Clinical postoperative surveillance of breast carcinoma]. Recenti Prog Med 2002; 93:637–641.
9. Levin M. Breast cancer: issues in risk reduction, screening and surveillance, early identification and therapy planning. Drug News Perspect 2003; 16:395–398.
10. Truong PT, Olivotto IA, Whelan TJ, Levine M. Clinical practice guidelines for the care and treatment of breast cancer: 16. Locoregional post-mastectomy radiotherapy. CMAJ 2004; 170:1263–1273.
11. Smith TJ, Davidson NE, Schapira DV, et al. American Society of Clinical Oncology 1998 update of recommended breast cancer surveillance guidelines. J Clin Oncol 1999; 17:1080–1082.
12. American Society of Clinical Oncology. 1997 update of recommendations for the use of tumor markers in breast and colorectal cancer. Adopted on November 7, 1997 by the American Society of Clinical Oncology. J Clin Oncol 1998; 16:793–795.
13. Bast RC, Jr., Ravdin P, Hayes DF, et al. 2000 update of recommendations for the use of tumor markers in breast and colorectal cancer: clinical practice guidelines of the American Society of Clinical Oncology. J Clin Oncol 2001; 19:1865–1878.
14. Benson AB, III, Desch CE, Flynn PJ, et al. 2000 update of American Society of Clinical Oncology colorectal cancer surveillance guidelines. J Clin Oncol 2000; 18:3586–3588.
15. Smith RA, von Eschenbach AC, Wender R, et al. American Cancer Society guidelines for the early detection of cancer: update of early detection guidelines for prostate, colorectal, and endometrial cancers. Also: update 2001—testing for early lung cancer detection. CA Cancer J Clin 2001; 51:38–75.
16. American Society of Clinical Oncology. Clinical practice guidelines for the use of tumor markers in breast and colorectal cancer. Adopted on May 17, 1996 by the American Society of Clinical Oncology. J Clin Oncol 1996; 14:2843–2877.
17. Cooper GS, Yuan Z, Chak A, and Rimm AA. Geographic and patient variation among Medicare beneficiaries in the use of follow-up testing after surgery for nonmetastatic colorectal carcinoma. Cancer 1999; 85:2124–2131.
18. Desch CE, Benson AB, III, Smith TJ, et al. Recommended colorectal cancer surveillance guidelines by the American Society of Clinical Oncology. J Clin Oncol 1999; 17:1312.

19. Graham RA, Wang S, Catalano PJ, Haller DG. Postsurgical surveillance of colon cancer: preliminary cost analysis of physician examination, carcinoembryonic antigen testing, chest x-ray, and colonoscopy. Ann Surg 1998; 228:59–63.

20. Pfister DG, Johnson DH, Azzoli CG, et al. American Society of Clinical Oncology treatment of unresectable non-small-cell lung cancer guideline: update 2003. J Clin Oncol 2004; 22:330–353.

21. American Society of Clinical Oncology. Clinical practice guidelines for the treatment of unresectable non-small-cell lung cancer. Adopted on May 16, 1997 by the American Society of Clinical Oncology. J Clin Oncol 1997; 15:2996–3018.

22. Valk PE, Pounds TR, Tesar RD, Hopkins DM, Haseman MK. Cost-effectiveness of PET imaging in clinical oncology. Nucl Med Biol 1996; 23:737–743.

43   When Is Enough, Enough?

Edward C. Benzel, md, Michael P. Steinmetz, md, Ann M. Henwood, rn, msn, L. Brett Babat, md, and Anis O. Mekhail, md

Contents

1. INTRODUCTION

Many factors are involved in the decision-making process regarding the management of spinal tumor patients. Metastatic spine disease poses clinical and ethical dilemmas that are arguably second to none in all of medicine. Many considerations complicate this decision-making process. These include change in the quality of life, life expectancy (and its uncertainty), treatment costs, structural integrity of the spine, and the patient's fears and expectations. Each of these are addressed and are considered as they pertain to the decision-making process regarding the question, "When is enough, enough?"

In most cases, surgery in the setting of spinal metastasis is palliative: that is, cure is not possible. The goal of palliative medicine is to relieve suffering (mainly pain) and provide stability (if appropriate). The pioneers of modern hospice care were the Irish Sisters of Charity, founded by Sister Mary Aikenhead. In 1879, they opened Our Lady's Hospice for the Dying in Dublin. However, it was Dame Cicely Saunders (nurse, social worker, and physician) of Great Britain, who introduced the principle of relief from suffering rather than medical intervention for disease management, now known as palliative care *(1,2)*. According to Dunn *(1)*, Medicare Hospice Benefit eligibility criteria dictates that hospice care should begin when an individual has 6 mo or less of life expectancy, assuming the disease would run its usual course. Palliative care programs were born of the economic need and social concern

for those individuals who did not fit the Medicare Hospice Benefit criteria (i.e., individuals who had terminal illness but had >6 mo to live).

In 1975, Balfour Mount, a surgeon, introduced the term palliative care on the opening of a new consulting service and in-patient unit at the Royal Victoria Hospital in Montreal. He reported to Dunn that the word *hospice* in French was ultimately a word associated with negative meaning such as "institutional care for the indigent dying" *(1)*. In its place, the Latin word *pallium* was selected. In Latin this word means to cloak or cover, but in the Oxford English Dictionary the word palliate means to alleviate, mitigate, to lessen pain, and to give temporary relief *(1)*. When discussing patients with spinal tumors, more specifically those with cancer that has metastasized to the spine, palliation may be an important option. For some patients, surgery may be curative, for others, it can only be palliative.

The World Health Organization defines palliative care in general terms "the active total care of patients whose disease is not responsive to curative treatment *(3)*. Control of pain, of other symptoms, and of psychological, social, and spiritual problems is paramount. The goal of palliative care is achievement of the best quality of life for patients and their families" *(4)*. At this time, the literature is quite sparse regarding palliative surgery recommendations or standards. Miner et al. *(5)* conducted a review of the surgical palliative literature. They included articles published from 1990 to 1996. The 348 citations were evaluated according to the following elements and the percentage of articles in which the element was addressed: physiological response to the intervention (69%), survival (64%), morbidity and mortality (61%), need to repeat the inter-

From: *Current Clinical Oncology: Cancer in the Spine: Comprehensive Care.*
Edited by: R. F. McLain, K-U. Lewandrowski, M. Markman, R. M. Bukowski,
R. Macklis, and E. C. Benzel © Humana Press, Inc., Totowa, NJ

vention (59%), quality of life (17%), pain control (12%), and cost (2%). The elements most difficult to quantify (quality of life, pain control, and cost) were observed the least frequently in the 348 citations. However, they are also the elements that should be given the greatest consideration during the decision-making process for palliative surgery.

Very general recommendations for palliative surgery are mentioned in the surgical literature. Ball et al. *(6)* have outlined the five essential roles of surgical palliation as are paramount in regards to spinal metastasis: (1) initial evaluation of the disease, (2) local control of the disease, (3) control of discharge or hemorrhage, (4) control of pain, and (5) reconstruction and rehabilitation. In addition, The American College of Surgeons has drafted a Statement of Principles Guiding Care at the End Life. In light of the information available, the question remains, "When is enough, enough?" for the patient undergoing palliation spine surgery.

2. LIFE EXPECTANCY AND QUALITY OF LIFE

Two major factors deserve much attention when managing patients with metastatic spine tumors. These are life expectancy and quality of life. The two are now mutually exclusive and are often considered together, as described next. The life expectancy of a patient with metastatic spine cancer is affected by many variables. These include tumor burden and its control, tumor histology, and the patient's clinical history. Some tumors take a more "benign course" than others. Many surgeons would consider a 6-mo life expectancy to be acceptable for the recommendation for aggressive therapy. Others may feel that 3 mo is adequate, while still others would restrict this type of therapy to those with a reasonable estimated life expectancy of 1 yr or more. However, the patient may consider 1 mo or even less, to be a reasonable amount of time for a chance at an improved quality of life. Quality of life must be a major determinant of treatment strategy, and cannot be overemphasized. However, the physician and patient must remain realistic in their goal to improve quality of life. If a patient presents with severe back pain owing to vertebral body tumor involvement, but has only 3 mo to live, it would not be appropriate to perform a large spine operation in which the patient could not be expected to be free of postoperative pain until 3 mo after surgery. One must be reasonable and not be unduly pessimistic or optimistic during the decision-making process. The patient and the patient's family, as well as the treating physician, must all be realistic, and most importantly, honest about outcome, life expectancy, and quality of life.

An interesting prospective, randomized study by Sugarbaker et al. *(7)* assessed the quality of life following palliative surgery in 26 patients with extremity sarcoma. Interventions for the two groups were either extremity amputation and chemotherapy or limb-sparing surgery, radiation therapy, and chemotherapy. To the researchers' surprise, the patients who underwent amputation and potentially more life-threatening procedures had a higher quality of life. This underscores the importance of refraining from projecting preconceived notions about the quality of life onto patients who may be candidates for palliative surgery. It is vital that all options be taken into consideration, including

the extremes of aggressive surgery and no treatment at all. This requires open, honest discussions between the surgeon, the patient, and the patient's family. The patient's expectations and goals should be fully realized. This must be reflected in the final treatment plan.

Since the Sugarbaker et al. *(7)* study 30 yr ago, health-related quality of life instruments have been developed and applied to patients with cancer and chronic disease, generally to compare treatment outcomes in the context of clinical trials *(5)*. They came to the conclusion that no single "health related quality of life instrument would fit all the recommended conditions or is suitable in all clinical situations," though appropriate instruments may be helpful in identifying the optimal surgical procedure. For decision-making in the palliative surgery setting, such instruments are best used in conjunction with other indicators of quality of life, especially when the patient's situation is borderline and the decision-making process is complicated.

3. COST

Cost must be considered during the decision to perform an operation or other aggressive management paradigmt. The performance of an operation in a patient with metastatic spine cancer increases the cost of care substantially, often in excess of $100,000. Obviously, both life expectancy (*see* Subheading 2.) and bone integrity (*see* Subheading 6.) are important in this process, as is the operation that is selected. Simple operations are less costly than more extensive ones. The addition of spinal instrumentation greatly increases the cost of any procedure. Although cost is extremely important, individual patient characteristics should be considered first. If instrumentation is indicated, it should be utilized.

As Miner et al. *(5)* revealed, of the 348 citations reviewed, only 2% discussed cost with regard to palliation surgeries. Little is known about the effectiveness or cost of various ends of life therapies *(8)*. There are no current articles discussing surgical palliation for spine metastasis and cost. When considering a simple or complex palliative spine surgical procedure, cost vs benefit, and the overall health of the patient must be considered. Considered factors specific to the cancer patient should include: age, immunosupression, anorexia, cachexia, nutrition, steroid use, pulmonary function, hypocoaguability, deep vein thrombosis, and wound healing issues *(9)*. Ultimately, management of the tumor burden, type of surgery selected, implant selection, and co-morbidities will affect cost of care, as well as pain and suffering. The latter considers elements such as emotional (uncertainty, anxiety, low mood, communication breakdown costs), social (lifestyle disruption, role change, stigma), and physical distress (symptoms) *(5)*. The surgeon, the patient, and the patient's family must weigh cost against benefit on a case-by-case basis. Ultimately, what is best for the patient is chosen *(10)*.

4. PATIENT FEARS AND EXPECTATIONS

The primary concern and focus during the decision-making process should be the patient, as well as the patient's family. The terminal patient has many fears and expectations that may not be appreciated by the treating physician. The patient is often not as afraid of dying as of the unknown and of pain. Kushner discusses these issues in great detail *(11)*. His work demonstrated that terminal patients are predominantly afraid of two things: pain and abandonment. Therefore, open, honest discussions between the patient, the patient's family, and the treating physician should be the first priority. The patient's expectations and fears should be truly acknowledged. Moreover, the surgeon should clearly explain the extent of the patient's disease and prognosis. This should be coupled with the most appropriate treatment for the patient. Not necessarily all possible treatments for many would not be appropriate. The management of pain and the encouragement and involvement of family, as well as the inclusion of significant physician involvement and support of the patient is of paramount importance. A network including the patient, the patient's family, treating physician, social worker, palliative medicine and personnel should be assembled when appropriate.

Realistic expectations are imperative. The patient must verbalize regarding his/her mortality and understand the terminal nature of his/her disease, as well as understand and appreciate the realistic life expectancy. Neither the patient nor their family can make realistic decisions if this information is not shared with them. This involves a significant and, often times, emotionally draining informed decision-making process, where the patient and the patient's family confront the patient's mortality, life expectancy, and realistic expectations. A realistic description of the quality of life after a possible spine operation, as well as a realistic appraisal of the possible complications should be provided. If surgery will not fulfill the expectations, a large reconstructive procedure may not be appropriate.

The patient and the patient's family should understand that the primary goals of treatment are pain relief, function preservation, and quality-of-life extension. If there are indications for surgery, the patient clearly appreciates them, whether they are pain, instability, or neurological deficits. They should also appreciate the risks of surgery, the chance of achieving its goals, and long term consequences.

5. SURGEON EXPECTATIONS

In treating the patient with spinal metastasis, the surgeon is influenced by many variables. These include compassion, intellectual stimulation, financial factors, and feelings of helplessness. One should not fall into the trap of assuming that "when nothing else is working, surgery will." Surgeons must be honest with themselves and their patients while recognizing and preventing futile attempts at surgical intervention. Many surgical avenues are open and available to the spine surgeon. Almost all, from the simplest to the most complete, are essentially "possible" in almost every patient. The surgeon's frame of thinking should change from "What surgery can I do?" to "What surgery should I do, if any?" for the particular patient. Just because an operation can be performed, even with the patient's best interest in mind, it may lead to the patient experiencing increased suffering (i.e., pain, neurological deficit) during his/her final days of life. The informed decision-making process is much more than an informed consent. It involves an ongoing

dialogue and interchange. The potential for patient and family denial must be considered, further emphasizing the need for honesty. The treating physician must also be cognizant of the five phases of the patient's response to death and dying: (1) denial and isolation, (2) anger, (3) bargaining, (4) depression, and (5) acceptance *(12)*. Determining the stage the patient is experiencing plays a vital role in the decision-making process.

One must be very careful to ensure that the patient's denial does not permit them to unrealistically appraise the situation. A physician may state that the patient has a "chance to improve quality and length of life," whereas the patient hears "chance for cure." The physician must always maintain a high index of suspicion that the patient is not receiving the appropriate message under these circumstances.

6. BONE INTEGRITY

Bone integrity plays a major role in the decision-making process in patients with metastatic spine cancer. Metastatic cancer frequently affects multiple spinal levels, diminishing the structural integrity of any construct. One must be concerned about the possibility of myelophistic disease (extensive and often occult tumor involvement of multiple spinal segments), as well as osteoporosis. These issues affect cases in which spinal implants are planned and in those in which they are not. Often, a focal level of pathology is identified, for example, a midthoracic pathologic fracture. A relatively short segment construct (i.e., pedicle screw fixation two levels above and below the fracture) may be initially planned. Poor bone quality or myelophistic disease may dictate significantly extending the length of the dorsal construct. This may then necessitate an extensive spinal reconstruction. This procedure is likely beyond the patient's expectations and the surgeon's goals and, furthermore, may substantially add to the cost of caring for the patient. All may then agree that "enough is enough" and manage the patient with other conservative measures, such as bracing.

The issue of bone quality may also come into play when considering more "conservative" procedures in patients with spinal metastasis. Perhaps a simple two-level laminectomy may be appropriate for the management of spinal metastasis in a patient with myelopathy. Even though deformity or a fracture are not present, one may be required to provide stabilization (i.e., instrumentation) to prevent deformity progression and worsening neurological status following decompression. This is often performed without a fusion. Again, one must return to quality of life issues to determine if an extensive operation is appropriate.

7. CASE

In order to illustrate and illuminate many of the factors addressed in the prior pages, a complex case, from a decision-making perspective, is presented.

Mrs. B is a 76-yr-old woman with a history of moderately differentiated brochogenic carcinoma. She had undergone a right upper lobectemy 3 yr before presentation, followed by chemotherapy and radiation. Her spine was included in the radiated field, and had been subjected to 4000 rads, a maximal dose. She was referred by her oncologist for a

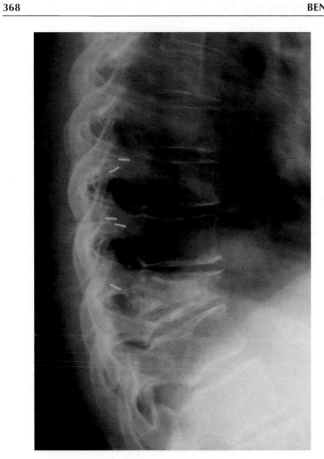

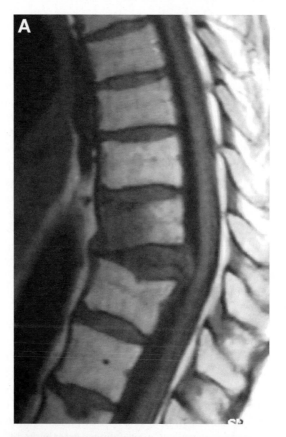

Fig. 1. Lateral X-ray of the thoracic spine. There is collapse of the T9 and T10 vertebral bodies with focal kyphosis.

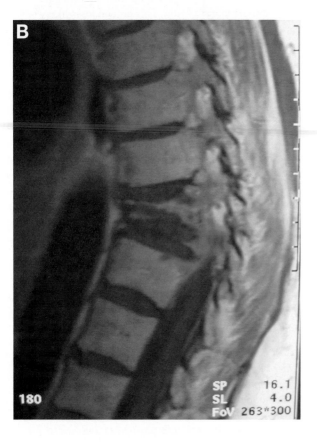

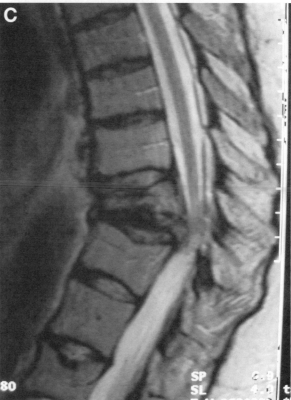

Fig. 2. (A) T1-weighted sagittal magnetic resonance imaging of the thoracic spine. The T9 and 10 vertebral bodies are involved with tumor. (B) There is evidence of gadolinium enhancement. (C) T2-weighted imaging demonstrated spinal cord compression.

history of mid-thoracic spine pain that radiated ventrally into her right chest wall. Plain radiographs and magnetic resonance imaging (MRI) demonstrated recurrence of her tumor, with metastasis to T9 and 10 (Figs. 1 and 2).

Physical examination revealed no neurological deficit or pathological reflexes. Her upper and middle thoracic spine was tender to palpation, primarily in the midline. Her previous medical history was, otherwise, remarkable for two myocardial infarctions and hypothyroidism. Her oncologist indicated that she had a life expectancy of 6 to 12 mo. Her radiation oncologist reiterated that she had already received a maximal radiation dose—with one proviso. If she were to develop intractable pain that could not be otherwise effectively managed, she could receive additional radiation—with the understanding that it would likely lead to irreversible spinal cord dysfunction.

Although Mrs. B knew that her cancer had recurred, she was not aware of her life expectancy when queried. Furthermore, she did not understand that the tumor had involved her spine. To have a common starting point from which to reach a treatment plan, both of these issues were directly addressed. A conference was held with the patient, the patient's family, her medical and radiation oncologists, and the treating spine surgeon. An open, honest discussion regarding the extent of the patient's disease and, more importantly, her prognosis ensued. After the patient and her family understood the true underlying general issues, the involvement of the spine by the tumor was addressed. It was iterated that given the extent of pre-existing spinal canal compromise, as well as the progressive nature of her cancer, it was likely that, without surgical intervention, she would develop a neurological deficit in the near future. Additionally, given the extent of bony destruction by tumor, it was probable that she would have further collapse of the involved vertebrae. Neurologically, catastrophic instability would likely result.

To surgically address these issues, a decompression and ventral and dorsal reconstruction would be required. This would necessitate operating through a previously irradiated field, with its attendant increased risk of infection and wound problems. Blood loss could be expected to be significant, and the surgery long, placing strain on the patient's already compromised heart. Her bone quality was mediocre, making fixation less secure. This would potentially require a lengthening of an already significant construct.

An extensive discussion was held with Mrs. B and her family. After the aforementioned factors were clearly outlined and the significant risks and potential benefits of surgery defined, the potential for significant postoperative pain, neurological deficit, and possible death were outlined. With the understanding of the patient's prognosis, the surgeon's expectations were clarified. Indeed, surgery would be very risky and would require an extensive ventral/dorsal procedure. The patient's fears and expectations were then addressed. Mrs. B explained that her greatest fears were paralysis and pain. She felt that her quality of remaining life would be severely affected by losing neurological function. She would be willing to undergo an extensive procedure in an attempt to preserve neurological function. The patient realized that neurological function preservation and the

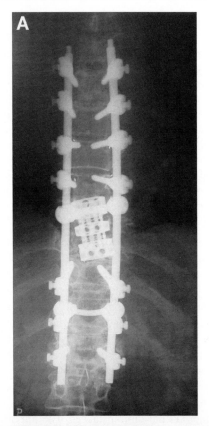

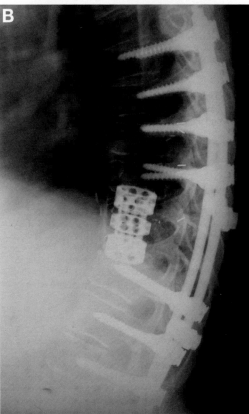

Fig. 3. (**A**) Anterior/posterior and (**B**) lateral X-rays of the thoracolumbar spine following surgery. The patient underwent T9–T10 corpectomy with the placement of an interbody cage. She also underwent T5–L5 pedicle screw fixation.

prevention of painful pathological fractures were the ultimate goals of surgery. It was made abundantly clear to her that "cure" was not possible. Finally, the significant risks of surgery were well defined. All were in agreement that surgery was the "most appropriate" treatment strategy for Mrs. B. She underwent a successful T9 and 10 corpectomy via an extrapleural thoracotomy. A cage packed with autograft was placed in the interbody space. The patient then underwent a dorsal approach and stabilization with pedicle screws from T5–L1. The patient remained neurologically intact and survived an additional 16 mo without neurological compromise or construct failure.

8. CONCLUSION

The surgeon and other treating physicians must not fall into the trap of thinking that surgery will work when other treatment strategies have not. The surgeon must ask "Can I help, and at what cost?" This entire process requires team play. The team includes the patient, the patient's family, other health care professionals and consultants, and the treating physician. All must have the same information and strive for the same goals and expectations. They must be honest and respect each other. The team, and especially the surgeon, must consider realistic life expectancies and, perhaps most importantly, should honestly consider what they would want for themselves or a family member under similar circumstances. The importance of the informed decision-making process, in which the patient, the patient's family, and the treating physician come to a mutual decision, is emphasized.

REFERENCES

1. Dunn GP. The surgeon and palliative care. Surg Oncol Clin N Am 2001; 10:7–24.
2. Dunn GP, Milch RA. Introduction and historical background of palliative care: where does the surgeon fit in? J Am Coll Surg 2001; 193:325–328.
3. World Health Organization. Cancer Pain Relief and Palliative Care: Report of a WHO Expert Committee. Technical Report Series No. 804. Geneva, Switzerland: World Health Organization; 1990:11.
4. Pronovost P, Angus, DC. Economics of end-of-life care in the intensive care unit. Crit Care Med 2001; 29:N46–N51.
5. Miner TJ, Jauues DP, Tavaf-Motamen H, Shriver CD. Decision-making on surgical palliation based on patient outcome data. Am J Surg 1999; 177:150–154.
6. Ball AB, Baum M, Breach NM, et al. Surgical palliation. In: Derek D, Hanks, GWC, MacDonald N, eds. Oxford Textbook of Palliative Medicine. Oxford, England: Oxford Press; 1998:282–297.
7. Sugarbaker PH, Barofsky I, Rosenberg SA, et al. Quality of life assessment of patients extremity sarcoma trials. Surgery 1982; 91:17–23.
8. Nazzaro JM. Metastatic spinal lesions. In: Benzel EC, (ed). Spine Surgery: Techniques, Complication Avoidance, and Management. Churchill: Livingstone; 1999:679–695.
9. Langenhoff, BS. Quality of life as an outcome measure in surgical oncology. Br J Surg 2001; 88:643–652.
10. Pearce S, Kelly D, Stevens W. "More than just money" –widening the understanding of the costs involved in cancer care. J Adv Nurs 2001; 33:371–379.
11. Kushner H. When Bad Things Happen to Good People. New York, NY: Schocken Books; 1981.
12. Kubler-Ross E. On Death and Dying. New York, NY: MacMillan Publishing Co; 1969.

Index